W0106301

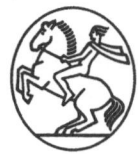

Therapy of Malignant Brain Tumors

Edited by
Kurt Jellinger

Springer-Verlag Wien New York

Prof. Dr. Kurt Jellinger

Ludwig Boltzmann Institute of Clinical Neurobiology
Lainz Hospital, Vienna, Austria

With 111 Figures

ISBN-13:978-3-7091-8878-1   e-ISBN-13:978-3-7091-8876-7
DOI: 10.1007/978-3-7091-8876-7

Foreword

The tumors of the brain similar to other pathological changes of that particular organ claim for a separate position in scientific medicine regarding biology, morphology, features of clinical manifestation, diagnostics and therapy. During the past years due to rapid progress in basic neurosciences and medical biotechnics the situation of the neuroclinician in front of brain tumors has been dramatically changed. The prerequisites for early and accurate diagnosis as well as for successful treatment also of malignant neoplasms have increased and remarkably improved. At the same time the information necessary for an appropriate pragmatic use of the available cognitive methods and therapeutic means increased along the same scale and is permanently being critically modified or changed due to fundamental new insights which come up in always shorter intervals. These facts necessitate the preparation of publications in which the state of the art is presented in possible completeness, systematic order and proper disposability for rational management and therapeutic strategies.

The primary aim of the present book is to serve these purposes. With 8 chapters the collective of competent authors deal on the biology, pathology and immunology of malignant brain tumors of adults and of children including relevant basic and recent data of experimental research; further on the available methods of therapy: neurosurgery, radiology and chemotherapy, the fundamental principals of their efficacy and the differing models of single respective combined application, in comprehensive critical form. In all contributions a well-matched balance and complementarity between mediation of the relevant basic knowledge and information about the given practical experiences and results of thorough evaluation is achieved. The present publication appears suitable to promote future competent management and broader better results in the complex field of multimodal brain tumor therapy.

For the exemplary realization of the challenging concept of this book which also presents an equally high standard of contributions from the scientific and the didactic point of view, the editor, Prof. Dr. K. Jellinger, merits great appreciation. I would like to wish this publication the proper full success through all field of the clinical neurosciences.

Vienna, November 1986   F. Seitelberger

Contents

2 Neurosurgery of Malignant Brain Tumors 91
By D. Voth

6 Principles of Chemotherapy in Brain Neoplasia 277
By Mary K. Gumerlock and E. A. Neuwelt

1

*Pathology of Human Intracranial Neoplasia**

K. Jellinger

Ludwig Boltzmann Institute of Clinical Neurobiology, Lainz Hospital, Vienna, Austria

I. Introduction

Intracranial neoplasms (ICN) are divided into primary growths derived from the central nervous system (CNS) and other structures within the cranial cavity, and secondary or metastatic tumors. Although ultimately classified according to the cell of origin, primary intracranial growths can be broadly subdivided into a) neuroectodermal neoplasms arising from the CNS tissue and b) those tumors derived from other structures within the cranial cavity. The natural history of ICN is not only related to their cytology, anatomical pattern, extent and growth behavior, but also to their location or site within the cranial cavity, and the reaction of the host with respect to increased intracranial pressure, cerebral barrier functions, blood flow, and immunological response.

With the exception of some genetically determined neoplastic syndromes, *e.g.* neurofibromatosis, tuberous sclerosis, Lindau's syndrome, etc, the etiology of tumors of the human CNS is largely unknown, and the causes may be multiple: maldevelopment, genetic factors, chromosomal aberrations, trauma, viruses, chemical compounds and immunological dysfunctions have been considered as etiological factors, but despite extensive experimental work it has not so far been possible to come to a positive conclusion. Various types of ICN, in particular neuroepithelial tumors, but also mesenchymal, meningeal and vascular neoplasms have been induced in animals by chemical carcinogens, oncogenic viruses or irradiation, but although recent epidemiologic studies suggested a link between occupational exposure to chemicals and increased incidence of ICN[262, 388], no environmental carcinogen has been identified as a causative agent in human brain tumors, and it is doubtful whether one of the factors inducing animal CNS tumors can at present be held responsible for producing human neoplasms. However, animal models using such agents and successful transplantation of human and experimental brain tumors or tumor cell lines into animals have proved to be

---

* Dedicated to Prof. Dr. F. Seitelberger on the occasion of his 70th birthday.

valuable in the elucidation of oncogenic mechanisms, of biological and growth behavior of human ICN. In recent years, significant progress in the understanding of the origin, development and response to treatment of human ICN has been achieved upon the informations obtained in animal model system. Morphologic and biologic features of experimental and basic neurooncology have been reviewed recently[359, 440, 457]. The present chapter gives an overview of the pathology of human ICN with critical reference to their general biology, modern problems of classification and grading, and, finally, will provide a description of the individual neoplasms by their incidence, usual sites of origin, gross features, histological, ultrastructural, and immunohistochemical appearance, and biological behavior.

II. Basic Principles of Neurooncology

1. General Biology of Brain Tumors

In general pathology, a distinction is made between benign, malignant, and intermediate tumors depending on their histological and biological degrees of differentiation which separate highly differentiated, moderately and poorly differentiated, and undifferentiated or anaplastic forms. The histological appearance of most tumors correlates well with their biological behavior and allows one to estimate the prognosis for patients harboring these neoplasms. Histological and cytological anaplasia is featured by both phenotypic and genotypic (karyotypic) heterogeneity of tumor cell populations and is associated with aggressive biological behavior, rapid tumor growth, and decreased patient survival. The *morphological criteria of malignancy* are: a) anaplasia, *i.e.* dedifferentiation, the histological and cytological features of which are dense cellularity, increased numbers of mitoses, nuclear hyperchromasia and pleomorphism, cellular pleomorphism, regressive changes including necrosis, indicating rapid tumor growth, and mesenchymal and vascular proliferation, b) invasiveness, *i.e.* invasive growth, extensive migration and spread through the adjacent tissue, c) tumor recurrence which develops from active or "dormant" tumor cell populations not removed or destroyed by cytoreductive therapy, and d) metastatic spread. The factors controlling tumor growth and growth kinetics, including chalones, tumor angiogenesis factor, immune surveillance, etc, are still poorly understood[421]. Solid tumors are composed of three populations of cells in terms of their kinetic behavior[182, 185]: the proliferating pool A of actively dividing cells, the "dormant" pool B or resting cells with remaining propensity of division, and the pool C of sterile or dead cells. The balance between the proliferating and nonproliferating cell compartments are governed by a large number of variables, *e.g.* tumor cell mass, growth kinetics, rate of cell loss, biochemical and immunological properties, cellular recovery capability, etc[182].

The above criteria of general oncology are basically valid for human brain tumors, the rates of proliferation of which have been found to be comparable with those observed in other types of cancer. Assuming a DNA synthesis of 15 hours, the average potential doubling time for glioblastoma and anaplastic astrocytoma is 10 days, for ependymoma 9 days, for well-differentiated astrocytoma and meningioma 36 and 34 days, respectively, which is comparable to melanoma (14 days), malignant lymphoma (16 days) and sarcoma (23 days), while colorectal carcinoma (2.5 days), squamous cell carcinoma (6.8 days), and undifferentiated bronchial carcinoma (2.5 days) appear generally to show more rapid proliferation[421]. However, ICNs show a number of special biological and pathophysiological features which particularly influence their behavior and prognosis. They are basically related to a) the particular development and neoplastic properties of brain tumors, b) their intracranial localization with particular reactions of the target organ.

a) Intrinsic brain tumors are suggested to develop from neoplastic transformation of preexisting differentiated cells within certain areas or fields[475], preferentially in the subependymal plate, subcortical regions and other main loci of continuous glia- and neurogenesis[255, 289, 368]. This transformation may be both monoclonal and multiclonal[118] and is suggested to result from a series of progressive multistep mutational events in which the transforming cells develop altered biological properties in a characteristic sequence[235]. There is increasing evidence that structural alterations of DNA in the chromatin are the primary events in the multistep process of malignant transformation by chemical carcinogens[235, 492]. Experimental neurooncology has confirmed the Willis theory that whole fields are affected by carcinomatous stimuli with continuing dedifferentiation and that brain tumors would enlarge not only by multiplication but also by progressive neoplastic transformation of cells at the periphery of the field[255, 289]. The dividing tumor cells percolate through a "dormant" environment of nondividing neurons and slowly proliferating, normal glia cells[101]. Well-differentiated neuroectodermal tumors are rarely encapsulated and, in most cases, they diffusely infiltrate the surrounding tissue. Despite their low growth rate, they may eventually kill the host especially when they are located in vital or deep areas inaccessible to surgery. Malignant brain tumors show a special form of invasiveness, since they are capable of extensive migration and spread through the surrounding brain with only minimal destruction of the preexisting tissue. Although invasiveness is considered as a major determinant for the malignant behavior in anaplastic gliomas[141, 283], remarkably little is known about the cellular and molecular biology of this process. Recent in vitro studies have shown invasiveness of human glioma cell lines characterized by progressive and irreversible replacement and destruction of normal tissue[95, 253]. In view of these facts, the criteria of "radical surgical resection" and of the "recurrence" of most intrinsic brain tumors need critical reconsideration. While total resection of a systemic cancer is frequently possible, "radical" surgical resection of brain tumors usually might remove 90 to 99% of the tumor, corresponding to a 2 log kill, which in many malignant neoplasms is not enough to allow the body's own natural immune mechanisms to kill the remaining tumor[396].

b) Although brain tumors defined by histological and cytological criteria, some major types, e.g. malignant gliomas, constitute morphologically, biochemically, immunologically and biologically heterogenous groups of neoplasms[283]. The manifestation of heterogeneity is diverse and includes genotypic (different marker chromosomes, DNA content) and phenotypical characteristics, e.g. differential growth rates, differences in expression of biochemical markers and surface antigens, and differential experimental tumorigenity and sensitivity to antitumor agents[163, 283, 397, 473]. There is extensive inter- and intraglioma cell line antigenic heterogeneity with complex correlations between morphology and different genotypical and phenotypical characteristivs, with existence of stable subpopulations of antigenically null or complex cells[473]. Neoplastic cell populations exhibit a dynamic state of flux between differentiation and anaplasia. Cellular differentiation is determined by the ontogenic memory of the cell clone originally hit and is associated with a decycling of the proliferating populations. Anaplasia results from the recruitment of proliferating cells from the nonproliferating pool and the progressive selection of clonogenic subpopulations that make up a heterogeneous neoplasm[368]. In contrast to *in vitro* systems that usually enhance cell differentiation[366], it is evident, that, *in vivo*, the balance of forces in the malignant state in general favors anaplasia over differentiation, a trend that is found also on tissue cultures of recurrent gliomas[152, 231], and on sequential transplantation of human gliomas that produce a gradual loss of heterogeneity[283, 389]. The existence of tumor subpopulations differing in fundamental neoplastic properties also provides a framework for the well-known capacity of cancer behavior to change during the course of disease, a phenomenon called "tumor progression"[125, 163]. Increased and more rapid patterns of growth observed in various brain tumors can be regarded a special form of "focal progression" in neoplasms[125, 387] which may occur both spontaneously or secondary to antineoplastic treatment. It is considered to result from selection of cell clones and subpopulations of tumor cells due to their instability, changes in cytokinetic balance and genetic expression, predominancy and overgrowth of primitive anaplastic cell populations with enhanced proliferation capacity, and other unknown variables. The search for both regulatory factors that may control the basic instability between the proliferating and nonproliferating pools of neoplastic cell population and of the pathways of differentiation and dedifferentiation in neoplastic development will be significant for the understanding of tumor biology[368].

c) In contrast to many other organs where normal function can continue undisturbed for a longer period of time in relation to the size of a neoplasms, the dependence of normal brain function upon the precise functional interrelationships and regional differentiation of functions, results in ICNs occurring in different specific sites in giving rise to permanent and progressive deficits. The growth of ICNs is confined to an eventually closed compartment which, in addition to their primary destructive effects, may induce secondary complications due to their space-occupying nature. In addition to the morphological criteria of biological behavior related to tumor morphology, the intracranial location of ICNs may produce clinical malignancy due to their site within the brain, increased intracranial pressure, and disturbances of the blood-brain barrier (BBB) and cerebral blood flow, etc. The pathology and pathophysiology of increased intracranial pressure and of their supratentorial and infratentorial lesions are well documented[339, 440, 495].

d) Metastatic spread of most intrinsic brain tumors is limited to transliquoral seeding throughout the neuraxis[109, 202, 324, 362], while metastases outside the CNS are considered to be rare in the majority of brain tumors, particularly involving the lungs, skeletal system, lymph nodes and liver[213, 244, 334, 362], about 40% occurring in children[71, 177]. Although CNS tumors can spread spontaneously beyond the confines of the CNS, most instances of extraneural metastases occur after craniotomy or CSF shunting procedures[71, 177, 213]. The pathogenesis of systemic metastases is related to breakage of the BBB, whether at surgery or tumor invasion into vascular channels or with systemic-cerebrospinal fluid shunting, dissemination of tumor cells via systemic circulation, arrest within distinct target organs, exit through the vascular walls and formation of metastases[71, 213, 267]. Malignant CNS tumors are known to invade veins and to be able to grow in extracranial sites[24]. In addition to spread of CNS tumors through craniotomy via head and neck lymphatics[104], there is also lymphatic drainage of CSF into extracranial tissues[282], but there have been examples of a variety of CNS neoplasms that have spontaneously spread to head and neck lymphatics and to distant sites throughout the body[177, 189, 362, 434].

2. Microvasculature and Blood-Brain Barrier (BBB)

Major distinguishing features of most brain tumors are abnormalities of their microvasculature with hyperplasia and an endothelial proliferation, most prominent in malignant CNS neoplasms, changes in the BBB within the tumor and in adjacent tissues, often associated with brain edema, and changes in blood-to-tissue transport which are of particular interest for the clinical course, diagnosis, and treatment of ICNs. The mechanisms of brain edema formation are poorly understood[23]. In the normal brain, the capillaries consist of a continuous lining of endothelial cells joined by tight junctions; they lack gaps and fenestrae, and have few pinocytotic vesicles. This combination constitutes the BBB by which the passage of protein and other large molecules from the blood to the brain is restricted. Blood vessels in malignant brain tumors differ physiologically from those in normal brain due to loss of their barrier features with increased permeability to protein[451]. Structural abnormalities in tumor vessels include vascular hyperplasia, with large sinusoids, glomeruloid structures composed of dense cells of hyperplastic capillaries, most prominent in anaplastic gliomas and adjacent areas of necrosis, and in border zone areas. These complex structures are composed of immature or regenerating capillaries or mature vessels[471]. The vascular endothelium reveals fenestrations, occasional discontinuities (gaps), junctional abnormalities, and an increased number of pinocytotic vesicles[269, 283, 456]. In various human brain tumors, e.g. gliomas, meningiomas, craniopharyngiomas, lymphomas, papillomas, metastatic carcinomas, schwannomas, and vascular tumors, and in experimental gliomas, microvessels with endothelial gaps, fenestrae, and active pinocytosis have been observed[92, 172, 269, 283, 451, 456]. It is significant, however, that these ultrastructural abnormalities are not found in all vessels, since large proportions of the microvasculature within a tumor and in the adjacent peritumoral regions may deviate only slightly from normal[471] or show completely normal ultrastructure[425]. The outer layers of the vessel wall are formed by pericytes and pleomorphic tumor cells which are surrounded by one or several basement membranes and often show extremely large perivascular spaces[471]. Quantitative studies in glioma models reveal a three-to sixfold increase in pinocytotic vascular density[92], about 30% of the tumor vessels have fenestrations, while the proportion of tumor vessel profiles with abnormal junctions ranges from 32–69%[425]. Although the role of pinocytotic vesicles in vascular transport is controversial and the junctional permeability is also poorly understood, these stuctural abnormalities in tumor vessel walls may represent permeability routes that permit the escape of serum constituents into the tumors and from there into the surrounding brain. Studies with the extracellular protein tracer horseradish peroxidase in experimental brain tumors confirmed the *in vivo* permeability of tumor vessel endothelium, either through gaps between the endothelial cells via broken tight junctions or endothelial fenestration or, more frequently, by pinocytotic transport across intact endothelial cells[151]. As one might expect from the uneven distribution of abnormal vessels and variations in their ultrastructural changes between different brain tumor models and tumor regions, malignant brain tumors exhibit regional variability in vascular permeability. Both human gliomas and tumor models show evidence of a nonuniform permeability varying from severe extravasation of HRP to complete impermeability, the average relative proportion of an individual tumor that is permeable to HRP ranging from 50 to almost 100%[283]. Recent evidence suggests that brain tumors, particularly small ones, and the adjacent brain may have regions in which the BBB is partially or wholly intact. Experimental studies indicate that in the central bulk of tumor the blood flow is reduced and the BBB disrupted, while along the edge of the tumor, the blood flow approaches normal and the BBB damage is minimal[283, 313]. Although accumulation of serum protein is seen in both the tumor and in the peritumoral brain, the extravasation of protein and tracers occurs only across the tumor vessels but not or only in insignificant amounts in the peritumoral zone. Edema, in consequence, originates mainly in the tumor from where it spreads into the brain tissue. The observation of intact BBB in the adjacent brain is similar to other types of vasogenic edema, *e.g.* induced by cold or stab wounds[233]. On the other hand, the evidence of nonuniform permeability and vascular hyperplasia with prominent neovascularization in peripheral tumor regions suggests an association with variable contrast enhancement in preoperative and postoperative CT scans[63, 70, 265, 432].

Vascularization of a neoplasm is a prerequisite for its continuous growth. Neovascularization occurring in all types of brain tumors including metastatic carcinomas, but most prominent in anaplastic gliomas, has been related to a soluble tissue angiogenesis factor (TAF). There is evidence that neoplasms occurring in a variety of sites, including gliomas and meningiomas, may secret angiogenesis factors, which promote the formation and growth of new blood vessels. Since glioma cells have been shown to secrete factors stimulating the proliferation of endothelial cells, smooth muscle, fibroblasts, and glial cells, some tumors may produce factors that stimulate the growth of both tumor cells and blood vessels simultaneously, indicating biological interactions between tumor and vascular mesenchyma[283].

In some brain tumors, particularly gliomas, neoplastic transformation of vascular to mesenchymal elements may result in the formation of mixed glioma-sarcomas[294, 405]. These mechanisms can be understood in the light of recent observations that activation of transforming genes may be included by the DNA of various human neoplasms and results in the *in vitro* transfer of genetic information coding for malignant transformation (transfection) in mouse fibroblasts[348] or *in vivo* induction of murine sarcoma following transplantation of a human ovarian cystadenocarcinoma in nude mice[148], suggesting horizontal transmission of malignancy to putatively normal differentiated stromal cells. Another possibility for the development of mixed tumor cell populations would be a biclonal transformation of cells of different lineage in the CNS[368]. The possibility of metaplasia from neoplastic glial to mesenchymal cells, characterized by antigenic loss of GFAP and other biochemical differentiation markers of neuroepithelial cells and by the expression of proteins not associated with differentiated glia, such as collagen and fibronectin, has recently been tentatively revived, with the suggestion that some neoplastic glial cells are able to express both GFAP and fibronectin[218].

Some recent papers on the prognostic factors related to the survival of patients with malignant gliomas suggested that among other histological criteria, both tissue necrosis and a greater degree of neovascularization may carry a poorer outcome, both being indicators of malignant biological behavior of tumors[68, 85, 130, 135].

3. Immunological Responses

The relations between the brain, brain tumor and the immune system are still poorly understood. Despite the widely held view that the brain is a site of partial immunological privilege[453], and previous suggestions that brain tumors are therefore unlikely to give rise to an immune response, in recent years evidence has accumulated for:

a) The shearing of antigenicity between the CNS and immune systems, and the antigenic cross-reactivity between human brain tumor cells of both neuroepithelial (gliomas, PNETs, schwannomas) or nonneurogenic origin (meningioma, angioblastoma, metastases) and hematopoietic/lymphoid cells[58, 283, 340, 473].

b) Complex disturbances of immunoregulation with impairment of both humoral and cellular immunological reactivity in patients harboring primary ICNs that particularly have been shown to have a marked decrease in cell-mediated immunity[39, 52, 136, 232, 314, 453]. It has been suggested that the origin of immunologic impairment lies in a specific interaction between primary brain tumors and the immune system[34].

c) On the other hand, mononuclear lymphocytic infiltrations similar to that observed in allergic encephalitis are observed by conventional histogical techniques in 30–60% of both well and poorly differentiated gliomas and their microenvironment[39–41, 59, 69, 152, 311, 328, 341, 352, 382, 420, 433, 453, 480], as well as in and around sarcomas, cerebral metastases[39, 152, 328, 352, 382], in germ cell tumors[199, 315], meningiomas[181, 226], and other intracerebral tumors[34]. Mononuclear cell infiltrates, similar to those in other solid or systemic extraneural malignancies[16, 37, 42, 449] are not only present in perivascular regions within or adjacent to the Virchow-Robin spaces[39–41, 51, 328, 433], but also within the tumor tissue and the parenchyma of the adjacent brain[203, 453]. Using monoclonal antibodies and lymphocyte markers, these infiltrates have been shown to include macrophages[420, 480] and T-lymphocytes of predominently suppressor/cytotoxic cell phenotype[297, 315, 453] or mixed suppressor/cytotoxic or helper cell phenotype[453], while very few B lymphocytes are present within anaplastic gliomas[470]. They are suggested to reflect an expression of host-tumor interaction, with inherent lymphocyte populations potentially exerting functional impact in the mediation of immunosuppression within the CNS. Although there is no ultrastructural evidence of a cytotoxic effect of mononuclear cells on adult glioma cells, they may show a marked cytotoxic effect on cultivated glioma cells which is inhibited by blocking factors, and no correlation of mononuclear infiltrates or decreased T-cell function to cellular immunity against autologous tumor or soluble immune complexes in patient's sera could be verified[39, 480]. The presence of increased suppressor/cytotoxic cells infiltrating brain tumors and their microenvironment with simultaneous decrease in peripheral blood suppressor/cytotoxic cells[453] may be explained by selective depletion of active functional subsets from the peripheral blood due to active migration of systemic effector cells into the target organ as a neoplastic site, resulting in a modulation of the host response to a neoplastic challenge originating in the CNS. The presence of suppressor/cytotoxic cells in brain tumors may reflect suppression of immunologic activity rather than a cytotoxic attack. Suppressive factors have been identified not only in the serum but also in cyst fluid from patients with cystic anaplastic gliomas[232]. Lymphocytes of different sites have been found either to inhibit or to enhance tumor cell proliferation, whereby the functional activites of the mononuclear cells seem to depend on the stage of tumor progression[37, 42].

The question of the biological value of mononuclear infiltration in brain tumors in terms of malignant behavior, tumor burden, histological cell type, and patient outcome or survival is still unresolved. Some investigations of mononuclear infiltrates in systemic neoplasms correlate infiltration with a lower incidence of metastasis and enhanced survival independent of other factors[37, 199]. T-lymphocytes are insufficient for defense against tumor cells, but may help to destroy circulating cancer cells and to prevent their setting and proliferating to metastases[42], which may explain the relative rarity of extraneural spread of primary intracranial tumors. On the other hand, an interaction between lymphoid cells and some malignant glioma lines has been suggested to enhance cell coat production which many account for an apparent suppressor effect and thus malignant behavior[283]. It appears that human glioma cells may escape cellular immune attack through the presence of a mucopolysaccharide coat that impairs the generation of lymphocytes in response to certain glioma lines in vitro[96]. Such cell-surface-associated hyaluronidase-sensitive sulphated glycosaminoglycans have been observed in a variety of brain tumors, particularly gliomas, and show progressive decrease with increasing anaplasia, suggesting a progressive cellular degeneration[38, 145]. Glycoproteins are synthesized by glioma cells in vitro and are deposited in glial basement membranes in vivo. Cell coat production is enhanced by the interaction of glioma cells with a macromolecular factor released by human peripheral blood mononuclear cells in culture. This interaction is suggested to constitute an unusual mechanism by which inflammatory cells may nonspecifically suppress the generation of cell-mediated immune response in gliomas and may cause resistance of human glioma cells to natural killer activity of lymphocytes[96, 490, 491].

There are conflicting data on the relationship of mononuclear infiltration in glial tumor evolution in terms of patient survival. Most studies have been unable to substantiate any link between the presence and extent of lymphocytic invasion with enhanced survival[68, 69, 152, 296, 311, 382], or even saw shorter survival[352], although in some series increased malignant potential appears paradoxically related to increased levels of mononuclear infiltration. Glioblastomas show a lower incidence and intensity, than well differentiated or anaplastic gliomas[39-41, 203, 352] and brain metastases[152, 328, 382], despite the apparent associated evidence for prolonged survival in the presence of mononuclear infiltrates[41, 51, 328, 433]. Increased occurrence of lymphocytic infiltrates in recurrent gliomas may be related to disorders of the BBB. While preoperative steroid treatment has been shown not to severely influence the frequency but to reduce the intensity of these infiltrates[41], a decreased incidence of lymphocyte invasion has been observed following radiation and chemotherapy[137, 382]. The immunobiological significance of these findings with regard to tumor-host interaction within the CNS and tumor behavior needs further elucidation. However, the recognition that the cellular immune response is impaired in patients with certain brain tumors is particularly significant as it is mainly the cellular immune response which is of primary importance for the eradication of solid tumors *in vivo*[42, 96, 136, 453].

III. Classification and Grading

Rapid progress in diagnosis and treatment of brain tumors using increasingly sophisticated methods demands a common and uniform or, at least comparable, concept of CNS tumors in order to be able to compare the effectiveness of the diagnostic and therapeutic strategies. There have been attempts to classify the ICNs on the basis of their histopathology or of their CT appearance[190, 225, 432] and to correlate their clinical evolution and natural history with the site, morphology or cytokinetic behavior of the neoplasm. The taxonomy of neoplasms has to consider both their histogenesis and (de)differentiation. The histogenesis of malignant tumors is determined by their cells of origin, their initial state of differentiation and the phenotypic and genotypic changes they undergo as the neoplasm evolves. General approaches to classification of CNS tumors are embodied in the two major classification systems:

1. The *embryogenetic* system emphasizes the cytologic similarities between neoplastic cells and their embryonal counterparts in normal development[17]. Tumors are viewed as arising from immature cells that may undergo further differentiation as the tumor evolves[370], and attempts have been made to classify the tumors in terms of the different stages which the cells pass through during oncogenesis. Despite considerable criticism this scheme has remained the cornerstone on which subsequent classifications have been based, although many attempts have been made to modify[362, 270, 495, 499]. Many authors refer to the classification of Russel & Rubinstein[370] (Tab. 1).

2. In contrast, several numerical *grading systems* were introduced, based on the histologic and cytologic anaplasia[229, 353]. Tumors are viewed as arising from mature, differentiated cells that undergo progressive dedifferentiation as the tumor evolves. Following the grading of epithelial tumors elsewhere in the body

Table 1. Brain tumor classification (modified after [370])

A. Tumors of the glial series
    I. Astrocytic group
      1. Astrocytoma
      2. Astroblastoma
      3. Polar spongioblastoma
      4. Glioblastoma multiforme
    II. Oligodendroglia
      Oligodendroglioma
    III. Ependyma and homologues
      1. Ependymoma—subependymoma
      2. Choroid plexus papilloma
      3. Colloid cyst

B. Pineal parenchyma
    I. Pinealoblastoma
    II. Pinealocytoma

C. Retina (primitive epithelium)
    I. Retinoblastoma

D. Tumors of the neuron series
    I. Medulloblastoma
    II. Medulloepithelioma
    III. Neuroblastoma
    IV. Ganglioneuroma and ganglioglioma

E. Tumors of meninges and related tissues
    I. Benign meningioma
      1. Syncytial
      2. Transitional
      3. Fibroblastic
      4. Angioblastic
    II. Malignant meningeal tumors
      1. Malignant meningioma
      2. Primary sarcoma of the meninges and brain

F. Congenital tumors of maldevelopmental origin
    I. Teratoma and teratoid tumors
    II. Dermoid and epidermoid cyst
    III. Craniopharyngioma
    IV. Intrasellar cysts
    V. Lipoma
    VI. Ectopias and hamartomas of neural tissue
    VII. Dysgenetic syndromes associated with tumor formation
      1. Von Hippel-Lindau disease
      2. Tuberous sclerosis
      3. Von Recklinghausen's neurofibromatosis
      4. Neurocutaneous melanosis and melanosis and melanoma of the leptomeninges
      5. Hamartomatous lesions of the CNS

introduced by Broder[49] as a means of coding lesser or higher anaplasia among specimens of a single tumor type, several attempts have been made to apply a system of grading by ascending degrees of malignancy to neuroectodermal tumors or even to all CNS neoplasms. Kernohan *et al.*[229] formulated a four-tiered classification separating a well differentiated glioma grade I, a more cellular and anaplastic grade II, and the gliomas grade III and IV that were synonymous with the glioblastoma multiforme. Its subdivision into grade III and IV was based on the number of mitotic figures, the percentage of malignant cells, the extent of necrosis and vascular proliferation, and the degree of pleomorphism. A three-tiered system proposed by Ringertz[353], dividing the gliomas into benign, intermediate, and malignant or anaplastic, has been widely used[68, 302, 309], although the Kernohan classification is still employed by many pathologists. It must be emphasized that neither conceptual scheme accounts for all features of CNS tumors, and both viewpoints may be relevant to the histogenesis of malignant gliomas and other brain neoplasms.

A combination of histological classification and of different degrees of malignancy using a rather arbitrary grading of various types of CNS tumors as suggested expression of their biological behavior and dignity has been proposed by Zülch[498]. This coding system separating benign, semibenign, semimalignant and malignant neoplasms and attributing to some tumor types one or more "grades" of malignancy was correlated with the average survival times after tumor resection. A more detailed grading system which avoided the forcing of established tumor entities into rigid grades[499] has been the precursor of the grade coding system added to the WHO classification[497]. A more simplified classification and grading system for the most frequent types of brain tumors using four degrees of malignancy is given in Table 2.

As the result of collaboration of different schools and centers grouped around a reference center, the World Health Organization (WHO) has proposed a new "Histological classification of tumors of the CNS"[496, 497]. Its main purpose was to create a uniform international nomenclature considering both the histological type and degree of malignancy and to provide guidelines enabling the biological behavior of a given oncotype to be evaluated uniformly as a prerequisite for a joint evaluation procedure in diagnosis and therapy (Table 3). This WHO classification has been shown to have several shortcomings and misunderstandings which have been critically reviewed and commented upon[19, 26, 56, 143, 152, 202, 225, 357, 426]. In view of recent results of special investigationd methods, in particular of the use of specific cell and tissue markers, a modified version has been proposed by the Austrian Society of Pathology (Table 4). Recently, a classification for childhood brain tumors based upon revision of the WHO nomenclature of all brain tumors has been proposed by the Committee on Pathology at the Pediatric Brain Tumor Workshop (Table 5). In line with recent concepts of neurooncology, these revised WHO classifications include, among others, the concept of primitive neuroectodermal tumors (PNET) originating from the neoplastic transformation of primitive neuroectodermal cells of the subependymal zone irrespective of their localization[356]. These new classifications do not include any pragmatic grading system of degrees of malignancy which had been added to previous classification[229, 288, 496, 499], because a numerical "grading" of different types of

Table 2. Classification and grades of human intracranial tumors (modified after[288, 497])

Tumor	Grade I benign	Grade II semi-	Grade III semi-	Grade IV malignant
Angioblastoma	+ + +			
Choroid plexus papilloma	+ + +		+	
Craniopharyngioma	+ + +			
Chordoma	+ + +	+ +	+	
Epidermoid	+ + +			
Gangliocytoma(-glioma)	+ + +	+ +	+	
Meningioma	+ + +		+	
Neurilemmoma	+ + +		+	
Paraganglioma	+ + +			
Pineocytoma	+ + +	+ +		
Pituitary adenoma	+ + +	+		
Subependymoma	+ + +			
Pilocytic astrocytoma	+ + +		+	
Astrocytoma		+ +	+	
Oligodendroglioma		+ +	+	
Ependymoma	+ +	+ + +	+	+
Germinoma				+ + +
Glioblastoma				+ + +
Lymphomas			+	+ + +
Medulloblastoma + PNET				+ + +
Pinealoblastoma				+ + +
Sarcoma				+ + +
Metastases				+ + +

Explanation: + + + usual; + + less frequent; + rare.

tumors as a suggested expression of their biological behavior appears extremely difficult and may be misleading, since they should be different for each tumor. In addition, the specific criteria usually are not clearly stated, which gives the impression that grades have sometimes been applied in an arbitrary fashion[26, 56, 152, 202, 426]. Although cellular data, such as increased cellularity, the presence and nature of mitotic figures, and pleomorphism of tumor cells, and tissue data, such as necrosis and vascular proliferation, are used to determine the degree of malignancy, none of these features is an absolute indication of malignancy, and may be misleading, especially when working with limited or insufficient material, e.g. in small stereotaxic biopsies or cytologic smears[1, 152, 211]. Other methods establishing criteria of determining biological malignancy and prognosis include the evaluation of numerous histological variables, e.g. used in the evaluation of 3,300 childhood brain tumors[144], or an automated tumor image analysis of gliomas using morphometric, densitometric and mitotic parameters[237, 275, 354, 416]. However, these approaches, used to get prognostically relevant information by cytopathologists and hematopathologists, require a great deal of further substantiation before they can be applied for general use in the study of CNS neoplasms.

Table 3. Histological classification of tumors of the central nervous system (World Health Organization[496, 497])

	Grade
I. Tumors of neuroepithelial tissue	
A. Astrocytic tumors	
1. Astrocytoma	II
a) Fibrillary	
b) Protoplasmic	
c) Gemistocytic	
2. Pilocytic astrocytoma	I
3. Subependymal giant cell astrocytoma (ventricular tumor of tuberous sclerosis)	I
4. Astroblastoma	II–IV?
5. Anaplastic (malignant) astrocytoma	III
B. Oligodendroglial tumors	
1. Oligodendroglioma	II
2. Mixed oligo-astrocytoma	II
3. Anaplastic (malignant) oligodendroglima	III
C. Ependymal and choroid plexus tumors	
1. Ependymoma	I
Variants:	
a) Myxopapillary ependymoma	I, II
b) Papillary ependymoma	I
c) Subependymoma	I
2. Anaplastic (malignant) ependymoma	III, IV
3. Choroid plexus papilloma	I
4. Anaplastic (malignant) choroid plexus papilloma	III, IV
D. Pineal cell tumors	
1. Pineocytoma (pinealocytoma)	I–III
2. Pineoblastoma (pinealoblastoma)	IV
E. Neuronal tumors	
1. Gangliocytoma	I
2. Ganglioglioma	I, II
3. Ganglioneuroblastoma	III
4. Anaplastic (malignant) gangliocytoma and ganglioglioma	III, IV
5. Neuroblastoma	IV
F. Poorly differentiated and embryonal tumors	
1. Glioblastoma	
Variants:	
a) Glioblastoma with sarcomatous component (mixed glioblastoma and sarcoma)	IV
b) Giant cell glioblastoma	
2. Medulloblastoma	
Variants:	
a) Desmoplastic	
b) Medullomyoblastoma	IV
3. Medulloepithelioma	
4. Primitive polar spongioblastoma	
5. Gliomatosis cerebri	?

Table 3 (continued)

	Grade
II. Tumors of nerve sheath cells	
A. Neurilemmoma (schwannoma, neurinoma)	I
B. Anaplastic (malignant) neurilemmoma (schwannoma, neurinoma)	II
C. Neurofibroma	I
D. Anaplastic (malignant) neurofibroma	III, IV
(neurofibrosarcoma, neurogenic sarcoma)	
III. Tumors of meningeal and related tissues	
A. Meningioma	
1. Meningotheliomatous (endotheliomatous,	
syncytial, arachnotheliomatous)	
2. Fibrous (fibroblastic)	
3. Transitional (mixed)	I
4. Psammomatous	
5. Angiomatous	
6. Hemangioblastic	
7. Hemangiopericytic	II
8. Papillary	II, III
9. Anaplastic (malignant) meningioma	II, III
B. Meningeal sarcomas	
1. Fibrosarcoma	III, IV
2. Polymorphic cell sarcoma	III, IV
3. Primary meningeal sarcomatosis	IV
C. Xanthomatous tumors	
1. Fibroxanthoma	?
2. Xanthosarcoma (malignant fibroxanthoma)	?
D. Primary melanotic tumors	
1. Melanoma	IV
2. Meningeal melanomatosis	IV
E. Others	
IV. Primary malignant lymphomas	III, IV
V. Tumors of blood vessel origin	
A. Hemangioblastoma (capillary hemangioblastoma)	I
B. Monstrocellular sarcoma	IV
VI. Germ cell tumors	
A. Germinoma	II, III
B. Embryonal carcinoma	IV
C. Choriocarcinoma	IV
D. Teratoma	I
VII. Other malformative tumors and tumor-like lesions	
A. Craniopharyngioma	I
B. Rathke's cleft cyst	
C. Epidermoid cyst	
D. Dermoid cyst	
E. Colloid cyst of the third ventricle	
F. Enterogenous cyst	I?
G. Other cysts	

Table 3 (continued)

	Grade
H. Lipoma	
I. Choristoma (pituicytoma, granular cell "myoblastoma")	
J. Hypothalamic neuronal hamartoma	
K. Nasal glial heterotopia (nasal glioma)	
VIII. Vascular malformations	
A. Capillary telangiectasia	
B. Cavernous angioma	
C. Arteriovenous malformation	
D. Venous malformation	I
E. Sturge-Weber disease (cerebrofacial or cerebrotrigeminal angiomatosis)	
IX. Tumors of the anterior pituirary	
A. Pituitary adenomas	
1. Acidophil	I
2. Basophil (mucoid cell)	I
3. Mixed acidophil-basophil	I
4. Chromophobe	I
B. Pituitary adenocarcinoma	III
X. Local extensions from regional tumors	
A. Glomus jugulare tumor	?
(chemodectoma, paraganglioma)	See
B. Chordoma	similar
D. Chondrosarcoma	tumors
E. Olfactory neuroblastoma (esthesioneuroblastoma)	elsewhere
F. Adenoid cystic carcinoma (cylindroma)	in the
G. Others	body
XI. Metastatic tumors	
XII. Unclassified tumors	

Tumors of the nervous system are also included in the coded nomenclature of the "International Classification of Diseases for Oncology" (ICD-O)[482], an enlargement of chapter II (neoplasias) of the 9th revision of the "International Classification of Diseases" (ICD-9) which developed from the morphological part of the "Manual of Tumor Nomenclature and Coding" (MOTNAC)[273] and is identical to the morphological part of the "Systematized Nomenclature of Medicine" (SNOMED)[431]. It includes a systemic index of tumors using a five-tiered code for the histologic diagnosis, where the first four figures indicate morphology (M) and the fifth position after a bracked indicates the degree of malignancy ("behavior coding"). The latter separates benign (0), intermediate (1), primary malignant (3) and secondary malignant (6) tumors. In addition, a four-tiered coding for the degree of differentiation is used, separating well, moderately, poorly differentiated and anaplastic tumors. Brain and nervous system tumors are coded

Table 4. Classification of tumors of the CNS (after [56])

I. **Neuroepithelial**
  A. Astrocytic
    1. Astrocytoma
      a) Fibrillary
      b) Protoplasmic
      c) Gemistocytic
      d) Mixed
      e) Others
    2. Pilocytic astrocytoma
    3. Subependymal giant cell astrocytoma
    4. Astroblastoma
    5. Meningocerebral pleomorphic xanthoastrocytoma
    6. Anaplastic astrocytoma
  B. Oligodendroglial and mixed oligoastrocytic
    1. Oligodendroglioma
    2. Anaplastic oligodendroglioma
    3. Oligoastrocytoma
    4. Anaplastic oligoastrocytoma
  C. Ependymal
    1. Ependymoma
      a) Classical
      b) Myxopapillary
      c) Papillary
      d) Foramen Monroi type
      e) Subependymoma
      f) Others
    2. Anaplastic ependymoma
    3. Ependymoblastoma (see 1. H. 2. b ii)
  D. Glioblastomatous
    Glioblastoma
      a) Multiforme
      b) Giant cell ("monstrocellular" glioblastoma)
      c) Glioblastoma with sarcomatous component (gliosarcoma)
      d) Others
  E. Choroid plexus tumors
    1. Choroid plexus papilloma
    2. Malignant plexus papilloma (choroid plexus carcinoma)
  F. Pineal cell tumors
    1. Pinealocytoma (pineocytoma)
    2. Pinealoblastoma (see 1. H. 2.)
  G. Neuronal and mixed neuronal, glial
    1. Gangliocytoma
    2. Anaplastic gangliocytoma
    3. Ganglioglioma
    4. Anaplastic ganglioglioma
    5. Neuroblastoma and ganglioneuroblastoma (see I. H. 2. b iii)
  H. Embryonal
    1. Medulloepithelioma

Table 4 (continued)

2. Primitive neuroectodermal tumor (PNET) and medulloblastoma (PNET of cerebellum) and pinealoblastoma (PNET of pineal parenchyma); desmoblastic (additional term for tumors with prominent mesenchymal components)
    a) Without differentiation
    b) With differentiation
        i) Glial (astrocytic and/or oligodendroglial)
        ii) Ependymal (ependymoblastoma)
        iii) Neuronal (neuroblastoma, ganglioneuroblastoma)
        iv) Bipotent or pluripotent
3. Medullomyoblastoma
4. Primitive polar spongioblastoma
5. Others

I. Others

II. Meningeal and mesenchymal
A. Meningioma
  1. Benign
     a) Meningiomatous
     b) Fibrous
     c) Transitional and mixed
     d) Psammomatous
     e) Angiomatous
     f) Hemangioblastic
     g) Others
  2./3. Intermediate and malignant
     a) Hemangiopericytic
     b) Papillary
     c) Anaplastic (malignant)
     d) Others
B. Primary melanocytic
  1. Meningeal melanocytoma
  2. Malignant melanoma
  3. Meningeal melanosis
  4. Malignant meningeal melanoblastoma
  5. Neurocutaneous melanosis
  6. Others
C. Mesenchymal
  1. Benign
     a) Hemangioblastoma (Lindau tumor)
     b) Others
  2. Malignant
     a) Primary meningeal sarcomatosis
     b) Sarcoma with glial (glioblastomatous) component
     c) Others

III. Primary malignant lymphomas

IV. Germ cell tumors

V. Malformative tumors
1. Craniopharyngioma
2. Others

Table 4 (continued)

VI. Tumors of the neurohypophysis
1. Granular cell tumor (choristoma)
2. Others (astrocytic tumors)

VII. Metastatic tumors

VIII. Unclassified tumors

IX. Tumor-like
1. Cysts
   a) Epidermal cyst
   b) Dermoid cyst
   c) Colloid cyst of third ventricle
   d) Enterogenous cyst
   e) Rathke's cleft cyst
   f) Others
2. Neuronal hamartoma of the hypothalamus
3. Nasal glial heterotopia (nasal "glioma")
4. Ecchordosis
5. Lipoma
6. Vascular malformations
8. Others

as M 938–958, and other intracranial tumors as M-935–937, using IDC-O preferred terms (IPT), IAS (acceptable synonyms), and ISF (special forms), with additional T-terms for topography [191, 194, 339, 482]. A ten-tiered code allows a complete identification of topographic site (4 figures), morphologic type (4 figures), degree of malignancy (1 figure), and stage or differentiation (1 figure) of a tumor. As an example, medulloblastoma of the cerebellum is coded as M-9470/3, T 191.6, while metastatic medulloblastoma is coded as M-9470/6. However, the 9th revision of ICD in many respects does not agree with the current classifications of brain tumors, *e.g.* the different types of astrocytoma are coded as M-9400/3 (astrocytoma NOS), M 9401/3 (anaplastic), M 9410/3 (protoplasmic), M-9411/3 (gemistocytic), M-9420/3 (fibrillary), M-9421/3 (pilocytic), M-9383/1 (subependymal large cell astrocytoma), etc. The diagnostic index issued 1973 and 1976 by the German Societies of Neurology and Neurosurgery (NDV) uses a seven-tiered code, indicating the nosological diagnosis (4 figures), location (2 figures), and site of involvement (1 figure).

Each of the currently used classifications provides information about the "prominent" cell population in a brain tumor, while grading systems provide ease in recognizing the ends of the prognostic spectrum (benign versus malignant). Although most of these classifications agree in principle, they often contain differing designations for one and the same tumor type, while some neoplasms of the brain are absent from these classifications. Not all tumors found in the CNS are easily to classify. Moreover, each classification and grading system fails to evaluate formally the effects of prognosis of many important factors, *e.g.* a) the localization or site in

Table 5. Modified WHO classification of brain tumors in children (from [357])

I. **Tumors of neuroepithelial tissue**
  A. Glial tumors
    1. Astrocytic tumors
      a) Astrocytoma (fibrillary, protoplasmic, gemistocytic, pilocytic and xanthomatous)
      b) Anaplastic astrocytoma
      c) Subependymal giant cell tumors (tuberous sclerosis)
      d) Gigantocellular glioma
    2. Oligodendroglial tumors
      a) Oligodendroglioma
      b) Anaplastic oligodendroglioma
    3. Ependymal tumors
      a) Ependymoma
      b) Anaplastic ependymoma
      c) Myxopapillary ependymoma
    4. Choroid plexus tumors
      a) Choroid plexus papilloma
      b) Anaplastic choroid plexus tumor (carcinoma)
    5. Mixed gliomas
      a) Oligoastrocytoma
        1.Anaplastic oligoastrocytoma
      b) Astroependymoma
        1.Anaplastic ependymoastrocytoma
      c) Oligoastroependymoma
        1.Anaplastic oligoastroependymoma
      d) Oligoependymoma
        1.Anaplastic oligoependymoma
      e) Subependymoma-subependymal glomerate astrocytoma
      f) Gliofibroma
    5. Glioblastomatous tumors
      a) Glioblastoma multiforme
      b) Giant cell glioblastoma
      c) Gliosarcoma
    7. Gliomatosis cerebri

  B. Neuronal tumors
    1. Gangliocytoma
    2. Anaplastic gangliocytoma
    3. Ganglioglioma
    4. Anaplastic ganglioglioma

  C. "Primitive" Neuroepithelial tumors
    1. "Primitive" neuroectodermal tumor, not otherwise specified (NOS)
    2. "Primitive" neuroectodermal tumor, with
      a) Astrocytes
      b) Oligodendrocytes
      c) Ependymal cells
      d) Neuronal cells
      e) Other (melanocytic, mesenchymal)
      f) Mixed cellular elements

Table 5 (continued)

      3. Medulloepithelioma
         a) Medulloepithelioma, NOS
         b) Medulloepithelioma with:
            1.Astrocytes
            2.Oligodendrocytes
            3.Ependymal cells
            4.Neuronal cells
            5.Other (melanocytic, mesenchymal)
            6.Mixed cellular elements
   D. Pineal cell tumors
      1. "Primitive" neuroectodermal tumor (see C) (pineoblastoma)
      2. Pineocytoma

II. Tumors of meningeal and related tissues
   A. Meningiomas
      1. Meningioma, NOS
      2. "Papillary" meningioma
      3. Anaplastic meningioma
   B. Meningeal sarcomatous tumors
      1. Meningeal sarcoma, NOS
      2. Rhabdomyosarcoma or leiomyosarcoma
      3. Mesenchymal chondrosarcoma
      4. Fibrosarcoma
      5. Others
   C. Primary melanocytic tumors
      1. Malignant melanoma
      2. Melanomatosis
      3. Melanocytic tumors, miscellaneous

III. Tumors of nerve sheath cells
   A. Neurilemmoma (schwannoma, neurinoma)
   B. Anaplastic neurilemmoma (schwannoma, neurinoma)
   C. Neurofibroma
   D. Anaplastic neurofibroma (neurofibrosarcoma, neurogenic sarcoma)

IV. Primary malignant lymphomas
Classify according to local current standards

V. Tumors of blood vessel origin
   A. Hemangioblastoma
   B. Hemangiopericytoma
   C. Neoplastic angioendotheliosis-angiosarcoma

VI. Germ cell tumors
   A. Germinoma
   B. Embryonal carcinoma
   C. Choriocarcinoma
   D. Endodermal sinus tumor
   E. Teratomatous tumors
      1. Immature teratoma

Table 5 (continued)

---

    2. Mature teratoma
    3. Teratocarcinoma
  F. Mixed

VII. Malformative tumors
  A. Craniopharyngioma
  B. Rathke's cleft cyst
  C. Epidermal cyst
  D. Dermoid cyst
  E. Colloid cyst of third ventricle
  F. Enterogenous or bronchial cyst
  G. Cyst, NOS
  H. Lipoma
  I. Granular cell tumor (choristoma)
  J. Hamartoma
    1. Neuronal
    2. Glial
    3. Neuronoglial
    4. Meningioangioneurinomatosis

VIII. Tumors of neuroendocrine origin
  A. Tumors of anterior pituitary
    1. Adenoma
    2. Pituitary carcinoma
  B. Paraganglioma

IX. Local extensions from regional tumors
  Type to be specified according to primary diagnosis

X. Metastatic tumors

XI. Unclassified tumors

---

the brain, b) the extent of tumors and their growth tendency. c) Individual histological features[68, 69, 85, 130, 144, 296, 308, 309], and major kinetic differences[129 a, 182, 183, 185, 421]. d) clinical expression and e) the age of the patient.

One major aspect of the classifications of CNS tumors that did not receive sufficient attention is the site of the brain tumor. The WHO classification refers the interested reader to the "ICD"[194, 482], but does not sufficiently emphasize site designations. Designation of tumor site is important, as it appears to be related to prognosis. It is well-established, *e.g.*, that a child with a cerebellar astrocytoma has a better prognosis than a child with a histologically similar tumor located in the cerebrum. Therefore, recently proposed designation of site[26, 357] is listed in Table 6. For example, the cerebellar astrocytoma would have the diagnosis "astrocytoma (pilocytic), Ih". This proposed list does not give a minute breakdown of anatomical sites, but outlines the major sites, general acceptance of which would provide a practical guide to localization of ICNs.

Table 6. Location of tumors interfacing with the nervous system (from [26, 357])

Site	Designation
Central nervous system	I
Hemispheres	a
Frontal	
Parietal	
Temporal	
Occipital	
Thalamus and basal ganglia	b
Hypothalamus	c
Optic nerve	d
Ventricles	e
Pineal region	f
Brain stem	g
Cerebellum	h
Spinal cord	i
Peripheral nervous system	II
Meninges	III
Intradural	
Extradural	
Pituitary gland	IV
Suprasellar region	V
Orbit (eye)	VI
Skull and/or vertebral column	VII

Another staging of cancer of the brain, recommended by the American Joint Committee for Cancer Staging[272] applies to the TNM classification and considers histopathology, histological grading, anatomic sites, TNM staging and performance state of the host. The staging includes: 1.0 histopathology, evaluating the 11 major types of brain tumors (astrocytomas, oligodendrogliomas, ependymal and choroid plexus tumors, glioblastomas, medulloblastomas, neurilemmomas, hemangioblastomas, neuronal tumors, sarcomas, and malignant lymphomas); 1.2 histologic grading with 4 degrees (G): well-differentiated, moderately well-differentiated, no mitoses, poorly differentiated, frequent mitoses, and very poorly differentiated, frequent mitoses, necroses and marked pleomorphism; 2.0 anatomy (primary and metastatic sites), 3. staging (3.1. clinical-diagnostic; 3.2. surgical evaluation, 3.3. postsurgical treatment pathologic staging, 3.4. retreatment staging including recurrences, and 3.5. autopsy staging); 4.0 TNM classification, separating supratentorial and infratentorial primary tumors (T), nodal involvement (N), distant metastasis (M), 5. postsurgical residual tumor (R), 6. stage grouping, and 7. performance status of the host (H). In practice, this combined staging system has not been widely used so far, although its application for medulloblastomas of the posterior fossa has proven prognostics relevance[258].

There is general agreement that, at present, there is obviously no "ideal" classification of CNS neoplasms which will depend on a full characterization of pathological variables and their influence on prognosis. Currently available information about these variables remains incomplete, even for traditional histologic and cytologic features, and certainly for those studied by the newer methods, including electron microscopy, immunocytochemistry, cytogenetics, flow cytophotometry[3, 116, 416] and various quantitative and automatized image analyses[62, 152]. The acquisition of these pathologic data will depend on maximizing the amount of information obtained at each stage that excised tissue or cytologic imprint material is evaluated, assembling these data, and making the appropriate clinicopathologic correlations.

Suggestions for improvement of the mechanism to test the biologic significance of pathologic findings in CNS neoplasms in order to get better information on the biologic behavior and prognosis recommend a systematic approach using standardized techniques[62, 202]. They include a) minimizing tissue sampling problems which are especially critical for CNS neoplasms because of the great intratumor heterogeneity of these lesions, since fractions of the tumor sent to pathology examination may not be the representative for the neoplasm as a whole, b) improvement of tissue handling and processing in order to get optimal results, c) improvement of tissue examination. Routine tissue examination is generally done by light microscopy using routine and special stains including immunohistochemistry and study of specific markers, and electron microscopy, while other modern techniques, including tissue culture, immunology, and cytokinetics will provide additional insights into the dynamic aspects of tumor growth and biology. However, the principal diagnostical tool in clinical neurooncology still remains the traditional light microscopic examination of either cytological and/or tissue preparations of material removed at operation, either by craniotomy, burr hole biopsy or more recently, by CT guided stereotaxic biopsy. Often, material is used for rapid preparations—smears, imprint cytology or frozen sections— which can give helpful information during the course of operation. The diagnostic accuracy of smear or imprint cytology methods in experienced hands is about 93–94% and, hence, is almost as high as that of obtained on paraffin sections using routine staining methods[1, 477], but various are pitfalls awaiting the inexperienced and unwary.

The use of biologic characteristics of a) the survival associated with the individual histologic features and b) clustering of histologic and clinical features in the construction of a classification system and the survival associated with individual clusters might also improve the prognostic value of the currently available pathologic diagnostic system[68, 69, 85, 130, 144, 191, 191a, 296, 308, 309].

IV. Epidemiology

Intracranial neoplasms (ICN) account for 5–10% of all tumors in all age groups, but for 20–40% of all malignancies in childhood, thus representing the third and second most common groups of neoplasms, respectively[462]. International population surveys indicate an annual incidence for primary ICN varying between 5 and 15.8 per 100,000[82, 195, 196] and of secondary malignant ICN between 2.8 and 11.1

(mean 8–9) per 100,000 population[207, 388]. From the national survey of ICN in the USA, during 1973/74, the annual incidence for all age groups was estimated at 16,000 for primary ICN (58% gliomas, 20% meningiomas, 14% adenomas, 7% neurinomas), and 17,400 for secondary ICN, *i.e.* 8.2 and 8.3/100,000 US population[459]. Similar or even higher annual incidence of CNS neoplasms was reported in other countries[82, 121]. The annual incidence of ICN for children under age 15 years is 2–3/100,000[84, 262, 388, 488]. Comparison of international death rates for the years 1967–1974 revealed an average age-adjusted death rate for ICN of 5.8 to 7.5 per 100,000 per year[388]. In the USA there are about 400,000 deaths from cancer each year and 40,000–100,000 (13–30%) are associated with CNS involvement[493]. It is estimated that in 1983 10,800 deaths were caused by primary ICN and about half of them by malignant gliomas, a mortality equal to that predicted for the non-Hodgkin's lymphomas[73]. Primary ICN account for 1.0–2.7% of all autopsy deaths and for 9–10% of all malignancies seen in autopsies of all age groups, but for 50–55% of all malignant neoplasms in autopsy deaths between age 10 and 19 years[462]. IC metastases are observed in 12–34% of all autopsy cases with solid malignancies[178, 207].

Statistics on the prevalence of the different types of brain tumors vary considerably depending from the type of material (surgical or postmortem), the age distribution, geography, and diagnostic criteria[339, 388, 462, 488]. The reported incidence of brain tumors in children and adults, and in all age groups is summarized from several series from the literature and our own material (Table 7). The common topographic distribution of the major types of ICN is listed in Table 8.

V. Special Neurooncology

The present description of intracranial neoplasms follows the standard approach of the WHO classification[496] and its two recent revisions[56, 357]. It is based not only upon light microscopic features but also immunocytochemical and electron microscopic findings of the tumors[10, 20–22, 45, 67, 81, 93, 98, 152, 195, 202, 230, 288, 299, 339, 345, 359 a, 362, 366, 370, 445, 450, 452, 470, 494–499]. Although recognizing the heterogeneity of both individual cell morphologic features and tissue patterns of many tumors within the same diagnostic category, we maintained the convention of placing a neoplasm within a specific category on the basis of the predominant cell type, while neoplasms formed by different cell types are referred to as mixed tumors, *e.g.* oligoastrocytoma or gliosarcoma. Grade coding to denote the degree of histological malignancy and description of typical tumor sites are referred to if necessary.

1. Tumors of Neuroepithelial Tissue

They are derived from neuroepithelial elements and include: A) glial tumors; B) pineal cell tumors; C) neuronal tumors; D) "primitive" neuroectodermal tumors (PNET).

Table 7. Age-related incidence of intracranial neoplasms (percent)

Type of tumor	A. Children (0–15 years) 26 series/mean	B. Adults (> 15 years) 10 series/mean	C. All age groups 23 series/mean
1. Neuroepithelial	58.6–88.0/80.0	20.2–67.0/48.0	25.5–68.0/50.2
Gliomas	48.0–67.0/55.4	20.0–65.0/46.2	25.0–62.0/45.0
Astrocytomas	20.5–52.4/37.6	2.4–26.7/12.8	4.1–24.0/19.0
Oligodendrogliomas	0.6– 2.0/ 0.9	1.0– 7.8/ 4.0	1.1–10.0/ 3.3
Ependymomas	3.8–22.7/11.1	0.3– 3.3/ 1.9	0.9– 5.4/ 4.0
Glioblastomas	0.0–20.3/ 4.4	6.8–54.2/27.9	6.4–53.5/17.1
Gliomas, others	0.0– 1.6/ 1.1	0.0– 2.3/ 0.5	0.0– 8.8/ 1.4
Plexus papillomas	0.0– 7.6/ 1.3	0.0– 0.5/ 0.3	0.0– 0.7/ 0.5
Pineal tumors	0.2– 3.5/ 1.7	0.1– 2.4/ 0.6	0.2– 4.4/ 0.9
Neuronal tumors	0.0– 3.4/ 0.9	0.0– 0.2/ 0.1	0.0– 0.5/ 0.3
Medulloblastomas	10.6–34.4/21.3	0.1– 1.3/ 0.9	0.5– 4.5/ 3.6
2. Meningeal/mesenchymal	0.0– 9.0/ 4.6	10.0–28.3/21.6	8.1–32.0/19.6
Meningiomas	0.4– 4.6/ 1.7	9.7–23.5/19.0	8.1–26.0/15.8
Sarcomas	0.0– 6.0/ 1.8	0.1– 1.2/ 0.8	0.0– 3.8/ 1.4
Lymphomas	0.0– 0.8/ 0.1	0.0– 2.4/ 0.8	0.0– 3.6/ 0.7
Angioblastomas	0.0– 3.0/ 1.1	0.3– 4.8/ 1.8	0.3– 3.1/ 2.4
3. Nerve sheath tumors (neurinoma, neurofibroma)	0.0– 1.1/ 0.4	2.2–15.4/ 6.0	1.7–13.8/ 4.6
4. Germ cell tumors	1.0– 3.2/ 1.7	0.0– 0.4/ 0.1	0.0– 1.6/ 0.8
5. Malformative tumors	0.0–13.8/ 7.2	0.0– 6.1/ 2.2	0.1– 9.4/ 3.2
Craniopharyngioma	0.0– 9.8/ 6.2	0.0– 5.9/ 1.8	0.8– 7.6/ 2.6
Others	0.0– 4.9/ 1.0	0.5– 1.2/ 0.4	0.1– 1.8/ 0.8
6. Pituitary adenomas	0.0– 1.5/ 0.5	4.0–14.0/ 8.5	3.1–18.0/ 8.2
7. Regional tumors	0.0– 3.2/ 0.3	0.0– 1.1/ 0.4	0.0– 3.2/ 0.6
8. Metastatic tumors	0.0– 3.8/ 0.4	5.4–24.4/10.9	4.1–29.6/ 9.4
9. Others	0.0–16.7/ 2.4	0.0–23.9/ 0.3	0.0– 2.5/ 0.8
10. Unclassified	0.0– 8.5/ 2.1	0.0– 5.6/ 1.2	0.0–12.5/ 1.8
Total (literature and personal series)	7,120	13,500	52,000

A. References[84, 146, 212, 388, 488]. B. References[10, 195, 212, 370, 388, 440, 462, 494, 498, 499]. C. References[10, 195, 212, 230, 339, 370, 388, 459, 462, 494, 498].

Table 8. Topographic distribution of intracranial tumors in children and adults

Location	Type of tumor (prominent)	
	Adults	Children
Cerebral hemispheres	astrocytoma	astrocytoma
	astrocytoma, anaplastic	astrocytoma, anaplastic
	glioblastoma	ependymoma
	meningioma	mixed gliomas
	metastases	oligodendroglioma
	oligodendroglioma	
	ependymoma	
	lymphoma	
Basal ganglia	astrocytoma	astrocytoma
	oligodendroglioma	oligodendroglioma
	glioblastoma	
	metastases	
Corpus callosum	astrocytoma	astrocytoma
	astrocytoma, anaplastic	astrocytoma, anaplastic
	glioblastoma	oligodendroglioma
	oligodendroglioma	lipoma
	lymphoma	
	lipoma	
Lateral ventricles	ependymoma	ependymoma
	meningioma	choroid plexus papilloma
	subependymoma	
	chor. plexus papilloma	
Third ventricle	colloid cyst	ependymoma
	ependymoma	choroid plexus papilloma
Optic nerve chiasm	meningioma	astrocytoma, pilocytic
	astrocytoma, pilocytic	
Diencephalon	astrocytoma, pilocytic	astrocytoma, pilocytic
	astrocytoma, anaplastic	
Pineal region	germ cell tumors	germ cell tumors
	pineocytoma	pineoblastoma
	hamartoma	pineocytoma
	astrocytoma	hamartoma
Cerebellum	angioblastoma	medulloblastoma
	astrocytoma, pilocytic	astrocytoma, pilocytic
	metastases	angioblastoma
		dermoid cyst
Cerebello-pontine angle	schwannoma	ependymoma
	meningioma	choroid plexus papilloma
	epidermoid cyst	
	glomus jugulare tumor	
Fourth ventricle	meningioma	ependymoma
	schwannoma	choroid plexus papilloma
	subependymoma	
Sellar region	pituitary adenoma	craniopharyngioma
	meningioma	germ cell tumors
	craniopharyngioma	
	germ cell tumors	

A. Glial Tumors or Gliomas (ICD-0 M-9380/1–3, ICD-9: 225.0 NDV: 1814000)

This largest group of intracranial neoplasms accounting for 45–55% of the brain tumors in both children and adults is derived from different types of neuroglial cells found in the CNS astrocytes, oligodendrocytes, ependymal or mixed populations. The taxonomy is organized along both the predominant "cell of origin" and anatomical or regional lines, while the degree of dedifferentiation is expressed by the designation whether a tumor is or is not anaplastic. Many clinico-pathological studies and evaluations of treatment protocols, however, still use numerical coding systems separating three or four degrees of malignancy (see Table 9).

1. Astrocytic Tumors

a) Astrocytoma (M-9400/1–3, ICD-9: 237.5 NDV: 1809000)

This tumor constituting some 20–30% of all gliomas and affecting all age groups is composed predominantly of astrocytes with variable numbers of intracytoplasmic intermediate filaments demonstrated by antisera to glial fibrillary acidic protein (GFAP), the major protein component of glial intermediary filaments and a marker for astrocytic differentiation[45, 93, 154, 283, 445, 450].

Its histologic classification into various subgroups (fibrillary, protoplasmic, pilocytic gemistocytic, xanthomatous) depends on the appearance of the individual tumor cells and on the patterns they form with each other and with other tissue elements. Because of regional histological variability and the uncertain relationship of histological pattern and biological behavior, these tumors are often simply designated "astrocytoma". However, if there is preponderance of one histologic pattern, the appropriate adjective should be used.

The major topographic sites include a) *cerebral hemispheres* appearing as diffuse and ill defined, solid or cystic tumors of fibrillary, protoplasmic or mixed cellular type. They represent about 25–30% of intracranial tumors in both children and adults[84, 362, 370]. They may invade the leptomeninges and occasionally undergo dedifferentiation into anaplastic astrocytoma or glioblastoma. Growth kinetic data on isomorphic astrocytomas indicate a mean labeling index of < 1.0–1.27%, a growth fraction of 1–3%, a cell cycle time of 48 days and a potential doubling time of 36 days[182, 183, 185, 421], which are undoubtedly very different from those of anaplastic astrocytomas and glioblastomas (Table 10). Recurrent astrocytomas rather often show an increase in histological malignancy, as was observed in about two-thirds of recurrent astrocytomas of the cerebral hemispheres[200, 205]. Only about 40% of recurrent isomorphic or moderately differentiated astrocytomas are histologically unchanged at second biopsy and/or autopsy, while the majority shows increased signs of anaplasia and may finally develop into anaplastic (high-grade) astrocytomas or show the features of glioblastoma (Table 11). Recurrent gliomas with large cell populations often display transition into and preponderance of small anaplastic cells with increased aggressiveness[141, 185–187, 200]. This progressive dedifferentiation has been confirmed by *in vitro* studies of recurrent gliomas that showed increased growth intensity and kinetics[152, 231], and serial transplantation of gliomas[283, 389], while organotypic cultures of glioblastoma reveal progressive astrocytic differentiation with increased formation of glial fibrils, indicating the astrocytic origin of most glioblastomas[366]. b) *Brain stem tumors*, occupying the

Table 9. Major histologic grade coding systems for gliomas

A. *Four-Tiered Grading Systems*[229, 230, 288, 499]

Grade I: (benign): isomorphic, differentiated tissue picture of low cellularity, no pleomorphism, no hyperchromatic nuclei, no or rare mitotic activity, no or only minimal regressive tissue changes, restricted to cystic or mucoid transformation.

Grade II: (semibenign): moderate cellularity, slight pelomorphism, mild nuclear hyperchromasia, occasional mitotic activity, no or only mild vascular proliferation, no necroses.

Grade III: (semimalignant): moderate to marked hypercelluarity and pleomorphism, but cellular origin of many neoplastic cells still recognizable (positive immunoreaction with specific markers, *e.g.* GFAP); hyperchromatic nuclei, high mitotic activity, vascular proliferation and rare necroses.

Grade IV: (malignant): extreme hypercellularity, marked cellulary and nuclear pleomorphism, hyperchromatic nuclei; cytologic origin of most neoplastic cells no more recognizable (no or only little immunoreaction with specific marker, *e.g.* GFAP), abundant mitotic activity, necroses with or without a pseudopalisading: marked vascular proliferation and mesenchymal reaction.

B. *Three-Tiered Grading System*[302, 353]

Grade I: (isomorphic, benign): differentiated tissue picture of low to moderate cellularity, no or only slight pleomorphism, no mitoses, vascular proliferation or necroses.

Grade II: (intermediate): less well differentiated tissue pattern, moderate hypercellularity, moderate pleomorphism, iso-orhyperchromatic nuclei, moderate number of mitoses, vascular proliferation, no or only few necroses.

Grade III: (anaplastic): dedifferentiated picture, marked hypercellularity, extreme cellular and nuclear pleomorphism, abundant pathologic mitoses, true necroses and massive capillary endothelial proliferation.

C. *Histologic Criteria of Astrocytomas* used by the US-BTSG (Brain Tumor Study Group) (see[68, 308, 309])

I. *Astrocytoma:* moderate to high cellularity, slight pleomorphism, no hyperchromatic nuclei, no vascular proliferation, no necroses.

II. *Anaplastic astrocytoma:* moderate hypercellularity, moderate pleomorphism, hyperchromatic nuclei, vascular proliferation, no necroses.

III. *Glioblastoma multiforme:* Marked hypercellularity, pleomorphism, hyperchromatic nuclei, necroses with or without pseudopalisading (*required*), vascular proliferation (*not required*). In this classification, the key criterion used to distinguish glioblastoma from anaplastic astrocytoma is *necrosis*.

---

region traversed by the aqueduct of Sylvius and the fourth ventricle, particularly affect children and adolescents, where they account for 8–12% of all brain tumors[84, 240]. They show diffuse invasive growth causing diffuse enlargement of the brain stem with frequent invasion of the fourth ventricle or cerebellum. Their histology resembles fibrillary astrocytoma with many tumors showing various degrees of anaplasia with areas ranging from isomorphic to anaplastic astrocytoma, while others show hemorrhage and necrosis characteristic of glioblastoma[362, 370]. Tumor spread has been found to be dependent on the site of origin and the histologic grade of malignancy[271].

Prognosis of supratentorial astrocytomas is related to the morphological grade of malignancy and to specific histologic features indicating tumor behavior. Low-grade (isomorphic) tumors show 5-year survivals of 30–50%, with average survival rates after surgery of 48 months and long-term survival up to over 10 years[84, 210, 248, 308, 391], and variable improvement by radiation[135, 398, 399]. Brain stem astrocytomas have a poor prognosis with 5-year survival rates between 25 and 35% which have not been considerably improved despite aggressive radiation and chemotherapy[35, 36, 84].

b) Pilocytic Astrocytoma (M-9421/1; ICD-9: 192.9: NDV; 1807000)

The pilocytic pattern, previously referred to as spongioblastoma[498], is composed of elongated cells with unipolar or bipolar processes that tend to form parallel bundles adjacent to loosely structured microcystic areas. Rosenthal fibers and eosinophilic intracytoplasmic droplets are usually found; they contain densely packed glial filaments[98, 152] but are mostly either GFAP-negative or partially positive[154, 406]. This tumor is most common in children and is generally localized in midline structures, particularly in the cerebellum, diencephalon and optic nerve, while the cystic type of "juvenile" pilocytic astrocytoma of the cerebral hemispheres, also referred to as "Bergstrand tumor"[249] accounts for less than 10% of cerebral gliomas[135, 329].

Cerebellar astrocytomas, representing about 12% of brain tumors in children, are the second most common cerebellar tumor affecting both the midline and the hemispheres[84, 144, 362]. They are usually solid and noninvasive and often contain large cysts. Histologically, several types have been described[144, 146, 147, 370]: a) the classical type similar to the "juvenile" type of pilocytic astrocytoma of the third ventricle with compact areas of strongly fibrillated fusiform cells alternating with spongy and microcystic areas, and b) a much less frequent diffuse type characterized by an equal distribution of glial fibrils, uniform cells and small, evenly dispersed cavities which is similar to diffuse cerebral astrocytoma. Gilles *et al.*[143, 144] attempted to define prognostic microscopic features: They found that the presence of microcysts, leptomeningeal deposits, Rosenthal fibers, and oligodendroglial foci (type A, present in about 70%) indicated an excellent prognosis (10-year-survival rate of 94%), whereas perivascular pseudorosettes, high cell density, necrosis, mitoses, and calcification (type B present in about 20%) suggested a poor prognosis (10-year-survival rate of 29%). However, by 15 years the "diffuse" astrocytoma has a 70% survival, and by 25 years only a 38% survival, whereas the "juvenile" astrocytoma after radical excision remains relatively recurrence-free. Malignant transformation of pilocytic astrocytomas is extremely rare[30, 55, 236]. In general,

Table 10. Some kinetic data of human brain tumors

Type	References	LI (labeling index) % mean (range)	GF (growth fraction) %	Tc (cell cycle time) hours/days	Cell loss fraction %	Tp (potential) tumor doubling time/days
Glioblastoma in vivo	182, 185, 186, 187, 421	9 (4.4-17) (5.1-15)	0.15-0.3 (0.21-0.58)	2-3 d (39-87 hours) 5-10 days	80-85%	3-8 6.1-15
	254a		0.6 6.07[b]	36-151 hours		
	303a	4,8 ± 0,3[a] 5.2 (2-11)				
in vitro						9-10
Gliosarcoma	182		0.23-0.25	83-89 hours		
	303a	7.8 ± 1.5[a]				
Anaplastic Astrocytoma in vivo	182, 185, 186, 187	4.7 (2.3-8.7) (2.6-10.9)	6.07 0.09-0.25 0.01-0.12			
	421, 254a			6.5-13 days (154-316 hours) 1.9-2.2 days (43.9-53 hours)		7-10
in vitro	182					
Astrocytoma well differentiated	182, 185	1.27 (0.4-1.9) <1.0 (0.3-1.7)	0.01-0.03 (< 1%)	48 days (1,154 hours)		36-51 50.3
	303a, 254a					
Ependymoma	182	5.2 (2-11)				9
Medulloblastoma	184, 421 (n = 4)	12.0 ± 1.3 8.0*	0.3-0.35 10-18.2[b]	2-3 days (22.2-30.6 hours)	74-97%	9.4/69
	169*, 254a, 66a					

Meningioma	421, 254a	1.4 (1.2–1.6)	0.5–1,0[b]	34
Meningioma malignant	129a, 303a	<1.0[a]	<1.0[b]	
Hemangiopericytoma,	129a	9.0–13.6[a]	9.9 (4.1–15.5)[b]	
recurrent	129a, 292a	2.0[a]	1.3[b]	
Neurinoma	421	0.2	0.3–1.14[b]	
Malignant schwannoma		23		
Neuroblastoma		13.5 ± 7.5		3.5
Metastasis	66a, 182, 355a	6.3–13.6	20–>50.0[b]	108 hours
Undiff. bronch. cancer				2.5
Colorectal cancer				3.1
Sigma cell cancer	421			6.8
Melanoma	254a		18.52	14
Lymphoma				16
Sarcoma				24

[a] Bromodeoxyuridine uptake
[b] Kc-67 mouse monoclonal anti-proliferation antibody (66a, 254a, 292a, 355a)

pilocytic astrocytoma differs in its biological beavior[152] and shows a much better outcome than other isomorphic astrocytomas. Hence, in the WHO classification they were coded as grade I, while the other astrocytomas were coded as WHO grade II[496, 497], but subarachnoid spread of histological benign cerebellar astrocytomas may occur[14, 200].

c) Astroblastoma (M-9430/3; ICD-9: 192.9, NDV: 1809000)

This rare tumor occurring in cerebral hemispheres of young adults shows a perivascular arrangement of radiating cellular processes forming pseudorosettes and a corresponding ultrastructure showing the coexistence of varied maturity astrocytic cells and their compact arrangement around fenestrated blood vessels[247]. It is considered a subtype of protoplasmic astrocytoma with intermediate malignancy that has to be separated from both ependymomas and anaplastic astrocytomas, although some "astroblastomas" reported in the literature may represent ependymal tumors with swollen, perivascular, GFAP-positive, astrocyte-like cells[152, 153]. Astroblastomatous structures are occasionally seen in anaplastic astrocytomas and glioblastomas, too.

d) Subependymal Giant Cell Astrocytoma (in Tuberous Sclerosis) (M-9384/1; ICD-9: 225.9 NDV: 1808000)

This periventricular, usually circumscribed tumor is composed of giant, often fusiform cells with various degrees of astrocytic and/or neuronal differentiation[359a]. A perivascular arrangement may be conspicuous, and calcification is frequent. The tumor arises from the medial part of the floor of the lateral ventricle and may occlude the foramen of Monro it typically occurs in young patients as part of the tuberous sclerosis complex[46, 304]. There is no known malignant transformation, or transliquoral seeding of this tumor.

e) Xanthomatous Astrocytoma (ICD-9: 191.9; NDV: 1800000)

Meningocerebral xanthoastrocytoma, referred to as pleomorphic xanthoastrocytoma (PXA) is a tumor that occurs primarily in children and young adults[228]. They are primarily supratentorial tumors growing in the superficial cortex with extensive invasion of the leptomeninges. Histologically, they are featured by cellular pleomorphism with many large, atypical, and lipidized cells containing cytoplasmic GFAP-positive material and showing the ultrastructural features of fibrillary astrocytes, supporting the proposed subpial astrocytic origin of PXA. Despite their bizarre cellular pleomorphism, these tumors show a favorable outcome[149, 228], but malignant transformation of recurrent tumor with bad outcome has been observed[332, 469]. It has to be distinguished from "heavily lipidized malignant gliomas"[22] constituting a rare subgroup of giant cell glioblastomas with poor prognosis[139] and from granular cell glioblastoma[241a]

f) Anaplastic Astrocytoma (M-9401/3; ICD-9: 192.9; NDV: 1808000)

A tumor formed by astrocytes demonstrating various degrees of pleomorphism, increased cellularity, and variable numbers of mitotic figures, anaplastic astrocytoma akin to WHO grade III may show vascular endothelial proliferation but no or only rare foci of necrosis which are not of the pseudopalisading type[68, 69, 309, 357]. Anaplastic astrocytomas occur in 10–20% of the patients entering in major clinical glioma trials[68, 309], but there is evidence that some degree of anaplasia is present in 40–80% of astrocytomas[370, 381]. These changes may develop at any stage of the life history of the tumor, and a fairly large number of anaplastic forms may develop from previously differentiated neoplasms (Table 11). This has been well demonstrated by histological and tissue culture studies from recurrent astrocytomas[11, 152, 200, 205, 231]. Cytologic heterogeneity in anaplastic astrocytomas is also seen *in vitro* in permanent glioma-derived cell lines showing distinct morphologic patterns, while after serial passage to nude mice an in organotypic cultures a gradual loss of heterogeneity in such tumors is more common[283, 366].

Although attempts to identify histologic criteria that could separate anaplastic astrocytomas into subgroups differing in their biologic behavior and clinical behavior had only limited success[69, 230, 353] an association of specific histologic features with tumor behavior appears more promising[68, 85, 130, 144, 308, 309, 435], and some specific histologic variables have been shown to serve as prognostically significant markers: While no correlation with survival was found for estimation of nuclear pleomorphism and cell density or the presence of secondary structures (perivascular or subpial growth patterns), vascular endothelial proliferation and increased mitotic activity were found to be correlated with significantly shorter survival in one series of anaplastic astrocytomas[130]. Among 10 histologic variables investigated in 150 cases of anaplastic astrocytoma[68], the only significant prognostic variable was vascular proliferation showing inverse relation to the length of survival. However, there were significant internal positive relations between gemistocytes and bizarre cells or perivascular lymphocytes, and cellularity versus small cells and necroses. In most current studies, anaplastic astrocytoma is distinguished from glioblastoma multiforme by the rather frequent and strong expression of the astrocytic marker GFAP by tumor cells and, particularly by the absence of frank necroses[68, 130, 218, 308, 309] and by major cell kinetic differences, *e.g.* a much lower labeling index and growth fraction, longer cell cycle time and potential tumor doubling time (Table 10).

Prognostic evaluation of supratentorial astrocytomas displayed average postoperative survival in anaplastic forms to be about half of those in patients with low-grade (well differentiated) tumors[248, 391]. On the other hand, it is well established that anaplastic astrocytoma carriers are significantly different in age, duration of preoperative symptoms and outcome showing 50 to 100% longer survival than those with glioblastoma irrespective the type of treatment[68, 69, 141, 210, 215, 308, 309, 336, 394, 397, 398, 430, 435, 457]. As biological entities, the anaplastic astrocytoma and glioblastoma may be more individual than is often assumed, although some of the anaplastic astrocytomas would become glioblastoma in time. Although rapid anaplasia may occur spontaneously in supratentorial gliomas of adolescents and young adults[362, 387], there may be a small number of gliomas at risk of an adverse response to antitumor treatment with anaplastic change of phenotype due to "focal progression" in tumor with preponderance and overgrowth of small anaplastic cell populations. In two series of anaplastic gliomas treated with adjuvant radiation and chemotherapy such enhancement of anaplasia possibly related to treatment was seen in 3 and 4.7% respectively[61, 208].

Table 11. Morphologic dedifferentiation in relapsing supratentorial gliomas (from[2, 11*, 205])

Primary tumor	Recurrence		No change	Increased anaplasia	Glioblastoma
Astrocytoma	first	482	192 ± 39.8%	285 ± 59.2%	5 ± 1.0%
	second	71	15 ± 21.0%	44 ± 62.0%	12 ± 17.0%
	third	18	—	9 ± 50.0%	9 ± 50.0%
Anaplastic astrocytoma	first	240	148 ± 61.7%	—	92 ± 38.3%
	second	28	15 ± 53.6%	—	13 ± 46.4%
Oligodendroglioma	first	51	38 ± 74.5%	13 ± 25.5%	—
	second	18	7 ± 38.9%	10 ± 55.6%	1 ± 5.5%
	third	4	1 ± 25.0%	3 ± 75.0%	—
Anaplastic oligodendroglioma	first	8	4 ± 50.0%	—	4 ± 50.0%
	second	2	—	—	2 ± 100%
Ependymoma*	first	65	50 ± 77%	14 ± 21%	1 ± 3%
	second	19	6 ± 32%	10 ± 53%	3 ± 15%
	third	2	—	2 ± 100%	—
Anaplastic ependymoma*	first	11	10 ± 90%	—	1 ± 10%

2. Oligodendroglial Tumors

They comprise 5–12% of all gliomas and 5–7% of all intracranial neoplasms, and occur at any age, chiefly in adults. Prominent sites are the cerebral hemispheres, particularly frontal, with a tendency towards diffuse infiltration of the cerebral cortex and frequent invasion of the leptomeninges, while tumors in the posterior fossa are rare[269a, 296, 325]. Although oligodendroglial tumors present a spectrum of histological anaplasia, recent classification assign two grades, *i.e.* "typical" oligodendroglioma and mixed oligoastrocytoma (see mixed gliomas), and their anaplastic variants, while others use three or four grades[296, 312, 391, 269a].

a) Oligodendroglioma (M-9451/0; ICD-9: 191.9; NDV: 1806000)

Well-differentiated oligodendroglial tumors have a uniform histological appearance, featured by a monotony of round cells with small regular nuclei with moderate prominent nucleoli, clear cytoplasm, and scant mitotic activity. This monotony tends to be broken up by a distinctive network of blood vessels which often imparts a rather lobulated pattern to the tumor. A distinctive feature is the "fried-egg" or "honeycomb" appearance due to the occurrence of artefactual perinuclear halos. Despite the presence of carbonic anhydrase C in normal adult oligodendrocytes and of myelin basic protein in infant oligodendrocytes, neither of these markers has been found in oligodendrogliomas[45, 470]. Ultrastructurally, the tumor cells have rounded nuclei and a well-defined scanty rounded or angular cytoplasm with poor organelles and no glial fibrils, but occasional crystalloid inclusions[98, 299]. There is a tendency for the vessels to undergo mucoid or hyaline degeneration, and calcification is present in some 90% of the tumors; it may be so heavy that it can be seen in plain X-rays of the skull.

b) Anaplastic Oligodendroglioma (M-9451/3; ICD-9: 191.9; NDV: 1805000)

The anaplastic variant, representing about 30% of all oligodendrogliomas is a markedly densely cellular tumor with pleomorphic nuclei, more prominent nucleoli, frequent mitotic activity, vascular proliferation and occasional giant cells[22]. Although some of these tumors present with necrotic foci and therefore histologically merge with the glioblastoma[362, 392, 498], most anaplastic forms fall short of this state, although their *in vitro* behavior is *similar* to glioblastoma[152].

   Prognosis of oligodendrogliomas is similar to that of astrocytomas[205, 269a, 312]; relationship between histological features and clinical malignancy are not clear, although some grading systems pretend to correlate with prognosis[269a, 296, 391, 408]. Longer survival was seen when the neoplasm has a low cell density, microcystic changes and no necrosis, than in oligodendrogliomas with high cellularity, necrosis and microcystic changes, whereas other histological variables (number of mitotic figures, calcification or perivascular lymphocytic infiltration) appear not to be factors of prognostic value[269a, 296]. Average survival of isomorphic tumors with low cell density is about 8 years with survivals up to over 25 years, and 5-year survivals of 70%, of intermediate forms about 4–5 years, with 40% 5-year survival, but only 17 months for anaplastic tumors[269a]. Recurrence after surgery is seen in about 50% with rather little tendency towards anaplasia, about 75% of recurrences showing similar histological features as the primary tumor, while multiple recurrences and relapsing anaplastic neoplasms show stronger tendency towards dedifferentiation (Table 11). The transition from benign to malignant behavior may not occur for many years. Invasion into the meninges and dissemination through the CSF pathway is well recognized and was observed in two thirds of recurrent oligodendrogliomas at biopsy and/or autopsy[200, 202, 362]. Remote extracranial metastasis has been described[99, 177, 213].

Many oligodendrogliomas contain cells with astrocytic characteristics including positive GFAP reaction, and "gliofibrillary" oligodendrocytes contain bundles of filaments which are strongly positive for GFAP[154, 165]. These subtypes with GFAP-containing cells are considered to be of oligodendroglial origin, while lesions with a significant component of neoplastics astrocytes should be regarded as mixed oligoastrocytomas, which are tumors of two distinctive and nontransitional cell populations (see mixed gliomas).

3. Ependymal Tumors

a) Ependymoma (M-9391/1; ICD-9: 191.1; NDV: 1815000)

They constitute 4–6% of all intracranial tumors and are more common in childhood. They typically project from an ependymal surface, most commonly the floor of the fourth ventricle or lateral and third ventricles, but also arise in the cerebellopontine angle, the region of the central canal of the spinal cord, or from the filum terminale. About two thirds are infratentorial, and about one third supratentorial[9, 84, 195, 240, 362]. Grossly, circumscribed and well-defined solid or cystic, and partially encapsulated growth, their histology shows high cellularity with regular patterns composed predominantly of ependymal cells often expressing GFAP[45] that form rosettes (structures resembling the central canal of the spinal cord), canals (structures resembling ventricular walls), and perivascular pseudorosettes (arrangements of cells with processes oriented toward the wall of a blood vessel, the gliovascular structure). The perivascular pseudorosette is the most common feature, while structures resembling central canals or ventricular linings are diagnostic but infrequent, but this tumor may exhibit a diverse range of histologic patterns that make diagnosis difficult[357]. Tumor cells may contain eosinophilic intracytoplasmic granules and PTAH-positive structures, called blepharoblasts, the basal end bodies of cilia along the free borders of ependymal cells. At the ultrastructural level, tumor cells contain zonulae adherentes, cilia with either the normal 9 + 2 configuration of their axial filament complex or with an abnormal internal configuration, and microvilli[98, 128, 299, 345, 366]. These tumors may contain cartilage, calcium deposits or dysplastic bones.

Ependymomas are grouped according to microscopic criteria into several groups: a) *classical* type with solid cellular or ependymal architecture; b) *papillary* (M-9393/1) with epithelial arrangement of papillae and tubules which, in places, especially when situated in the fourth ventricle, may mimic the features of choroid plexus papilloma. A distinction between these two based on the presence of PTAH-positive processes and a typically glial stroma may be misleading, since GFAP has been demonstrated in choroid plexus papillomas with the implication that these tumors can develop glial characteristics[365]; c) *myxopapillary* type (M-9341/1) which occurs virtually exclusively in the region of cauda equina and originates from the filum terminale or the conus medullaris. It is composed of ependymal cells often arranged in a perivascular papillary manner around central cores of cellular hyaline connective tissue. There is highly vascular stroma, and mucin is often demonstrable in the cytoplasm of tumor cells and in blood vessel walls. This material may be so prominent that the architecture is blurred[414]. Ultrastructure includes the presence of few cilia, of complex intercellular digitations, and of abundant basement membrane material, attributable to the normal structure of the filum terminale, where ependymal cells are directly apposed to connective tissue derived from the leptomeninges[299, 366]. d) The *foramen Monro* type (M-9391/1) that usually lacks the typical gliovascular structures and frequently shows cells that by light microscopy resemble oligodendrocytes but have their ultrastructural features of ependymal cells[223].

In general, these varying pathologic subtypes do not have prognostic features, although some tissue patterns, such as subependymal pattern with clustering of cells, regions of high fibrillarity, perivascular pseudorosettes, calcifications, foci of increased cellularity, etc, may have a relationship to the patient survival[192]. Recurrent ependymomas of the posterior fossa almost never show a tendency towards anaplasia, which is more often observed in supratentorial ependymomas that may undergo progressive dedifferentiation (Table 11)[2, 9, 200, 205]. CSF seeding occurs in about 20%, more often in infratentorial ependymomas[84, 373].

b) Subependymoma (Subependymal Glomerulate Astrocytoma) (M-9383/1; ICD-9: 191.9; NDV: 1815000)

This variant of ependymoma in which the fibrillary subependymal glia is the dominant cell[74, 128], by others is considered as a mixed tumor consisting of astrocytes and ependymal cells and, hence, is classified as a mixed glioma[357]. The tumors arise beneath the lining of the fourth or lateral ventricles, and contain clusters of nests of nuclei interspersed in a background of fine or coarse fibrils. Nuclei are usually uniform, and there is only slight to moderate pleomorphism. Vacuoles, mineralization, and microcysts may be present. Ultrastructural studies disclose presence of glial filaments, microvilli, and zonulae adherentes[299, 349]. These tumors are often small, asymptomatic nodules incidentally discovered at autopsy, but large symptomatic examples particularly in the fourth ventricle may also occur[67, 219, 349, 376]. There is no known anaplastic subset of this tumor.

c) Anaplastic Ependymoma (M-9392/3; ICD-9: 191.9; NDV: 1815000)

Tumors showing the typical features of ependymomas, but presenting anaplastic features such as nuclear atypica, high nuclear/cytoplasmic ratio, increased cellularity, multiple nuclei, a marked increase in number of mitotic figures, necrosis and vascular endothelial proliferation, occur in both children and adults and account for about 5 to 10% of all ependymomas[9, 370, 495], but may range from 15–86%[471a]. They are more commonly located in the supratentorial region and, in 20–60% are associated with spreading along the CSF pathways or spinal cord seeding, while some of them show extraneural metastases[84, 177, 213, 373]. Anaplastic ependymoma is to be distinguished from "ependymoblastoma", an extremely unusual tumor of primitive origin with characteristic histologic and ultrastructural features[171, 254a, 360], now grouped among the PNETs[56, 357, 364].

The prognosis of ependymomas varies with the age of the patient, location and malignancy grade of the tumor. The overall 5-year survival in children with intracranial ependymoma is approximately 30%, and combination treatments have improved prognosis with 10-year survival rates of 20 and 74%, for high and low grade tumors, respectively[36, 84], whereas adults with this tumor usually show a much better prognosis[152, 192].

4. Mixed Gliomas

Mixed gliomas containing a conspicuous mixture of two or three types of glial cells, in most classification are grouped within other main categories, while Rorke et al.[357] spearated them as a distinct group, occurring in the brains of both children and adults, more often in the cerebral hemispheres of young patients.

a) Oligoastrocytoma (M-9382/1–3; ICD-9: 191.9; NDV: 1806000)

Oligoastrocytoma contains a conspicuous admixture of oligodendroglial cells and astrocytes. The oligodendroglial cells may be sparse or abundant with expression of GFAP. Either component (oligodendroglia or astrocytic) may predominate, and the name may be modified accordingly. Anaplastic oligoastrocytoma shows anaplasia of either component. These tumors are found most commonly in the cerebral hemispheres of adults. Their biology is similar to "pure" glial tumors, but many of them may present cytological problems in the further evolution with respect to their malignancy potentials.

b) Ependymoastrocytoma

This very rare type contains perivascular pseudorosettes in addition to astrocytes. The astrocytic component must be external to the perivascular pseudorosettes, as the radially oriented eosinophilic fibrils within the pseudorosettes are often PTAH- and GFAP-positive. Ependymal rosettes may be present, and ultrastructural studies confirm the ependymal nature of the cells[223]. Anaplastic forms may occur.

c) Oligoastroependymoma

This rare type contains distinct regions with each of the three glial cell types. Patches of oligodendroglial cells, with or without interspersed perivascular pseudorosettes and regions of astrocytes are all present.

d) Oligoependymoma

Oligoependymoma contains prominent patches of oligodendroglia and perivascular pseudorosettes without an appreciable astrocytic component.

e) Gliofibroma (ICD-9: 225.0; NDV: 1814000)

Gliofibroma is a rare tumor of infancy and childhood composed of intermingled well differentiated astrocytes and fibroblasts[127, 350]. The two cell types are often surrounded by the same basal lamina, collagen and reticulin fibers with abundant gliofibrils, and are suggested to develop from pluripotent cells or hamartoma-like lesions developing into glial and mesenchymal cells[350]. The tumor usually displays no evidence of anaplasia.

5. Glioblastomatous Tumors

The WHO classification proposed the grouping of glioblastoma and medulloblastoma into one category called "poorly differentiated and embryonal tumors", which has been found to be inappropriate for many reasons[26, 56, 152, 203, 339, 357]. Glioblastoma is now widely accepted as an extreme manifestation of dedifferentiation on part of glioma cells, mostly astrocytes[366], but occasionally tumors with other histologic features are said to evolve into glioblastoma[495, 498]. Hence, a compromise suggestion was to make "glioblastoma" a separate category[56, 357].

a) Glioblastoma Multiforme (M-9440/3; ICD-9: 191.9; NDV: 1811000)

This highly malignant neoplasm, representing 15–20% of all intracranial tumors and about 50% of all gliomas, may occur in all parts of the brain[203, 380]. It is found most commonly in the cerebral hemispheres in adults with a peak age of 45 to 55 years, while it accounts for only 7–8% of all intracranial tumors in childhood[203]. Often deeper structures are involved with butterfly-like growth through the corpus callosum, while the tumor is rare in the cerebellum and brain stem[78, 161, 203, 370, 390], part of which have been interpreted as pilocytic astrocytomas with regressive cellular atypias[152]. Glioblastoma is often large and apparently well circumscribed, with highly variegated and multicolored surface, white-yellow necroses and hemorrhages. Microscopically, the tumor shows high cellularity, marked pleomorphism, high mitotic rate, extensive, often serpiginous areas of necrosis bordered by glial cells that give the appearance of pseudopalisading, and marked hypervascularity with endothelial proliferation and glomeruloid structures composed of dense coils of hyperplastic vessels. There is a tremendous variability in the histologic appeararance between different areas of the same tumor and between the tumor of different patients which are composed of very diverse cells that sometimes resemble one or more of the glial cell types (fibrillary astrocytes, gemistocytes, large bizarre glia, and small anaplastic cells, etc), but more often are only recognizable as neoplastic cells without GFAP immunoreactivity[68, 141, 154, 203, 362]. Cytologic heterogeneity is present also *in vitro* in permanent glioma-derived cell lines showing stable but distinct morphologic patterns of growth which can be characterized as fibroblastic, glial, fascicular etc, while after serial passage to nude mice and in organotypic cultures a gradual loss of heterogeneity in such tumors is more common[283, 366].

The spectrum of cytologic heterogeneity is even further expanded by radiation and chemotherapy which introduce additional extremes of nuclear size, pleomorphism, giant cells and necroses[65, 137, 208, 384, 385, 476]. Glioblastoma multiforme is a controversial term. Many examples are probably derived by anaplasia of a preexisting glioma, and about 25–30% exhibit morphologic evidence of having arisen from such a preexisting astrocytoma[370, 380, 381, 383]. The astrocytic origin of most glioblastomas has been well demonstrated *in vivo* and *in vitro* by electron microscopy, immunocytological demonstration of the astrocytic differentiation marker GFAP, and in organotypic tissue cultures showing progressive differentiation towards astrocytomas[45, 98, 218, 283, 299, 366, 450]. Other tumors, the so-called "primary" glioblastomas, are suggested to arise as anaplastic and poorly differentiated neoplasms *de novo* from a primitive stem cell, the glioblast, there being no evidence of a preexisting better-differentiated glioma[203, 370]. In the studies of the US-BTSG (Brain Tumor Study Group), the relation between anaplastic astrocytoma and glioblastoma was 175 to 1,265, *i.e.* glioblastomas representing 88% of the total[68]. In spite of the glioblastomas' well recognized morphologic diversity, the pathologic substrate of aggressiveness of this malignant glioma is related largely to the proliferation of a population of small anaplastic cells, showing a positive correlation versus cellularity and mitoses[68, 141]. The prevalence of small cell types was also evident in most infiltrated regions and metastatic foci, whereas in cases with predominant composition of large and gemistocytic cells, only limited infiltration of brain tissue and no metastatic spread was seen. Small cells as the principal cell types in CNS implants of glioblastomas[489], in cerebrospinal fluid cytology of glioblastomas[211], and in extraneural metastases have also been noted[104, 189, 213]. These small anaplastic cell populations have the highest labeling index and aneuploidy, whereas large, bizarre, and multinucleated or gemistocytic cells are rather indolent[186]. Internal correlation between histological variables disclosed statistically significant association between the presence of small cells versus cellularity, between cellularity versus necrosis and vascular proliferation on one hand, and between the presence of gemistocytes and bizarre large cells, and between these giant cell populations and perivascular mononuclear lymphoid infiltrates[68, 152, 433]. The prognostic significance of these perivascular lymphocytes exhibiting a predominantly suppressor/cytotoxic phenotype (see page 7) has not been defined although they have been proposed to be[41, 42, 51, 328] or not to be associated with a more favorable prognosis[68, 69, 152, 203, 311, 382]. Inverse relation between the degree of histologic malignancy and the patient's age usually are associated with inverse relation between the age and both duration of survival and of preoperative symptoms[42, 382, 458], but the cause of the strong negative relationship between age and survival in patients with anaplastic astrocytoma/glioblastoma cannot be explained fully by the histologic variables of these neoplasms[68]. Cytokinetic studies in glioblastoma revealed an average labeling index of 9% (range 4.4–17%) similar to metastases and much higher than in anaplastic astrocytoma, a growth fraction averaging 30% (range 21–58%), *i.e.* one third of the viable cells are in active proliferation, a cell cycle time of 2–3 days, and a tumor turnover time (potential doubling time) of 3–8 days assuming no cell loss (Table 10). While glioblastoma cells proliferate rapidly, a cell loss of about 85% maintains tumor doubling time at at approximately 40 to 55 days and, considering a 3-log kill, effective tumor regrowth time will be 7 to 11 weeks[182, 183]. The rate of tumor growth in glioblastoma probably correlates better with the growth fraction (ratio of proliferating cells to total cell number) than with the cell cycle time. This fact and the marked heterogeneity in anaplastic gliomas with various degrees of drug-sensitivity, and the development of therapeutic resistance are important prognostic variables[68, 183, 283, 358, 359, 454, 457].

Although most of the glioblastomas are macroscopically well circumscribed, approximately 2–3% are multicentric[25, 203, 370], *i.e.* they arise at some distance from each other in which no evidence is found for dissemination by any of the known pathways, and between which no microscopic continuity can be demonstrated[60], while a larger number are multifocal. However, in most of these cases the multiple foci can be accounted for microscopically by the metastatic spread of neoplastic cells through the CSF spaces or the intervening brain parenchyma. Glioblastomas show invasive tendency with involvement of the leptomeninges and/or the ventricular system, seen in 10 to 15% of the biopsy specimens and in more than one-third of the autopsies[203, 362], with subsequent metastatic spread through the neuraxis[109, 119]. Diffuse invasive and multifocal growth and generalized CSF spreading may be enhanced with increased survival time due to aggressive treatment[65, 208]. In a personal autopsy series of 321 anaplastic supratentorial gliomas (including 217 glioblastomas), CSF dissemintion was seen in 24.7% at was less frequent in cases with spontaneouse course (13.5%) than after surgery (32%), postoperative radiation (31%), chemotherapy (42%) or multimodality treatment (27.5%), but its incidence was not related to the survival time or type of treatment[208]. By contrast, metastases of malignant gliomas outside the CNS are rare, but glioblastomas form about 25% of all intracranial tumors with remote metastases[177, 203]. However, the incidence of remote extracranial metastases of anaplastic gliomas may increase with prolonges survival. Among about 2,000 gliomas, we observed 13 cases (0.65%) with metastases outside the neuraxis (lymph nodes, lungs, liver, bone), five of which were among the recent series of 321 autopsies (1.5%). Only 4 of these patients had surgery alone, all the others had adjuvant radiation and/or chemotherapy; survival ranged from 7 to 32 months[208]. These and other data[177] indicate that the danger of remote extraneural metastases in glioblastoma may increase with therapy-induced prolongation of survival of the tumor host.

b) Giant Cell (Monstrocellular) Glioblastoma (M-9481/3; ICD-9: 191.9; NDV: 1811000)

The giant cell subset of glioblastoma, previously referred to as "monstrocellular sarcoma"[498] is set apart because it contains bizarre, often multinucleated giant cells that show the ultrastructural and immunocytochemical evidence (GFAP expression) of astrocytes[102, 366]. The giant cells may be ordered in regular fascicular arrays or can be junbled in the stroma often containing abundant amounts of reticulin. Otherwise, the tumor displays the features and prognosis of a glioblastoma multiforme, although some giant cell gliomas, due to the biologically less aggressive behavior of the bizarre cells[185, 186], may have a somewhat better outcome[68, 141, 152]. On the other hand, these large bizarre cells may arise as an effect of radiation and/or chemotherapy (?)[65, 137, 208, 384, 385].

c) Glioblastoma with Sarcomatous Component (Gliosarcoma) (M-9442/3; ICD-9: 191.9; NDV: 1813000)

Neoplastic transformation of mesenchymal elements, resulting in the formation of mixed gliosarcomas are observed in about 8% of all glioblastomas[294]. In most mixed tumors, the sarcomatous components have the characteristics of either fibrosarcoma or angiosarcoma[331, 362, 383, 405], although in rare instances they take the form of a chondrosarcoma[351] or rhabdomyosarcoma[21]. The origin of the sarcomatous elements from hyperplastic vascular endothelium suggested by morphological and animal transplantation studies has recently found support by the demonstration of factor-VIII reactive antigen (F VIII/RAg) and Ulex europeus I (UEA I) antigen in both the lumen-lining vascular cells in both glioma and sarcomatous parts of gliosarcoma, in glomeruloid structures and, with decreasing intensity, in adjacent sarcoma cells. Electron microscopy shows admixture of glial and mesenchymal tumor cells which show the features of either fibrosarcoma or angiosarcoma; *in vitro* studies demonstrate a separate growth of glial and mesenchymal cells with a divergent migratory speed[152, 405]. Hence, at least part of the sarcomatous components in most gliosarcomas is considered to originate from vascular endothelial proliferation and to represent the final stage of a transformation process starting with capillary hyperplasia[383, 405].

The prognosis of all types of glioblastoma is poor, with spontaneous historical median life span of 4–6 months that has been improved by tumor resection plus aggressive radiation and chemotherapy to 12–18 months, with 35 to 50% one-year survival and 10 to 20% 2-year survival[68, 210, 215, 308, 374, 399, 454, 457]. Patients harboring glioblastomas predominantly composed of small cell populations often show shorter survivals than those with giant cell lesions[69]. This corresponds to cytogenetic studies showing that patients harboring anaplastic gliomas with labeling index over 5%, despite aggressive treatment, usually die within 6 months, while those with an LI of less than 5% may survive more than one year[182].

d) *Gliomatosis cerebri* (M-9381/3; ICD-9: 191.9; NDV: 1812000)

This rare neoplastic process of the CNS which can only be diagnosed with certainly at necropsy is characterized by diffuse gliomatous proliferation in widespread distribution or located in multiple sites of the nervous system, affecting the forebrain, hindbrain or spinal cord. Neoplastic glial cells of diverse origin and patterns are infiltrating normal nervous tissue with destruction of myelin, but only slight damage to neurons and axons. The neoplastic cells may range from isolated single isomorphic or pleomorphic cells to widespread, diffuse or nodular involvement by cells of single or several lineages. According to immunocytochemical studies, it is composed predominantly of neoplastic cells of astrocytic origin in all stages of development, small undifferentiated elements, transitional forms from oligodendroglia to astroglia, and oligodendroglial cells[12]. This type of neoplasia is suggested to arise diffusely over wide or multiple fields of cells that have undergone simultaneous neoplastic transformation.

6. Choroid Plexus Tumors

a) *Choroid Plexus Papilloma* (M-9390/0; ICD-9: 225.0; NDV: 1816000)

This intraventricular tumor representing less than 1% of all intracranial growths, is mostly harbored by children in the lateral and fourth ventricles (about 40% each), with only 10% occurring in the third ventricle. The globular, cauliflower-like mass is usually composed of a single layer of low columnar or cuboidal cells lying upon a basement membrane that covers a delicate vascular connective tissue core, and thus recapitulates the histologic appearance of the normal choroid plexus. There are numerous branching papillary formations; cytoplasm is pale and vacuolar, and mucus secreting columnar cells may occur[370]. Plexus cells do not contain glial fibers, but small foci of ependymoma with glial fibrils and positive for GFAP have been detected in plexus papillomas[437]. Expression of carbonic anhydrase as a plexus-specific marker is found[278]. While S-100 protein immunoreactivity is prominent in well differentiated neoplasms, some are also positive for cytokeratin (CKER), neuron specific enolase (NSE), GFAP, and carcinoembryonic antigen (CEA), the latter being associated with a more aggressive pattern[83a]. Ultrastructural features include maintenance of the apical-based polarity of the neoplastic cells with various numbers of surface microvilli but devoid of cilia and thus distinguishable from ependymomas, and the presence of a uniform and continuous basement membrane outlining the basal plasmalemma, and of large aggregates of glycogen granules. These characteristics are typical of epithelium involved in fluid transport and may explain the well-known fact that these tumors participate in the formation of cerebrospinal fluid[138, 279, 291, 299]. Even through these tumors are histologically mature, they may seed throughout the CSF pathways. Prognosis after total resection is good, although hydrocephalus may develop[84, 257, 291].

b) Anaplastic Choroid Plexus Papilloma (Carcinoma) (M-9390/3; ICD-9: 191.5; NDV: 1816000)

Unlike the benign papilloma, this malignant tumor is characterized by cellular pleomorphism, loss of the regular papillary structure, mitoses, multinucleated cells, and may invade the surrounding brain. It may arise in any ventricle or site of choroid plexus in both adults and children, most frequently in the lateral ventricles, either *de novo* or by anaplasia in a choroid plexus papilloma, about 20% of which show varying degrees of anaplasia that may increase with time[47, 153, 362]. Ultrastructural findings are compatible with choroid plexus differentiation[284], the cells being similar to the underdeveloped type III cells[279]. These tumors can produce transliquoral seeding and also extraneural metastases[83a, 362]. Immunocytochemistry shows positive expression of CEA and often of CKER, while S-100, GFAP and NSE are negative[83a].

B. Pineal Cell Tumors

Tumors of the pineal region are rare, comprising from 0.4 to 6.59% (average 1–2%) of all intracranial neoplasms, with a substantially higher incidence in Japan than in the West[239, 386, 448]. They are separated into two major groups: a) teratomatous or germ cell tumors, the commonest form of malignancy to involve this region, which is listed under "germ cell tumors" (see p. 59), b) those derived from the neuroepithelial anlage of the gland itself, *i.e.* the pineal parenchymal tumors, which can be separated into two groups: 1) pineocytoma, and 2) pineoblastoma. Separation of these two types is important as their biologic behavior is different, but distinction may be difficult, as transitional forms are frequent or the patterns may coexist, and both types may differentiate.

a) Pineocytoma (Pinealocytomas) (M-9361/1; IDC-9: 237.1; NDV: 1817000)

This rare, usually circumscribed and noninvasive tumor, occurring at any age, is derived from and composed of relatively mature cells of the pineal parenchyma displaying a lobular pattern. Its uniform appearance resembles that of the normal pineal gland; the cells have polar processes that radiate toward a blood vessel, forming distinct rosettes that are reminiscent of neuroblastoma. Neoplastic cells may range in size from small to large. Some of these tumors show distinctive neuronal or astrocytical or divergent neuronal and astrocytic differentiation with the histologic features of pineocytoma with ganglion cells or astrocytes, or both[239, 413] with expression of both neuronal and astrocytic cell markers[322]. They may contain large rosettes that appear different from the Homer-Wright type[47], and their centers may contain mature ganglion cells, ultrastructurally featured by numerous dense core vesicles and synaptic complexes[299, 366]. Others may show an admixture of neoplastic astrocytes or of gangliogliomatous elements forming the picture of ganglioglioma of the pineal[167, 363], while others have a prominent papillary component and flower-like structures indicating transition to pineoblastoma or retinoblastoma, which is associated with malignant behavior[446].

b) Pineoblastoma (Pinealoblastoma) (M-9362/3; ICD-9: 191.8; NDV: 1817000)

This rare and highly cellular tumor mostly involving infants is composed of poorly differentiated cells resembling medulloblastoma. It may display retinoblastomatous differentiation with rosettes of the Flexner-Wintersteiner variety and/or fleurettes, flower-like arrangements of cells undergoing photoreceptor differentiation[299]; ultrastructural study also reveals club-shaped cilia with a 9 + 0 microtubular pattern[422]. Therefore, this tumor is regarced as a "primitive" neuroectodermal tumor arising from the neuroepithelial anlage of the pineal[357]. Its differentiation is poor and it often displays infiltrative growth with frequent spread in CSF. The prognosis of pineal tumors is poor, and children with pineoblastoma often have disseminated disease at presentation and survive for a shorter period in contrast to those with pineocytoma, where tumor disseminates later in the course and survival may be prolonged[83, 133, 357].

C. Neuronal Tumors

Four types of tumors, each of which contains mature-appearing ganglion cells, constitute this category of neoplasms.

a) Gangliocytoma (M-9490/0; ICD-9: 225.0; NDV: 1819000)

This extremely rare tumor composed almost entirely of ganglion cells, some of which contain two or more nuclei, has an inconspicuous glial background but often a prominent mesenchymal component. Neurofilament protein (NFP) may be abundant, while NSE is not specific for neuronal tumors; the glial component is GFAP positive. Electron microscopy confirms the neuronal and glial features of the cells[366, 400]. The tumors occur most commonly in the cerebral hemispheres in childhood and may show cyst formation and/or calcification. They are slowly growing neoplasms with a generally good prognosis.

Dysplastic gangliocytoma of the cerebellum or Lhermitte-Duclos disease[264] is a hamartomatous lesion, and more likely a malformation than a true neoplasm, but may present as a mass lesion during late childhood. Affected folia may or may not be enlarged; microscopically it is featured by diffuse scattering of abnormal large neurons thought to be derived from granule cells[6, 356]. It is often associated with malformations (megalencephaly, hemihypertrophy, etc); familial occurrence is known.

b) Anaplastic Gangliocytoma (M-9490/1)

Anaplastic gangliocytoma is a tumor composed almost entirely of ganglion cells which displays anaplastic features.

c) Ganglioglioma (M-9505/1; ICD-9: 237.5; NDV: 1819000)

This rare tumor is composed of both ganglion cells and neoplastics glia, usually astrocytes. The ganglion cell component may be arranged diffusely or forms clusters, and there may be a prominent connective tissue component. Perivascular lymphomonocytes are common. These tumors, like the gangliocytoma, predominantly affect children and young adults, and are located at the bottom of the third ventricle, hypothalamus, or temporal lobe. They are often cystic; immunocytochemical and electron microscopic features are as outlined for gangliocytoma[98]. They tend to grow slowly and have a good prognosis[217].

d) Anaplastic Ganglioglioma (M-9490/3; ICD-9: 191.9)

In the anaplastic form, anaplasia generally affects the glial component and may manifest features of glioblastoma multiforme.

D. Embryonal Tumors

They comprise an important and, often, a diagnostically challenging group of primitive neoplasms in different locations that most commonly occur in childhood and in which a correlation can be drawn between the various tumor types and the sequential stages of neurocytogenesis in the forebrain and hindbrain (Table 12). They may arise in the cerebrum, cerebellum, pineal gland, or elsewhere in the CNS and, aside from "undifferentiated" cells, these tumors, regardless of site of origin, may show variable forms of differentiation: neuronal, glial, ependymal (ependymoblastoma), neural tube (medulloepithelioma), melanin, mesenchymal, muscle cell, olfactory epithelial cell (esthesioneuroblastoma), retinal and/or pineal differentiation. Some tumors may contain more than one mature or immature cell type. Enlarging the term "primitive neuroectodermal tumor" (PNET), introduced by Hart and Earle[157], this designation has since been used in a wider sense, including brain tumors with a predominent undifferentiated small cell component and a variable degree of focal neuronal, glial and/or mesenchymal differentiation, previously classified as central neuroblastoma, cerebellar medulloblastoma, primitive polar spongioblastoma, ependymoblastoma, and pinealoblastoma[26, 27, 356, 357]. Two entities are relatively common, *i.e.* medulloblastoma and retinoblastoma (not included in this classification), while others are rare. Cerebral PNETs have been

Table 12. Correlation of normal stages of neurocytogenesis with embryonal central nervous system tumors (from [367])

Stages of neurocytogenesis		Normal cell type	Equivalent tumor
Forebrain	first	primitive ventricular (matrix, neuroepithelial) cell	cerebral medulloepithelioma
	second	neuroblast	cerebral neuroblastoma
	third	glioblast (spongioblast)	polar spongioblastoma
		ependymoblast	ependymoblastoma
Cerebellum	cell rests in posterior medullary velum	undifferentiated "medulloblast"	medulloblastoma
	external granular layer		

reported to comprise 2.1–2.8% of supratentorial tumors in childhood[53, 132]. The classification of these primitive tumors, not literally included in the WHO classification, is controversial. A recent revised WHO classification for childhood brain tumors[357] deletes a number of documented histologic entities and separates three major groups of PNETs which appears somewhat oversimplified[364]:

1. "Primitive" Neuroectodermal Tumors NOS (Not Otherwise Specified) (ICD-9: 191.9; NDV: 1800000)

They occur most commonly in the midline region of the cerebellum but may be located anywhere in the CNS, including the pineal gland, and tend to spread widely within the CNS through CSF pathways and rarely metastasize outside the nervous system. They are composed of poorly differentiated neuroepithelial cells that consist of small chromatin-rich nuclei and a minimal rim of cytoplasm without GFAP or NFP reaction, and electron microscopy shows undifferentiated cells with large nuclei and nucleoli and scanty cytoplasm with inconspicuous organelles. Occasionally, the cells form Homer-Wright rosettes; mitotic figures are frequent, and there may be variable fibrovascular stroma, foci of necroses and multinuclear tumor cells. These tumors without differentiation include a) some forms of medulloblastoma (PNET of the cerebellum), and b) pineoblastoma (PNET of the pineal parenchyma).

2. PNET with Differentiation

a) Glial (Astrocytic, Oligodendroglial)

They contain poorly differentiated neuroepithelial and neoplastic glial cells that may resemble immature forms or express GFAP and display the ultrastructural features of astroglia or oligodendroglia. Neuroepithelial and glial cells may be separated by a "stroma", with indistinct or sharply defined transitional fields. These tumors may include medulloblastoma with glial differentiation, primitive gliomas[132, 157, 347], while others show maturation to both astrocytoma and ependymoma[117].

b) Ependymal (Ependymoblastoma)

These rare ependymal cell tumors are highly cellular composed of small to medium-sized poorly differentiated neuroepithelial cells with a uniform cytologic appearance, frequent mitotic figures, and numerous diagnostic ependymal rosettes and tubules[298]. GFAP reaction may or may not be positive, but differentiation is restricted to glial precursor cells with the differentiating features of ependymal cells. Ultrastructural features include elongated junctional devices, rosette-like arrangements, microvilli, cilia, and basal bodies[171]. There are cells less differentiated than 3-week embryonal ependymal cells representing a stage in the differentiation of the primitive medulloepithelial cell to mature ependyma[254b]. In addition to abundant ependymoblastic rosettes ependymal rosettes are also present, but the absence of pleomorphism, giant cells, multinucleation and pseudopalisades, and the scanty proliferation of vascular endothelial cells are features that delineate this tumor from

48

an anaplastic ependymoma[298]. The median age of the patients is 2 years; prognosis is poor, and leptomeningeal spread is frequent.

c) Neuronal (Neuroblastoma) (M-9500/3; ICD-9: 191.9; NDV: 1800000)

These rare neuronal tumors are made up of poorly differentiated neuroepithelial cells and a variable number of mature ganglion cells showing positive NFP and NSE reactions[445, 447]. Ultrastructural studies reveal presence of clear or dense core vesicles, synapses, cilia with 9 + 0 pattern, and blunt cytoplasmic processes that contain abundant actin filaments, microtubules or large clear vesicles resembling growth cones or developing nerve cells[33, 98, 299, 320, 338, 484]. These childhood tumor are often histologically indistinguishable from peripheral neuroblastomas.

d) Choroid Plexus

Recently, a benign form of a cerebral undifferentiated round cell tumor with formation of glandular parts of papillary epithelial structures was reported, indicating PNET with differentiation towards choroid plexus[197].

e) Others (Melanocytes, Mesenchymal)

Rarely, PNETs may contain cells with melanin pigment. They are primarily located within the cerebellar vermis, referred to as melanotic "medulloblastoma"[100] (see p. 50). Others show mesenchymal components[13, 33, 97], components of mature or immature striated or smooth muscle[419, 458]. The precise nature of this "medullomyoblastoma" is controverse (see p. 50). The pluripotent nature of pimitive neuroectodermal tumors is also reflected by the occasional focal differentiation towards Schwann cells[134].

3. Medulloblastoma, NOS, and with Differentiation
(see below)

Since a more precise classification of embryonal CNS tumors will emerge sooner or later, the present description will follow another modified WHO classification referring to the classically documented histological entities[56] which separates the following groups:

a) Medulloepithelioma (M-9501/3; ICD-9: 191.9; NDV: 1801000)

This rare tumor in infancy and childhood most often arises in the cerebral hemispheres, but also may occur in brain stem, cerebellum[198, 221, 344, 379], or peripheral nerve[305]. Its histologic appearance of columnar cells forming stratified tubular or papillary structures that rest upon a sharply delimiting PAS-positive membrane recapitulates the embryonic neural tube. The ultrastructure of the cells which have minimal cytoplasm with few organelles and no cilia or microvilli and primitive cell-junctions is basically that of the fetal neural tube[344]. Morphologic variations with astrocytic, oligodendroglial, ependymal, neuronal, or mixed cellular differentiation reflect the multipotential nature of this most primitive embryonic tumor[13, 379]. The tumor follows a biologically malignant course, generally disseminating widely throughout the CSF pathways; survival averages 6 months.

b) Medulloblastoma (PNET of the Cerebellum) (M-9470/3; ICD-9: 191.9; NDV: 1801000)

This malignant tumor of the posterior fossa accounts for 3–5% of all intracranial neoplasms in all ages, but for 20–25% of all brain tumors in childhood, with an age peak around 5 years; about 80% of all medulloblastomas occurring before 15 years of age. Sites of predilection are midline, cerebellar vermis and fourth ventricle, or the cerebellar hemispheres, the latter being more frequently involved in older children and adults. Grossly soft, fleshy and often well demarcated, the cerebellar medulloblastoma is a heterogenous neoplasm that usually exhibits a variety of histologic features[144, 152, 356, 361]. It generally consists of small round to oval-appearing cells with hyperchromatic, carot-shaped nuclei and scanty cytoplasm, arranged in dense or diffuse sheets, parallel rows or forming Homer-Wright rosettes. Mitotic figures are frequent. Reticulin fibers occur when the meninges are invaded or in the "*desmoplastic* variant"[369] or "circumscribed arachnoid sarcoma of cerebellum"[124], showing a mosaic-like pattern of pale cellular island surrounded by strands of fibrous tissue rich in reticulin. Their ultrastructure shows round undifferentiated cells with little cytoplasm and few organels[98, 361, 366], but rather often neuronal and astrocytic differentiation does occur[117, 164, 299, 356, 367]. Today, medulloblastoma is regarded as an embryonic neuroectodermal tumor with variable glial and neuronal differentiation potential[356, 364], supposed to be derived from embryonic cells in the posterior or anterior medullary velum and from multipotential external granular layer cells, areas specifically involved in the development of the cerebellum during fetal life. From clinical, epidemiological, experimental and recent growth analysis data it seems reasonable that medulloblastomas, particularly those of the midline, may originate in the cerebellum during the period of active development of the cerebellum[84, 115, 169, 303, 367, 500]. Medulloblastomas have been induced in rodents by injection of oncogenic viruses during the pre- and neonatal period[303, 500], and recent clinical growth analyses of this tumor in young children extrapolated the origin of medulloblastoma to about 16–17th week of gestation[169]. Cell kinetic characteristics of medulloblastoma, showing a labeling index of 8–14%, cell cycle time of 22.2–31.6 hours, S phases of 26.3–27%, a cell loss fraction of 74 and 97%, and a potential tumor doubling time ranging from 9.4 to 69 days[169, 184] are similar to glioblastoma, while the growth fraction of 12% in medulloblastoma is higher than in glioblastoma (Table 10). The capacity of medulloblastoma for divergent cellular differentiation, in particular its bipotentiality along glial and neuroblastic lines is well documented *in vitro* and *in vivo*[164, 366], also based on ultrastructural demonstration of features characteristic of neurons and astroglia[72] and immunohistochemical demonstration of neuron-specific (neurofilament protein NFP, and neuron-specific enolase ENS) and astrocytic markers GFAP[64, 166, 250, 330, 333, 356]. While many medulloblastomas are GFAP negative[154], signs of astrocytic differentiation, *i.e.* GFAP-immunoreactive cells, are particularly seen in the "desmoplastic" variant[166] usually found in young adults with a frequent superficial location in the cerebellar hemispheres. This variant, interpreted either as an extracerebellar growth pattern of medulloblastoma[369] or as a mixed mesenchymal-ectodermal tumor[152] has been claimed to carry a better prognosis after total resection than the classical medulloblastoma[75, 152]. Other histological features indicating a better prognosis include fibrillar areas, areas of decreased density and glial differentiation[241]. For the current SIOP medulloblastoma study, histological examination performed by the Brain Tumor Reference Center at Zurich considers the different forms and degrees of cellular (neuronal and glial) differentiation, cellular and nuclear pleomorphism, mitotic rate, necroses, vascular and stromal reaction, and the results of immunocytochemical studies[64].

Other possible variants of medulloblastomas containing mature or immature striated or smooth muscle fibers ("medullomyoblastoma") or pigmented cells containing melanosomal melanin[43, 428] are interpreted as either differentiated forms of PNETs which may show vertical differentiation along glial and rhabdomyoblastic lines, as differentiated medulloblastomas with a myogenic potential[97] or mixed neuroepithelial-mesenchymal neoplasms developing from the pluripotential neural crest-derived "ectomesenchymal" cells[403, 407, 419, 458, 464], while others regard them as teratoid tumors[80, 356, 364]. Therefore, they are listed as a separate group of primitive tumors[56], and should be separated from pure rhabdomyosarcomas which may also occur in the cerebellar vermis of children (see p. 56). "*Melanotic medulloblastoma*" (M-9363/0), or melanotic neuroectodermal tumor in infancy or melanotic progonoma may occur both in the cerebellar vermis and also in extracranial sites, particularly the maxilla.

Medulloblastoma is known for its tendency to seed the subarachnoid space, both locally and distally, with frequent dissemination throughout the spinal cord and other CNS, and extraneural metastases of medulloblastomas are well documented, and in some series approach an overall incidence of 5–30%[84, 177, 236], over one-third being metastatic to the bone marrow[418].

Modern classification systems for PNETs of the posterior fossa using an adapted TNM staging with postoperative MAPS (metastasis, age, pathology, surgery) classification[258] have proven prognostic relevance, while the currently performed SIOP medulloblastoma study uses a new histologic evaluation. Despite its previously poor prognosis, recent treatment standards including surgery, aggressive radiation and multiple agent chemotherapy are encouraging and allow reasonably to expect 5-year survival of 50–70% and 10-year survival of 30 up to over 40%[35, 36, 84, 210], whereas only 20–25% of the patients with PNETs survive 5 years[132].

c) Pineoblastoma (PNET of Pineal Parenchyma)
(see p. 44)

d) PNET with Differentiation

aa) glial (astroglial and/or oligodendroglial)—see primitive gliomas
ab) ependymal—see ependymoblastoma
ac) neuronal—Central neuroblastoma (M-9470/3; ICD-9: 191.9; NDV: 1800000)

Primary intracerebral neuroblastoma is an uncommon tumor of the CNS usually occurring in the first decade of life. This rapidly growing tumor arises in the cerebrum and cerebellum as a solid, firm and lobulated or cystic lesion sharply deliminated from the surrounding brain tissue. It consists of densely packed, small, poorly differentiated cells, with variable numbers of immature or mature ganglion cells, Homer-Wright rosettes, and axonal processes demonstrable with silver impregnations. Immunoperoxidase stains for NFP and NSE are usually positive[445, 447]. Abundant fibrous connective tissue stroma is present in a desmoplastic variant, often resembling desmoplastic medulloblastoma[179, 463]. Ultrastructurally, clear and dense core vesicles, synapses, cytoplasmic processes with neurofilaments and abundant actin filaments, cilia with 9 + 0 pattern, microtubules and clear vesicles resembling growth cones or developing nerve cells of monopolar and bipolar type have been observed[15, 222, 320, 338, 366, 400, 442, 463, 484, 485]. These central tumors are often histologically indistinguishable from the peripheral neuroblastoma which is among the most common of childhood neoplasms. The tumors exhibit a wide spectrum of cellular differentiation both towards ganglion cells of the multipolar type (ganglioneuroblastoma) and along neuroglial lines[15, 91, 372, 442] supporting the concept of a pluripotential cell of origin. According to their degree of cellular differentiation, they show a wide range from low- to high-grade malignancy which seems to correlate with their biological behavior[28, 320, 442]. Most cerebral neuroblastomas show high-grade malignancy, and have poor prognosis, with frequent recurrences and cerebrospinal, or rare, extraneural, metastases. Five-year postoperative survival is about 30%, but rare cases showing evidence of neuronal maturation[28, 29, 320, 442] or towards ganglioglioma[463] have a rather long survival.

ad) Central neurocytoma (ICD-9: 225.0; NDV: 1818000)

   This extremely rare tumor, which, by conventional light microscopy is virtually identical with oligodendrogliomas, on the basis of electron microscopic features, has been interpreted as neuronal, the cells representing small well-differentiated nerve cells rather than primitive neuroblasts[158, 320, 443a]. The tumor is mainly located in the fornix, septum pellucidum or corpus callosum.

e) Medullomyoblastoma (M-9472/3; ICD-9: 191.9 NDV: 1801000) (see p. 50)

f) Primitive Polar Spongioblastoma (M-9423/3; ICD-9: 191.9; NDV: 1803000)

This extremely rare tumor in children and adolescents is composed of elongated bipolar cells arranged in rhythmical parallel palisades, and arises at ventricular walls, particularly the third ventricle. It has been aligned with the third stage of cytogenesis in the forebrain, which is initiated by the migration of primitive spongioblasts from the primitive ventricular epithelium and has been compared with the palisading of the migrating spongioblasts. It should not be confused with the considerably more frequent pilocytic astrocytoma and shows a poor prognosis with a tendency towards seeding the CSF pathways[370].

2. Tumors of Nerve Sheath (Nerve Sheath Cells)

Although nerve sheath tumors, by definition, represent neoplasms of the peripheral nervous system[57], they are conventionally also placed among CNS growths[356, 496]. They are classified as a) neurilemmomas (schwannomas) and neurofibromas[106, 481], and their anaplastic variants.

A. Neurilemmoma (Schwannoma, Neurinoma) (M-9560/0; ICD-9: 225,8; NDV: 1818000; 3801000)

Schwannomas, considered to consist almost exclusively of and originating from Schwann cells, account for 6–8% of all intercranial growths, and mainly occur in adults. They may arise from all cranial nerves and nerve roots, but their major sites are the cerebello-pontine angle (acoustic neurinoma), and less frequently, the trigeminal, 9th and 10th cranial nerves. They are encapsulated, firm, sometimes cystic lesions that may displace or compress adjacent brain structures without invasive growth. Dense cellular areas arranged in drifts, whorls or forming true palisades (Antoni type A pattern) alternate with more loosely structured areas with honeycomb appearance that may contain lipid and foam cells (Antoni type B pattern). Nerve fibers can usually be found stretched over the capsule but not within the tumor. Ultrastructure shows uniform proliferation of Schwann cells with a continuous basal lamina, long slender processes, often showing mesaxon formation, and bundles of tiny intracytoplasmic filaments[108, 299] and more or less conspicuous proliferation of collagen fibers, and fibrous long-spacing banded collagen suggested to be formed by Schwann cells[86]. Both human and experimental tumors derived from Schwann cells have been shown to possess S-100 protein and other markers characteristic of neural tissue[93, 468].

B. Neurofibroma (M-9540/0; ICD-9: 225.8; NDV: 3802000)

This localized or diffuse tumor, grossly indistinguishable from neurinoma, consists of Schwann cells, perineurial and intermediate cells, including endoneurial fibroblasts and transitions between the several kinds of neoplastic cells[174, 256, 467, 481]. There are loosely arranged collagen fibers and mucoid material with an intersecting pattern of wavy fascicles in which neurites may be demonstrable. Antoni A and B patterns may rarely be seen. Ultrastructural studies show that these axons are surrounded by neoplastic Schwann cells but also by perineurial cells, both containing S-100 protein, while the endoneurial fibroblasts contain no S-100 protein[174, 465, 481]. These tumors forming solitary or multiple lesions of nerve roots usually occur as a component of von Recklinghausen's neurofibromatosis. Three subtypes are separated[246]; the encapsulated plexiform type I, the diffuse type II without capsule; and type III containing tactile-like corpuscles which are composed of perineurial-like cells[409, 467] showing S-100 protein immunoreactivity[465].

In exceptional cases melanin pigment is found in both schwannomas[285, 466] and neurofibromas[335, 424]. Ultrastructural studies in both pigmented human schwannomas and neurofibromas[335] and in experimentally induced pigmented malignant schwannomas[417] demonstrating melanosomes within Schwann cell cytoplasm give support for production of melanin by neoplastic Schwann cells.

C. Anaplastic Nerve Sheath Tumors (M-9540/3; ICD-9: 225.2; NDV: 3853000, 3858000)

They include anaplastic neurilemmomas and neurofibromas (neurofibrosarcoma, neurogenic sarcoma), rare malignant counterparts of nerve sheath tumors, showing infiltrative growth. Transformation of a neurofibroma into a sarcoma is a well recognized complication of von Recklinghausen's disease.

3. Tumors of Meningeal and Related (Mesenchymal) Tissues

This group includes a) the different types of meningiomas, b) primary melanocytic, and c) meningeal sarcomatous tumors.

A. Meningiomas (M-9530/0)

This term is restricted of a neoplasm found only in the meninges, or meningeal rests, as occasionally observed in the skull, along peripheral nerves, or in the skin. Meningiomas account for 10–19% of all intracranial tumors; they occur at any age, but most frequently in adults, while their incidence in children is less than 2%[84]. Sites of predilection are the cerebral convexity and falx (50–60%), olfactory grove, sphenoid ridge and suprasellar region (25–40%), posterior fossa and tentorium (15%); multiple sites are rare. They are smooth, lobulated masses that tend to be broadly attached to the dura, although they may be intraventricular or in the spinal epidural space. Although they may adhere to the pial surface, invasion of the brain is exceptional in the histologically well-differentiated lesions. Adjacent bone can be involved with tumor or may exhibit osteoblastic response. Meningiomas display a variety of histologic patterns, the majority of which have no or little prognostic significance; they show similar ultrastructure with uniform composition of arachnoid cells with complex interdigitations of plasma membranes and collagen[67, 226, 299]. Most classifications separate the common major subtypes of meningiomas, such as a) meningotheliomatous (syncytial—M-9531/0), b) fibroblastic (fibrous—M-9532/0), c) transitional or mixed (M-9537/0), d) psammomatous (M-9533/0), e) angiomatous (M-9534/0), f) hemangioblastic (M-9535/0), g) hemangiopericytic (M-9536/3), h) papillary (M-9538/1), h) anaplastic or malignant (M-9530/3); the groups a–e) classified as benign; f–h) as intermediate or malignant[56], while the revised classification by Rorke et al.[357] only separates 3 major groups:

1. Meningioma NOS (M-9530/0; ICD-9; 225.2; NDV: 1825000)

This category includes the common major subtypes: the most frequent meningotheliomatous (syncytial) type (about 60%) is formed by sheets of polygonal cells with indistinct borders. Nuclei are oval, have a delicate chromatin pattern and small nucleolus, and closely resemble arachnoid cap cells. Cytoplasmic invagination into nuclei (pseudoinclusions) and true intranuclear inclusions are common. The fibroblastic (fibrous) type (about 6%) is formed by spindel-shaped cells that resemble fibroblasts in interwoven fascicles within a dense collagen network. Fibrous connective tissue in these tumors may be calcified. Arachnoid whorl-like structures are seen in either of these two subtypes. The transitional pattern is a combination of syncytial and fibrous elements, the former often forming lobules or whorls (about 20% of all tumors). The psammomatous subtype is one in which the bulk of the mass is composed of psammoma bodies with or without calcification most frequently occurring in the spinal cord of elderly females. The previous "angiomatous" type, accounting for about 8%, includes three different variants[152, 214, 226]: a) highly vascularized, but otherwise typical meningiomas of syncytial or transitional type; b) the hemangioblastic type which is identical with the hemangioblastoma (Lindau's tumor) of the cerebellum, but arises in the supratentorial space, and c) the hemangiopericytic variant which has the morphologic features of hemangiopericytoma arising elsewhere in the body[106]. Both the latter variants should be reasonably grouped among the tumors of blood vessel origin (see pp. 58 ff.).

2. "Papillary" Meningioma (M-9538/1; ICD-9: 237.5 NDV: 1825000))

This rare type has a distinctive appearance because of the orientation of neoplastic cells to blood vessels, producing radiating perivascular structures similar in some respects to that of the ependymoma. Reticulin fibers are seen within these radiations. The nuclei are round and resemble those in other meningioma, but may be slightly more hyperchromaticed and there are rather frequent mitotic figures. Although the lesion may not have overt microscopic features of malignancy, recurrence and late distant metastases are frequent, the latter observed in about 30% of the cases[362].

3. Anaplastic Meningioma (M-9530/3; ICD-9: 192.1; NDV: 1824000)

This diagnosis is assigned to lesions that have either a) clearcut histologic evidence of anaplasia or b) anaplastic features that develop over time in a previously well-differentiated tumor. While most recurrent meningiomas do not significantly change their histologic appearance, about 12% show increased cellularity and mitotic activity, indicating increased growth rate[214]. Their labeling index is significantly increased and may be higher than in anaplastic astrocytoma[129a] (Table 10). In contrast to the typical meningioma, the anaplastic lesions show hypercellularity, pleomorphism, higher mitotic rates and, sometimes, elongated cells assume a more sarcomatous appearance, although they remain plump and lack the well-defined fascicular arrangement of the fibrosarcoma, the development of which from previously typical meningioma has been observed in less than 3%[180, 214]. In the anaplastic type, representing 1.4% to 10%, necrosis may be prominent, and invasion of the cerebral parenchyma is frequent.

The recurrence rate of meningiomas after total removal has been estimated from 5–21%, while it is twice as high after partial removal[214]. There are no definite difference in the recurrence rates and intervals between the various histologic subtypes except for anaplastic meningiomas and meningeal hemangiopericytomas which show significantly higher frequency and shorter intervals of recurrence[200, 214]. The features of hypercellularity, increased mitotic activity and cortical invasion are useful criteria in suggesting recurrence, while nuclear pleomorphism, necroses, increased vascularity, and the presence of mitotic figures alone are of no or only little prognostic value. Hence, most histologic features in typical meningiomas are not considered predictive for the biological behavior of a given tumor[214, 226]. Infiltration of the cerebral cortex is one of the histologic features commonly cited as denoting malignant biologic behavior of a meningioma.

4. Meningio-Angiomatosis

This rare benign condition of probable malformative origin is morphologically characterized by a) diffuse meningovascular proliferation with diffuse invasion of the cerebral cortex by both meningiomatous areas and blood vessels, and b) leptomeningeal calcification. These lesions, often associated with neurofibromatosis are considered rather of hamartomatous than of a true neoplastic nature[226, 362] and have been reviewed by Halper *et al.*[154a].

B. Primary Melanocytic Tumors

Among 220 primary pigmented tumors of the CNS and meninges, 63% were diffuse or multifocal melanoblastomas, 37% solitary pigmented tumors, and 26% associated with neurocutaneous melanosis[18]. They can be separated into:

a) Meningeal melanocytoma (M-9368/3; ICD-9: 192.1; NDV: 1825000)

This rare tumor is formed of nests of melanocytes that represent rare benign, hamartomatous growths, located in the cerebellum, cerebrum of spinale cord; these solitary benign tumors are extremely rare and, occasionally, have been referred to as melanocytic meningiomas[226, 266].

b) Meningeal melanosis (melanomatosis) (M-2511/1–3; ICD-9: 192.9)

The nervous system of infants or children with certain phacomatosis such as basal cell nervus syndrome may contain diffuse meningeal or parenchymal perivascular nests of melanocytes that more commonly represent hamartomatous, nonspace-occupying growths[404].

c) Primary malignant melanoma (M-9363/3; ICD-9: 192.3)

This rare neoplasm may occur in the leptomeninges as a focal event or diffusely or as multiple tumors in the cerebral hemispheres and posterior fossa as an isolated event or, more frequently, in association with cutaneous or ocular nevi belonging to the group of neurocutaneous melanosis[443]. Intracranial lesions associated with skin lesions are usually present in childhood and present as diffuse or focal proliferation of malignant melanocytes.

d) Malignant meningeal melanoblastosis (primary melanoblastosis of the meninges)

It is characterized by diffuse involvement of the intracranial and intraspinal spaces, part of them associated with neurocutaneous melanosis[113], while others show multiple tumor growth without diffuse melanoblastosis[18]. Tumor cells express S-100 protein. Metastatic melanoma has to be excluded. Primary meningeal melanoblastosis is not associated with any clinical or radiological features; premortem diagnosis may be obtained by cytological examination of the CSF using electron microscopical identification of pigment granules[4]. The prognosis of this highly malignant neoplasm is poor[18].

e) Other melanocytic tumors

Miscellaneous melanocytic tumors include the so-called pigmented meningioma[266] and other melanin containing tumors which have been related to cutaneous nevocellular nevi or occur in other neoplasmic of neuroepithelial origin.

C. Meningeal Sarcomatous Tumors

The sarcomatous neoplasms of the meninges previously have been listed as variants like fibrosarcoma, polymorphic cell sarcoma, primary meningeal sarcomatosis, etc, but as mesenchymal markers become widely used, this group will be more logically subdivided. At present, the following types are distinguished:

1. Meningeal Sarcoma and Primary Meningeal Sarcomatosis (M-9539/3; ICD-9: 192.1; NDV: 1846000)

These rare types of diffuse proliferation within the subarachnoid space of undifferentiated small or pleomorphic mesenchymal cells mainly occur in children and young adults, and are to be distinguished from anaplastic meningioma[59]. They may arise multifocally, and frequently invade the brain and, most frequently, the spinal cord. Their prognosis is poor.

2. Fibrosarcoma (M-9530/3; ICD-9: 192.1; NDV: 1841000)

Mesenchymal tumors composed of spindle cells, reticulin, and collagen, with a well-differentiated fascicular pattern or cellular disarray and anaplasia, may occur at any age and arise from the dura, the leptomeninges, but rarely may occur within the brain[321, 362]. Based on morphological and histochemical findings, some of the tumors are considered as being of meningothelial origin and might be included to malignant meningiomas[321]. Fibrosarcomas are not uncommon secondary malignancies following cranial irradiation, showing usually a very long latency between 2 and 24 years[201, 362, 441, 460], although some may also arise after short latency periods[321].

3. Sarcoma with Glio(blastomatous) Component ("Sarcoglioma")

While most mixed glio-sarcomas arise from neoplastic transformation of mesenchyma in anaplastic gliomas, primary dural fibrosarcoma or meningeal sarcoma may induce "secondary" gliomas[254, 362].

4. Rhabdomyosarcoma (M-8900/3; NDV: 4810000) and Leiomyosarcoma

Rare malignant tumors composed of striated muscle may occur primarily in the cerebral hemispheres of adults and in the posterior fossa of children[48, 323]. These mesenchymal neoplasms showing rhabdomyoblastic differentiation similar to in normal myogenesis[168] can be identified by ultrastructural demonstration of myofilaments and immunohistochemical expression of myosin and desmin myoglobin as tumor markers[94, 436]. Rare meningeal rhabdomyosarcoma[407] is to separated from meningeal extension of rhabdomyosarcomas from parameningeal sites of the head and neck[32]. Primary intracranial leiomyosarcoma is exceedingly rare[7, 299].

5. Mesenchymal Chondrosarcoma (M-9220/3)

This rare mesenchymal tumor represents a multilobulated mass attached to the dura, preferentially occurring in the anterior fossa of children. It consists of predominantly mesenchymal cells with islands of cartilaginous differentiation and, thus, resembles soft tissue chondrosarcomas elsewhere[106], but may be difficult to diagnose if no cartilagineous differentiation is present. It may be confused with a neuroepithelial tumor, as cells may form Homer-Wright-like rosettes, but mesenchymal character becomes evident by the use of trichrome stains. The tumor has a poorer prognosis than chondrosarcoma (see p. 64), trends to recur and may invade the brain[378].

6. Xanthosarcoma

These rare supratentorial tumors occurring particularly in children and young adults, are composed of large and lipidized or fusiform cells, similar to fibrous xanthomas of skin and soft tissues, but their frequent expression of GFAP has documented their astrocytic nature. Therefore, they are now classified as xanthoastrocytomas[228] (see p. 32).

4. Primary Malignant Lymphomas (M-9591/3; ICD-9: 192.9; NDV: 1843000)

Primary malignant lymphomas affecting the CNS without evidence of extraneural involvement, previously referred to as reticulum cell sarcoma/microglioma[375], represent 0.5–1.5% of all intracranial neoplasms and 1–2% of the malignant lymphomas of all sites[162, 204, 206, 209]. Since they are morphologically and immunologically identical to the non-Hodgkin's lymphomas elsewhere in the body, they are classified according to specific lymphoma classifications[155, 162, 206, 209, 260]. They occur at all ages with a peak in the 6th and 7th decade. Immunocompromised patients including transplant recipients[162, 206, 224] and AIDS patients are known to have a high risk of CNS lymphomas[142, 263, 411]. Grossly, they represent single or multiple solid lesions often resembling malignant gliomas or metastases or they display diffuse, encephalitis- or edema-like changes. Preferred sites of involvement are the cerebral hemispheres, basal ganglia, posterior fossa, and corpus callosum presenting as butterfly tumors, while 20% show multiple lesions. Primary involvement of the spinal cord and cauda is rare[209, 280]. Among 130 primary lymphomas of the CNS we only saw one example of isolated involvement of the spinal cord. The histology of CNS lymphomas is that of diffuse non-Hodgkin's lymphomas with perivascular or diffuse infiltration of the brain tissue and frequent spread into meninges and ventricles. The predominant subtypes are immunoblastomas (43%) and immunocytomas (about 40%), less frequent are lymphoblastomas (about 12%) including the primary Burkitt type[160, 206, 209, 238]; follicular center lymphomas of the centroblastic-centrocytic type are rare, but have been observed among primary cerebral lymphomas[150]. Ultrastructural, histochemical and immunological studies show that the majority of the intracranial lymphomas are of B-cell origin[112, 150, 206, 209, 250, 260, 337, 439], much like their extraneural counterparts, while primary T-cell lymphomas of the brain appear to be exceedingly rare[114, 274]. However, surface marker heterogeneity has been observed in both primary CNS and generalized lymphomas[126, 209, 346].

Although most primary CNS lymphomas remain confined to the brain and meninges and although their initial response to radiation and chemotherapy is good[162, 204, 206, 209, 270, 287], the overall prognosis particularly of the high-grade NH-lymphomas of the brain, *i.e.* immunoblastomas and lymphoblastomas, is poor, with 50% survivals of 6–8 months and one-year survival rates of 10–20%, while the low-grade immunocytomas after aggressive treatment show better prognosis with 50% survival of 18 months and two-year survival rates of 35–40% and occasional survival up to or over 10 years[204, 209, 270, 375]. Primary CNS lymphomas are to be distinguished from secondary CNS involvement in systemic lymphomas ranging from 10 to 34% with highest incidence in high-grade NH-lymphomas (see p. 66).

5. Tumors of Blood Vessel Origin

Tumors derived from blood vessels overlap in part with the angiomatous tumors conventionally included with meningiomas, while vascular malformations (angiomas) forming a separate group in the WHO classification[496] are *not* neoplasms and therefore should be excluded.

A. Hemangioblastoma (M-9161/1; ICD-9: 228.0; NDV: 1826000)

These tumors of endothelial cell origin account for approximately 2% of intracranial neoplasms, and most commonly occur in the cerebellum but may be found in brain stem, cerebrum and spinal cord. They occur at all ages, mainly in adults, and may be part of Lindau's syndrome or of von Hippel-Lindau disease. The solitary or multiple growths are solid or cystic; in the cerebellum cysts with mural nodules may occur. The supratentorial tumors are globoid, highly vascularized and often, but not always, attached to the dura and, therefore have been previously designated as "angioblastic meningiomas"[180, 362, 370]. Histologically, both cerebellar and extracerebellar hemangioblastomas are composed of small blood vessels that are separated by stromal cells with clear and foamy cytoplasm containing neutral lipids[345]. Ultrastructural and immunohistochemical studies demonstrating endothelial markers have confirmed the endothelial origin of vascular tumor cells[77, 175], while the origin of the stroma cells is still not known. The currently favored possible site of origin are pericytes[77, 395] and endothelial cells[175], but many stroma cells have cylindrical processes containing intermediate filaments possibly derived from vasoformative cells[401] which have to be separated from processes of GFAP-positive reactive astrocytes[107]. "Reactive" glioma around a typical hemangioblastoma is to be distinguished from a mixed capillary hemangioblastoma and glioma ("angioglioma"), considered as a tumor of mixed glial and vascular tissue origin[44]. Prognosis of hemangioblastomas after resection is good, but the hazard of recurrence is well known, and malignant spread may occur[293].

Primary *angiosarcoma* (malignant hemangiodendothelioma) in the human brain showing the morphologic features of soft tissue angiosarcoma[106] is exceedingly rare[286], although similar vascular neoplasms have been experimentally induced by sarcoma virus[343]. Recently, a primary multifocal angiosarcoma of the spinal meninges after chordotomy was observed[245].

B. Hemangiopericytoma (M-9536/0; ICD-9: 237.5; NDV: 18250000)

The structure and ultrastructure of this vascular tumor which may or may not be attached to dura and, therefore has been include with hemangiopericytic variant of meningiomas, are identical with that of hemangiopericytomas arising that elsewhere in the body[67, 87, 106, 299, 317]. Histologically, in these firm and solid tumors, the endothelium of the capillary channels is separated by a basement membrane from masses of cells with oval nuclei, variable chromatin and poorly defined cell boundaries, displaying negative immunoreactions with endothelial markers[45]; perivascular and pericellular reticulin is abundant and mitoses are frequent. Meningeal hemangiopericytomas which represent 3–4% of meningeal tumors, tend to be aggressive in their growth, show a high recurrence rate with short intervals, invade adjacent tissues and may produce extracranial metastases[214, 295, 342, 370].

C. Neoplastic "Angioendotheliosis (Angioendotheliomatosis)" (NAE)—Intravascular Lymphomatosis

A rare lethal systemic neoplasia composed of intravascular proliferation of cells showing various degrees of nuclear atypia and mitotic activity which has been thought to be of endothelial origin[131, 319]. Tumors of this type occur with similar involvement of skin and/or visceral structures, while others may involve predominantly or exclusively the CNS. The latter have been designated "cerebral angioendotheliosis" or "neoplastic angioendotheliosis of the CNS"[319, 429], where tumor cells within cerebral blood vessels and associated areas of ischemia are found predominantly in the cerebral hemispheres. This intravascular proliferation has been considered part of a widely disseminated neoplasia of the endothelium or as intravascular spread from an unrecognized focus of primary malignancy, some having the histological and ultrastructural appearance of lymphomas[8, 98, 486]. In some typical cases of NAE there are extravascular large-cell lymphomas in other organs, while others showed evidence of autoimmune disorders[472]. Recent immunocytochemical and ultrastructural studies indicate that NAE is not a malignant endothelial cell neoplasm but a leukocyte-derived malignancy representing intravascular malignant lymphomatosis which may represent a primary manifestation and/or a major secondary form of disseminated malignant lymphoma[72a, 472].

6. Germ Cell Tumors

Accounting for 1–2% of intracranial neoplasms with highest frequence in Japan[216, 239, 326], these tumors occur most often in the pineal or other midline regions (suprasellar, hypothalamic) and are most commonly found in children and young adults. They tend to extent into neighboring structures and may seed along the CSF pathways. Their classification follows that of testicular tumors[300, 362, 393].

A. Germinoma (M-9064/3; ICD-9: 191.9; NDV: 1839000)

These tumors which are histologically and ultrastructurally indistinguishable from the testicular seminoma or ovarian dysgerminoma represent 50–75% of the CNS germ cell tumors with predilection to the pineal and suprasellar regions. They are more common in males[84, 199, 326, 423]. They are composed of large spheroidal or vesicular cells with one or two large eosinophilic nucleoli, ultrastructurally showing clear chromatin with a rope-like nucleolus and varying amounts of glycogen and annulated lamellae, while the stroma shows prominent invasion of T-lymphocytes[159, 299, 315]. Fibrous and granulomatous reactions, including multinucleated giant cells, and inflammatory elements are similar to the pathology found in testicular and ovarian germinomas; the intensity of the inflammatory immune reaction appears to be of some prognostic relevance[199].

B. Embryonal Carcinomas (M-9070/3; ICD-9: 191.9; NDV: 1839000)

These less frequent tumors are composed of cells of primitive epithelial appearance, often with clear cytoplasm growing in a variety of patterns: acinar, tubular, papillary, and solid. Both alpha-fetoprotein (AFP) and human chorionic gonadotropin (HCG) may be demonstrable[220, 234].

C. Choriocarcinoma (M-9100/3) and Endodermal Sinus Tumor (M-9071/3)

These rare and highly malignant tumors are more primitive than the germinomas; choriocarcinoma is composed of elements identical with syncytiotrophoblasts and cytotrophoblasts. The endodermal sinus tumor (yolk sac carcinoma) has several patterns, the most common of which is characterized by a reticular arrangement of primary epithelial cells, distinctive papillary structures resembling the endodermal sinuses of the rodent placenta, and hyaline globules, both intracellular and extracellular[67, 199, 393]. These tumors which are strongly positive for AFP and may also contain human HCG[5] occur in the pineal region; they are highly invasive and metastasis outside the CNS is well documented[326, 438].

D. Teratomas (M-9080/0–3; ICD-9: 239.6; NDV: 1839000)

Teratoid tumors are rare childhood lesions located in the pineal or sellar region, third or lateral ventricles or elsewhere in the intracranial space, often as lobular or multicystic lesions which histologically express the totipotentiality of a germinal cell[67]. They include a) *mature teratomas* composed of exclusively mature elements resembling tissues derived from two or more of the embryonic germ layers, b) *immature teratomas* containing immature structures resembling those of the embryo, but mature elements including neuroectodermal tissue being present in many of the cases, and c) *teratocarcinomas* which are basically teratomas in which one or more epithelial component may exhibit anaplasia[67, 316, 370, 402]. The outcome of immature teratomas and teratocarcinomas is poor, and malignant forms may show extraneural metastases[402]. Most germ cell tumors occur in pure form, but each may also be mixed with one or more types, *e.g.* germinomas are associated with features of endodermal sinus tumor[67, 455] or as intrasellar mixed germ-cell tumor[327].

7. Malformative Tumors

The WHO classification includes craniopharyngioma and tumor-like lesions which, in contrast to another classification[357] may also be separated into a) malformative tumors and b) tumor-like lesions[56].

A. *Craniopharyngioma* (M-9350/1; ICD-9; 237.0; NDV: 1831000)

Craniopharyngiomas, accounting for 3% of all ICN in all ages, but for 6–10% in children[362], typically occur in the suprasellar or intrasellar regions and grow into the hypothalamus or third ventricle. Grossly, they are largely cystic or partially solid, with a firm capsule, while two histological features are recognized: stratified squamous epithelium, frequently lining a cyst, and ameloblastomatous (adam-antinomatous) tissue forming more solid areas. Keratin pearls may be among the areas of squamous epithelium; calcification, ossification and inflammatory re-actions are common. Cystic cavities, lined by keratinizing squamous epithelium, may be indistinguishable from epidermoid cysts[362]. The adjacent brain tissue often shows astrogliosis and Rosenthal fibers. Successful total surgical removal depends on the locations and size of the tumor, but approximately 50% of the surgically treated patients will have tumor recurrence, and thus may require radiotherapy. Carcinomatous changes are uncommon.

B. *Rathke Cleft Cyst* (M-3340/0; ICD-9: 253,9; NDV: 1839000)

These rare cystic lesions usually arise within the sella and are lined by cuboidal, often ciliated, epithelium identical with the lining of small cysts frequently found between the pars anterior and the infundibular process.

C. *Epidermoid and Dermoid Cyst* (M-3341/0 and M-9084/0; ICD-9: 225.0; 225.3; NDV: 1838000; 1839000, 2838000)

These cystic lesions, representing about 1% of all ICNs, arise at any age in several particular locations of the cranial cavity, including the diploe; the cerebellopontine angle and the suprasellar regions being frequent sites[67, 370]. Epidermoid cysts are lined by keratin-producing squamous epithelium; the contents are brittle, white and pearly, and the cysts are referred to as pearly tumors or cholesteatoma. A dermoid cyst is lined by keratin-producing squamous epithelium and contains skin appendages. It frequently occurs in a midline location and may communicate with the skin via a sinus tract. The contents are smeary or cheesy and may include hair and rarely teeth. Malignant degeneration of both epidermoid and dermoid cysts, and transliquoral seeding have been recorded[67, 362].

D. *Colloid Cysts of the Third Ventricle (Paraphyseal) or Neuroepithelial Cyst* (M-9395/0; ICD-9: 225.0; NDV: 1839000)

Cysts occurring in the region of the foramen of Monro, near the choroid plexus, are lined by ciliated columnar or cuboidal epithelium that may become flattened under pressure, and there may be secretory epithelial cells. Ultrastructurally, the cells are joined by desmosomes, the luminar surface bears irregular microvilli, some cells are ciliated, others contain droplets of mucus, and cytoplasmic filaments may be seen[98, 170]. The origin of these cysts is debatable. They are interpreted either as paraphysial cysts or as derived from endodermal structures, most possibly from respiratory endothelium[170] or from neuroepithelial structures, either from choroid plexus epithelium[310] and/or ependyma[259].

E. Enterogenous and Respiratory Cyst (M-2666/0; ICD-9: 225.0; NDV: 1839000)

These rare cysts are lined by mucin-secreting (enterogenous) or ciliated respiratory epithelium, or show transition from pseudostratified ciliated columnar epithelium with goblet cells to papillary stratified squamous pithelium, histological features essentially identical to squamous papillomas of the nasal cavity. These cysts can occur in the subarachnoid space of the brain stem[380] or in the spinal cord in association with dysraphic lesions[259].

F. Other Cysts

Other cysts include arachnoid cysts, subarachnoidal and intraparenchymatous neuroepithelial cysts[140], ependyma-lined cysts, and neuroglial-lined cysts, the latter occurring in the pineal gland[259].

G. Lipoma (M-8850/0; ICD-9: 225.0; NDV: 1827000)

Lipomas or lipomatous hamartomas[54] are rare localized masses of adipose tissue, representing less than 0.5% of all ICNs, found over the corpus callosum (about 50%), the quadrigeminal plate, hypothalamus, and spinal cord. They are suggested to arise either from vascular or pluripotent arachnoid cells[129, 156], and are often asymptomatic, but may be associated with dysraphic states or other CNS malformations[54].

H. Granular Cell Tumors (Choristoma) (M-9320/0; ICD-9: 225.0: NDV: 1836000)

These rare nodular lesions composed of cells with eosinophilic cytoplasm resembling the granular myoblastoma elsewhere in the body[106], are located in the pars nervosa of the pituitary gland and tuber cinereum[188, 277]. They are composed of groups of large granulated cells which ultrastructurally contain characteristic granules partially surrounded by vacuoles which are different from those in the alveolar soft tissue sarcoma often metastasizing to the brain[106]. The ultrastructure of these granule cells and their strong expression of S-100 protein and other peripheral nerve myelin proteins[301, 307, 424] strongly support their derivation from Schwann cells. Adenohypophyseal neuronal choristoma is rare[377].

Rare *intracerebral granular cell tumors* in the cerebral hemispheres show some morphologic features identical with noncerebral granular cell tumors, but recent immunohistochemical and ultrastructural data strongly suggest that they are derived from neoplastic astrocytes[97a, 241a].

I. Hamartomas (M-9351/0)

These malformations include neuronal, glial and neuronoglial forms.

1. Hypothalamic Neuronal Hamartoma (M-9251/0; ICD-9: 225.0; NDV: 1839000)

Neuronal hamartoma is a rare collection of mature neurons arranged in disordered manner, most common in or near the hypothalamus (misplaced tuber nuclei), which may be associated with endocrinopathy (precocious puberty). Similar neuronal hamartomas may also occur elsewhere in the brain[362, 377].

2. Glial Hamartoma (Nasal Glioma) (M-2616/0; ICD-9: 225.1; NDV: 3808000)

Glial hamartoma is a malformation with an admixture of neuroglia and connective tissue composed of disorganized glial elements in and abundant fibrillar matrix, arising most commonly in the ventral subarachnoid space at the level of the infundibulum and optic tract, while ectopic astrocytic lesions may also occur in the nasal cavity or mastoid[67, 318].

3. Meningioangioneurinomatosis

A local proliferation of arachnoidal cells, blood vessels, and Schwann cells often associated with other features of neuroectodermal dysplasia, this lesion may occur at any level and may present as a mass lesion before the first year of life[103].

8. Tumors of Neuroendocrine Origin

A. Pituitary Tumours

Neoplasms of the anterior pituitary represent about 10% of all intracranial tumors and mainly occur in adults.

1. Pituitary Adenomas (M-8270/0; ICD-9: 227.3; NDV: 1832000–1836000)

Adenomas of the anterior pituitary have been classically diagnosed by light microscopy with the use of routine stains and special histochemical techniques for the demonstration of alpha and beta cells. The conventional nomenclature recognizing chromophobe (about 78%), eosinophilic (15%), basophil (mucoid cell) (5–6%), and mixed adenomas showing diffuse, sinusoidal or papillary patterns is incomplete and biologically obsolete, and can now only be used in a descriptive manner. Immunohistochemical techniques are required for an accurate classification of these tumors by identification of hormones produced by the tumor cells [110, 111, 242, 243, 276, 371]. The following designations are more appropriate: a) prolactin (PRL) cell adenomas including chromophobe and acidophil tumors causing amenorrhoea (28–30%); b) growth hormone (GH) cell tumors secreting somatotropic hormone (STH) (16–25%) akin to previous acidophil and mixed tumors; c) mixed GH-PRL cell adenoma (2–5%); d) adrenocorticotroph (ACTH) cell adenoma (15–20%), histologically simulating chromophobe, mucoid or amphopil, PAS-positive tumors; e) undifferentiated or null cell adenoma (oncocytic and nononcocytic), ultrastructurally filled with densely packed mitochondria and representing about 10–25%, and f) unclassified plurihormonal adenomas (1–3%). Pituitary adenoma cells may be densely or sparsely granulated on electron microscopy and in many cases the size of the granules, reflects the type of hormone secretion[299]. However, electron microscopic evaluation is not as reliable as immunohistochemical characterization of the hormonal activity of the cells[193]. Recurrence rate of pituitary adenomas after total resection ranges from 6 to 20%, but like other endocrine lesions, neither the aggressiveness of the lesion nor its recurrence tendency can be predicted reliably from light or electron microscopy[167].

2. Pituitary Carcinoma (M-8140/3)

Rarely, an adenocarcinoma can arise in the anterior lobe of the pituitary, showing anaplasia and obvious mitotic activity, although mitoses may be seen in normal adenomas. Anaplastic growths may remain confined to the sella and suprasellar areas or may be extensively invasive of bone, disseminated in the subarachnoid space, or metastatic to distant organs[67, 90, 120].

9. Local Extension from Regional Tumors

This group of regional tumors which may extend into the cranial cavity, listed in the WHO classification of CNS tumors[496], is not included in other recent classifications[56, 357] or listed under the heading "other tumors" (IDC-0; M 935-937) and classified as similar neoplasms elsewhere in the body. They include olfactory and glomus tumors, chordomas, and other tumors arising from different parts of the bone and paranasal sinuses.

A. Paraganglioma (Chemodectoma) (M-8690/0; ICD-9: 237.3; NDV: 3804000)

Paraganglioma showing a histology similar to the carotid body with occasional large neurons, may arise in the head and neck or the glomus jugulare, and usually extends into the cranial cavity, *e.g.* posterior fossa and pontocerebellar angle, from a contiguous site[252, 268]. The same of tumor may also arise in the pineal, pituitary or cauda equina region, and ultrastructure shows neuronal differentiation with numerous dense core vesicles[268, 461]. Immunohistochemistry shows NSE and various transmitters (serotonin, leuenkephalin, substance P. etc)[461]. Malignant transformation is rare.

B. Chordoma (M-9370/1–3; NDV: 1829000)

This rare gelatinous, lobated tumor of intraosseous notochordial origin usually arises at the base of the skull (clivus), but may also occur in the spinal cord. It is composed of cords of plant-like vesiculated cells with vacuolar cytoplasms. Their ultrastructure is similar to the ecchordosis physaliphora, both lesions showing morphologic features of both epithelial and mesenchymal origin[176], and both keratin and tissue polypeptide antigen (TPA) are constantly expressed by both lesions, while they are negative in chondrosarcomas[66, 290, 415]. These facts support the concept that chordomas arise from heterotopic notochordial remnants in the craniovertebral canal[66, 176]. Mucoid degeneration and calcification are frequent. Despite its benign histologic features, the poor prognosis of this lesions results from its propensity to local invasion and destruction, and malignant transformation with dissemination may occur[478].

C. Chondroma, Osteochondroma, Chondrosarcoma (M-9220/0–3; ICD-9: 213.0; NDV: 6811000, 6832000)

The rare intracranial cartilage cell tumors accounting for 0.2% of intracranial growths are attached to the dura of the convexity of the falx or arise from the base of the skull. They have a chondroid appearance with or without calcification. The majority are chondromas, most frequently arising from the base of the skull; less frequent are chondrosarcomas, most frequently arising in the parasellar or cerebellopontine angle/petrous bone areas. This well-differentiated tumor with few myxoid or mesenchymal components and a predominance of the cartilaginous elements tends to recur and invade the brain, but has a better prognosis than mesenchymal chondrosarcoma mainly arising above the skull base[89]. The so-called *chondroid chordomas*, based on immunohistochemical evidence, are suggested to be be cartilagineous in nature and to represent well-differentiated chondrosarcomas[50].

D. Olfactory Neuroblastoma (Esthesioneuroblastoma) (M-9523/1–3; ICD-9: 225,5; 160.0; NDV: 3808000)

Rare neuroepithelial tumors of the olfactory epithelium in children and adults arise in the nasal cavity and may invade the cranial cavity and disseminate through the CSF pathways. They are composed of primitive neuroepithelial cells forming neuroblastic rosettes and can show different degrees of neuronal differentiation, according to which three types are distinguished: a) olfactory neurocytoma (esthesioneurocytoma), b) olfactory neuroblastoma (esthesioneuroblastoma), and c) olfactory neuroepithelioma (esthesioneuroepithelioma). The ultrastructural features of olfactory neuroblastoma are the presence of membrane-bound neuro-secretory granules in cytoplasmic processes, synaptic formations and bulbous expansions reminiscent of axonal growth cones similar to neuroblastomas arising from the adrenals or sympathetic system[76, 173, 288]. Immunocytochemistry includes positive NSE expression in irregular clusters of tumor cells, with S-100 being present in peripheral cells forming a marginal network, while GFAP positive cells are rarely present[79]; it further shows an abnormal neurofilament synthesis[444], and the presence of biogenic amines[173]. These tumors may occasionally contain melanin[88] or mixed neuroblastoma and undifferentiated carcinoma[292].

10. Metastatic Tumors (M-8000/6; ICD-9: 198.3; NDV: 1851000–1859000)

Metastatic involvement of the CNS and its coverings can be expected in 13–25% (range 3–50%) of all patients harboring solid tumors[207, 493], in 10 to 34% of those with malignant lymphomas, with highest incidence in high-grade non-Hodgkin's lymphomas[204, 206, 270], and in 45–85% of patients with leukemia[206]. The incidence of metastatic lesions among intracranial neoplasm averages 15–30%, with a range from 5–15% in clinical series and from 14 to 63% in autopsy series[178, 195, 207]. The most common primary sites of solid neoplasms are lung (60–65%), kidney and urinary tract (6–10%), gastrointestinal (GI) tract (5–8%), and skin (melanoma) (5–7%), these five groups accounting for 65–90% of all metastatic cerebral growths in the brain. The highest tendency towards CNS metastases is known for malignant melanomas (40–92%), germ cell tumors (choriocarcinoma, gonadal germ cell tumors) (50–60%) and broncho-pulmonary carcinomas (40 to over 50%), with highest incidence in small-cell carcinoma and undifferentiated forms[31, 178, 207]; next are breast carcinoma (40–50%), renal carcinoma (about 20%), head and neck tumors (20–25%), thyroid, liver and pancreatic, and GI carcinomas (2–15% each), while other malignancies, including female genital and prostatic carcinomas have no or only little tendency to invade the brain.

Metastatic growth may be located at any site of the CNS, forming solitary or multiple, well circumscribed nodules or diffuse invasive lesions of the brain, leptomeninges and dura. Dural involvement is seen in 10–18% of patients with solid tumors, most often with breast carcinoma (over 50%), prostatic and gastric carcinomas and, very frequently, in leukemias. Brain metastases may occur as solitary lesions (15–25%) and, more often, as multiple lesions of variable size and location. About 75% are supratentorial, with rather uniform involvement of both cerebral hemispheres, affecting both the gray and white matter. The deep cerebral structures, including basal ganglia, and the cerebellum are equally involved in about 30% each; isolated involvement of the brain stem is seen in 5–10%, while metastatic involvement of the pituitary occurs in 1–6% of all solid tumors, most often in breast carcinoma [31, 178]. Metastatic involvement of the meninges is seen in 15–60% of all patients with solid tumors, in about 40% of malignant lymphomas, in up to 90% of acute leukemias [178, 206, 207]. While in 60% of the cases, meningeal carcinosis is associated with solid brain metastases, "pure" meningeal carcinosis can be expected in 5–12% of all patients harboring solid malignancies, most often with lung, breast, gastric carcinomas, and melanomas [211]. Meningeal involvement in both solid neoplasms, lymphomas and leukemias may be focal or diffuse, and in about 60% is associated with involvement of the cranial nerve roots and invasion of the brain parenchyma due to spreading via the pia-glial barrier. A rare form of CNS involvement is "diffuse" brain carcinosis with diffuse perivascular infiltration and spread to the inner and outer CSF pathways. It has been observed in about 5% of brain metastases, particularly with small cell and adenocarcinoma of lung, breast carcinoma and melanoma [295, 207].

CNS involvement in leukemias and malignant lymphomas also includes a) solid cranial and dural deposites, accounting for about 1% of intracranial metastases [206], b) neoplastic pachymeningosis seen in 50–90% of autopsy cases; c) meningeal involvement, seen in 50–93%, most frequently in acute leukemias and high-grade lymphomas, with or without involvement of cerebral parenchyma; d) diffuse meningoencephalosis due to combined meningeal and parenchymal involvement is also most frequent in acute leukemias and high-grade non-Hodgkin's lymphomas, while solid intracranial deposits with tumor formation are much less frequent in both malignant lymphomas (2–10%) and leukemias (1–5%), where chloromas more frequently arise from the skull, paranasal sinuses or dura and may invade the brain [206]. Metastatic involvement of the CNS and its coverings in solid neoplasms, lymphomas and leukemias due to a) hematogenous spread, b) direct (continuous) invasion from affected adjacent from structures; and c) via trans-liquoral spreading (see [204, 206]).

11. Unclassified Tumors

A small number of tumors, when examined by standard light microscopic techniques, cannot be placed in one of the above categories and will remain "unclassified". Immunocytochemical methods and electron microscopy may assist in defining the nature of some tumors and would reduce their number to a minimum, but a fraction may remain nameless even after all avenues of investigation have been exhausted. For these rare cases a preliminary descriptive diagnosis will be provided.

References

1. Adams JH, Graham DI, Doyle D (1981) Brain biopsy—the smear technique for neurosurgical biopsies. Chapman & Hall, London
2. Afra D, Müller W, Slowik F, Wilcke O, Budka H, Turoczy L (1983) Supratentorial lobar ependymomas; reports on the grading and survival periods in 80 cases, including 40 recurrences. Acta Neurochir (Wien) 69: 243–251
3. Ahyal A, Zimmermann A, Spaar FW (1983) Flow fluorescence-cytometry DNA in meningiomas; studies on surgically removed tumor specimens compared with their cells in primary tissue cultures. Surg Neurol 20: 195–205
4. Aichner F, Schuler G (1982) Primary leptomeningeal melanoma: Diagnosis by ultrastructural cytology of cerebrospinal fluid and cranial computed tomography. Cancer 50: 1751–1756
5. Allen JC, Nisselbaum J, Epstein F, Rosen G, Schwartz MK (1980) Alphafetoprotein and human chorionic gonadotropin determination in cerebrospinal fluid. An aid in the diagnosis and management of intracranial germ-cell tumors. J Neurosurg 51: 369–374
6. Ambier M, Pogacar S, Sidman R (1969) Lhermitte-Duclos disease (granule cell hypertrophy of the cerebellum): Pathological analysis of the first familial cases. J Neuropathol Exp Neurol 28: 622–647
7. Anderson WR, Cameron JD, Tsai SH (1980) Primary intracranial leiomyosarcoma. J Neurosurg 53: 401–405
8. Ansell J, Bhawan J, Cohen S, Sullivan J, Sherman D (1982) Histiocytic lymphoma and malignant angioendotheliomatosis. One disease or two? Cancer 50: 1506–1512
9. Arendt A (1975) Ependymomas. In: Vinken PJ, Bruyn GW (eds) Handbook of clinical neurology, vol 18. Elsevier, Amsterdam New York, pp 105–150
10. Arendt A (1977) Histologisch-diagnostischer Atlas der Geschwülste des Zentralnervensystems und seiner Anhangsgebilde. Fischer, Jena
11. Arendt A (1982) Histopathologie von Gliomrezidiven. Zbl allg Path pathol Anat 126: 499–504
12. Artigas J, Cervos-Navarro J, Iglesias JR, Ebhardt G (1985) Gliomatosis cerebri: clinical and histological findings. Clin Neuropathol 4: 135–148
13. Auer RN, Becker LE (1983) Cerebral medulloepithelioma with bone, cartilage and striated muscle. J Neuropathol Exp Neurol 42: 256–267
14. Auer RN, Rice GPA, Hinton GG, Amacher AL, Gilbert JJ (1981) Cerebellar astrocytoma with benign histology and malignant clinical course. J Neurosurg 54: 128–132
15. Azzarelli B, Richards DE, Anton AH, Roesmann U (1977) Central neuroblastoma—Electron-microscopic observations and catecholamine determinations. J Neuropathol Exp Neurol 36: 384–397
16. Bagshawe KD (1976) Risk and prognostic factors in trophoblastic neoplasia. Cancer 58: 1375–1378
17. Bailey P, Cushing H (1926) Classification of tumors of the glioma group on a histogenetic basis with a correlated study of prognosis. Lippincott, Philadelphia
18. Bamborschke S, Ebhardt G, Szelies-Stock B, Dreesbach HA, Heiss WD (1985) Review and case report: Primary melanoblastosis of the leptomeninges. Clin Neuropathol 4: 47–55

19. Barnard RO (1982) The classification of tumors of the central nervous system. Neuropathol Appl Neurobiol 8: 1–10

20. Barnard RO (1986) The pathology of brain tumours. In: Bleehen NM (ed) Tumours of the brain. Springer, Berlin Heidelberg New York Tokyo, pp 1–18

21. Barnard RO, Bradford R, Scott T, Thomas DCT (1986) Gliomyosarcoma: Report of a case of rhabdomyosarcoma arising in a malignant glioma. Acta Neuropathol (Berl) 69: 23–27

22. Barnard RO, Logue V, Reaves PS (1976): An atlas of tumours involving the central nervous system. Baillière & Tindall, London

23. Bartkowski HM (1984) Peritumoral edema. Prog Exp Tumor Res 27: 179–190

24. Battista AF, Bloom W, Koffman H, Feigin I (1961) Autotransplantation of anaplastic astrocytomas into the subcutaneous tissue of man. Neurology 11: 977–981

25. Batzdorf U, Malamud N (1963) The problem of multicentric gliomas. J Neurosurg 20: 122–136

26. Becker LE (1985) An appraisal of the World Health Organization classification of tumors of the central nervous system. Cancer 56: 1858–1864

27. Becker LE, Hinton D (1983) Primitive neuroectodermal tumors of the central nervous system. Hum Pathol 14: 538–550

28. Bennett JP, Rubinstein LJ (1984) The biological behavior of primary cerebral neuroblastoma: A reappraisal of the clinical course in a series of 70 cases. Ann Neurol 16: 21–27

29. Berger MS, Edwards MSB, Wara WM, Levis VY, Wilson CB (1983) Primary cerebral neuroblastoma. Long-term follow-up and therapeutic guidelines. J Neurosurg 59: 418–423

30. Bernell WR, Kepes JJ, Seitz EP (1972) Malignant recurrence of childhood cerebellar astrocytoma. J Neurosurg 37: 470–475

31. Bernstein U, Schreiber D, Schweider J (1982) Tumormetastasen im Zentralnervensystem. Eine prospektive Studie. Zbl Allg Pathol Anat 126: 53–63

32. Berry MP, Jenkin RDT (1981) Parameningeal rhabdomyosarcoma in the young. Cancer 48: 281–288

33. Biggs PJ, Powers JM (1984) Neuroblastic medulloblastoma with abundant cytoplasmic actin filaments. Arch Pathol Lab Med 108: 326–329

34. Bilzer TH, Stavrou D (1985) Cell-mediated immune response during progressive glioma growth. In: Voth D, Krauseneck P (eds) Chemotherapy of gliomas. de Gruyter, Berlin New York

35. Bloom HJG (1982) Intracranial tumor: Response and resistance to therapeutic endeavors. Int J Rad Oncol Biol Phys 8: 1083–111

36. Bloom HJG (1986) Treatment of brain gliomas in children. In: Bleehan NM (ed) Tumours of the brain. Springer, Berlin Heidelberg New York, pp 121–140

37. Bloom HJG, Richardson WW, Field JG (1970) Host resistance and survival in carcinoma of the breast: A study of 104 cases of medullary carcinoma in a series of 1,411 cases of breast cancer followed for 20 years. Brit Med J 3: 181–188

38. Böck P, Jellinger K (1981) Detection of glycosaminoglycans in human gliomas by histochemical methods. Acta Neuropathol (Berl) Suppl 7: 81–84

39. Böker DK (1982) Lymphocytic infiltration in human intracranial tumors. Morphologic evidence for a host-immune reaction and comparison with the leukocyte migration test. Clin Neuropathol 1: 113–120

40. Böker DK, Gullotta F (1985) Mononuclear infiltrates in human brain tumours: possible morphological equivalence of an immunological defence reaction. In Voth D, Krauseneck P (eds) Chemotherapy of gliomas. De Gruyter, Berlin, pp 87–92

41. Böker DK, Kalff R, Gullotta F, Weekes-Seifert S, Möhrer S (1984) Mononuclear infiltrates in human intracranial tumors as a prognostic factor. Influence of preoperative steroid treatment. I. Glioblastoma. Clin Neuropathol 3: 143–147

42. Boekstegers A, Grundmann E (1985) What a new in natural killer cells? Path Res Pract 180: 536–552

43. Boesel CP, Suhan JP, Sayers MP (1978) Melanotic medulloblastoma. Report of a case with ultrastructural findings. J Neuropathol Exp Neurol 37: 531–543

44. Bonnin JM, Pena CE, Rubinstein LJ (1983) Mixed capillary hemangioblastoma and glioma. Redefinition of the "angioglioma". J Neuropathol Exp Neurol 42: 504–516

45. Bonnin JM, Rubinstein LJ (1984) Immunocytochemistry of central nervous system tumors: Its contribution to neurosurgical diagnosis. J Neurosurg 60: 1121–1133

46. Bonnin JM, Rubinstein LJ, Papasozomenos SCH, Marangos PJ (1984) Subependymal glial cell astrocytoma. Significance and possible cytogenetic implications of an immunohistochemical study. Acta Neuropathol (Berl) 62: 185–193

47. Bont A, Blackwood W, Mair WGP (1980) The separation of pineocytoma from pineoblastoma. Cancer 45: 1408–1418

48. Bradford R, Crockard HA, Isaacson PG (1985) Primary rhabdomyosarcoma of the CNS (case report). Neurosurg 17: 101–104

49. Broder AC (1926) Carcinoma. Grading and practical application. Arch Path (Chic) 2: 376

50. Brooks JJ, LiVolsi VA, Trojanowski JQ (1986) Does chondroid chordoma exist? Acta Neuropathol (Berl) in press

51. Brooks WH, Markesberry WR, Gupta GD, Roszman TL (1978) Relationship of lymphocyte invasion and survival of brain tumor patients. Ann Neurol 4: 219–224

52. Brooks WH, Roszmal TL (1980) Cellular immune responsitiveness of patients with primary intracranial tumours. In: Thomas DGT, Graham DI (eds) Brain tumours. Butterworth, London Boston, pp 121–132

53. Bruno LA, Rorke LB, Norris DG (1981) Primary neuroectodermal tumors of infancy and childhood. In: Humphrey GB, Dehner LP (eds) Pediatric oncolocy, I. M Nijhoff, The Hague Boston, pp 265–267

54. Budka H (1974) Intracranial lipomatous hamartoma ("intracranial lipomas"). Acta Neuropathol (Berl) 28: 205–222

55. Budka H (1975) Partially resected and irradiated cerebellar astrocytoma of childhood: malignant evolution after 28 years. Acta Neurochir (Wien) 32: 139–146

56. Budka H (1984) Tumoren des Zentralnervensystems. In: Österr Ges Pathol (Hrsg) Histologische Tumorklassifikation. Springer, Wien New York, S 140–146

57. Budka H, Jellinger K, Lassmann H, Weiser G (1974) Tumoren des peripheren Nervengewebes. In: Österr Ges Pathol (Hrsg) Histologische Tumorklassifikation. Springer, Wien New York, S 147–149

58. Budka H, Majdic O, Knapp W (1985) Cross-reactivity between human hemopoietic cells and brain tumors as defined by monoclonal antibodies. J Neuro-Oncol 3: 173–179

59. Budka H, Pilz P, Guseo A (1975) Primary leptomeningeal sarcomatosis. Clinico-pathological report of six cases. J Neurol 211: 77–93

60. Budka H, Podreka I, Reisner TH, Zeiler K (1980) Diagnostic and pathomorphological aspects in glioma multiplicity. Neurosurg Rev 3: 233–241

61. Budka H, Podreka I, Zaunbauer F (1979) Overgrowth of a primitive cell population in operated recurrent gliomas: The possible cell population and radiotherapy. In: Paoletti P, Walker MD, et al. (eds): Multidisciplinary aspects of brain tumor therapy. Elsevier/North-Holland, Amsterdam New York, pp 357–362

62. Burger PC (1985) The "ideal" classification of pediatric central nervous system neoplasms. Cancer 56: 1865–1868

63. Burger PC, Dubois PJ, Schold SC Jr, Smith KR Jr, Odom GL, Crafts DC, Giangasparo F (1983) Computed tomographic and pathologic studies of the untreated, quiescent, and recurrent glioblastoma multiforme. J Neurosurg 58: 159–169

64. Burger PC, Grahmann F, Bliestle A, Kleihues P (1986) Differentiation in the medulloblastoma—an immunohistochemical study (abstr). Clin Neuropathol 5: 110

65. Burger PC, Mahaley MS, Dudka L, Vogel FS (1979) The morphologic effects of radiation administered therapeutically for intracranial gliomas: A postmortem study of 25 cases. Cancer 44: 1256–1272

66. Burger PC, Makek M, Kleihues P (1986) Tissue polypeptide antigen (TPA) staining of the chondroma and notochordal remnants. Acta Neuropathol (Berl) 70: 269–272

66 a. Burger PC, Shibata T, Kleihues P (1986) The use of monoclonal antibody Ki-67 in the identification of proliferating cells. Application to surgical neuropathology. Amer J Surg Pathol 10: 611–617

67. Burger PC, Vogel SF (1982) Surgical pathology of the nervous system and its coverings, 2nd edn. J Wiley, New York

68. Burger PC, Vogel SF, Green SB, Strike TA (1985) Glioblastoma multiforme and anaplastic astrocytoma. Pathologic criteria and prognostic implications. Cancer 56: 1106–1111

69. Burger PC, Vollmer R (1980) Histologic factors of prognostic significance in the glioblastoma multiforme. Cancer 46: 1179–1186

70. Cairncross JG, Pexman JHW, Rathbone MP, del Maestro RF (1985) Postoperative contrast enhancement in patients with brain tumor. Ann Neurol 17: 570–572

71. Campbell AN, Chan HS, Becker LE, Aneman A, Park TS, Hoffmann HJ (1984) Extracranial metastases in childhood primary intracranial tumors. Cancer 53: 979–981

72. Camins MB, Cravioto HM, Epstein F, Ransohoff J (1980) Medulloblastoma: An ultrastructural study. Evidence for astrocytic and neuronal differentiation. Neurosurg 6: 398–411

73. Cancer statistics 1983. CA Cancer Clin 33: 9–25

74. Casentini L, Gullotta F, Möhrer U (1981) Clinical and morphological investigations on ependymomas and their tissue cultures. Neurochir (Stuttg) 24: 51–56

75. Chatty EM, Earle KM (1971) Medulloblastoma: A report on 201 cases with emphasis on the relationship of histologic variants to survival. Cancer 28: 977–983

76. Chaudry AP, Haar JG, Koul A, Nickerson PA (1978) Olfactory neuroblastoma (esthesioneuroblastoma). A light and ultrastructural study of two cases. Cancer 44: 564–579

77. Chaudry AP, Montes M, Cohn GA (1980) Ultrastructure of cerebellar hemangioblastoma. Cancer 42: 1834–1850

78. Chin HW, Maruyama Y, Tibbs P, Markesberry W, Young B (1984) Cerebellar glioblastoma in childhood. J Neuro-Oncol 2: 79–84

79. Choi HSH, Anderson PJ (1984) Immunohistochemical diagnosis of olfactory neuroblastoma. J Neuropathol Exp Neurol 44: 18–31

80. Chowdmury C, Roy S, Mahapara AK, Bhatia R (1985) Medullomyoblastoma, a teratoma. Cancer 55: 1495–1500

81. Coakham HB, Garson JA, Brownell B, Kemshead JT (1985) Diagnosis of cerebral neoplasms using monoclonal antibodies. In: Rose FS, Fields WS (eds), Neuro-Oncology. Karger, Basel

82. Codd MB, Kurland LT (1985) Descriptive epidemiology of primary intracranial neoplasms. In: Rose FS, Fields WS (eds) Neuro-Oncology. Karger, Basel

83. Coffin CM, Mukai K, Dehner LP (1983) Glial differentiation in medulloblastomas; Histogenetic insight, glial reaction, or invasion of the brain? Amer J Surg Pathol 7: 555–565

83 a. Coffin CM, Wick MR, Brain JTT, Dehner LP (1986) Choroid plexus neuroplasms. Clinicopathologic and immunohistochemical studies. Amer J Surg Pathol 10: 394–404

84. Cohen MF, Duffner PK (eds) (1984) Brain tumors in children. Principles in diagnosis and treatment. Raven Press, New York

85. Cohandon F, Aouad N, Rougier A, Vital C, Rivel J, Dartigues JF (1985) Histologic and non-histologic factors correlated with survival time in supratentorial astrocytic tumors. J Neuro-Oncol 3: 105–111

86. Conley FK, Rubinstein LJ, Spence AM (1976) Studies on experimental malignant nerve sheath tumors maintained in tissue and organ culture systems. II. Electron microscopy observations. Acta Neuropathol (Berl) 34: 293–310

87. Cosatto JO, Font RL (1982) Hemangiopericytoma of the orbit. Human Pathol 13: 210–218

88. Curtis JL, Rubinstein LJ (1982) Pigmented olfactory neuroblastoma. A new example of melanotic neuroepithelial neoplasm. Cancer 49: 2136–2143

89. Cybolski GR, Russell EJ, D Angelo CM, Bailey OT (1985) Falcine chondrosarcoma: Case report and literature review. Neurosurgery 16: 412–416

90. De Abrera VSE, Burke W, Bleasel KR, Bader L (1973) Carcinomas of the pituitary gland. J Pathol 109: 335–343

91. Dastur DK (1983) Cerebral ganglioglio-neuroblastoma: an unusual brain tumor of the neuron series. J Neurol Neurosurg Psych 45: 139–142

92. Deane BD, Lantos PL (1981) The vasculature of experimental brain tumors, Part 1 and 2. J Neurol Sci 49: 55–66, 67–77

93. De Armond SJ, Eng LF (1984) Immunohistochemistry: Techniques and application to neurooncology. Progr exp Tumor Res 27: 92–117

94. De Jong ASH (1984) Myosin and myoglobin as tumor markers in the diagnosis of rhabdomyosarcoma. Amer J Surg Pathol 8: 521–528

95. De Ridder LI, Laerum OD, Mørk SV, Bigner DD (1986) Invasiveness of human glioma cell lines in vitro: Relation to tumorigenicity in atypic mice. Acta Neuropathol (Berl) 71:

96. Dick SJ, Macchi B, Papazoglou S, Oldfield EH, Kornblith PL, et al. (1983) Lymphoid cell-glioma cell interaction enhances cell coat production by human gliomas; Novel suppressor mechanisms. Science 220: 739–741

97. Dickson DW, Hart MN, Menezes A, Cancilla PA (1983) Medulloblastoma with glial and rhabdomyoblastic differentiation. J Neuropathol Exp Neurol 42: 639–647

97 a. Dickson DW, Suzuki KI, Kanner R, Weitz S, Horoupian DS (1986) Cerebral granular cell tumor: Immunohistochemical and electron microscopic study. J Neuropathol Exp Neurol 45: 304–314

98. Dolman CL (1984) Ultrastructure of Brain Tumors and Biopsies. A diagnostic atlas. Praeger, New York Philadelphia

99. Dohrmann GJ, Farwell JR, Flannery JT (1978) Oligodendrogliomas in children. Surg Neurol 10: 21–25

100. Drut R, Jones MC (1983) Melanotic medulloblastoma of infancy: A case report with immunohistochemical study and literature review. Morf Norm Patol 7: 53–62

101. Duffy PE (1983) Astrocytes: Normal, reactive, and neoplastic. Raven Press, New York

102. Duffy PE, Huang Y, Rapport MM, Graf L (1980) Glial fibrillary acidic protein in giant cell tumors of brain and other gliomas. Acta Neuropathol (Berl) 52: 51

103. Duhaime AC, Schut L, Rorke LB, Bruce DA, Sutton LN (1984) The MEAN disease. Karger, Basel, pp 154–164 (Concepts in pediatric neurosurgery, vol V)

104. El-Gindi S, Salama M, El-Heaway M, Farag S (1973) Metastases of glioblastoma multiforme to cervical lymph nodes. J Neurosurg 38: 631–634

105. Elkon D, Hightower SI, Lim MI, Cantrell RW, Constable WC (1979) Esthesioneuroblastoma. Cancer 44: 1087–1994

106. Enzinger FM, Weiss SW (1983) Soft tissue tumors. Mosby, St Louis Toronto London

107. Epstein JI, White CL, Mendelsohn G (1984) Factor VIII related antigen and glial fibrillary acidic protein immunoreactivity in the differential diagnosis of central nervous system hemangioglastomas. Am J Clin Pathol 81: 285–292

108. Erlandson RA, Woodruff JM (1982) Peripheral nerve sheath tumors: An electron-microscopic study of 43 cases. Cancer 49: 273–287

109' Erlich SS, Davis RL (1978) Spinal subarachnoid metastases from primary intracranial glioblastoma multiforme. Cancer 42: 2854–2864

110. Esiri MM, Adams CBI, Burke C, Umberdown R (1983) Pituitary adenomas: Immunohistology and ultrastructural analysis of 118 tumors. Acta Neuropathol (Berl) 62: 1–14

111. Ezrin C, Kovacs, Horvath E (1982) Pathology of the adenohypophysis. In: Bloodworth JMB (ed) Endocrine pathology: general and surgical, 2nd edn. William & Wilkins, Baltimore, pp 100–132

112. Ezrin-Waters C, Klein M, Deck J, Lang AE (1984) Diagnostic importance of immunological markers in lymphoma involving the central nervous system. Ann Neurol 16: 668–672

113. Fallace WJ, Okawara SH, McDonald JV (1984) Neurocutaneous melanosis with extensive intracerebral and spinal cord involvement. Report of two cases. J Neurosurg 61: 782–785

114. Fan KJ, Pezeshkpour F (1986) Immunoperoxidase study of primary central nervous system lymphomas. Acta Neuropathol (Berl) in press

115. Farwell JR, Dohrmann GJ, Flannery JT (1984) Medulloblastoma in childhood: an epidermiological study. J Neurosurg 61: 657–664

116. Feichter G, Schwechheimer K, Goertler K (1983) Assistierte impulszytometrische Beurteilung bei der Routine-Diagnostik von Meningeomen und Gliomen. Pathologe 4: 294–302

117. Feigin I, Epstein F, Mangiardi J (1983) Extensive advanced maturation of medulloblastoma to astrocytoma and ependymoma. J Neuro-Oncol 1: 95–108

118. Fialkow PJ (1979) Clonal origin of human tumors. Rev Med 30: 135–143

119. Firsching R, Schröder R, Köning W, Frowein RA (1985) Spinale Abtropfmetastase beim cerebralen Glioblastom/Gliosarkom. Nervenarzt 56: 629–634

120. Fleischer AS, Reagan T, Ransohoff J (1972) Primary carcinomas of the pituitary gland with metastasis to the brain stem. J Neurosurg 36: 781–784

121. Fogelholm R, Uutela T, Murros K (1984) Epidemiology of central nervous system neoplasms. A regional survey in Central Finland. Acta Neurol Scand 69: 129–136

122. Folkman J (1984) What is the role of endothelial cells in angiogenesis? Lab Invest 51: 601–604

123. Folkman J (1985) Tumor angiogenesis. In: Klein G, Weinhouse S (eds) Advances in cancer research, vol 43. Academic Press, New York, pp 175–203

124. Foerster O, Gagel O (1938) Das umschriebene Arachnoidalsarkom des Kleinhirns. Z Ges Neurol Psych 164: 565

125. Fould L (1969) Neoplastic development, vol 1. Academic Press, London New York

126. Freedman AS, Byod AW, Anderson KC, Fisher DC, Pinkus GS, Schlossman SF, Nadler-LM (1985) Immunologic heterogeneity of diffuse large cell lymphomas. Blood 65: 630–637

127. Friede RL (1978) Gliofibroma: A peculiar neoplasia of collagen forming glia-like cells. J Neuropathol Exp Neurol 38: 300–313

128. Friede R, Pollak A (1978) The cytogenetic basis for classifying ependymomas. J Neuropathol Exp Neurol 37: 103–118

129. Frydl Y (1985) Intrakranielle Lipome und Xanthome. Med Welt 36: 375–381

129 a. Fukui M, Iwaki T, Sawa H, Inoue T, Takeshita I, Kitamura K (1986) Proliferative activity of meningiomas as evaluated by bromodeoxyuridine uptake examination. Acta Neurochir (Wien) 81: 135–141

130. Fulling KH, Garcia DM (1985) Anaplastic astrocytoma of the adult cerebrum: Prognostic value of histologic features. Cancer 55: 928–931

131. Fulling KH, Gersell DJ (1983) Neoplastic angioendotheliosis. Histologic, immunohistochemical, and ultrastructural findings in two cases. Cancer 51: 1107–1118

132. Gaffney CC, Sloane JP, Bradley NJ, Bloom HJG (1985) Primitive neuroectodermal tumours of the cerebrum. Pathology and treatment. J Neuro-Oncol 3: 23–33

133. Gallassi E, Tognetti F, Frank F, Gaist G (1984) Extraneural metastases from primary pineal tumors. Review of the literature. Surg Neurol 21: 497–504

134. Gambarelli D, Hassoun J, Choux M, Toga M (1982) Complex cerebral tumor with evidence of neuronal, glial and Schwann cell differentiation: A histologic, immunocytochemical and ultrastructural study. Cancer 49: 1420–1428

135. Garcia DM, Fulling KH (1985) Juvenile pilocytic astrocytoma of the cerebrum in adults. A distinctive neoplasm with favorable prognosis. J Neurosurg 63: 382–386

136. Gately MK, Glaser M, Carron RM, Dick SJ, Dick MD, Mettetal RW, Kornblith PL (1982) Mechanisms by which human gliomas may escape cellular immune attack. Acta Neurochir (Wien) 64: 175–197

137. Gerstner L, Jellinger K, Heiss WD, Wöber G (1976) Morphological changes in anaplastic gliomas treatet with radiation and chemotherapy. Acta Neurochir (Wien) 36: 117–138

138. Ghatak NR, McWhorter JM (1976) Ultrastructural evidence for CSF production by a choroid plexus papilloma. J Neurosurg 45: 409–415

139. Gherardi R, Baudrimont M, Nguyen JP, Gaston A, Cesaro P, et al. (1986): Monstrocellular heavily lipidized malignant glioma. Acta Neuropathol (Berl) 67: 28–32

140. Gherardi R, Lacombe MJ, Poirier J, Roucayrol AM, Wechsler J (1984) Asymptomatic encephalic intraparenchymatous neuroepithelial cysts. Acta Neuropathol (Berl) 63: 264–268

141. Giangasparo F, Burger PC (1983) Correlations between cytologic composition and biologic behavior in the glioblastoma multiforme. A postmortem study of 50 cases. Cancer 52: 2320–2333

142. Gill PS, Levine AM, Meyer PR, Boswell WD, et al. (1985) Primary CNS lymphoma in homosexual men: Clinical, immunologic and pathologic features. Amer J Med 78: 742–748

143. Gilles FH (1985) Classification of childhood brain tumors. Cancer 56: 1857–1859

144. Gilles FH, Leviton A, Hedley-Whyte ET, Jasnow M (1983) Childhood brain tumors update. Human Pathol 14: 834–845

145. Giordana MT, Bertelotto A, Migheli A, Pezzotta S, et al. (1982) Glycosaminoglycans in human cerebral tumors. Acta Neuropathol (Berl) 57: 299–305

146. Gjerris F, Harman A, Klinken L, Reske-Nielsen E (1978) Incidence and long-term survival of children with intracranial tumours treated in Denmark 1935–1959. Brit J Cancer 38: 442–451

147. Gjerris F, Klinken L (1978) Long-term prognosis in children with benign cerebellar astrocytoma. J Neurosurg 24: 125–135

148. Goldenberg DM, Pavia RA (1982) In vivo horizontal oncogenesis by a human tumor in nude mice. Proc Natl Acad Sci USA 79: 2389–2392

149. Gomez JG, Garcia JH, Colon LE (1985) A variant of cerebral glioma called pleomorphic xanthoastrocytoma. Neurosurg 16: 703–706

150. Grant JW, Jones DB (1984) Immunohistochemistry of lymphomas affecting the nervous system. Neuropathol Appl Neurobiol 10: 310

151. Groothuis DR, Molnar P, Blasberg RG (1984) Regional blood flow and blood-to-tissue transport in five brain tumor models. Implications for chemotherapy. Prog Exp Tumor Res 27: 132–153
152. Gullotta F (1981) Morphological and biological basis for the classification of brain tumors, with a comment on the WHO-classification 1979. In: Krayenbühl H (ed) Advances and technical standards in neurosurgery, vol 8. Springer, Wien New York, pp 123–165
153. Gullotta F, de Melo AS (1979) Das Karzinom des Plexus chorioideus. Neurochir (Stuttg) 22: 1–9
154. Gullotta F, Schindler F, Schmutzler R, Weeks-Seifert A (1965) GFAP in brain tumor diagnosis: possibilities and limitations. Path Res Pract 180: 54–60
154 a. Halper J, Scheithauer BW, Okazaki H, Laws ER, Jr (1986) Meningio-angiomatosis. A report of six cases with special reference to the occurrence of neurofibrilary tangles. J Neuropathol Exp Neurol 45: 426–446
155. Hanak H, Radaszkiewicz T (1984) Tumoren des lymphatischen Systems. In: Österr Ges Pathol (Hrsg) Histologische Tumorklassifikation. Springer, Wien New York, pp 133–135
156. Hara M, Kawachi S, Hirano A (1981) Lipoma of the superior medullary velum with Schwann cells. Acta Path Jpn 31: 825–833
157. Hart MN, Earle KM (1973) Primitive neuroectodermal tumors of the brain in children. Cancer 32: 890–897
158. Hassoun J, Gambarelli D, Grisoli F, Pellet W, Salomon G, Pellissier JF, Toga M (1982) Central neurocytoma. An electron microscopic study of two cases. Acta Neuropathol (Berl) 56: 151–156
159. Hassoun J, Gambarelli D, Pellissier JF, Henin D, Toga M (1981) Germinomas of the brain. Light and electron microscopic study. Acta Neuropathol (Berl) 37: 105–108
160. Hegedüs K (1984) Burkitt-type lymphoma and reticulum cell sarcoma, an unusual mixed form of two intracranial primary malignant lymphomas. Surg Neurol 21: 23–29
161. Hegedüs K, Molnar P (1983) Primary cerebellar glioblastoma multiforme with an unusual long survival. J Neurosurg 58: 589–592
162. Helle TL, Britt RH, Colgy TU (1984) Primary lymphoma of the central nervous system. J Neurosurg 60: 94–103
163. Heppner GH, Shapiro WR, Rankin JK (1981) Tumor heterogeneity. In: Humphrey GB, et al. (eds) Pediatric oncology, vol 1. Nijhoff, The Hague Boston London
164. Herman MM, Rubinstein LJ (1984) Divergent glial and neuronal differentiation in a cerebellar medulloblastoma in an organ culture system. Acta Neuropathol (Berl) 65: 10–24
165. Herpers MJHM, Budka H (1984) Glial fibrillary acidic protein (GFAP) in oligodendroglial tumors: gliofibrillary oligodendroglioma and transitional oligoastrocytomas as subtypes of oligodendrogliomas. Acta Neuropathol (Berl) 64: 265–272
166. Herpers MJHM, Budka H (1985) Primitive neuroectodermal tumors including the medulloblastoma: glial differentiation signaled by immunoreactivity for GFAP is restricted to the pure desmoplastic medulloblastoma ("arachnoidal sarcoma of the cerebellum"). Clin Neuropathol 4: 12–18
167. Herrick K, Rubinstein LJ (1979) The cytological differentiating potential of pineal parenchymal neoplasms (true pinealomas). Brain 102: 289–320
168. Hinton DR, Halliday WD (1984) Primary rhabdomyosarcoma of the cerebellum. A light, electron microscopic, and immunohistochemical study. J Neuropathol Exp Neurol 43: 439–449
169. Hirakawa K, Suzuki K, Ueda S, Handa J (1986) Fetal origin of medulloblastomas as manifested by growth analyses. Acta Neuropathol (Berl) 70: 227–234

170. Hirano A, Ghatak NR (1974) The fine structure of colloid cysts of the third ventricle. J Neuropathol Exp Neurol 33: 333–341

171. Hirano A, Ghatak NR, Zimmerman HM (1973) The fine structure of ependymoblastoma. J Neuropathol Exp Neurol 32: 144–152

172. Hirano A, Matsui T (1975) Vascular structures in brain tumors. Human Pathol 6: 611–621

173. Hirano T, Aida T, Moriyama M, Asano G, Suzuki I, Yuge K (1985) Primary neuroblastoma of the nasal cavity and review of literature. Acta Pathol Jpn 35: 183–191

174. Hirose T, Sano T, Hizawa K (1986) Ultrastructural localization of S-100 protein in neurofibroma. Acta Neuropathol (Berl) 69: 103–110

175. Ho KL (1984) Ultrastructure of cerebellar capillary hemangioblastoma I. Weibel-Palade bodies and stroma cell histogenesis. J Neuropathol Exp Neurol 43: 592–608

176. Ho KL (1985) Ecchordosis physaliphora and chordoma; a comparative ultrastructural study. Clin Neuropathol 4: 77–86

177. Hoffman HJ, Duffner KP (1985) Extraneural metastases of central nervous system tumors. Cancer 56: 1778–1782

178. Hojo S, Hirano A (1982) Pathology of metastases effecting the Central nervous system. In: Takakura K, Sano K, Hojo S, Hirano A (eds) Metastatic tumors of the central nervous system. Igaku-Shoin, Tokyo New York

179. Horten BC, Rubinstein LJ (1976) Primary cerebral neuroblastoma. Brain 99: 735–756

180. Horten BC, Urich H, Rubinstein LJ, Montague S (1977) Malignant meningiomas and hemangiopericytomas. J Neurol Sci 31: 387–410

181. Horten BC, Urich H, Stefoski D (1979) Meningiomas with conspicuous plasma cell-lymphocytic components. Report of five cases. Cancer 41: 258–264

182. Hoshino T (1981) Cellular aspects of human brain tumors (gliomas). In: Fedoroff, Hertz. (eds) Advances in cellular neurobiology, vol 2. Academic Press, New York, pp 167–209

183. Hoshino T (1984) A commentary on the biology and growth kinetics of low-grade and high-grade gliomas. J Neurosurg 61: 895–600

184. Hoshino T, Kobayashi S, Townswend JJ, Wilson CB (1985) A cell kinetic study on medulloblastoma. Cancer 55: 1711–1713

185. Hoshino T, Wilson CB (1979) Cell kinetic analyses of human malignant brain tumors (gliomas). Cancer 44: 956–962

186. Hoshino T, Wilson CB, Ellis WG (1975) Gemistocytic astrocytes in gliomas: An autoradiographic study. J. Neuropathol Exp Neurol 34: 263–281

187. Hoshino T, Wilson CB, Muraoka I (1979) The stathmokinetic (mitostatic) effect of vincristine and vinblastine in human gliomas. Acta Neuropathol (Berl) 47: 21–25

188. Houtteville JP, Lechavalier B, Lecog PJ, Wesley C, Escourolle R (1976) Pituicytome à cellules granulaires (choristome) de la tige pituitaire Rev Neurol (Paris) 137: 589–604

189. Hulbanni S, Goodma PA (1976) Glioblastoma multiforme with extraneural metastases in absence of previous surgery. Cancer 37: 1577–1583

190. Iglesias JR, Kazner E, Aruffo C, Esparza J (1985) CT diagnosis of brain tumours: Semiautomatical type-specific diagnosis with the help of a personal computer. In: Lamke HU, Rhodes ML, et al. (eds) Computer assisted radiology. Springer, Berlin Heidelberg New York Tokyo, pp 443–448

191. Iglesias JR, Sanchez MJ, Sendra A, Mohnhaupt A (1983) Computer model of archive and diagnosis of brain tumours based on the WHO classification. EDV in Medizin und Biologie 14: 40–44

191 a. Iglesias JR, Pfannkuch F, Aruffo C, Kazner E, Cervos-Navarro J (1986) Histopathologic diagnosis of brain tumors with the help of a computer: Mathematical fundaments and practical application. Acta Neuropathol (Berl) 71: 130–135

192. Ilgren EB, Stiller CA, Hughes HT (1984) Ependymomas: A clinic and pathological study. Part II. Survival features. Clin Neuropathol 3: 122–127
193. Ironside JW, Jefferson AA, Timperley WR (1986) Growth hormone-secreting pituitary adenoma of mixed cell type: a histological, ultrastructural and immunocytochemical study. Clin Neuropathol 5: 28–33
194. Jacob W, Scheida D, Wingert F (eds) (1978) ZNS-Tumor-Histologie-Schlüssel ICD-0-DA. International classification of diseases for oncology. Springer, Berlin Heidelberg New York
195. Jänisch W, Güthert H, Schreiber D (1976) Pathologie der Tumoren des Zentralnervensystems. VEB Fischer, Jena
196. Jänisch W, Fennwarth B, Lagemann G (1967) Zur Epidemiologie der Geschwülste des Zentralnervensystems. Dtsch Z Nervenheilk 191: 80–90
197. Janzer RC, Kleihues P (1985) Primitive neuroectodermal tumor with choroid plexus differentiation. Acta Neuropathol (Berl) 4: 93–98
198. Jellinger K (1972) Cerebral medulloepithelioma. Acta Neuropathol (Berl) 22: 95–101
199. Jellinger K (1973) Primary intracranial germ cell tumors. Acta Neuropathol (Berl) 25 291–306
200. Jellinger K (1977) Zur Histopathologie von Hirntumorrezidiven. Zbl Neurochir 38: 307–324
201. Jellinger K (1977) Human central nervous system lesions following radiation therapy. Zbl Neurochir 38: 199–220
202. Jellinger K (1978) Pathology of brain tumours with relation to prognosis. Zbl Neurochir 39: 285–300
203. Jellinger K (1978) Glioblastoma multiforme. Acta Neurochir (Wien) 42: 5–32
204. Jellinger K (1983) Primäre und sekundäre Lymphome des ZNS. In: Seitz D, Vogl P (Hrsg) Verh Dtsch Ges Neurol, vol 2. Berlin Heidelberg New York, S 14–48
205. Jellinger K (1983): Histologische Klassifikation und therapie-bedingte Veränderungen. In: Krauseneck P, Mertens HG (Hrsg) Therapie maligner Neoplasien des Gehirns. Perimed, Erlangen, S 15–24
206. Jellinger K (1983) Maligne Lymphome und Leukämien im Zentralnervensystem. Verh Dtsch Ges Path 67: 556–573
207. Jellinger K (1984) Häufigkeit und Charakteristik der zerebralen Karzinommetastasen. In: v Heyden HW, Krauseneck P (Hrsg) Hirnmetastasen. Zuckschwerdt, München Bern Wien, S 49–79 (Akt Oncol 13)
208. Jellinger K (1985) Therapy-induced changes in anaplastic gliomas and brain tissue. In: Voth D, Krauseneck P (eds) Chemotherapy of gliomas. De Gruyter, Berlin New York, pp 151–176
209. Jellinger K (1986) Primary non-Hodgkin's lymphoma of the CNS. J Neuro-Oncol (in press)
210. Jellinger K (1986) Present limits of conventional treatment of malignant brain tumors. In: Hatanaka H (ed) Boron neutron capture therapy of tumors. Nishimura-Elsevier, Tokyo Amsterdam New York, pp 309–347
211. Jellinger K, Grisold W, Weiss R (1986) Zytologische Differenzierung von Malignomzellen des Liquor cerebrospinalis. In: Kölmel W, Dommasch H (Hrsg) Liquorzytologie. Edition Medizin, Weinheim S 137–175
212. Jellinger K, Machacek E (1982) Rare intracranial tumours in infancy and childhood. In: Voth D, Gutjahr P, Langmaid C (eds) Tumours of the central nervous system in infancy and childhood. Springer, Berlin Heidelberg New York, pp 44–52
213. Jellinger K, Schuster H (1977) Extraneurale Metastasierung anaplastischer Gliome. Zbl Allg Path Pathol Anat 121: 526–534
214. Jellinger K, Slowik F (1975) Histological subtypes and prognostic problems in meningiomas. J Neurol 208: 279–298

215. Jellinger K, Volc D, Grisold W, Flament H, Weiss R (1983) Kombinationsbehandlung maligner Gliome. Wien Klin Wschr 95: 407–415
216. Jennings MT, Gelman R, Hochberg F (1985) Intracranial germ-cell tumors, Natural history and pathogenesis. J Neurosurg 63: 155–167
217. Johannsson JH, Rekate HL, Roessmann U (1981) Gangliogliomas pathological and clinical correlation. J Neurosurg 54: 58–63
218. Jones TR, Ruoslahti E, Schold SC, Bigner DD (1982) Fibronectin and glial fibrillary acidic protein expression in normal human brain and anaplastic human gliomas. Cancer Res 42: 168–177
219. Jooma R, Torrens MJ, Bradshaw J, Brownell B (1985) Subependymomas of the 4th ventricle. Surgical treatment in 12 cases. J Neurosurg 62: 508–512
220. Jordan RM, Kendall JW, McClung M, Kammer H (1980) Concentration of human choriostic gonadotrophies in the cerebrospinal fluid of patients with germinal cell hypothalamic tumors. Pediatrics 65: 121–124
221. Karch SB, Urich H (1972) Medulloepithelioma: Definition of an entity. J Neuropathol Exp Neurol 31: 27–53
222. Katenkamp D, Stiller D, Holzhausen HJ (1983) Morphologie des Neuroblastoms. Zbl Allg Path Anat 127: 207–218
223. Kawano N, Yada K, Aikara M, Yagishita S (1983) Oligodendroglioma-like (clear cells) in ependymoma. Acta Neuropathol (Berl) 62: 141–144
224. Kay HEM (1983) Immunsuppression and the risk of brain lymphoma. New Engl J Med 308: 109
225. Kazner E, Wende S, Grumme TH, Lanksch W, Stochdorph D (1981) Computertomographie intrakranieller Tumoren aus klinischer Sicht. Springer, Berlin Heidelberg New York
226. Kepes JJ (1982) Meningiomas: biology, pathology and differential diagnosis. Masson, New York
227. Kepes JJ, Rubinstein LJ (1981) Malignant gliomas with heavily lipidized (foamy) tumor cells: a report of three cases and report with immunoperoxidase study. Cancer 47: 2451–2459
228. Kepes JJ, Rubinstein LJ. Laurence F (1979) Pleomorphic xanthoastrocytoma: a distinctive meningocerebral glioma of young subjects with relatively favourable prognosis. Cancer 44: 1839–1852
229. Kernohan JW, Mahon RF, Svien HJ, Adson AW (1949) A simplified classification of the gliomas. Proc Mayo Clin 24: 71–74
230. Kernohan JW, Sayre GP (1952) Tumors of the central nervous system. In: Atlas of tumor pathology, fasc 35. Armed Forces Institute of Pathology, Washington, DC
231. Kersting G (1973) Tissue culture of recurrent gliomas. In: Modern aspects of neurosurgery, vol 3. Excerpta Medica, pp 122–124
232. Kikuchi K, Neuwelt EA (1983) Presence of immunosuppressive factors in brain tumor cyst fluid. J Neurosurg 59: 790–799
233. Klatzo I (1967) Neuropathological aspects of brain edema. J Neuropathol Exp Neurol 26: 1–14
234. Klee GC, Go VLW (1982) Serum tumor markers. Mayo Clin Proc 57: 129–132
235. Kleihues P, Rajewsky MF (1984) Chemical neuro-oncogenesis: Role of structural DNA modification, DNA repair and neural target cell population. Prog Exp Tumor Res 27: 1–16
236. Kleinmann GM, Schoene WC, Walshe TM III, Richardson EP (1978) Malignant transformation of benign cerebellar astrocytoma. J Neurosurg 52: 414–418
237. Klinken LH, Diemer NH, Gjerris F (1984) Automatized image analysis, histologic malignancy grading, and survival in patients with astrocytic gliomas. Clin Neuropathol 3: 107–112

238. Kobayashi H, Sano T, Li K, Hizawa K (1984) Primary Burkitt type lymphoma of the CNS. Acta Neuropathol (Berl) 64: 12–14

239. Koide C, Watanabe Y, Sato K (1980) A pathologic survey of intracranial germinoma and pinealoma in Japan. Cancer 45: 2119–2130

240. Koos WT, Miller M (1971) Intracranial tumors of infants and children. Mosby, St Louis

241. Kopelsen G, Linggood RM, Kleinman GM (1983) Medulloblastoma: the identification of prognostic subgroups and implications for management. Cancer 51: 312–319

241 a. Kornfeld M (1986) Granular cell glioblastoma: A malignant granular cell neoplasm of astrocytic origin. J Neuropathol Exp Neurol 45: 447–462

242. Kovacs K (1984) Light and electron microscopic pathology of pituitary tumors: Immunohistochemistry. In: McBlack P, *et al.* (eds) Secretory tumors of the pituitary gland. Raven Press, New York, pp 365–375

243. Kovacs K, Horvath E, Ryan N (1981) Immunocytology of the human pituitary. In DeLellis RA (ed) Diagnostic immunocytochemistry. Masson, New York, pp 17–35

244. Kretschmer H (1974) Die extrakranielle Metastasierung intrakranieller Geschwülste. Zbl Neurochir 35: 81–112

245. Kristoferitsch W, Jellinger K (1986) Multifocal spinal angiosarcoma after chordotomy. Acta Neurochir (Wien) 79: 145–153

246. Krücke W (1974) Pathologie der peripheren Nerven. In: Olivecrona H, Tönnis W, Krenkel W (Hrsg) Handbuch der Neurochirurgie, vol 7, Teil 3. Springer, Berlin Heidelberg New York

247. Kubota T, Hirano A, Sato K, Yamamota S (1985) The fine structure of astroblastoma. Cancer 55: 745–750

248. Kuhlendahi H, Miltz H, Wüllenweber R (1973) Die Astrozytome des Großhirns. Acta Neurochir (Wien) 29: 151–162

249. Kuhlendahi H, Stochdorph O, Hübner G (1975) Zur nosologischen Stellung und histologischen Herleitung des sogenannten Kleinhirnastrozytoms. Acta Neurochir (Wien) 32: 235–245

250. Kumimashi T, Washiyama K, Saito T (1986) Primary malignant lymphoma of the brain; An immunhistochemical study of 8 cases using a panel of monoclonal and heterologous antibodies. Acta Neuropathol (Berl) 71: 190–196

251. Kuminashi T, Washiyama K, Watanabe K, Sekiguchi K (1985) Glial fibrillary acidic protein in medulloblastomas. Acta Neuropathol (Berl) 67: 1–5

252. Lack EE, Cubilla AL, Woodruff JM (1979) Paragangliomas of the head and neck region: A pathological study of tumors from 71 patients. Human Pathol 10: 191–218

253. Laerum OD, Bjerkvig R, Steinsvag SK, de Ridder L (1984) Invasiveness of primary brain tumors. Cancer Metastasis Rev 3: 223–236

254. Lalitha VS, Rubinstein LJ (1979) Reactive glioma in intracranial sarcoma: a form of mixed sarcoma and glioma (sarcoglioma). Cancer 43: 246–257

254 a. Lang C, Möbius H-J, Schlote W (1986) The growth fraction of human gliomas as determined by the Ki-67 mouse monoclonal anti-proliferation antibody (abstr). 10 Int Congr Neuropath, Stockholm, abst # 869, p 431

254 b. Langford LA (1986) The ultrastructure of the ependymoblastoma Acta Neuropathol (Berl) 71: 136–141

255. Lantos PL (1980) Chemical induction of tumors in the nervous system. In: Thomas DGT, Graham DI (eds) Brain tumours. Butterworth, London Boston Sidney, pp 85–108

256. Lassmann H, Jurecka W, Lassmann G, Gebhart W, Matras H, Watzek G (1977) Different types of benign nerve sheath tumors. Light microscopy, electron microscopy and autoradiography. Virchows Arch (Pathol Anat) 375: 197–210

257. Laurence KM (1979) The biology of choroid plexus papilloma in infancy and childhood. Acta Neurochir (Wien) 50: 79–90
258. Laurent JP, Chang CH, Cohen ME (1985) A classification system for primitive neuroectodermal tumors (medulloblastoma) of the posterior fossa. Cancer 56: 1807–1809
259. Leech RE, Olafson RA (1977) Epithelial cysts of the neuaxis. Arch Path Lab Med 101: 196–202
260. Lennert K (1981) Histopathologie der Non-Hodgkin-Lymphome (nach der Kiel-Klassifikation). Springer, Berlin Heidelberg New York
261. Letendre L, Banks PH, Reese DF, Miller RN, Scanlon PW, Kiely JM (1982) Primary lymphoma of the central nervous system. Cancer 49: 939–943
262. Leviton A (1984) Principles of epidemiology. In: Cohen ME, Duffner PK (eds) Brain tumors in children. Raven Press, New York, pp 22–45
263. Lewy RM, Bredesen DE, Rosenblum ML (1985) Neurological manifestations of the acquired immunodeficiency syndrome (AIDS): Experience at UCSF and review of the literature. J Neurosurg 62: 475–495
264. Lhermitte J, Ducclos (1920) Sur un ganglioneurome diffuse du cortex du cervelet. Bull Ass Franç Étude Cancer 9: 99–106
265. Lilja A, Bergstrom K, Spannare B, Olsson Y (1981) Reliability of computed tomography in assessing histopathological features of malignant supratentorial gliomas. J Comput Assist Tomogr 5: 625–636
266. Limas C, Tio FO (1972) Meningeal melanocytoma ("melanotic meningiomas"). Its melanocytic origin as revealed by electron microscopy. Cancer 30: 1286–1294
267. Liwnicz BH, Rubinstein LJ (1979) The pathways of extraneural spread in metastasizing gliomas. A report of three cases and critical review of the literature. Hum Pathol 10: 453–467
268. Llena JF (1983) Paraganglioma in the cerebrospinal axis. In: Zimmerman HM (ed) Progress in neuropathology, vol 5. Raven Press, New York, pp 261–276
269. Long DM (1970) Capillary ultrastructure and the blood-brain barrier in human malignant brain tumors. J Neurosurg 32: 127–144
269a. Ludwig CL, Smith MT, Godfrey AD, Armbrustmacher VW (1986) A clinico-pathological study of 323 patients with oligodendrogliomas. Ann Neurol 19: 15–21
270. Mackintosh FR, Colby TV, Podolsky WJ, et al. (1982) Central nervous system involvement in non-Hodkin's lymphomas: Analysis of 105 cases. Cancer 49: 586–595
271. Mantravani RVP, Phatak R, Bellur S, Liebner EJ, Haas R (1982) Brain stem gliomas—an autopsy study of 25 cases. Cancer 49: 1294–1296
272. Manual for staging of cancer (1977) American joint committee on cancer staging and end results reporting. Amer J Cancer 10: 167–172
273. Manual of tumor nomenclature and coding (1968) American Cancer Society, New York
274. Marsh WL, Stevenson OR, Long HJM (1983) Primary leptomeningeal presentation of T-cell lymphoma. Cancer 51: 1125–1131
275. Martin H, Voss K, Hufhagl P, Frölkich K (1984) Automated image analysis of gliomas. An objective and reproducible method for tumor grading. Acta Neuropathol (Berl) 63: 160–169
276. Martinez AJ, Lee A, Moossy J, Maroon JC (1980) Pituitary adenomas: Cytopathological and immunohistochemical study. Ann Neurol 7: 24–36
277. Massie AP (1979) A granular pituicytoma of the neurohypophysis. J Path 129: 53–56
278. Masuzawa T, Sato F (1983) The enzyme histochemistry of the choroid plexus. Brain 106: 55–99
279. Matsushima T (1983) Choroid plexus papillomas and human choroid plexus. A light and electron microscopic study. J Neurosurg 59: 1054–1064

280. Mauney M, Sciotto CG (1983) Primary malignant lymphoma of the cauda equina. Amer J Surg Pathol 7: 185–190
281. Maunoury R, Vedrenne C, Constans JP (1975) Infiltrations lymphocytaires dans les gliomes humains. Acta Neuropathol (Berl) 21: 213–222
282. McComb JG (1984) Recent research into the nature of cerebrospinal fluid formation and absorption. J Neurosurg 59: 369–383
283. McComb RD, Bigner DD (1984) The biology of malignant gliomas—a comprehensive survey. Clin Neuropathol 3: 93–106
284. McComb RD, Burger PC (1983) Choroid plexus carcinoma. Report of a case with immunohistochemical and ultrastructural observations. Cancer 51: 470–475
285. McGravan WL, Sypert GW, Ballinger WE (1978) Melanotic schwannoma. Neurosurgery 2: 47–51
286. Mena H, Garcia JH (1978) Primary brain sarcomas. Light and electron microscopic features. Cancer 42: 1298–1307
287. Mendenhall NP, Thar TL, Agee OF, Harty-Golder B, Barringer WE III, Million RR (1983) Primary lymphoma of the central nervous system. Cancer 52: 1993–2000
288. Mennel HD (1985) Classification of supratentorial gliomas. In: Voth D, Krauseneck P (eds) Chemotherapy of gliomas. De Gruyter, Berlin New York, pp 3–17
289. Mennel HD, Invankovis S (1975) Experimentelle Erzeugung von Tumoren des Nervensystems. In: Handbuch der allgemeinen Pathologie, vol 6/7. Springer, Berlin Heidelberg New York , S 33–122
290. Miettinen M, Lehto VL, Dahl D, Virtanen I (1983) Differential diagnosis of chordome, chondroid, and ependymal tumors as aided by anti-intermediate filament antibodies. Amer J Pathol 112: 160–169
291. Milhorat TH, Hammock MK, Davis DA, Fenstermacher JD (1976) Choroid plexus papilloma. II. Ultrastructure. Child's Brain 2: 290–303
292. Miller DC, Goodman ML, Pilch BZ, Shi SR, Dickersin GR, Halpern H, Norris CM Jr (1984) Mixed olfactory neuroblastoma and carcinoma. A report of two cases. Cancer 43: 2019–2028
292 a. Möbius HJ, Lang C, Schlote W (1986) Zellproliferation in Meningeomen und Neurinomen. Quantitative immunhistochemische Untersuchungen (abstr). 31th Ann Meet Germ Assn Neuropath, Mainz, October 8–10, 1986. Zbl allg Path Path Anat (in press)
293. Mohan J, Brownell B, Oppenheimer DR (1976) Malignant spread of haemanglioblastoma: Report of two cases. J Neurol Neurosurg Psychiat 39: 515–525
294. Morant RA, Feigin I, Ransohoff J (1976) Gliosarcoma: a clinical and pathological survey of 24 cases. J Neurosurg 45: 398
295. Morild I, Bang G, Mörk S (1984) Hemangiopericytic meningioma with extracranial spread to multiple sites without intracranial recurrence. Clin Neuropathol 3: 128–130
296. Mørk SJ, Halvorsen TB, Lindegaard KK, Eide GE (1986) Oligodendroglioma. Histologic evaluation and prognosis. J Neuropathol Exp Neurol 45: 65–78
296 a. Mørk SJ, Lindegaard KF, Halvorsen TB, Lehmann EH, et al. (1985) Oligodendroglioma: incidence and biological behavior in a defined population. J Neurosurg 63: 881–889
297. Mørk SJ, Nyland H, Matre R, Ganz J (1985) Characterization of host mononuclear cells in gliomas (abstr). J Neuropathol Exp Neurol 44: 317
298. Mørk SJ, Rubinstein LJ (1985) Ependymoblastoma. A reappraisal of a rate embryonal tumor. Cancer 55: 1536–1542
299. Moss TH (1986) Tumours of the nervous system. An ultrastructural atlas. Springer, London Berlin Heidelberg New York Paris Tokyo
300. Mostofi FK, Sobin LH (1977) Histologic typing of testicular tumours. World Health Organization, Geneva

301. Mukai M (1983) Immunohistochemical localization of S-100 protein and peripheral nerve myelin proteins (P 2 protein, P 0 protein) in granular cell tumors. Am J Pathol 112: 139–146

302. Müller W, Schröder R (1968) Zur Diagnostik der Gliome. Neurochir (Stuttg) 11: 30–36

303. Nagashima M, Yasui K, Kimura J, Washizu M, Yamaguchi K, Mori W (1984) Induction of brain tumors by a newly isolated JC virus. Amer J Pathol 116: 455–463

303 a. Nagashima T, DeArmond SJ, Murovic J, Hoshino T (1985) Immunocytochemical demonstration of S-phase cells by anti-bromo-deoxyuridine monoclonal antibody in human brain tumor tissues. Acta Neuropathol (Berl) 67: 155–159

304. Nakamura V, Becker LE (1983) Subependymal giant cell tumor: Astrocytic or neuronal? Acta Neuropathol (Berl) 60: 287–299

305. Nakamura Y, Becker LE, Mancer K, Gillespie R (1982) Peripheral medulloepithelioma. Acta Neuropathol (Berl) 57: 137–142

306. Nakamura Y, Becker LE, Marks A (1983) Distribution of immunoreactive S-100 protein in pediatric brain tumors. J Neuropathol Exp Neurol 42: 136–145

307. Nakazato Y, Ishizeki J, Takahashi K, Yamaguchi H (1982) Immunohistochemical localization of S-100 protein in granular cell myoblastoma. Cancer 49: 1624–1628

308. Nelson DF, Nelson JS, Davis DR, Chang CH, Griffin TW, Pajak TF (1985) Survival and prognosis of patients with astrocytoma with atypical or anaplastic features. J Neuro-Oncol 3: 99–103

309. Nelson JS, Tsukada Y, Schoenfeld D, Fulling K, Lamarche J, Peress N (1983) Necrosis as a prognostic criterion in malignant supratentorial astrocytic gliomas. Cancer 52: 550–554

310. Netsky MG, Shuangshoti S (1975) The choroid plexus in health and disease. University Press of Virginia, Charlottesville

311. Neumann J (1985) Zur Frage der prognostischen Bedeutung perivasaler Rundzellinfiltrate bei Oligodendrogliomen. Neurochir (Stuttg) 28: 17–19

312. Neumann J, Kimpel I, Gullotta F (1978) Das Oligodendrogliom. Klinischer Verlauf in Bezug zum histologischen Grading. Neurochir (Stuttg) 21: 35–42

313. Neuwelt EA (1984) Therapeutic potential for blood-brain barrier modification in malignant brain tumors. Prag Exp Tumor Res 28: 51–66

314. Neuwelt EA, Kikuchi K, Hill S, Lipsky P, Frenkel EP (1983) Immune response in patients with brain tumors. Cancer 51: 248–255

315. Neuwelt EY, Smith RG (1979) Presence of lymphocysts surface markers on "small cells" in a pineal germinoma. Ann Neurol 6: 133–136

316. Norris HJ, Liskin JJ, Benson WL (1976) Immature malignant teratoma of the ovary. A clinical and pathologic study. Cancer 37: 2359–2372

317. Nunnery EW, Kahn LB, Reddick RL, Lipper S (1981) Hemangiopericytoma. A light microscopic and ultrastructural study. Cancer 47: 906–914

318. Oehmichen M (1971) Extracerebrale Gliome im Gesichtsbereich. Acta Neuropathol (Berl) 17: 321–330

319. Ojeda VJ (1982) Neoplastic angioendotheliosis of the spinal cord. Acta Neuropathol (Berl) 62: 164–166

320. Ojeda VJ, Stokes BAR, Lee MA, Thomas GW, et al. (1986) Primary cerebral neuroblastomas. A clinico-pathological study of one adolescent and five adult patients. Pathology 18: 41–49

321. Okeda R, Mochizuki T, Terao E, Matsutani M (1980) The origin of intracranial fibrosarcoma. Acta Neuropathol (Berl) 52: 223–230

322. Okeda R, Song SJ, Nakajima T, Matsutani M (1984) Pineocytoma. Observation of an autopsy cases by electron microscopy and cell markers. Acta Pathol Jpn 34: 911–918

323. Olson JJ, Menezes AH, Godersky JC, Laborsky JM, Hart M (1985) Primary intracranial rhabdomyosarcoma. Neurosurgery 17: 25–34

324. Packer JR, Siegel KR, Sutton LN, Litmann P, Bruce DA, Schut L (1985) Lepto-meningeal dissemination of primary central nervous system tumors of childhood. Ann Neurol 18: 217–221

325. Packer RJ, Sutton LN, Rorke LB, Zimmermann RA, Littman P, *et al.* (1985) Oligodendroglioma of the posterior fossa in childhood. Cancer 56: 195–199

326. Packer RJ, Sutton LN, Rosenstock JG, Rorke, *et al.* (1984) Pineal region tumors of childhood. Pediatrics 74: 97–102

327. Page RB, Plourde PV, Coldwell D, Heald JI, Weinstein J (1983) Intrasellar mixed germ-cell tumor. J Neurosurg 58: 766–770

328. Palma L, di Lorenzo N, Guidetti B (1978) Lymphocytic infiltrates in primary glioblastomas and redivius gliomas: Incidence, fate, and relevance to prognosis in 228 operated cases. J Neurosurg 49: 854–861

329. Palma L, Russo A, Mercuri S (1983) Cystic cerebral astrocytoma in infancy and childhood. Long term results. Child's Brain 10: 79–91

330. Palmer JO, Kasselberg AG, Netsky MG (1981) Differentiation of medulloblastoma. J Neurosurg 55: 161–169

331. Pasquier B, Couderc P, Pasquier D, Panh MH, N'Golet A (1978) Sarcoma arising in oligodendroglioma of the brain: A case with intramedullary and subarachnoid spinal metastases. Cancer 42: 2753–2758

332. Pasquier B, Kojder I, Labat F, Keddar E, Pasquier D, *et al.* (1985) Pleomorphic xanthoastrocytoma of young subjects. A report of 2 cases with discordant course and review of literature. Ann Pathol (Paris) 5: 29–44

333. Pasquier B, Lachard A, Pasquier D, Couderc P, Delpech B, Courel MN (1983) Protéine gliofibrillaire acide (GFA) et tumeurs nerveuses centrales. Étude immunohisto-chimique d'une série de 107 cas. Ann Pathol (Paris) 3: 203–211

334. Pasquier BV, Pasquier D, Colet A, Panh MH, Couderc P (1980) Extraneural metastases of astrocytomas and glioblastomas: Clinicopathological study of two cases and review of literature. Cancer 45: 112–125

335. Payan MJ, Gambarelli D, Keller P, Lacherd A, Garcin M, Vigouroux C, Toga M (1986) Melanotic neurofibroma. A case report with ultrastructural study. Acta Neuropathol (Berl) 148–152

336. Payne DG, Simpson WJ, Keen C, Plattis ME (1982) Malignant astrocytoma: Hyperfractionated and standard radiotherapy with chemotherapy in a randomized prospective clinical trial. Cancer 50: 2301–2306

337. Pearl GS, Chan WC, Bakay RAE, Wood JH (1985) Primary lymphoma of the central nervous system diagnosed by computerized scan-directed needle-biopsy with a frozen section immunoperoxidase techniques. Neurosurgery 16: 1–4

338. Pearl GS, Takei Y (1981) Cerebellar "neuroblastoma". Nosology as it relates to medulloblastoma. Cancer 47: 772–779

339. Pfeifer J (1984) Tumoren des Nervensystems. In: Remmele W (Hrsg) Pathologie, vol 4. Springer, Berlin Heidelberg New York Tokyo, S 247–287

340. Perentes E, Rubinstein LJ (1986) Immunohistochemical recognition of human neuroepithelial tumors by anti-Leu 7 (HNK-1) monoclonal antibody. Acta Neuropathol (Berl) 69: 227–233

341. Phillips JP, Eremin O, Anderson JR (1982) Lymphoreticular infiltrates in human brain tumors and in normal brain. Brit J Cancer 45: 61–69

342. Pitkethly DT, Hardman JM, Kempe LG, Earle KM (1970) Angioblastic meningiomas: Clinicopathologic study of 81 cases. J Neurosurg 32: 539–544

343. Pitts OM, Powers JM, Hoffman PM (1983) Vascular neoplasms induced in rodent central nervous system by murine sarcoma viruses. Lab Invest 49: 171–182

344. Pollak A, Friede RL (1977) Fine structure of medulloepithelioma. Neuropathol Exp Neurol 36: 712–725

345. Poon TP, Hirano A, Zimmerman H (1971) Electron microscopic atlas of brain tumors. Grune & Stratton, New York

346. Porwit-Ksiazek A, Christensson B, Lindemalm C, Mellstedt M, et al. (1983) Characterization of malignant and non-neoplastic cell phenotypes in highly malignant non-Hodgkin's lymphomas. Int J Cancer 32: 667–674

347. Priest J, Dehner LP, Sung JH, Nesbit ME (1981) Primitive neuroectodermal tumors (embryonal gliomas) of childhood. In: Humphrey GB, et al. (eds) Pediatric oncology, vol I. Nijhoff, The Hague Boston London, pp 247–264

348. Pulciani S, Santos E, Lauver AF, Long LK, Barbacid M (1982) Oncogenesis in human tumor cell lines: molecular cloning of a transforming gene from human blander carcinoma cells. Proc Natl Acad Sci USA 79: 2846–2849

349. Rea GL, Akerson RD, Rockswald GL, Smith SA (1983) Subependymoma 2½ years old boy. J Neurosurg 59: 1088–1091

350. Reinhardt V, Nahser NCH (1984) Gliofibroma originating from temporoparietal hamartoma-like lesions. Clin Neuropathol 3: 131–138

351. Richman AV, Balis GA, Moniscalco JE (1980) Primary intracerebral tumor with mixed chondrosarcoma and glioblastoma: Gliosarcoma or sarcoglioma? J Neuropathol Exp Neurol 39: 329–335

352. Ridley A, Cavanagh JB (1971) Lymphocytic infiltration in gliomas: Evidence of possible host resistance. Brain 94: 117–124

353. Ringertz N (1950) Grading of gliomas. Acta Path Microbiol Scand 27: 54–64

354. Robertson AJ, Anderson JM, Brown RA, Slidders W, Beck JS (1978) Grading of astrocytomas using a Quantimet 720 image-analyse computer. J Neurol Neurosurg Psychiat 31: 469–474

355. Roessmann U, Velasco ME, Gambetti P, Autilio-Gambetti L (1983) Neuronal and astrocytic differentiation in human neuroepithelial neoplasm. An immunohistochemical study. J Neuropathol Exp Neurol 42: 113–121

355a. Roggendorf W, Schuster Th, Peiffer J (1986) Immunhistologische Untersuchungen zum Proliferationsverhalten nicht glialer Hirntumoren (abstr). 31th Ann Meet Germ Assn Neuropath, Mainz, October 8–10, 1986. Zbl Allg Path Path Anat (in press)

356. Rorke LB (1983) The cerebellar medulloblastoma and its relationship to primitive neuroectodermal tumors. J Neuropathol Exp Neurol 42: 1–15

357. Rorke LB, Gilles F, Davis RL, Becker LE (1985) Revision of the World Health Organization Classification of brain tumors for childhood brain tumors. Cancer 56: 1869–1985

358. Rosenblum ML, Gerosa MA, Bodell WJ, Talcott RL (1984) Tumor cell resistance. Prog exp Tumor Res 27: 191–214

359. Rosenblum ML, Wilson CB (eds) (1984) Brain tumor biology. Karger, Basel (Prog exp tumor res, vol 27)

359a. Royds JA, Ironside W, Taylor CB, Graham DI, Timperley WR (1986) An immunohistochemical study of glial and neuronal markers in primary neoplasms of the central nervous system. Acta Neuropathol (Berl) 70: 320–326

360. Rubinstein LJ (1970) The definition of ependymoblastoma. Arch Path (Chic) 90: 35–45

361. Rubinstein LJ (1974) The cerebellar medulloblastoma. Its origin, differentiation, morphological variants, and biological behavior. In: Vinken PJ, Bruyn GW (eds) Handbook of clinical neurology, vol 18. North-Holland, Amsterdam, pp 167–193

362. Rubinstein LJ (1979) Tumors of the central nervous system. Atlas of tumor pathology, 2nd series, fasc 6. Armed Forces Institute of Pathology, Washington

363. Rubinstein LJ (1981) Cytogenesis and differentiation of pineal neoplasms. Human Pathol 12: 441–448

364. Rubinstein LJ (1985) Embryonal central neuroepithelial tumors and their differentiating potential. A cytogenetic view of a complex neurooncological problem. J Neurosurg 62: 795–805
365. Rubinstein LJ, Brucher JM (1981) Focal ependymal differentiation in choroid plexus papilloma. Acta Neuropathol (Berl) 53: 29–33
366. Rubinstein LJ, Herman MM (1979) Recent advances in human brain neurooncology. In: Smith WT, Cavanagh JB (eds) Recent advances in neuropathology, vol 1. Churchill-Livingstone, Edinburgh London New York, pp 179–223
367. Rubinstein LJ, Herman MM, Hanbery (1974) The relationship between differentiating medulloblastoma and dedifferentiating diffuse cerebellar astrocytoma. Cancer 33: 675–690
368. Rubinstein LJ, Herman MM, Vanden Berg SR (1984) Differentiation and anaplasia in central neuroepithelial tumors. Prog Exp Tumor Res 27: 32–48
369. Rubinstein LJ, Northfield DWC (1964) The medulloblastoma and the so-called arachnoidal cerebellar sarcoma. A critical reexamination of a nosological problem. Brain 87: 379–412
370. Russell DS, Rubinstein LJ, (1977): Pathology of tumours of the nervous system, 4th edn. Arnold, London
371. Saeger W (1981) Die Hypophyse. In: Doerr W, Uehlinger E, Seifert G (Hrsg) Spezielle pathologische Anatomie. Springer, Berlin Heidelberg New York
372. Sakaki S, Mori Y, Motozaki T, Nakagawa K, Matsuoka K (1981) A cerebral neuroblastoma with extracranial metastases. Surg Neurol 16: 53–59
373. Salacar OM (1983) A better understanding of CSF seeding and a brighter outlook of postoperatively irradiated patients with ependymomas. Int J Rad Oncol Biol Phys 9: 1231–1234
374. Salcman M (1980) Survival in glioblastoma: Historical perspective. Neurosurg 7: 435–439
375. Schaumburg HH, Plack CR, Adams RD (1972) The reticulum cell sarcoma-microglioma group of brain tumors. Brain 95: 199–212
376. Scheithauer BW (1978) Symptomatic subependymoma. J Neurosurg 49: 689–696
377. Scheithauer BW, Kovacs K, Randall RY, Horvath E, Okazaki H, Laws ER (1983) Hypothalamic neural hamartoma and adenohypophyseal neuronal choristoma: Their association with growth hormone adenoma of the pituitary gland. J Neuropathol Exp Neurol 42: 648–663
378. Scheithauer BW, Rubinstein W (1978) Meningeal and mesenchymal chondrosarcoma: Report of eight cases with review of the literature. Cancer 42: 2744–2752
379. Scheithauer BW, Rubinstein LJ (1979) Cerebral medulloepithelioma. Childs Brain 5: 62–71
380. Schelper RL, Kagan-Hallet KS, Huntington HW (1986) Brainstem subarachnoid respiratory epithelial cysts: Report of two cases and review of the literature. Hum Pathol 17: 417–422
381. Scherer JH (1940) The forms of growth in gliomas and their practical significance. Brain 63: 1–35
382. Schiffer D, Cavicchioli D, Giordana MT, Palmucci L, Piazza A (1979) Analysis of some factors affecting survival in malignant gliomas. Tumori 65: 119–125
383. Schiffer D, Giordana MT, Mauro A, Migheli A (1984) GFAP, F VIII/RAg, laminin, in gliosarcomas: an immunohistochemical study. Acta Neuropathol (Berl) 63: 108–116
384. Schiffer D, Giordana MT, Paoletti P, Soffietti R, Rarenzi L (1980) Pathology of human malignant gliomas after radiation and chemotherapy Acta Neurochir (Wien) 53: 205–216

385. Schiffer D, Giordana MT, Soffietti R, Sciolla R, Sannazzari GL, Vasario E (1984) Effects of radiotherapy on the astrocytomatous areas of malignant gliomas. J Neuro-Oncol 2: 167–175
386. Schindler E (1985) Die Tumoren der Pinealisregion. Springer, Berlin Heidelberg New York
387. Schmitt HP (1983) Rapid anaplastic transformation in gliomas of adulthood. "Selection" in neuro-oncogenesis. Path Res Pract 176: 313–323
388. Schoenberg BS (1983) The epidemiology of central nervous system tumors. In: Walker EA (ed) Oncology of the nervous system. Nijhoff, Boston Hague, pp 1–29
389. Schold SC Jr, Bullard DR, Bigner SH, Jones TR, Bigner DD (1983) Growth, morphology, and serial transplantation of anaplastic human gliomas in athymic mice. J Neuro-Oncol 1: 5–14
390. Schreiber D, Warzok R, Güthert H, Schneier J (1980) Tumoren des ZNS im Biopsie- und Autopsiegut. 4. Glioblastoma. Zbl Allg Pathol Pathol Anat 124: 416–423
391. Schröder R, Müller N, Bonis G, Vorreith M (1970) Statistische Beiträge zum Grading der Gliome. III. Astrozytome und Oligodendrogliome. Acta Neurochir (Wien) 18: 186–200
392. Schuier F (1976) Is there an anaplastic oligodendroglioma? J Neurol 213: 263–267
393. Scully RE (1979) Tumors of the ovary and maldeveloped gonads. Atlas of Tumor Pathology. Fascicle 16, series 2. Armed Forces Institute of Pathology, Washington, DC
394. Seiler RW (1982) Die undifferenzierten Astrozytome des Großhirns. Springer, Berlin Heidelberg New York
395. Seyama S, Ohta M, Nishio S, Matsushima T, Kitamura K (1982) Cells constitutin cerebellar hemangioblastomas. Ultrastructural study. Acta Pathol Jpn 32: 399–413
396. Shapiro WR, Byrne TH (1983) Chemotherapy of brain tumors basic concepts. In: Walker MD (ed) Oncology of the nervous system. Nijhoff, Boston Hague, pp 223–245
397. Shapiro JR, Shapiro WR (1984) Clonal tumor cell heterogeneity. Prog Exp Tumor Res 27: 49–66
398. Sheline GE (1983) Radiotherapy of adult primary cerebral neoplasm. In: Walker MD (ed) Oncology of the nervous system. Nijhoff, Boston Hague, pp 223–245
399. Sheline GE (1986) Normal tissue tolerance and radiation therapy of gliomas of the adult brain. In: Bleehan NM (ed) Tumours of the brain. Springer, Berlin Heidelberg New York Tokyo
400. Shimada H (1982) Transmission and scanning electron microscopic studies on the tumors of neuroblastoma group. Acta Pathol Jpn 32: 415–426
401. Shimura T, Hirano A, Llena JF (1985) Ultrastructure of cerebellar hemangioblastoma. Some new observations on the stromal cell. Acta Neuropathol (Berl) 67: 6–12
402. Shokry A, Janzer RC, von Hochstetter AR, Yaşargil MG, Hedinger C (1985) Primary intracranial germ-cell tumors. J Neurosurg 62: 826–830
403. Suangshoti S, O'Charoen (1983) Cerebellar neoplasm of mixed mesenchymal and neuroepithelial origin. J Neurosurg 59: 337–343
404. Slaughter JC, Dardman JM, Kempe LG, Earle KM (1969) Neurocutaneous melanosis and leptomeningeal melanomatosis in children. Arch Pathol 88: 298–304
405. Slowik F, Jellinger K, Gaszó L, Fischer J (1985) Gliosarcomas. Histological, immunohistochemical, ultrastructural, and tissue culture studies. Acta Neuropathol (Berl) 67: 201–210
406. Smith DA, Lantos PL (1985) Immunocytochemistry of cerebellar astrocytomas: with a special note on Rosenthal fibres. Acta Neuropathol (Berl) 66: 155–159
407. Smith MT, Armbrustmacher VM, Violett TW (1981) Diffuse meningeal rhabdomyosarcoma. Cancer 47: 2081–1086
408. Smith MT, Ludwig CL, Godfrev AD, Armbrustmacher VW (1983) Grading of oligodendrogliomas. Cancer 52: 2107–2144

409. Smith TW, Bhawan J (1980) Tactile-like structures in neurofibromas. An ultra-structural study. Acta Neuropathol (Berl) 50: 233–236
410. Smith TW, Davidson RI (1984) Medulloblastoma. A histologic, immunohistochemical and ultrastructural study. Cancer 54: 323–332
411. Snider WD, Simpson DM, Nielsen S, Gold JWM, Metroka CR, Posner JB (1983) Neurological complications of acquired immune deficiency syndrome: Analysis of 50 patients. Ann Neurol 14: 403–418
412. Sobel HJ, Markquet E, Schwarz R (1973) Is schwannoma related to granular cell myoblastoma? Arch Pathol (Chic) 95: 396–401
413. Sobel RA, Trice JE, Nielson SL, Ellis WG (1981) Pineoblastoma with ganglionic and glial differentiation. Acta Neuropathol (Berl) 55: 243–246
414. Sommeland PR, Scheithauer BW, Onofrio BM (1985) Myxopapillary ependymoma. A clinico-pathologic and immunocytochemical study of 77 cases. Cancer 56: 883–893
415. Sonoda H, Matsukado Y, Uemura S, Kaku M (1984) Tissue polypeptide antigen as a tumor marker of brain tumors. Neurol Med Chir 24: 655–662
416. Spaar FW, Blech M, Ahyal A (1986) DNA-flow fluorescence-cytometry of ependy-momas. Acta Neuropathol (Berl) 69: 153–160
417. Spence AM, Rubinstein LJ, Conley FK, Herman MM (1976) Studies on experimental malignant nerve sheath tumors maintained in tissue and organ culture systems. Acta Neuropathol (Berl) 35: 27–45
418. Spencer GD, Weiss RB, van Eys J, Cohen P, Edwards B (1984) Medulloblastoma metastatic to the marrow. J Neuro-Oncol 2: 223–235
419. Stahlberger R, Friede RL (1977) Fine structure of medullomyoblastoma. Acta Neuropathol (Berl) 37: 43–48
420. Stavrou D, Anzil AP, Weidenbach W, Rodt H (1977) Immunofluorescence study of lymphocytic infiltration in gliomas. J Neurol Sci 33: 275–282
421. Steel GG (1980) Growth kinetics of brain tumors. In: Thomas DGT, Graham DI (eds) Brain tumours. Butterworth, London Boston, pp 10–20
422. Stefanko SZ, Manschot WA (1979) Pinealoblastoma with retinoblastomatous dif-ferentiation. Brain 102: 321–332
423. Stefanko SZ, Talerman A, Mackay WM, Vuzevski VD (1979) Infundibular germi-noma. Acta Neurochir (Wien) 50: 71–78
424. Stefansson K, Wollmann R, Jerkovic M (1982) S-100 protein in soft-tissue tumors derived from Schwann cells and melanocytes. Am J Pathol 106: 261–268
425. Stewart PA, Hayakawa K, Hayakawa E, Farrell CL, de l'Maest RF (1985) A quantitative study of blood-brain barrier permeability. Ultrastructure in a new rat glioma model. Acta Neuropathol (Berl) 67: 96–102
426. Stochdorph O (1979) How to handle brain tumor classification. Adv Neurosurg 7: 381–384
427. Stout AP, Murray MR (1942) Neuroepithelioma of the radial nerve with a study of its behaviour in vitro. Rev Can Biol 1: 651–659
428. Sung JH, Mastri AR, Segal EL (1973) Melanotic medulloblastoma of the cerebellum. J Neuropathol Exp Neurol 32: 437–445
429. Sunohara N, Mukoyama M, Satoyoshi E (1984) Neoplastic angioendotheliosis of the central nervous system. J Neurol 231: 14–19
430. Sweet DL, Hendler FH, Hanlon K, Hekmatpanah J, et al. (1979) Treatment of grade III and IV astrocytomas with BCNU alone and in combination with VM-26 following surgery and radiation therapy. Cancer Treatm Rep 63: 1707–1711
431. Systematized nomenclature of medicine (1976) College of the American Pathologists, Chicago

432. Takeda N, Tanaka R, Yamazaki K (1980) Correlation of computed tomography with post-mortem histopathology of cerebral malignant glioma. Neuro Med Chir (Tokyo) 20: 603–611

433. Takeuchi J, Barnard RO (1976) Perivascular cuffing in astrocytomas. Acta Neuropathol (Berl) 35: 265–271

434. Takeuchi J, Handa H (1979) Spontaneous extracranial metastases of cerebral neuroblastoma. Surg Neurol 12: 337–339

435. Takeuchi K, Hoshino K (1977) Statistical analysis of factors affecting survival after glioblastomas multiforme. Acta Neurochir (Wien) 37: 57–73

436. Taratuto AL, Molina HA, Diez B, Zuccaro G, Monges J (1985) Primary rhabdomyosarcoma of brain and cerebellum. Report of four cases in infants: An immunohistochemical study. Acta Neuropathol (Berl) 66: 98–104

437. Taratuto M, Molina H, Menges J (1983) Choroid plexus tumors in infancy and childhood. Focal ependymal differentiation. Acta Neuropath (Berl) 59: 304–308

438. Tavcar D, Robboy SJ, Chapmann P (1980) Endodermal sinus tumor of the pineal region. Cancer 45: 2646–2651

439. Taylor CR, Russell R, Lukes RJ, Davis RL (1978) An immunohistochemical study of immunoglobulin content of primary central nervous system lymphomas. Cancer 34: 1293–1302

440. Thomas DGT, Graham DT (eds) (1980) Brain tumours: Scientific basis, clinical investigation and current therapy. Butterworth, London Boston

441. Tiberin P, Maor E, Zaizov R, Cohen Ij, et al. (1984) Brain sarcomas of meningeal origin after cranial irradiation in childhood acute lymphocytic leukemia. J Neurosurg 61: 772–776

442. Torres LF, Grant N, Harding BN, Scaravelli F (1985) Intracerebral neuroblastoma: Report of a case with neuronal maturation and long survival. Acta Neuropathol (Berl) 68: 110–114

443. Touraine A (1949) Les mélanoses neuro-cutanées. Ann Dermatol Venerol 9: 489–524

443 a. Townsend JJ, Seaman JP (1986) Central neurocytoma. A rare benign intraventricular tumor. Acta Neuropathol (Berl) 71: 167–170

444. Trojanowski JQ, Lee V, Pillsbury N, Lee S (1982) Neuronal origin of human esthesioneuroblastoma demonstrated with anti-neurofilament monoclonal antibodies. New Engl J Med 307: 159–161

445. Trojanowski JQ, Lee VMY, Schlaepfer WW (1984) An immunohistochemical study of human central and peripheral nervous system tumors, using monoclonal antibodies against neurofilaments and glial filaments. Hum Pathol 15: 248–257

446. Trojanowsky JQ, Tascos NA, Rorke LB (1982) Malignant pineocytoma with prominent papillary features. Cancer 50: 1789–1793

447. Tankos M, Linnolla RI, Chandra RS, Triche TJ (1984) Neuron-specific enolase in the diagnosis of neuroblastoma and other small, round-cell tumors in children. Hum Pathol 15: 575–584

448. Ueki K, Tanaka R (1980) Treatment and prognosis of pineal tumors. Experience of 110 cases. Neurol Med Chir (Tokyo) 20: 1–26

449. Underwood JCE (1974) Lymphoreticular infiltration in human tumours: Prognostic and biological implications. Brit J Cancer 30: 538–548

450. Velasco ME, Dahl B, Roessmann U, Gambetti P (1980) Immunohistochemical localization of glial fibrillary acidic protein in human glial neoplasms. Cancer 45: 484–494

451. Vick NA, Khandekar JD, Bigner DD (1977) Chemotherapy of brain tumors: The "blood-brain barrier" is not a factor. Arch Neurol (Chic) 34: 523–526

452. Vinores SA, Bonnin JM, Rubinstein LJ, Marangos PJ (1984) Immunohistochemical demonstration of neuron-specific enolase in neoplasms of the CNS and other tissues. Arch Pathol Lab Med 108: 536–540

453. Von Hanwehr RL, Hofman FM, Taylor CR, Apuzzo MLJ (1984) Mononuclear lymphoid populations infiltrating the microenvironment or primary CNS tumors. Characterization of cell subsets with monoclonals antibodies. J Neurosurg 60: 1138–1147

454. Voth D, Krauseneck P (eds) (1985) Chemotherapy of gliomas. De Gruyter, Berlin New York

455. Vuia O (1980) Embryonic carcinosarcoma (mixed tumor) of the pineal gland. Neurochir (Stuttg) 23: 47–54

456. Waggener JD, Beggs JL (1966) Vasculature of neural neoplasms. Adv Neurol 15: 27–49

457. Walker EA (ed) (1983) Oncology of the nervous system. Nijhoff, Boston Hague Sidney

458. Walter GF, Brucher JM (1979) Ultrastructural study of medullomyoblastoms. Acta Neuropathol (Berl) 48: 211–214

459. Walker EA, Robins M, Weinfeld FD (1985) Epidemiology of brain tumors: The national survey of intracranial neoplasms. Neurology 35: 219–226

460. Waltz TA, Brownell BL (1966) Sarcoma: A possible late result of effective radiation therapy for pituitary adenoma. J Neurosurg 24: 901–907

461. Warren WH, Lee I, Gould VE, Memoli VA, Wellington J (1985) Paragangliomas of the head and neck: Ultrastructural and immunohistochemical studies. Ultrastruct Pathol 8: 333–344

462. Warzok R, Güthert H (1978) Die Tumoren des Zentralnervensystems im Biopsie- und Autopsiegut. Zbl All Path Path Anat 122: 462–473

463. Warzok R, Jänisch W, Lang C (1983) Morphology and biology of cerebellar neuroblastomas. J Neuro-Oncol 1: 373–379

464. Warzok B, Jänisch W, Schreiber D (1982) Das Gliomedullomyoblastom. Zbl Allg Path Path Anat 126: 5–15

465. Watabe K, Kumanishi T, Ikuta F, Oyake Y (1983) Tactile-like corpuscles in neurofibromas: Immunohistochemical demonstration of S-100 protein. Acta Neuropathol (Berl) 61: 173–177

466. Webb JN (1982) The ultrastructure of melanotic schwannoma of the skin. J Pathol 137: 25–36

467. Weiser G (1978) Neurofibrom und Perineuralzelle. Elektronenoptische Untersuchung an neun Neurofibromen. Virchows Arch Pathol Anat 375: 73–81

468. Weiss SW, Langloss JM, Enzinger FM (1983) Value of S-100 protein in the diagnosis of soft tissue with particular reference to benign and malignant Schwann cell tumors. Lab Invest 49: 299–308

469. Weldon-Linne GM, Victor TA, Groothuis DR, Vick NA (1983) Pleomorphic xanthoastrocytoma. Ultrastructural and immunohistochemical study of a case with a rapidly fatal outcome following surgery. Cancer 52: 2055–2063

470. Weller RO (1986) The immunopathology of brain tumours. In: Bleehan NM (ed) Tumours of the brain. Springer, Berlin Heidelberg New York Tokyo, pp 19–33

471 a. Weller RO, Foy M, Cox S (1977) The development and ultrastructure of the microvasculature in malignant gliomas. Neuropathol Appl Neurobiol 397–322

471 b. West CR, Bruce DA, Duffner PK (1985) Ependymomas. Factors in clinical and diagnostic staging. Cancer 56: 1812–1816

472. Wick MR, Mills SE, Scheithauer BW, Cooper PH, Davitz MA, Parkinson K (1986) Reassessment of malignant "angioendotheliomatosis". Evidence in favor of its reclassification as "intravascular lymphomatosis". Amer J Surg Pathol 10: 112–123

473. Wikstrand CJ, Graham FC, McComb RD, Bigner DD (1985) Antigenic heterogeneity of human anaplastic gliomas and gliomaderived cell lines defined by monoclonal antibodies. J Neuropathol Exp Neurol 44: 229–241
474. Willis K, du Boulay GH, Teather B (1981) Initial findings in the computer-aided diagnosis of cerebral tumors using CT scan results. Brit J Radiol 54: 948–952
475. Willis RA (1967) Pathology of Tumours, 3rd edn. Butterworth, London
476. Willson N, Duffy PE (1974) Morphologic changes associated with combined BCNU and radiation therapy in glioblastoma multiforme. Neurology (Minneap) 24: 465–471
477. Wöber G, Jellinger K (1977) Diagnostischer Wert der Abtupfzytologie in der Neurochirurgie. Wien Klin Wsch 89: 122–126
478. Wold LE, Laws ER Jr (1983) Cranial chordomas in children and young adults. J Neurosurg 59: 1043–1047
479. Wong SW, Ducker TB, Powers JM (1979) Fulminating parapontine epidermoid carcinoma in a four-year-old boy. Cancer 37: 1525–1531
480. Wood G, Morantz RA (1979) Immunohistologic evaluation of the lymphoreticular infiltrate in human central nervous system tumours. J Nat Cancer Inst 62: 485–491
481. Woodruff JM, Horten BC, Erlandson RA (1983) Pathology of peripheral nerves and paragangliomas. In: Silverberg SG (ed) Principles and practice of surgical pathology. Wiley, New York, pp 1503–1520
482. World Health Organization (1977): Manual of the international statistical classification of diseases, injuries, and causes of death, 1975 revision. World Health Organization, Geneva
483. Yagashita S, Itoh Y, Chiba Y, Fujino H (1979) Primary rhabdomyosarcoma of the cerebrum. Acta Neuropathol (Berl) 45: 111–115
484. Yagashita S, Itoh Y, Chiba Y, Kuwano N (1982) Investigations on cerebellar "neuroblastoma" group. Acta Neuropathol (Berl) 56: 22–28
485. Yagishita S, Itah Y, Chiba Y, Yamashita T, Nakazima F, Kuwabara T (1980) Cerebellar neuroblastoma: A light and ultrastructural study. Acta Neuropathol (Berl) 50: 139–142
486. Yamamura Y, Akamizu H, Hirata T, Kito S, Hamada T (1983) Malignant lymphoma presenting with neoplastic angioendotheliosis of the central nervous system. Clin Neuropathol 2: 62–68
487. Yasuda K, Alderson T, Phillips J, Sikora K (1983) Detection of lymphocytes in malignant gliomas by monoclonal antibodies. J Neurol Neurosurg Psychiat 46: 734–737
488. Yates AJ, Decker LE, Sachs LA (1979) Brain tumors in childhood. Child's Brain 5: 31–39
489. Yung WA, Horten BC, Shapiro WR (1980) Meningeal gliomatosis. A review of 12 cases. Ann Neurol 8: 605–608
490. Zänker KS, Lederer T, Trappe A, Blümel G (1985) Escape phenomena of glioma cells to allogenic lymphocytes and rhythmically altered protein synthesis encoded by signal transfer. In: Voth D, Krauseneck P (eds) Chemotherapy of gliomas. De Gruyter, Berlin New York, pp 71–76
491. Zänker KS, Trappe A, Blümel G (1982) In-vitro resistance of cloned human glioma cells to natural killer activity of allogeneic peripheral lymphocytes. Brit J Cancer 46: 617–624
492. Zeller WJ, Ivankovic S, Habs M, Schmah D (1982) Experimental chemical productions of brain tumors. Amer NY Acad Sci 381: 250–263
493. Zimm S, Wampler GI, Stablein D (1981) Intracerebral metastases in solid tumor patients. Cancer 48: 384–394
494. Zimmerman HM (1969) Brain tumors: Their incidence and classification in man and their experimental reproduction. Ann New York Acad Sci 159: 337–359

495. Zülch KJ (1975) Atlas of gross neurosurgical pathology. Springer, Berlin Heidelberg New York
496. Zülch KJ (1979) Histological typing of tumours of the central nervous system. World Health Organization, Geneva (Intern histol classification of tumours, no 21)
497. Zülch KJ (1980) Principles of the New World Health Organization (WHO) classification of brain tumors. Neuroradiol 19: 59–66
498. Zülch KJ (1986) Brain tumors: their biology and pathology, 3rd edn. Springer, New York
499. Zülch KJ, Wechsler W (1968) Pathology and classification of gliomas. Basel New York (Progr neurol surg, vol 2, pp 1–84)
500. Zu Rhein GM, Varakis JN (1979) Prenatal induction of medulloblastomas in syrian golden hamsters by an human polyoma virus (JC). Natl Cancer Inst Monogr 51: 205–208

Author's address: Prof. Dr. K. Jellinger, Ludwig Boltzmann-Institut für Klinische Neurobiologie, Krankenhaus Wien—Lainz, Wolkersbergenstrasse 1, A-1130 Wien, Austria.

2

Neurosurgery of Malignant Brain Tumors

D. Voth

Department of Neurosurgery, University of Mainz School of Medicine, Mainz, Federal Republic of Germany

I. Introduction and Historical Retrospect

To Virchow[167] belongs the credit of identifying as tumors, tissue changes already described in the brain, and at the same time to have published an account of the characteristics of the gliomas and the first classification of the various types. It was only the knowledge of the neoplastic nature of the gliomas[127] which made possible surgical action with the aim of extirpation (Fig. 1), when at the end of the 19th century the stormy development of surgery in other parts of the body was being practised successfully[162]. The first reports about the removal of an intracerebral space-occupying lesion came from Wernicke and Hahn (1881)[183] and also from Bennett and Godley (1884)[16]. In both cases the diagnosis was made exclusively by clinical neurological methods. While Wernicke and Hahn found an abscess, Bennett and Godley actually found a glioma. They have the credit in English-speaking countries as being the first to operate on a clinically diagnosed and correctly located glioma.

Today neurosurgery is a highly specialized independent speciality, that offers outstanding results; however, in the field of glioma surgery one is at the same time painfully aware of the limits of purely surgical measures. The maxim applies here that only in certain cases does the surgical removal of a glioma mean a cure (*e.g.* with pilocytic astrocytomas, or choroid plexus papillomas), while for the majority of the remaining gliomas the recurrent rate is depressingly high and the cure rate after exclusively surgical treatment is terribly low.

II. General Neurosurgery

a) Diagnosis by Means of Noninvasive and Invasive Measures

Apart from the subtle collecting of *neurological findings,* diagnosis by *computer tomography* (CT) nowadays occupies the first place for identifying the site, extent

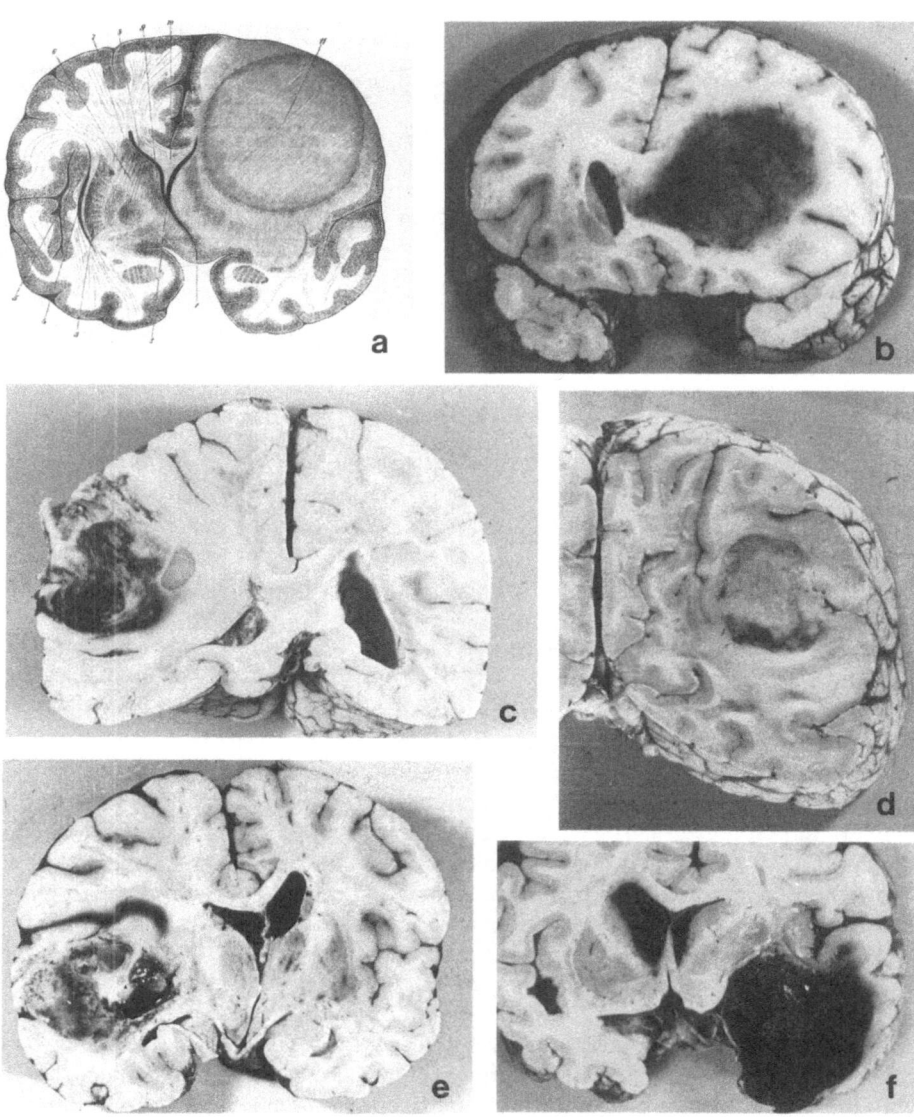

Fig. 1. *Supratentorial glioma.* **a** (after Nothnagel 1878) allows one to see clearly the characteristics of the tumor growth and the reaction of the surroundings. *1* Tuber cinereum, *2* ventric. tertius, *3* nucleus lentiformis, *4* claustrum, *5* insula, *6* Ausstrahlung der Basis, *7* corpus striatum, *8* ventric. lateralis, *9* thal. opticus, *10* corpus callosum, *11* tumor. **b–e** Malignant gliomas from various sites. **f** A "glioma apoplecticum" with rupture of hemorrhage into the ventricular system

and structure of an intracerebral lesion and further it enables one to suspect the type diagnosis with a probability of about 80% and more[7, 24, 25, 34, 70, 73, 79, 80, 87, 92, 98, 111, 121, 181, 182]. Electroencephalography, as well as radio-isotope diagnosis is now only of marginal significance. Among the imaging procedures recently developed is *nuclear magnetic resonance* (NMR) which has had and will have revolutionary significance for the diagnosis of intracerebral tumors particularly those in the posterior cranial fossa[12, 60, 109, 188]. In spite of very interesting results the value of *positron emission tomography* (PET) cannot be fully evaluated at the present time[40, 41, 66, 69, 74, 76, 96, 100, 158, 184]. Sonographic methods are only of significance as regards the diagnosis of tumor, but however, after posterior fossa craniotomies in childhood they allow follow-up of possible recurrence in medulloblastomas with a relatively greater degree of accuracy.

Cerebral angiography is still of significance, particularly as regards diagnosing the nature of a tumor, and also from the surgical point of view, in deciding whether the vascular system appears to be affected by the tumor, or if the vascular supply of the tumor is of any significance. The measurement of regional *cerebral blood flow* (rCBF) is possible today using 133-xenon inhalation methods, is not invasive and hence is atraumatic. However, any significance of this method in the setting of tumor surgery only applies in special situations. The possibility of the tomographic demonstration of the findings should be mentioned here. Finally, the significance of *evoked potentials,* especially in brain stem lesions, is emphasized[10, 42, 50, 53, 105, 112, 113, 134, 141, 143, 160, 161].

While all the previously mentioned methods are *noninvasive*, surgical measures are necessary for the continuous measurement of *intracranial pressure* (ICP).

1. Methods for Measurement of Intracranial Pressure

The intracranial pressure (ICP) is an important parameter for the postoperative supervision of a patient[8, 14, 20, 117, 154–156]. Apart from the *intraventricular measurement* developed by Lundberg[106] nowadays without exception *epidural measurement* is used. Both methods have their indications and contraindications.

Intraventricular Pressure Measurement

As a rule this is combined with the preliminary insertion of a *ventricular drain*. It is indicated in the first place in an obstructive hydrocephalus with the aim on the one hand, of relieving the pressure and on the other the possibility of continuous pressure measurement with closed drainage[36, 54, 135, 145, 148, 170]. The ventricular catheter which serves as the measuring tube is usually placed in the right frontal horn after making a suitably placed burr-hole and puncturing the ventricle with a Cushing cannula. It is then attached to a Statham element which functions as a receiver. This system is often found useful as it can serve for preliminary pressure-controlled drainage of the ventricle and also at the same time allows the removal of CSF samples and the injection of substances (Fig. 2). Intraventricular measurement of pressure is only suitable in large ventricles which are not displaced.

Epidural Pressure Measurement

In this procedure a pressure recorder (transducer) is placed between the skull bone and the dura [15, 21, 31, 44, 47, 103]. It is not necessary to open the subdural space. The danger of meningitis, which with Lundberg's method occurs with a probability of 0.5 to 2.0%, can be avoided by using epidural measurement. The measuring capsule is introduced through a small slit in the galea and through a burr hole after separating the dura, and the lead brought out of the wound through the galea. The

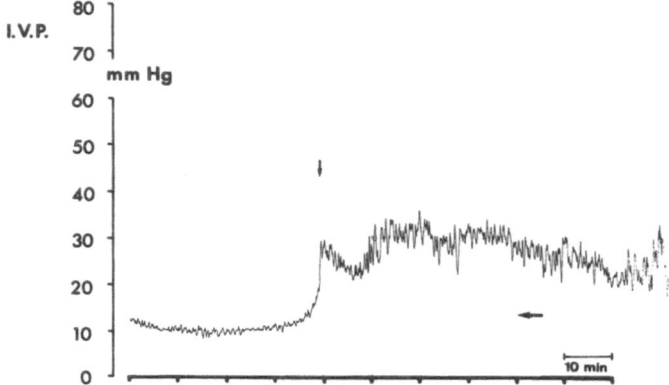

Fig. 2. *Intraventricular measurement of the ICP* by Lundberg's method. After releasing the ventricular drainage (↓) the pathologically high values fell rapidly to the normal range. This possibility of lowering the pressure, naturally does not exist with the epidural technique. (H.A. ♀ 10 years. Glioma of the hypothalamic region—occlusive hydrocephalus)

recorded values run parallel with the intraventricular measurements, nevertheless the method is technically not so satisfactory as Lundberg's method. The epidural method is especially indicated when the ventricles are small, compressed or displaced, as would be the case in unilateral space-occupying lesions in the hemispheres and also particularly in head injuries (Fig. 3).

2. Ventriculography with Positive Contrast Medium

Although the significance of this procedure is now confined to only a few slight problems [3, 5, 6, 18, 19, 27, 37, 93, 102] it should be briefly mentioned here. Nowadays it is done almost exclusively with modern contrast media such as metrizamide. The injection is made through a catheter placed in the lateral ventricle (preliminary ventricular drainage, intraventricular pressure measurement) after which the flow and the distribution of the contrast medium can be observed and radiologically documented.

Above all, stenosis or obstruction of the aqueduct can be shown, also paraventricular or intraventricular lesions in the fourth ventricle (Fig. 4) as well as disturbances of CSF outflow in the posterior fossa. The investigation no longer justifies a special operative approach to the ventricle, but however it can still be considered if there is already a ventricular drain *in situ*.

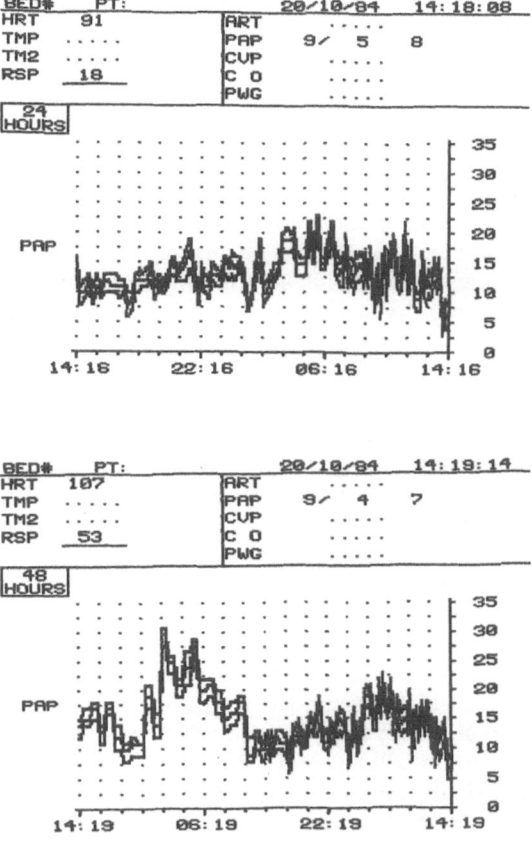

Fig. 3. *Epidural ICP measurement* with the Gaeltec transducer. In association with data storage it allows one to analyse any parameter which is desired. (A 14-year-old boy with an incipient obstructive hydrocephalus)

3. CT-Controlled Stereotactic Tumor Biopsy

This technique is of great significance in the planning of treatment[119, 120, 131, 152], nevertheless it is as yet possible at only a few centers. Its significance in relation to the classification of a tumor depends decisively on the experience of the particular neuropathologist. The method has a mortality of 1.1% and a transitory morbidity of 3%. The advantage of this method is the possibility of examining numerous small tissue samples from many biopsy sites[2, 85] and at the same time to reach critically situated lesions in the medulla oblongata, the basal ganglia or the pons, without undue risks. By a combined investigation with smears and with histological sections the method achieves an accuracy of 80% with precise classification of the tumor. In a further 6% the evidence of a tumor is confirmed but without definite classification and in a further 3% the possibility of a tumor is shown. Further statements are however not possible. We arrange to undertake a stereotactic biopsy in all cases where the tumor is in a critical location, frequently for a preoperative elucidation of the nature of the tumor and above all when there are unusual findings with other diagnostic procedures.

b) Preoperative and Postoperative Monitoring

The postoperative care of all patients after a brain tumor operation takes place under conditions of intensive supervision, and mostly also of intensive treatment. Necessary preoperative measures such as the insertion of a preliminary ventricular drainage or even the measuring of intracranial pressure can make it necessary to admit a patient to the intensive care ward even before the operation.

If the ICP reaches pathological levels, measures for lowering the pressure are indicated[43, 75, 114, 130, 136, 147, 169]. In the case of an obstructive hydrocephalus the drain should be opened to produce an immediate fall of pressure (Fig. 2). With epidural pressure measurement the possibility of relieving the pressure in this way does not exist. In these cases *edema prophylaxis* and treatment with dexamethasone and other corticosteroids can be used and osmotherapy if a rapid reduction of pressure becomes necessary, as well as controlled *hyperventilation*. In general, the patient should only be transferred to the general ward after the ICP has returned to normal. *Complications* such as a possible delayed epidural hemorrhage or a hemorrhage in the tumor resection cavity may be revealed by a rise of the ICP before there is any clinical evidence of deterioration.

The possibilities of the storage and evaluation of data by computer have not yet been adequately assessed as to their significance for intensive care (Fig. 3).

While it is not possible here to go into detail about the methods of monitoring and intensive care, it should still be emphasized that *anticonvulsive treatment* must always be given with existing convulsive attacks, and prophylactic anticonvulsants after a tumor resection from the day of the operation in all hemisphere lesions. A withdrawal of this prophylaxis should only take place under EEG control and after an interval of three months at the earliest.

c) Associated Perioperative Procedures and Palliative Operations

In many patients, apart from the removal of the tumor, it is necessary to do a certain supplementary or palliative procedure which are an essential part of neurosurgical procedures. These will be briefly described here.

1. Ventriculo-atrial Drainage

The possibility of an internal diversion of the CSF into the venous side of the circulation is indicated in certain types of hydrocephalus which persist in spite of the removal of tumor[1, 67, 77, 154]. It is *contraindicated* in malignant tumors, such as medulloblastoma or malignant ependymoma, where there is a tendency for dissemination through the CSF, as in these cases hematogenous spread is well known[71, 83, 174].

Among the numerous shunt systems available we favor the pattern of the Pudenz-Heyer with its use of the antisiphon device, which to a large extent avoids

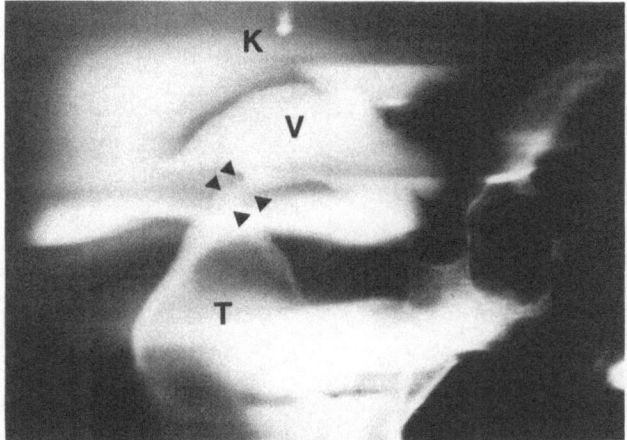

Fig. 4. *Ventriculography with positive contrast medium* (Metrizamide). Demonstration of a spherical tumor contour (*T*) in the fourth ventricle. The arrows indicate the dilated aqueduct. *V* third ventricle. *K* ventricular catheter. (A 6-year-old boy with a medulloblastoma)

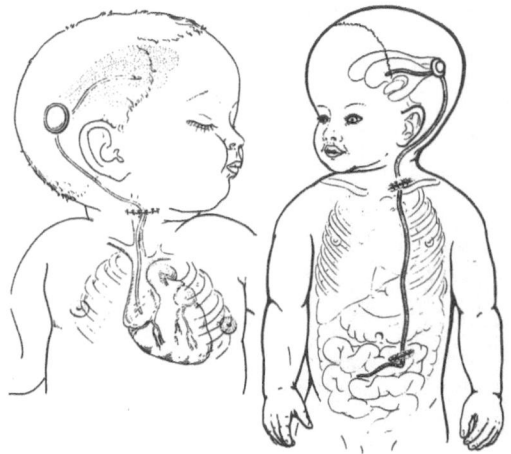

Fig. 5. Diagram of *internal ventricular drainage* (ventriculo-atrial and ventriculoperitoneal) We favor the Pudenz-Heyer-system with an antisiphon device

massive negative pressure within the ventricles. Nevertheless from the technical point of view other shunt systems are quite suitable. The ventricular catheter and the pump with its antisiphon device is always placed in the frontal region, as here the incidence of problems resulting from displacement of the catheter is minimal. The technical details of the procedure are shown in Fig. 4 and 5. Among *complications* can be mentioned the relatively frequent infection of the silicon material (in many series around 10%) and failure of the shunt which can appear after quite variable intervals of time.

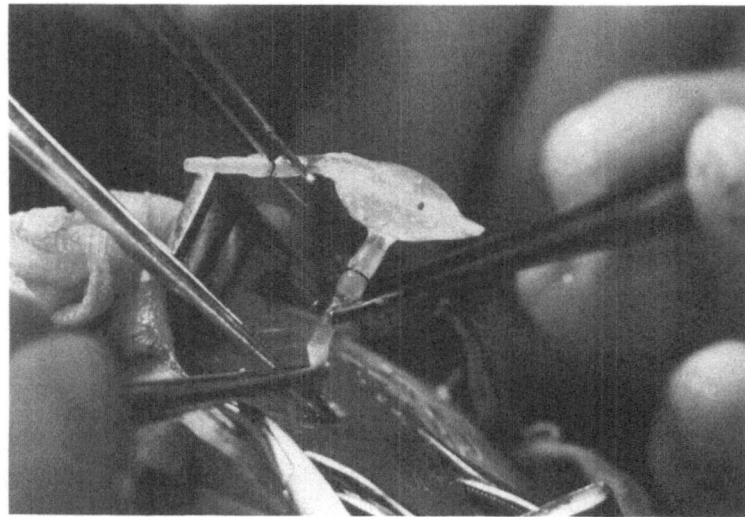

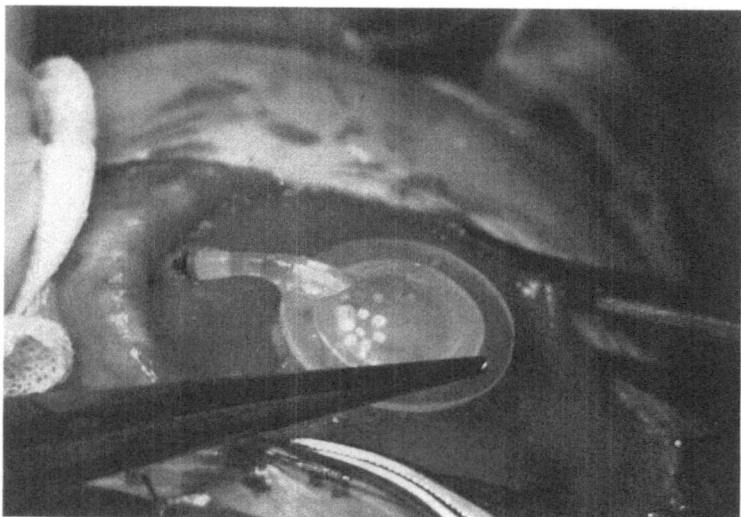

Fig. 6. Insertion of the pump of the Pudenz-Heyer system, without the antisiphon device. In the upper picture the ventricular catheter already inserted is fixed to the pump. In the lower picture the pump is precisely placed, while running off to the left is the cardiac catheter

2. Ventriculo-peritoneal Drainage

The indications for this form of internal drainage of the CSF are the same as for the methods described already[4, 68, 146]. Nevertheless we prefer it in older children and adults, mainly on account of the lower complication rate as regards blockage of the draining catheter. The operative procedure, as far as the placing of the ventricular catheter and the pump, is the same as with ventriculo-atrial drainage.

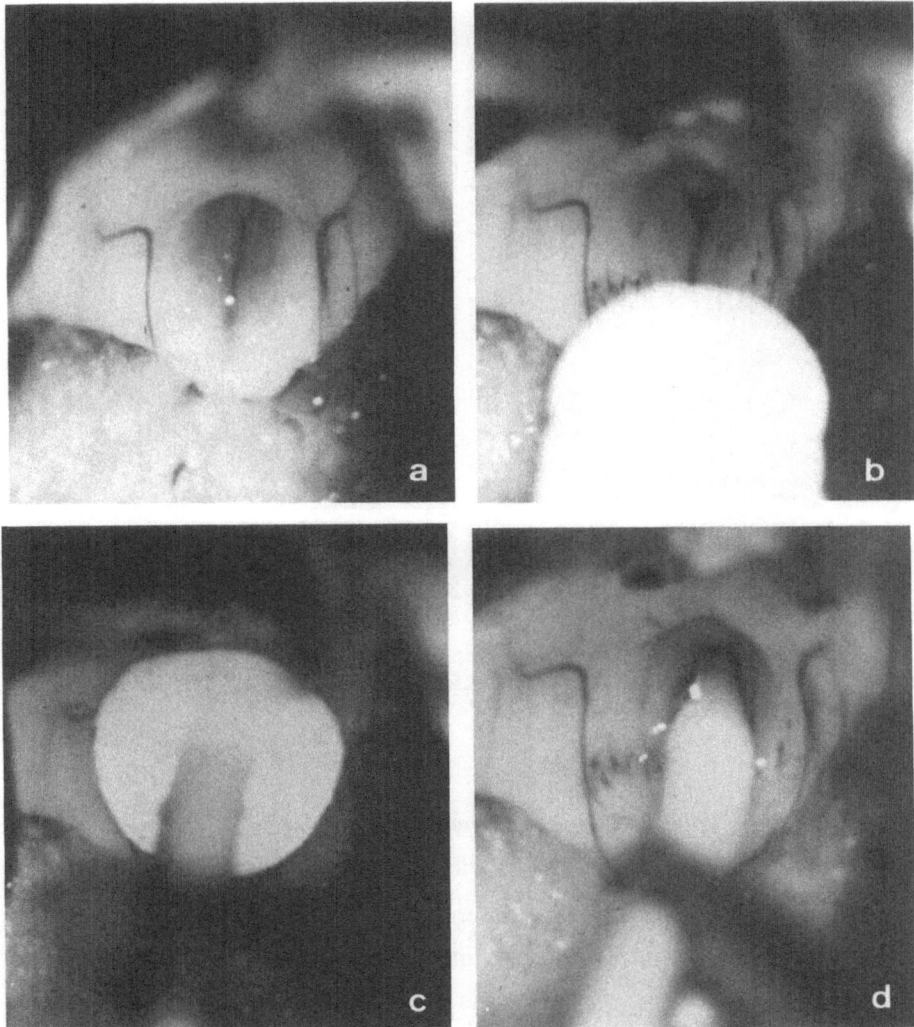

Fig. 7. *Ventriculo-cisternal drainage* according to Leksell (interventriculostomy). *a* Outlet of the aqueduct is displayed under the microscope. *b* and *c* Introduction of the lamellar catheter into the aqueduct and pushing it upwards into the anterior horn (*d*). This procedure must be done very carefully and without the use of any force

The peritoneal catheter is led into the upper abdomen for a distance of 20 to 25 cm through a small transrectal laparotomy and is then led subcutaneously up to the frontal operation field. We refuse to do a blind puncture of the peritoneal space.

Even with this internal drainage, shunt insufficiency is not uncommon. Among complications are recognized perforation of the abdominal hollow viscera (stomach, intestine, gall bladder, uterus) by the peritoneal catheter although the incidence is nervertheless very low.

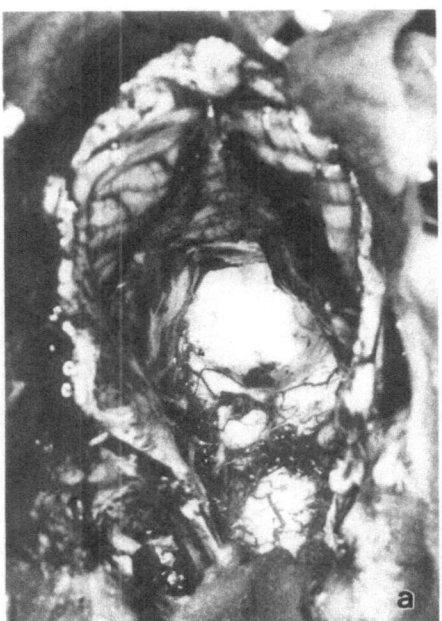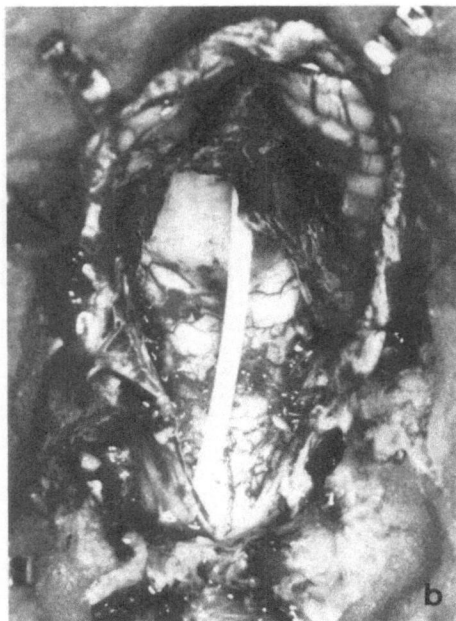

Fig. 8. Operation field after opening of the posterior fossa and resection of a midline cerebellar tumor, before *a* and after *b* insertion of a Leksell drainage. The lower end of the catheter is at the level of the second or third cervical vertebra

3. Ventriculo-cisternal Drainage (Interventriculostomy)

This procedure was suggested by Leksell[101] in 1949 for the treatment of aqueduct obstructions or stenoses. One may recommend that the original appallingly high mortality is temporarily forgotten[28, 35, 99, 123]. Since 1975 we have used a modified form of the technique in almost one hundred cases, without any complications[58, 173–175].

Indications: 1. In infratentorial tumors to reach the outlet of the aqueduct. 2. Possibility of a postoperative stenosis of the aqueduct. 3. Danger of recurrence after a subtotal resection of an infratentorial tumor and with marked malignancy. 4. When there is a risk of dissemination of the tumor (medulloblastoma, malignant ependymoma) in order to avoid a ventriculo-atrial or ventriculo-peritoneal drainage. The basis requirement is the exposure of the posterior fossa associated with the removal of the tumor.

Technique

After resection of the tumor, the microscope is used to expose the lower end of the aqueduct at the upper end of the fourth ventricle and a lamellar catheter is gently introduced (Fig. 7). It is then pushed forwards through the third ventricle and the foramen of Monro as far as the anterior horn. A definite resistance to any progress is then felt. The distal end is then placed in the spinal subarachnoid space at the level

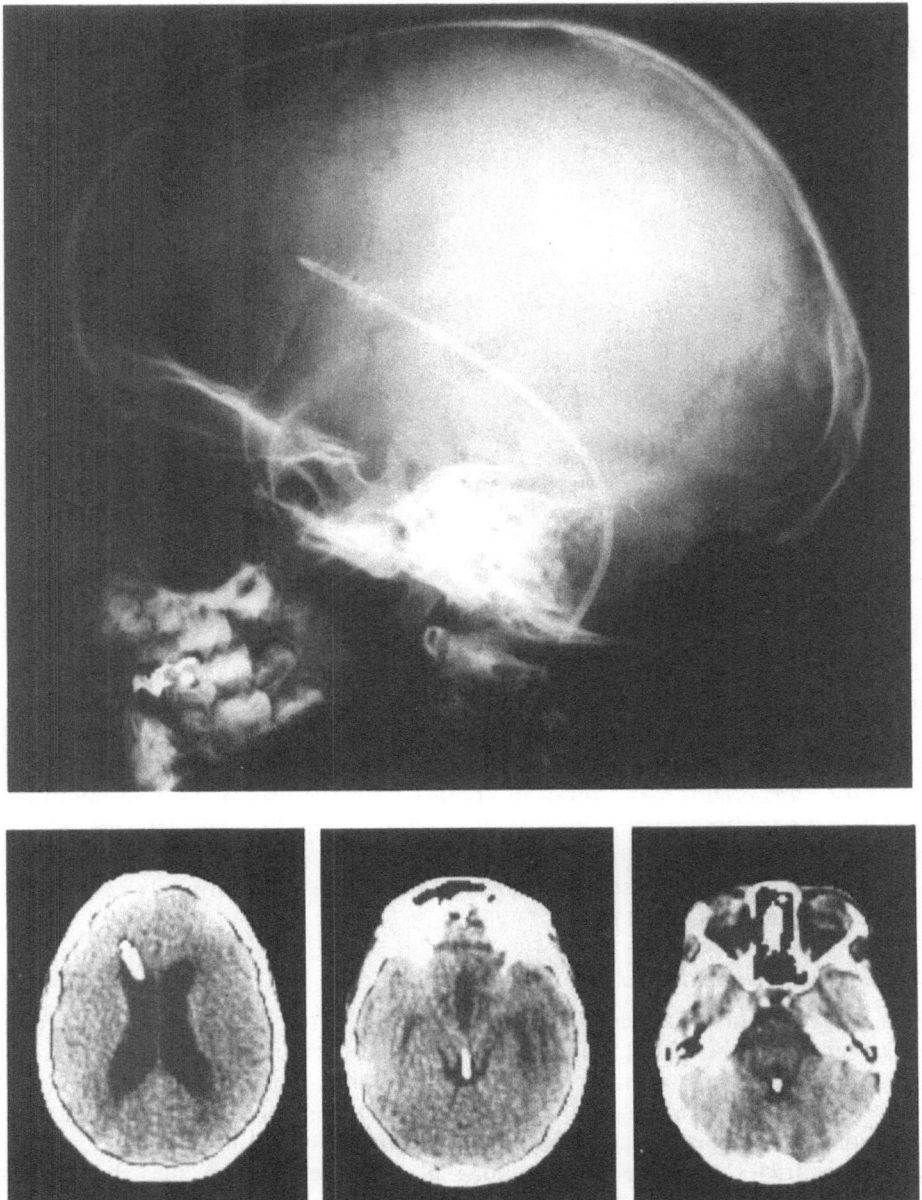

Fig. 9. *Leksell drainage* in a lateral radiograph and also in the CT (lower series of pictures). (Four and a half-year-old girl with a medulloblastoma)

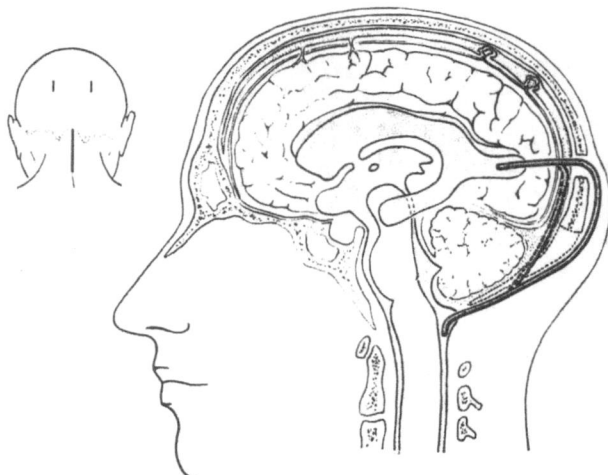

Fig. 10. *Ventriculo-cisternal drainage (Torkildsen)* bypasses stenoses or blockages of the fluid outflow in the third ventricle and the aqueduct. It can be put in one or both sides, with the catheter either epidural or subcutaneous (from Schürmann and Voth 1975)

of C 2 or C 3 (Fig. 8). Postoperative X-rays and CT control document the correct placing of the Leksell drain (Fig. 9).

The reliability of this procedure is absolute; we have not seen a displacement of the drain in a single instance. Even with recurrence of tumor the catheter can be surrounded on all sides by tumor, without its function becoming impaired. A patient can thus be spared any further palliative intervention, as the development of a further obstructive hydrocephalus due to recurrence of tumor can be avoided with certainty. *Side effects* were found in about 6% in the way of fleeting midbrain symptoms, persisting only a few days with diplopia and brief disturbances of co-ordination of eye movements.

Incidentally, a so-called "isolated fourth ventricle" can definitely be avoided by the insertion of Leksell drain[108].

4. Ventriculo-cisternal Drainage

This procedure may be briefly mentioned[42, 104, 165]. It is indicated when there is interference with the CSF flow in the third ventricle, the aqueduct of Sylvius and the fourth ventricle, when a direct attack on the lesion is not possible. However, we prefer the Leksell drainage in all cases in which the posterior fossa is opened. The Torkildsen drain forms a connection between the posterior horn of one or both lateral ventricles and the cisterna magna, and the catheter may be placed subcutaneously or epidurally. This procedure is shown diagramatically in Fig. 10. An advantage of this drainage is likewise its great functional reliability.

5. Implantation of an Ommaya Reservoir

This reservoir consists of a silicon capsule[126] to which is attached a ventricular catheter, which may not only be placed in one of the ventricles, in a tumor resection cavity, and the central tumor necrosis but it can also be put in an abscess cavity. As a rule it is introduced through a right frontal burr-hole and it thus provides a subcutaneously placed, rapidly available access to the ventricular system or to other intracranial cavities[17, 39, 45, 48, 84, 94, 140, 149].

This system can be used for the intrathecal administration of cytostatic drugs, when there is possible CNS involvement in a case of leukemia, in glioblastoma with central necrosis, or for drainage of intracranial cysts as well as occasionally for the administration of antibiotics in cases of fungus infections of the intracranial cavities[29].

Technique

The various types of these reservoirs are as a rule placed over a burr-hole in the desired position and are then joined up to the previously placed ventricular catheter. They are then fixed in the subcutaneous (subgaleal) space. The can be punctured percutaneously with fine needles as often as you wish. *Complications* are rare, but are possible however. We have had an infection rate of 9%[84]. With malignant tumors where radiotherapy is to be given the reservoir should always be outside the radiation field, as radiation can cause skin necrosis.

6. Preliminary Ventricular Drainage

This procedure has already been mentioned in connection with *intraventricular pressure measurement*. Various systems are available commercially, which besides the drainage catheter have a device for fixation to the skin of the scalp and, without exception, a one-way valve to prevent any reflux. Finally there is a collecting bag or graduated flask to collect the fluid which drains[43, 144, 147]. The drainage pressure is adjusted in most systems by fixation of the drainage tube or its end, at various heights. A system which we have developed[169] works with a one-way valve, whose opening pressure can be externally adjusted and varied between 50 and 100 mm of water.

The *indication* for ventricular drainage is firstly when there is an urgent and immediately required rapid release of pressure in a case of obstructive hydrocephalus, sometimes also for local treatment of the ventricular cavity in severe infections with an empyema of the ventricles[75, 114, 130, 136]. *Complications* can develop as a result of infection, with the development of meningitis. The drain should therefore not be left *in situ* for longer than eight days, or a maximum of ten days. Scrupulous attention to the entry point of the catheter in the galea with iodophores (not with antibiotics!) is an absolute requirement. Furthermore the ventricular catheter must be placed with as long a track as possible under the galea to its point of exit.

If a longer period drainage is necessary, then mentioned above the external drain must be exchanged for an internal one, such as a ventriculoperitoneal or ventriculo-atrial drainage.

7. Perioperative Administration of Antibiotics

Among the perioperative measures[62, 116] must also be included the administration of antibiotics, in the sense of perioperative *prophylaxis*. We have pointed out in detail the special conditions of neurosurgery[168, 171, 177, 180]. This treatment is, without exception, quite adequate if given as a "single dose" prophylaxis, but there is no indication for it in the case of a carefully planned intervention, such as a tumor resection. In this connexion nothing will be said about abscesses or contamination following trauma. A prophylactic, such as has been indicated, is sensible in all shunt operations, particularly as the incidence of infection has been described in many studies as around 10%, not only in Europe, but also in the USA and Japan. Here the use of "single dose" prophylaxis can definitely reduce the frequency of infection. We have reported in detail elsewhere about the details of treatment and the choice of antibiotic[180].

d) General Operative Technique

The principal of radical extirpation and removal "into healthy tissue" that is appropriate in many surgical specialties has not led to the expected cures in glioma surgery. Thus while the recurrence rate even in "benign" gliomas, such as astrocytoma II, turns out to be exceptionally high, that of the glioblastomas was well over 90%. Nowadays the attempt at a removal into healthy tissue is still regarded as reasonable for polar gliomas, such as those in the frontal or temporal lobes. In the same way gliomas of grade II malignancy and possibly even grade III in other parts of the brain should be resected with a safety margin of at least several millimeters, or better still up to one centimeter into the healthy tissue. Nevertheless functionally important areas of the brain will determine how radical the boundaries can be. This applies to Broca's and Wernicke's areas and possibly also for the motor cortex[30, 107, 125, 172, 179, 186].

With a glioblastoma WHO grade IV a possible radical extirpation reduces neither the recurrence rate from nearly 100% nor the recurrence-free interval. For that reason the operator should always give priority to the quality of survival rather than to the radical nature of the excision[11, 23, 26, 55, 78, 132, 139, 142, 187]. The pilocytic astrocytoma (WHO grade I), earlier called spongioblastoma, is the only truly *benign tumor* in the glioma series, apart from the rare *giant cell astroblastomas* (grade I) which without exception appear as intraventricular tumors, and the benign *plexus papillomas* (grade I). With pilocytic astrocytomas a radical removal should always be attempted if at all possible as this means the *cure* of the patient.

With the medulloblastomas (WHO grade IV) of the posterior fossa, the principal of maximal resection remains absolutely valid, whereas an attempt at a total extirpation to healthy tissue causes appalling mortality and besides, the concept is fictitious. We know that with these tumors the operation merely reduces the tumor cell population to a greater or lesser degree. Incidentally the survival rates in patients with an apparently total or actually only a partial resection, are not different after radiotherapy and chemotherapy. The pilocytic astrocytoma (grade I) of the posterior fossa should be removed as radically as possible and the same principle applies to the rarer ependymoma (grades II and III) although frequently it is not feasible on account of the involvement of the hindbrain. After exposure of the part of the brain involved with tumor, as a rule by an osteoplastic craniotomy, the operative procedure consists of an identification of the tumor according to its consistence, color and any changes of the preformed structures such as the surface appearance of the gyri and sulci (Fig. 11). Having regard to the findings of the

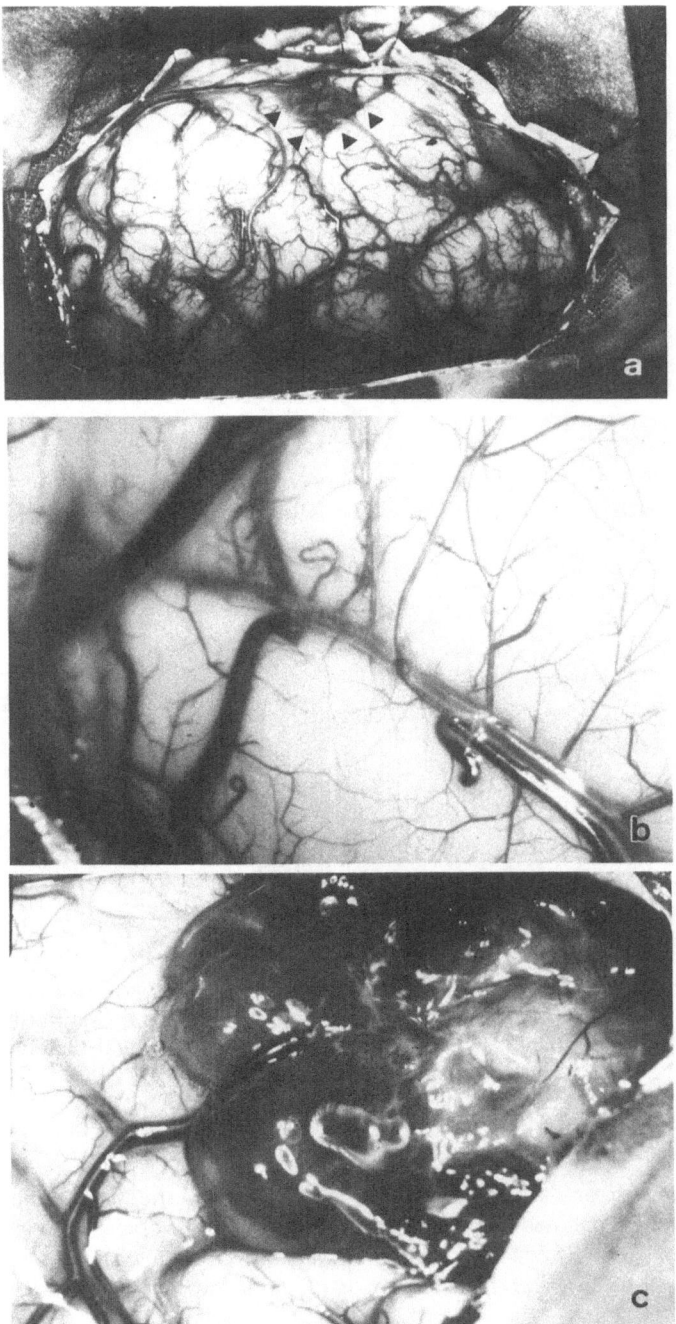

Fig. 11. *Cerebral hemisphere gliomas* which were visible on the surface after opening of the dura. *a* Glioblastoma (42-year-old woman). *b* Broadening of the gyri with obvious vascularity over an astrocytoma, (III) (24-year-old woman. *c* Benign glioma of the right frontal lobe in a 17-year-old girl. Such a clear cut demarcation of the tumor on the brain surface is very unusual

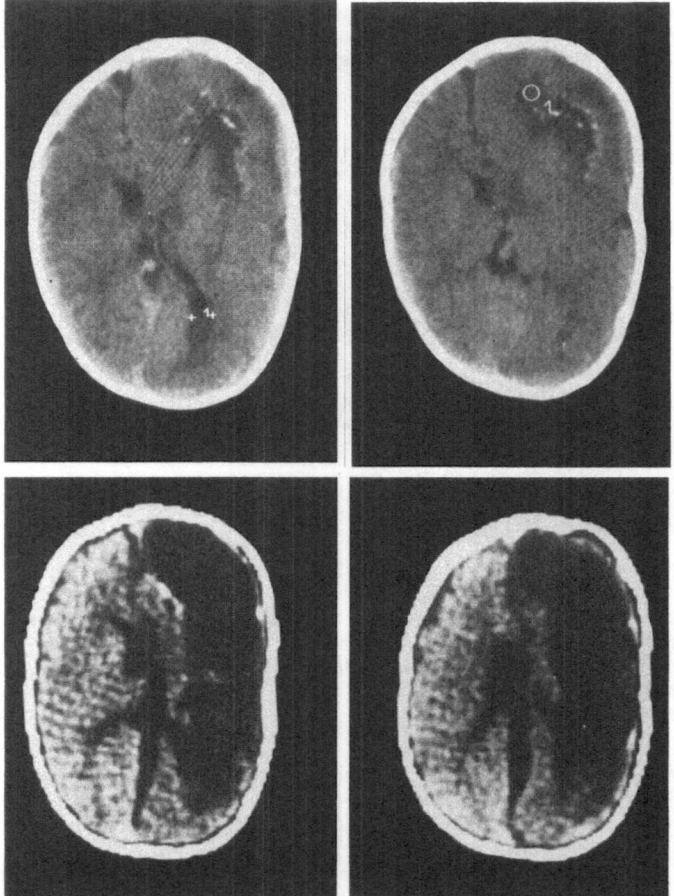

Fig. 12. CT pictures before (above) and after (below) a *subtotal hemispherectomy*. This 1-year-old girl presented preoperatively with an intractable epilepsy severe disability and marked retardation. After hemispherectomy the attacks ceased and the child developed rapidly and impressively

various diagnostic procedures, the tumor is located from the surface. The line of the resection is then decided and along it the superficial vessels are dealt with by electrocoagulation. Afterwards the resection is undertaken with the brain spatulas, working on all sides around the tumor, using endothermy or the laser[49, 82, 107, 115, 153, 164].

One proceeds in the same way for a lobectomy in polar tumors. A partial or total hemispherectomy is only rarely undertaken, usually for congenital tumors or severe epileptic attacks. For this operation it is worthwhile to follow a definite routine in the stages of the operation but the details of these different steps will not be dealt with any further here.

In 1984 we operated on a girl with a right-sided congenital glioma and uncontrollable epilepsy. After an extensive hemispherectomy (Fig. 12) she was free of attacks, showed an impressive spurt in her development and showed excellent motor function in the side of the body opposite to the resected hemisphere.

The control of bleeding from larger arteries is even today, still undertaken with metal clips. Otherwise the neurosurgeon largely avoids the use of intracranial metallic materials on account of the very marked artefacts in CT, and iron-containing implants on account of the difficulties with NMR tomography. In all other instances control of bleeding is possible with endothermy or the laser. With venous or diffuse bleeding from the tissues the laser likewise gives good service, but hemostasis with fibrin foam or collagen sponge and with fibrin glue may also be used. The use of embolization is not of any significance in the removal of gliomas. After a lobectomy or the enucleation of a tumor, hemostasis is undertaken and the cavity is filled with warm Ringer's solution. A water tight closure of the dura is always attempted, if necessary with the use of lyophilized heterologous dura or a free pedicled galeaperiosteal flap, with which the closure of larger defects can also be done without any difficulty. If there is a marked tendency to brain swelling the bone flap can be removed, in order to guarantee an adequate intracranial decompression. It can be kept sterile in the deep freeze for days, or even up to several weeks. Subcutaneous implantation under the skin of the abdomen is also possible.

It must still be emphasized that with lesions more deeply situated in the white matter consideration must be given during the operative procedure to the course of the fiber systems and the existing nuclear masses in order to keep the extent of any neurological deficit as small as possible. *The operative strategy should always be decided in advance, before the operation.*

e) Special Technical Aids

Surgery of the gliomas requires a great number of technical methods and aids, which are also of use in other neurosurgical procedures and in other specialities. These will be only briefly mentioned.

1. The Operating Microscope

The use of aids to magnification in surgery has greatly expanded in recent years [68, 90, 97, 118]. Microscopes with coaxial illumination offer the advantage of magnification and the optimal illumination of the operation field. Nowadays the operating microscope is an indispensible instrument for neurosurgeons and indeed, not only for the removal of lesions of the posterior cranial fossa or in deeply situated intraventricular tumors. Even the extirpation of gliomas and glioblastomas can be improved, to the extent that the procedure can preserve function and protect the tissues. The possibilities of photo documentation with miniature or with video cameras will only be mentioned.

2. Use of the Laser in Neurosurgery

In the last few years this technique has been successfully employed in neurosurgery. At the present time there are two laser systems in use, namely the CO_2 laser and Nd-YAG laser. Each of these systems has its own particular advantages. Thus the CO_2 laser has shown merits as a cutting instrument while the Nd-YAG laser shows its particular value rather in the coagulation of areas of tissue with severe bleeding. The combination of the laser with the microscope offers particularly good conditions for the use of this interesting method, which will certainly be important in the future [9, 13, 61, 163].

3. Electrocoagulation

In glioma surgery nowadays bipolar coagulation, introduced by Malis is used almost exclusively [51, 110]. Industry has developed a whole range of machines, which are continually being improved not only with regard to the comfort of the user, but also as regards its effectiveness, possibly by coupling the apparatus with a microcomputer [84].

4. The Use of Ultrasound

By the use of ultrasound the tissues can be broken up and liquified. The frequencies used are around 23 kHz. This apparatus originally used in opthalmology for cataract operations is nowadays quite widely used in neurosurgery [22, 38, 81]. The combination of the sound emitter with suction and irrigation equipment, which already exists with the CUSA apparatus, is an universally serviceable procedure by which, with no obvious contraindications tumors can be safely, quickly and carefully removed. Nevertheless the complete destruction of the tissue structure is depressing for the neuropathologist; the surgeon should not forget to obtain appropriate material for biopsy during the operation.

5. Microsurgical Instruments and Suture Material

The introduction of the operating microscope has led to a refinement, miniaturization and specialization of the instrumentarium, whereby for the first time the advantages of the magnification have been made really effective from the surgical point of view [32, 63–65, 89, 91, 138, 157, 172, 185].

III. Special Neurosurgery

The subdivision of the skull cavity into the supratentorial and infratentorial portions has its basis in clinical particularities. The supratentorial space is limited by the tentorial hiatus, which in space-occupying lesions can decisively influence the course of the illness by the development of midbrain herniation. The same holds true for the infratentorial space—the posterior fossa. In the presence of space-occupying lesions we are familiar with tonsillar herniation into the foramen magnum as well as—but very rarely however—midbrain herniation, as a result of shift of the brain structures rostrally.

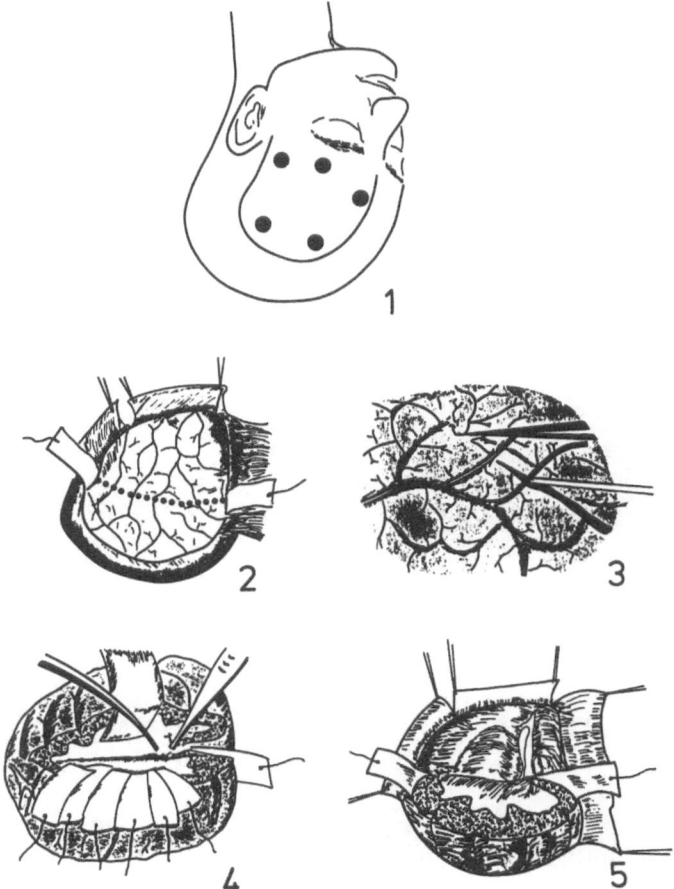

Fig. 13. Typical *frontal lobectomy* (diagramatic)

Furthermore, the two spaces are affected by particular types of tumor. Thus the glioblastoma multiforme is located almost exclusively above the tentorium whereas the medulloblastoma occurs mainly in the posterior cranial fossa.

Finally, the operative approaches are quite different for the two cavities; above the tentorium one uses mostly an osteoplastic flap, whereas infratentorially an osteoclastic craniotomy is used. For this reason the subdivision has proved useful for the neurosurgeon.

Extracerebral tumors such as craniopharyngioma, pituitary adenoma, meningioma and neurofibroma will not be discussed here.

a) Tumors of the Supratentorial Space

Tumors of the Cerebral Hemispheres

With polar tumors, for instance in the frontal, temporal and occipital lobes a partial or total lobectomy is indicated. It should keep to resection lines, which take notice

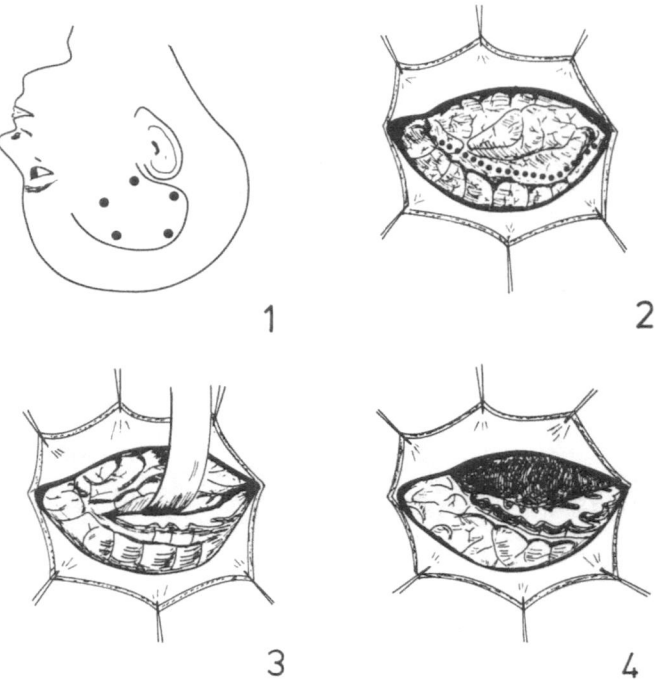

Fig. 14. Typical *temporal lobectomy* (diagramatic)

of important functional areas. Examples are shown in the illustrations (Figs. 13–15). The procedure applies above all to *gliomas of the lower grades of malignancy* (II and III).

With glioblastomas the principle of maximal resection applies, as with the highly malignant medulloblastomas. In order to keep any postoperative deficit as small as possible an operating using microsurgical technique is advisable. Tumors in the white matter should be exposed via a transcortical approach and enucleated. The protection of the vascular network can be ensured by using a linear transgyral incision, but with more deeply situated lesions a trans-sulcal approach is more convenient. Any gyri directly involved with the tumor are resected with it (Fig. 16).

The enucleation of tumors from the depths can be done with the CUSA-apparatus or with other suck and irrigate apparatus, without ultrasound.

By this method, which protects the tissues, even small tumors in the rostral basal ganglia can be "removed".

Intraventricular Lesions

Tumors of the lateral ventricles, according to their particular location, can be exposed and removed by means of a linear cortical excision (Fig. 19) in the frontal, temporal or occipital region. Here also the operating microscope, and the CUSA and the laser apparatus are a great advantage. Tumors of the third ventricle

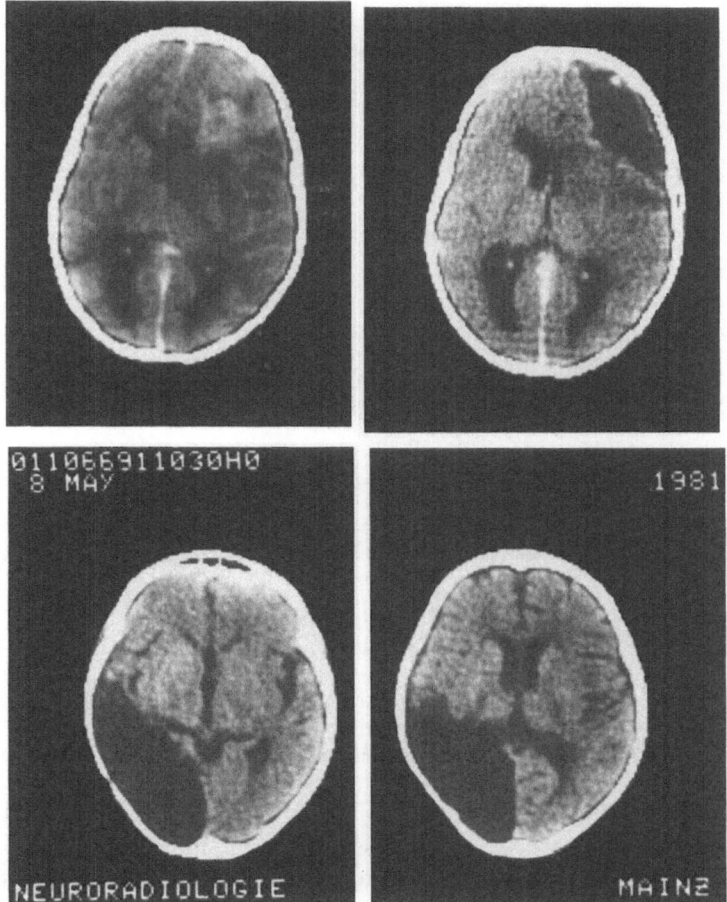

Fig. 15. Partial *frontal lobectomy* in the upper part of the picture (8-year-old girl, glioblastoma IV). CT findings before and after operation. The child died from a recurrence two years after the operation. Total occipital lobectomy. Postoperative CT pictures (below). Meanwhile this 15-year-old girl shows no evidence of recurrence of the ependymoma (II) after six years

(Fig. 17) can be exposed either by a frontal approach or by splitting the corpus callosum in the midline. When there is already hydrocephalus and a dilated lateral ventricle the transventricular frontal approach causes few problems, although the operator approaches the tumor from an oblique angle and often the foramen of Monro must be enlarged (Fig. 18). The approach through the corpus callosum has the advantage that one comes directly on the lesion and the orientation throughout appears easier. Which approach is to be used should be checked very carefully before the operation. Among the many factors to be considered are the size and extent of the lesion, whether it is symmetrical or asymmetrical, the extent of the ventricular dilatation, and the course of the internal veins, above all those in the

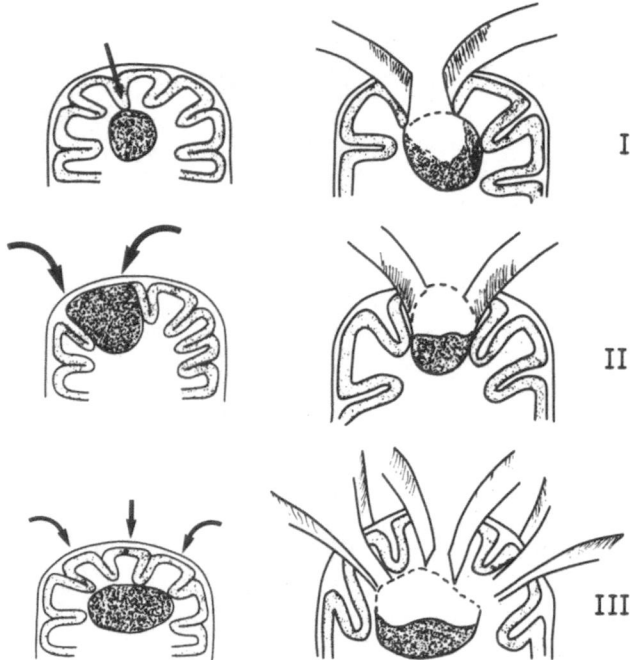

Fig. 16. *Microsurgical procedure* with transgyral approach, or by opening of the sulci. This procedure is particularly recommended for glioblastomas, in order to keep to a minimum during the intervention itself, any additional lesion with corresponding neurological deficit

septum pellucidum. We have the impression that the interhemispheric approach through the corpus callosum causes more stress to the patient than the transventricular approach [33, 46, 59, 137].

Midline Intrinsic Brain Tumors

Here must be mentioned the gliomas of the optic chiasm which, as a rule, are pilocytic astrocytomas (WHO I). They can also involve the floor of the third ventricle. While smaller lesions in the optic nerve and occasionally also in the chiasm and optic tract can be removed microsurgically, similar procedures when there is involvement of the hypothalamic region no longer offer much chance of success, apart from very small tumors. In this context the pituitary adenomas and craniopharyngiomas will not be discussed.

On the other hand the tumors of the quadrigeminal region are of interest (Fig. 20), especially those of the pineal [88, 122, 124, 150, 151]. These can sometimes be exposed by an occipital approach and resected. The clarification of their exact relationship to the lamine quadrigemina has become greatly facilitated by NMR tomography, especially as regards the distinction between pineal tumors and tumors of the midbrain. Two approaches (Fig. 21) are possible for removal of pineal tumors, namely supratentorially along the angle between the falx and the

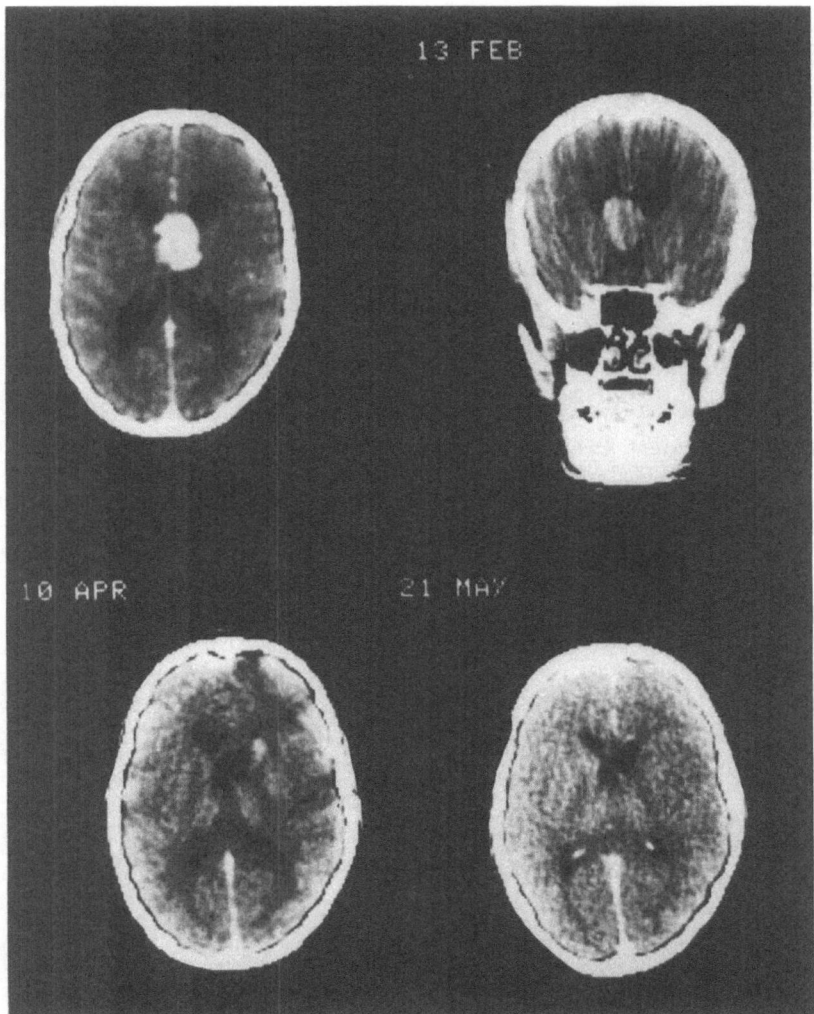

Fig. 17. *Tumour of the third ventricle* in a 14-year-old girl (astrocytoma III). After a right transventricular microsurgical removal the child remains free of recurrence after five years (with permission[172])

tentorium with splitting of the corpus callosum, or infratentorially, which nowadays is usually the approach which is favored. However, in the choice of an approach the extent and exact location of the tumor are of decisive importance[128, 129, 133, 159].

b) Tumors of the Posterior Fossa

Among the tumors of the cerebellar hemisphere and vermis (midline), there is at least one, the pilocytic astrocytoma (grade I) whose total resection results in a

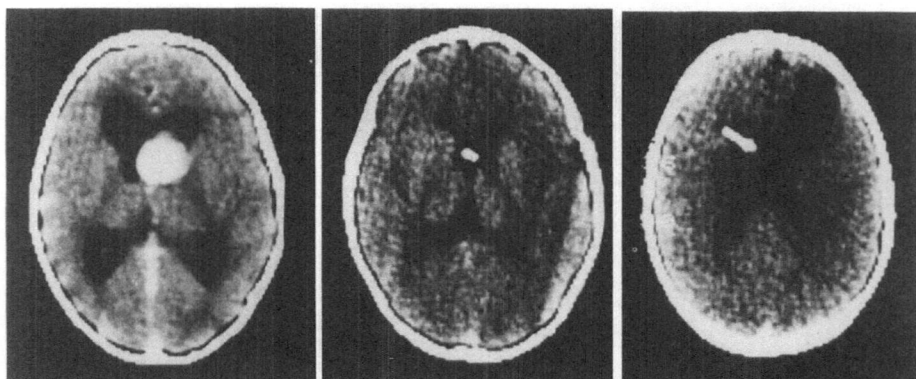

Fig. 18. *Intraventricular tumor* in the third ventricle and near the foramen of Monro. Removal via a right-sided transventricular approach. The later postoperative picture shows the successful removal of the lesion (part of picture); a ventricular catheter coming from the left side belongs to the ventriculoperitoneal drainage which was introduced before the operation. This was removed later (21-year-old man, giant cell astroblastoma I). After five years he remains free of recurrence

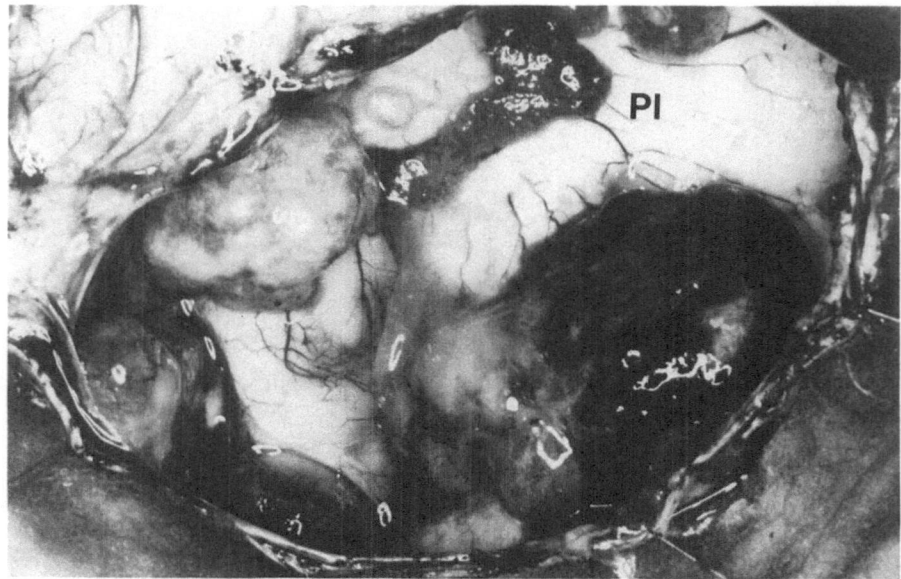

Fig. 19. *Intraventricular seeding from an ependymoma (III)* with formation of numerous patchy nodules of tumor. An 8-year-old boy with a left temporal ependymoma already resected twice, also treated with radiotherapy and chemotherapy. The child died two months after a third exploration in which the findings were as shown in the illustration. *Pl* choroid plexus

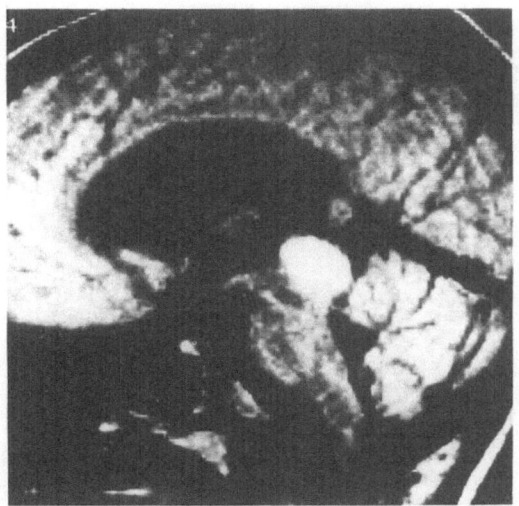

Fig. 20. *Tumor of the quadrigeminal region* shown by NMR tomography. 14-year-old girl. The tumor has been recognized for six years and has shown no progress

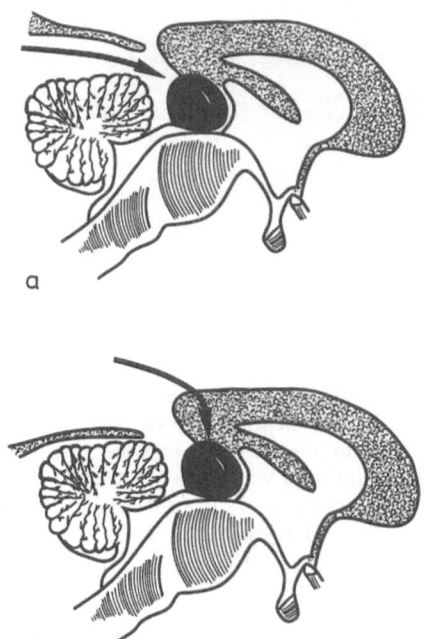

Fig. 21. Diagram of the *approach to the pineal* and quadrigeminal region

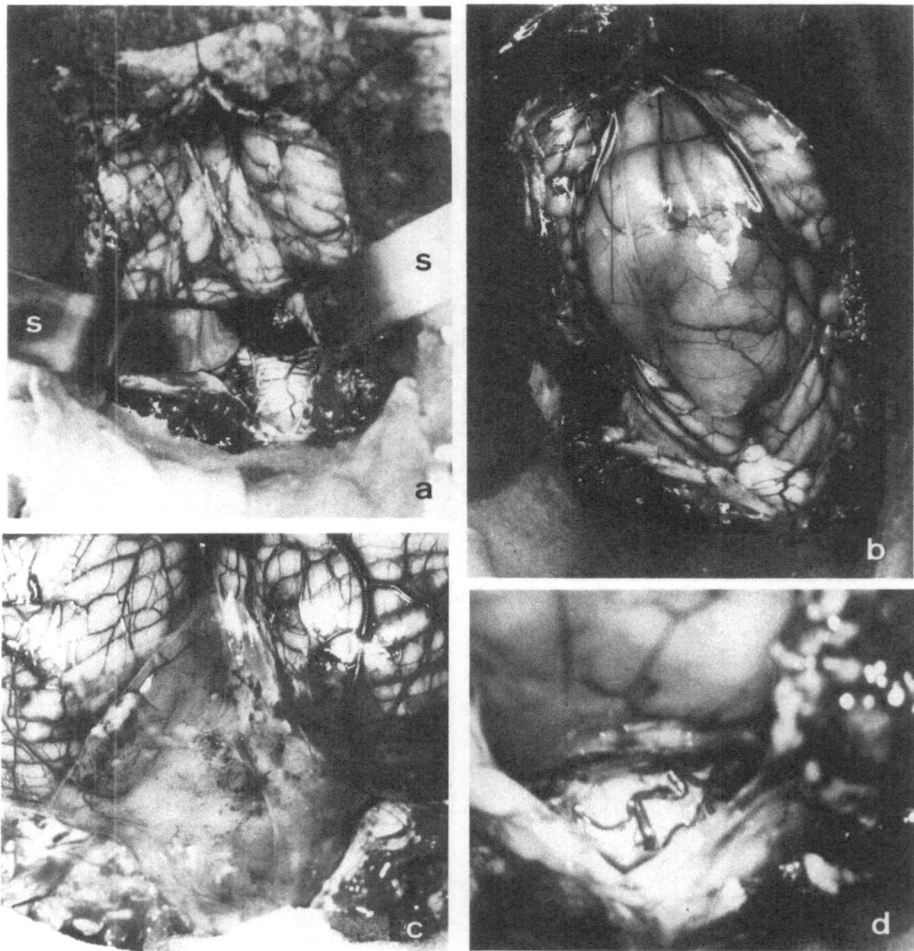

Fig. 22. *In midline lesions of the cerebellum* visible changes are often apparent immediately after opening the dura. *a* Between the cerebellar tonsils which are held aside with a spatula (*S*) a dark-colored tumor is visible (7-year-old girl, medulloblastoma IV). *b* Vermis greatly expanded by a glassy brownish tumor, which does not reach the tonsils (23-year-old woman, pilocytic astrocytoma I). *c* Tumor growing into the cisterna magna. The approach to the fourth ventricle is from below and not directly exposed (6-year-old boy. Medulloblastoma IV). *d* Waxy tumor of the hindbrain which here (lower picture) is growing out from the rhombencephalon near its transition to the medulla oblongata (19-year-old woman, pilocytic astrocytoma I)

successful cure. Resection in the cerebellar hemispheres are possible without any problems, but the rostral quadrant should be spared if at all possible in order to avoid producing considerable ataxic disturbances.

Even although sparing of the nuclei in the hemispheres, *e.g.* the dentate, emboliform, globose and fastigial is scarcely possible, the site of the nuclei and their

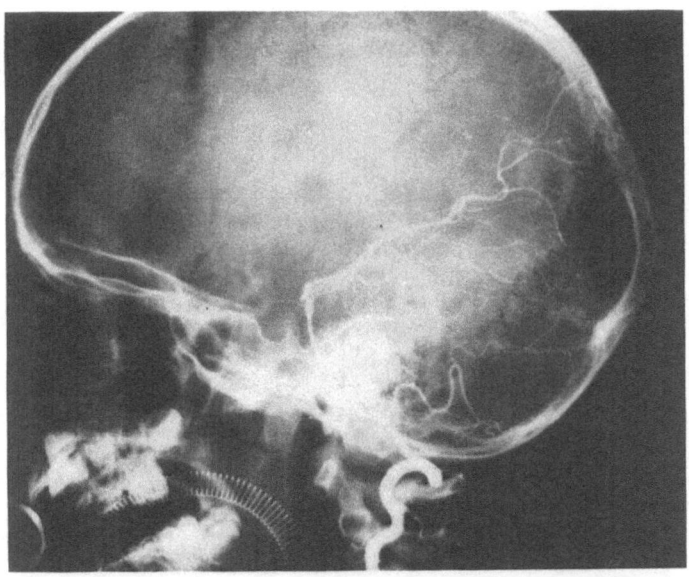

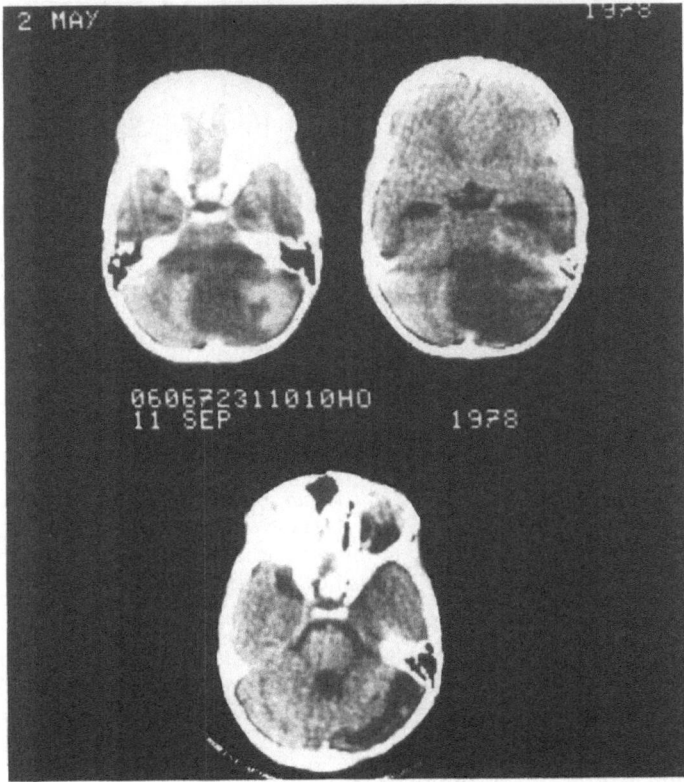

Fig. 23. Typical findings in a *tumor of the cerebellar hemisphere* (7-year-old boy, pilocytic astrocytoma (*I*). In the lateral angiogram signs of enlargement of the posterior fossa. In the preoperative CT (upper right) a large hypodense tumor of the right cerebellar hemisphere. After removal of tumor (lower right) expansion of the previously compressed part of the cerebellum and the brain stem. The child has already gone seven years without any recurrence

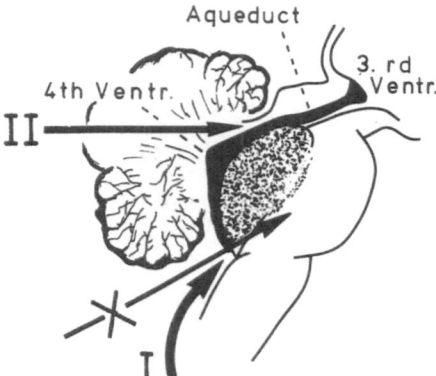

Fig. 24. *Diagram of the approach* in lesions growing in the floor of the rhomboid fossa. Any deviation in the hindbrain is dangerous

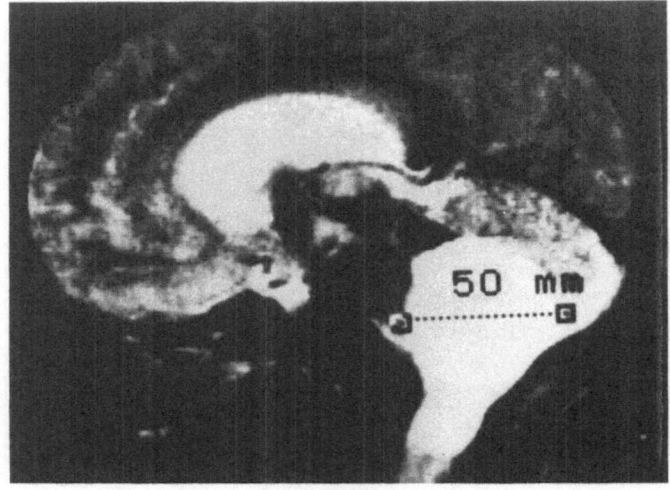

Fig. 25. *Large inoperable tumor of the hindbrain,* extending as far as the cervical cord (pilocytic astrocytoma I in an 8-year-old boy). The NMR tomogram showed the infiltration of the entire rhombencephalon which in this instance, made any extirpation of the tumor impossible. Smaller lesions however are quite removable

supposed location in relation to the position of the tumor must be considered in planning the operative approach. This is functionally important, as not uncommonly the nuclei are displaced and compressed and yet are still intact, not only anatomically but also functionally.

The enucleation of the tumor is carried out according to the criteria of the consistence and color of the tumor tissue, in the same way as with the supratentorial tumors (Fig. 22). If the tumor must be pursued into the cerebellar peduncles (the brachium pontis and conjunctivum or the restiform body) this is justified to a certain extent by the tumor, whose radical removal promises a cure, above all in the case of the pilocytic astrocytoma (Fig. 23). Removal of a medulloblastoma (grade IV) follows the maxim of a maximal, but not at any price a total, resection[56–58, 108, 172, 174]. If they are confined to the vermis, white matter or one or both cerebellar hemisphere, the "removal" is possible without difficulty. If they extend into the brachium conjunctivum or pontis and the restiform body, a too deep exploration is not expedient.

Lesions of the hindbrain are either primary tumors of the rhomboid fossa such as pilocytic astrocytomas in childhood, or secondary lesions growing in the hindbrain, mainly medulloblastomas (grade IV), juxtaventricular ependymomas (grade II–III) and finally also benign astrocytomas (grade I). Less common are choroid plexus papillomas of the fourth ventricle, which as a rule, respect borders of the floor of the fourth ventricle. Resection of tumor tissue in the hindbrain is basically possible but certainly numerous factors must be taken into consideration. The enucleation for instance of a small pilocytic astrocytoma, whose extent is well demonstrated by NMR tomography (Fig. 25) is microsurgically possible, as with the spinal manifestations of the tumor, sometimes with remarkably few side effects. It is important to establish the exact site of the lesion and its relation to the pyramidal tracts and the nuclei of the hindbrain as well as a very scrupulous procedure with microsurgical technique, the laser and the CUSA. The approach, according to the site, takes place either by splitting the vermis, or else from laterally. Unfortunately the most frequent "secondary tumors" in the hindbrain are the medulloblastomas spreading over the floor of the fourth ventricle and thus growing into the rhomboid fossa. They are approached first of all from caudally between the cerebellar tonsils after splitting the vermis or otherwise are exposed coming downwards from above when the anterior part of the rhomboid fossa is not yet infiltrated[72, 95]. It is important to work outwards from that part of the rhomboid fossa which is not infiltrated and thus to avoid penetrating too deeply into the hindbrain (Fig. 24). On account of the superficial position of many cranial nerve nuclei unwanted lesions can develop very quickly. The motor nuclei of the facial, abducens or trigeminal nerves can be affected in this way, as well as damage to the superficially situated vagus nucleus and more rarely even the hypoglossal nerve.

In conclusion one should stress the maxim known to all neurosurgeons, to take the greatest care of the blood supply of the hindbrain. It is most important to avoid any lesion of the AICA (anterior inferior cerebellar artery) and the PICA (posterior inferior cerebellar artery). The patency of the small pontine branches from the basilar artery can be decisive as regards the successful or fatal outcome of an operation. Exclusively intraventricular lesions of the posterior fossa are not very frequent. They include choroid plexus papillomas, more rarely paraventricular ependymomas and occasionally epidermoids. They are exposed by splitting the vermis. The removal of these lesions is technically quite simple.

IV. Significance of the Surgical Measures and Critical Assessment of Their Results

It is established that there are no particular technical problems associated with the removal of lesions of the cerebral and cerebellar hemispheres. Intraventricular

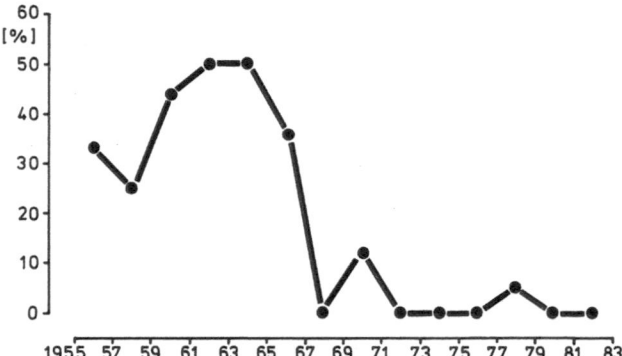

Fig. 26. *Perioperative mortality* (6 weeks post operationem, 1956–1983) for the operative removal of intrinsic brain tumors of the posterior cranial fossa (medulloblastoma IV, pilocytic astrocytoma I, ependymoma II and III etc). 196 patients, age < 15 years. The very high figures initially were the result of an attempted total resection of these lesions, especially with the medulloblastomas. Radical resection is only indicated in the case of pilocytic astrocytomas and this means a permanent cure. In all other lesions the principle of a maximal resection is the valid one. For many years the mortality in our clinical has been nil. Figures over 5% no longer correspond to international standards

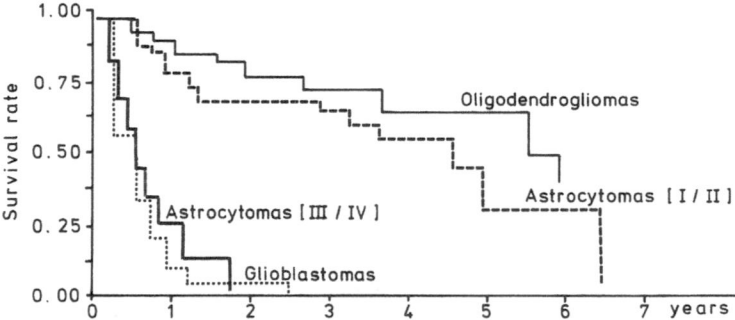

Fig. 27. Estimation of the possibility of survival of patients with gliomas treated *exclusively by operation*. It is evident that a cure is possible with intrinsic brain tumors, while in general the recurrence rate is variable depending on the type of tumor. The figures are taken from the material at the Neurosurgical Clinic in Mainz

tumors in the posterior fossa are quite easily removable, as they are in the supratentorial space. Finally even tumors in the rostral basal ganglia, the optic chiasm, in the midbrain as well as in the hindbrain are possibly totally or partially removable. There is no mistaking the progress that has been made with operative measures. A definite *multifactorial* parameter is the *perioperative mortality*. It fell, for instance, for interventions in the posterior fossa from values of around 50% to virtually nil (Fig. 26). A clinic whose corresponding mortality is over 5% does not satisfy the standard achieved internationally. Similar results can be achieved with supratentorial tumors, in which certainly the perioperative mortality is dependent on the type of tumor and above all on its location. Moreover these tumors mostly affect adults and not uncommonly older men, so that there tends to be a higher mortality. In spite of this the risks are also falling dramatically for supratentorial lesions. We now tend to take a *longer view of the chances of survival*. Here it is clearly shown in our patients, that the striking improvement in the operative results only related to the perioperative complications, whereas their life expectancy is determined by other factors entirely. Thus, the possibility of survival (Fig. 27) for patients with glioblastomas is unchanged at the 50% level at less than one year, and similarly for anaplastic astrocytomas WHO grade III or IV. The data are more favorable for patients with isomorphic astrocytomas (I and II) and with oligodendroglioma. With the exception of patients with pilocytic astrocytoma (grade I) and those uncommon cases of choroid plexus papilloma and subependymal giant cell astroblastoma, there are no chances of a lasting cure by means of operative measures alone.

This is a sobering thought, that even with the immense progress that has been made by neurosurgery in the one hundred years of its existence, it is unable to change very much. On the other hand it must stimulate us in our own surgical activity to look for methods and measures which will be able to improve the life expectancy of our patients.

References

1. Abraham J, Chandy J (1963) Ventriculo-atrial shunt in the management of posterior fossa tumors. J Neurosurg 20: 252–253
2. Adams H, Graham DI, Doyle D (1981) Brain biopsy. The smear technique for neurosurgical biopsies. Chapman & Hall, London
3. Agnoli I, Eggert HR, Zierski J, Seeger W, Kirchhoff D (1975) Diagnostische Möglichkeiten der positiven Ventrikulographie. Acta Neurochir (Wien) 31: 227–243
4. Albright AL 1984) The value of precraniotomy shunts in children with posterior fossa tumors. Clin Neurosurg 30: 278–285
5. Altenburg H, Walter W (1982) Die zentrale Ventrikulographie. In: Gund A, Koos W (Hrsg) Der Hirnstammtumor. G Thieme, Stuttgart
6. Altenburg H, Brandt M, König H-J (1982) Ventriculography as a diagnostic procedure in CNS tumors in childhood: Its indications and interpretations. In: Voth D, Gutjahr P, Langmaid C (eds) Tumours of the central nervous system in infancy and childhood. Springer, Berlin Heidelberg New York, pp 145–148
7. Ambrose J (1974) Computerized X-ray scanning of the brain. J Neurosurg 40: 679–684
8. Arnold H, Laas R (1980) Die Ursache der Plateauwellen: Kompression der sinusnahen Brückenabschnitte. Adv Neurosurg 9: 351–354
9. Ascher PW, Heppner F (1984) CO_2-laser in neurosurgery. Neurosurg Rev 7: 123–133
10. Barber C (ed) (1980) Evoked potentials. MTP Press, Baltimore
11. Bartal AD (1973) Extensive resection of primary malignant tumours of the left cerebral hemisphere. Surg Neurol 1: 337–342
12. Bauer R, Lauer O, Moerike K, Bauer U (1984) NMR-Tomographie des Kopfes, 1. Aufl.
13. Beck OJ (1984) Use of the Nd-YAG laser in neurosurgery. Neurosurg Rev 7: 151–158
14. Beks JWF, Journee HL, Albarda S, Flanderijn H (1976) The significance of ICP-monitoring in the post-operative period. In: Beks JWF, Bosch D, Brock M (eds) Intracranial pressure III. Springer, Berlin Heidelberg New York, pp 251–254

15. Beks JWF, Albarda S, Gieles ACM, Kuypers MH, Flanderijn H (1977) Extradural transducer for monitoring intracranial pressure. Acta Neurochir (Wien) 38: 245–250
16. Bennett AH, Godlee RJ (1884) Case of cerebral tumour. Lancet ii: 1090
17. Bleyer WA, Pizzo PhA, Spence AM, Platt WD, Benjamin DR, *et al.* (1978) The Ommaya-reservoir. Newly recognized complications and recommendations for insertion and use. Cancer 41: 2431–2437
18. Brachmann J, Fried H (1984) Die zentrale Ventrikulographie — Prä- und postoperative Befunde bei Tumoren des 4. Ventrikels. Zbl Neurochir 44: 267–273
19. Bradac GB, Simon RS, Grumme T, Schramm J (1977) Limitations of computed tomography for diagnostic neuroradiology. Neuroradiol 13: 243–247
20. Brawanski A, Gaab M (1980) Intracranial pressure gradients in the presence of various intracranial space-occupying lesions. Adv Neurosurg 9: 355–362
21. Brock M, Schmitz H-J (1982) The significance of continuous recording of intracranial pressure in children with brain tumours. In: Voth D, Gutjahr P, Langmaid C (eds) Tumours of the central nervous system in infancy and childhood. Springer, Berlin Heidelberg New York, pp 218–221
22. Brock M, Ingwersen I, Roggendorf W (1984) Ultrasonic aspiration in neurosurgery. Neurosurg Rev 7: 173–177
23. Bucy PC (1975) Treatment of supratentorial gliomas. In: Hekmatpanah J (ed) Gliomas—current concepts in histology, diagnosis and therapy. Springer, Berlin Heidelberg New York
24. Cail WS, Morris JL (1979) Localization of intracranial lesions from CT scans. Surg Neurol 11: 35–37
25. Caille JM, Salamon G (1980) Computerized tomography. Springer, Berlin Heidelberg New York
26. Chatel M, Menault F (1981) Bases biologiques des stratégies thérapeutiques des gliomes malins. Données oncologiques générales, place des moyens actuels et résultats, perspectives. Neurochir (Paris) 27: 299–303
27. Cronqvist S (1976) Ventriculography with amipaque. Neuroradiol 12: 25–32
28. Dandy WE (1969) The diagnosis and treatment of hydrocephalus resulting from structures of the aqueduct of Sylvius. Surg Gyn Obstet 31: 701–704
29. Diamond RD, Bennett JE (1974) A subcutaneous reservoir for intrathecal therapy of fungal meningitis. New Engl J Med 288: 186–188
30. Dietz H, Umbach W, Wüllenweber E (eds) (1982) Klinische Neurochirurgie. G Thieme Stuttgart New York
31. Dorsch NWC, Symon L (1975) A practical technique for monitoring extradural pressure. J Neurosurg 42: 249–257
32. Eggert HR, Gilsbach J, Sprich M, Schandelmaier C (1985) Quality of life following microsurgical removal of glioblastomas. In: Voth D, Krauseneck P (eds) Chemotherapy of gliomas. De Gruyter, Berlin New York, pp 215–217
33. Ehni G (1984) Interhemispheric and percallosal (transcallosal) approach to the cingulate gyri, intraventricular shunt tubes and certain deeply placed brain lesions. Neurosurgery 14: 99–100
34. Elke M, Wiggli U, Hünig R (1977) Praktische Gesichtspunkte zur Diagnose intracranieller Tumoren durch die Computertomographie. Radiologie 17: 157–170
35. Elvidge AR (1966) Treatment of obstructive lesions of the aqueduct of Sylvius by interventriculostomy. J Neurosurg 24: 11–23
36. Espaza J, Manrique A, Lobato RD (1980) Simultaneous epidural and intraventricular pressure measurement during the occurrence of supratentorial expanding lesions. In: Staubman K, Marmarou A, Mitter JD (eds) Intracranial pressure IV. Springer, Berlin Heidelberg New York, pp 377–380

37. Fitz CR, Harwood-Nash DC, Chuang S, Resjo IM (1978) Metrizamide ventriculography and computed tomography in infants and children. Neuroradiol 16: 6–9

38. Flamm ES, Ransohoff J, Wuchinich D (1978) Preliminary experience with ultrasonic aspiration in neurosurgery. Neurosurgery 2: 240–245

39. Fox JL (1967) Intermittend drainage of intracranial cyst via subcutaneous Ommaya reservoir. J Neurosurg 27: 272–273

40. Fox PT, Raichler ME (1984) Stimulus rate dependence of regional cerebral blood flow in human striate cortex, demonstrated by positron emission tomography. J Neurophysiol 51: 1109–1120

41. Frackowiak RJS, Lenzi GL, Jones T, Heather JD (1980) Quantitative measurement of regional cerebral blood flow and oxygen metabolism in man using ^{15}O and positron emission tomograph: Theory, procedure, and normal values. J Comput Assist Tomogr 4: 727–736

42. Fridman J, Zapulla R, Bergelson M, Greenblatt E, Malis L (1984) Morrell F, Hoeppner T (1984) Application of phase spectral analysis for brain stem auditory evoked potential detection in normal subjects and patients with posterior fossa tumors. Audiology 23: 99–113

43. Fuchs EL (1978) Quantitative CSF drainage in cases of posterior fossa tumors. Adv Neurosurg 5: 211–215

44. Gaab M, Knoblich OE, Dietrich K (1979) Miniaturisierte Methoden zur Überwachung des intrakraniellen Druckes. Techniken und klinische Ergebnisse. Langenbecks Arch Chir 350: 13–31

45. Galicich JH, Guido LJ (1974) Ommaya device in carcinomatous and leukemic meningitis. Surg Clin North Am 54: 915–922

46. Geffen G (1980) Comparison of the effects of transcortical and transcallosal removal of intraventricular tumours. Brain 103: 773–788

47. Gobiet W, Bock WJ, Liesegang J, et al. (1972) Longtime monitoring of epidural pressure in man. In: Brock M, Dietz H (eds) Intracranial pressure: experimental and clinical aspects. Springer, Berlin Heidelberg New York, pp 14–17

48. Goedhart ZD, Hekster REM, Matricali B (1978) Neurosurgical and neurological applications of the Ommaya reservoir system. Adv Neurosurg 6: 45–47

49. Goldhahn W-E, Goldhahn G (1978) Hirntumoren. A Barth, Leipzig

50. Greenberg RP, Ducker ThB (1982) Evoked potentials in the clinical neurosciences. J Neurosurg 56: 1–18

51. Greenwood J (1940) Two point coagulation. A new principle and instrument for applying current in neurosurgery. Am J Surg 50: 267–270

52. Grote E, Zierski J, Klinger M, Grohmann G, Markakis E (1978) Complications following ventriculo-cisternal shunts. Adv Neurosurg 6: 10–16

53. Grundy BL, Jannetta PJ, Procopio PT, Lina A, et al. (1982) Intraoperative monitoring of brain stem auditory evoked potentials. J Neurosurg 57: 674–681

54. Guillaume J, Janny P (1951) Manométrie intracranienne continue. Intérêt de la méthode et premiers résultats. Rev Neurolog (Paris) 84: 131–142

55. Gullotta F, Bettag W (1967) Long survival in glioblastoma. Acta Neurochir (Wien) 16: 122–128

56. Gutjahr P, Voth D, Neidhardt M (1978) Ergebnisse der kombinierten Behandlung (Operation, Radio- und Chemotherapie) bei 132 Kindern mit primären ZNS-Tumoren. Therapiewoche 28: 4346–4352

57. Gutjahr P, Voth D (1979) Treatment and prognosis of childhood brain tumours: experience with 140 cases. Verhdlg Deutsch Krebsges 2: 434–435

58. Gutjahr P, Voth D, Heidfeld J, Walther B, Kutzner J (1982) Infratentorial tumours—treatment and results in 109 children. In: Voth D, Gutjahr P, Langmaid C (eds) Tumours of the central nervous system in infancy and childhood. Springer, Berlin Heidelberg New York, pp 358–364

59. Gutjahr P, Freitag-Rozek H, Voth D (1982) Riesenzellastrozytom bei tuberöser Sklerose (Epiloia). Kinderarzt 13: 165–169

60. Habermehl A, Graul EH (1982) Kernspinresonanz-Tomographie. Dtsch Ärztebl 79: 17–29

61. Handa H, Takeuchi J, Yamagami T (1984) Nd-YAG-laser as a surgical tool. Neurosurg Rev 7: 159–163

62. Harnoss B-M (1978) Perioperative Antibiotika-Prophylaxe in der Chirurgie. Med Klinik: 205–208

63. Hassler W, Seeger W (1978) Microsurgery of tumors of the frontal white matter. Acta Neurochir (Wien) 44: 11–47

64. Hassler W, Gilsbach J, Birg W, Eggert H-R, Seeger W (1982) Computer tomographic findings of brain tumors projected on X-rays and scalp. Adv Neurosurg 10: 11–15

65. Hassler W, Harders A, Seeger W (1985) Microsurgical management of gliomas. In: Voth D, Krauseneck P (eds) Chemotherapy of gliomas. De Gruyter, Berlin New York, pp 177–188

66. Heiss WD, Pawlik G, Herholz K, Wagner R, Goldner H, Wienhard K (1984) Regional kinetic constants and cerebral metabolic rate for glucose in normal human volunteers determined by dynamic positron emission tomography of 18 F-2 Fluoro-2-deoxy-D-glucose. J Cereb Blood Flow Metab 4: 213–223

67. Hekmatpanah J, Mullan S (1967) Ventriculocaval shunt in management of posterior fossa tumours. J Neurosurg 26: 609–613

68. Hemmer R, Haensel-Friedrich G, Friedrich H (1977) The value of pre-operative shunt in posterior fossa tumours. Mod Probl Paediat 18: 48–50

69. Herholz K, Pawlik G, Wagner R, Wienhard K, Heiss WD (1984) Determination of regional glucose metabolism in patients with ischaemic infarct by positron emission tomography. In: Voth D, Glees P (eds) Cerebral vascular spasm. De Gruyter, Berlin New York, pp 315–332

70. Hinck V, Clifton GV (1981) A precise technique for craniotomy localization using computerized tomography. J Neurosurg 54: 416–418

71. Hoffmann HJ, Hendrick EB, Humphrey RP (1976) Metastasis via ventriculoperitoneal shunt in patient with medulloblastoma. J Neurosurg 44: 562–566

72. Hoffmann HJ, Hendrick EB, Humphrey RP (1983) Management of medulloblastoma in childhood. Clin Neurosurg 30: 226–245

73. Hounsfield GN (1973) Computerized transverse axial scaning (tomography). Part I. Description of the system. Brit J Radiol 46: 1016–1022

74. Huang S-C, Phelps ME, Hoffman EJ, Sideris K, et al. (1980) Noninvasive determination of local cerebral metabolic rate of glucose in man. Am J Physiol 238: E 69–E 82

75. Ingraham FD, Campell JB (1941) An apparatus for closed drainage of the ventricular system. Ann Surg 114: 1096–1098

76. Ito M, Lammertsma AA, Wise RJS, Frackowiak RSJ, et al. (1982) Measurement of regional cerebral blood flow and oxygen utilization in patients with cerebral tumours using ^{15}O and positron emission tomography: Analytical techniques and preliminary results. Neuroradiol 23: 63–74

77. Jane JA, Kaufman B, Nulsen F (1975) The role of angiography and ventriculovenous shunting in the treatment of posterior fossa tumours. Acta Neurochir (Wien) 28: 13–28

78. Jelsma R, Bucy PC (1967) The treatment of glioblastoma multiforme of the brain. J Neurosurg 27: 388–400

79. Kazner E, Wende S, Grumme Th, Lanksch W, Stochdorph O (1981) Computertomographie intrakranieller Tumoren aus klinischer Sicht. Springer, Berlin Heidelberg New York

80. Kazner E, Kretzschmar K (1982) Computer tomographic diagnosis of CNS tumours in childhood. In: Voth D, Gutjahr P, Langmaid C (eds) Tumours of the central nervous system in infancy and childhood. Springer, Berlin Heidelberg New York, pp 115–121

81. Kelman CD (1969) Phaco-emulsification and aspiration. A progress report. Am J Ophthalmol 67: 464–477

82. Kempe LG (1968/70) Operative neurosurgery. Springer, Berlin Heidelberg New York

83. Kessler LA, Dugan P, Concannon JP (1975) Systemic metastases of medulloblastoma promoted by shunting. Surg Neurol 3: 147–152

84. Kessel G, Schwarz M, Voth D (1985) The Ommaya reservoir and its significance for intrathecal cytostatic treatment. Surgical aspects and complications. In: Voth D, Krauseneck P (eds) Chemotherapy of gliomas. De Gruyter, Berlin New York, pp 209–212

85. Kiessling M, Anagnostopoulos J, Lombeck G, Kleihues P (1982) Diagnostic potential of stereotactic biopsy of brain tumours. A report of 400 cases. In: Voth D, Gutjahr P, Langmaid C (eds) Tumours of the central nervous system in infancy and childhood. Springer, Berlin Heidelberg New York, pp 247–256

86. Klein F (1984) Möller UNIVERSAL operation unit. Neurosurg Rev 7: 99–102

87. Kluge W, Sprung C (1982) Has computed tomography led to earlier diagnosis of brain tumors? Adv Neurosurg 10: 3–6

88. Konovalov AN (1984) Microsurgery of tumours of diencephalic region. Neurosurg Rev 6: 37–41

89. Koos W, Böck FW, Spetzler RF (1976) Clinical microneurosurgery. Stuttgart: Thieme

90. Krampe C (1984) Zeiss operating microscopes for neurosurgery. Neurosurg Rev 7: 89–97

91. Krauseneck P, Mertens HG (1983) Therapie maligner Neoplasien des Gehirns. Perimed, Erlangen

92. Kretzschmar K, Aulich A, Schindler E, Lange S, et al. (1978) The diagnostic value of CT for radiotherapy of cerebral tumours. Neuroradiol 14: 245–250

93. Kunze St (1977) Ventrikulographie mit positiven Kontrastmitteln. In: Diethelm L, Wende S (Hrsg) Handbuch med Radiologie XIV/2. Springer, Berlin Heidelberg New York

94. Kutzner J, Gutjahr P, Voth D, Kretzschmar K (1979) Schädelkalotten-Nekrose bei gleichzeitiger Strahlen-Chemotherapie mit Ommaya-Reservoir. In: Wannemacher M, Gauwerky F, Streffer Ch (Hrsg) Kombinierte Strahlen- und Chemotherapie. Urban & Schwarzenberg, München Wien Baltimore, S 177–179

95. Lamers JM (1983) Clinical and diagnostic appearance of tumors of the posterior fossa in childhood: results of a retrospective cooperative study. Adv Neurosurg 11: 175–180

96. Lammertsa A (1984) Positron emission tomography of the brain: Measurement of regional cerebral function in man. Clin Neurol Neurosurg 86: 1–11

97. Land WH, Muchel F (1981) Zeiss microscopes for microsurgery. Springer, Berlin Heidelberg New York

98. Lanksch W, Kazner E (1976) Cranial computerized tomography. Springer, Berlin Heidelberg New York

99. Lapras C, Poirier N, Deruty R, Bret P, Joyeux O (1975) Le cathétérisme de l'àqueduct de Sylvius. Neuro-Chir 21: 101–109

100. Leenders KL, Thomas DGT, Beaney RP, Brooks DJ (1985) Cerebral gliomas studied with positron emission tomography. In: Voth D, Krauseneck P (eds) Chemotherapy of gliomas. De Gruyter, Berlin New York, pp 101–110

101. Leksell L (1984) A surgical procedure for atresia of the aqueduct of Sylvius. Acta psychiatr (København) 24: 559–568
102. Leonardi M, Cecetto C, Fabris G (1977) Corrales selective ventriculography in the study of posterior fossa pathology. J Neurosurg Sci 21: 65–70
103. Levin AB (1977) The use of a fibre-optic intracranial pressure monitor in clinicl practice. Neurosurgery 1: 266–271
104. Lorenz R (1966) Komplikationen nach Torkildsen-Drainagen. Acta Neurochir (Wien) 14: 246–253
105. Lumenta CB, Krämer M, Bock WJ, Lappe M, Link A (1960) Brain stem auditory evoked potentials (BAEP) during and after posterior fossa operations. Adv Neurosurg 12: 247–252
106. Lundberg N (1960) Continuous recording and control of fluid pressure in neurosurgical practice. Acta Psych Neurol Scand [suppl] 149: 1–193
107. MacCarthy CS (1955) Surgical treatment of gliomas of the brain. J Internat Coll Surg 23: 290–297
108. Mahlmann E, Schwarz M, Voth D (1982) The "isolated fourth ventricle": Review of current concepts and report of three cases in children. In: Voth D, Gutjahr P, Langmaid D (eds) Tumours of the central nervous system in infancy and childhood. Springer, Berlin Heidelberg New York, pp 180–185
109. Mahlmann E, Kessel G, Voth D, Schwarz M, Kühnert A (1986) The significance of NMR-tomography for the treatment of supra- and infratentorial midline tumours. Neuropaediatrics 15—in press
110. Malis LI (1967) Bipolar coagulation in microsurgery. In: Donaghy RMP, Yaşargil MG (eds) Microvascular surgery. G Thieme, Stuttgart, pp 126–130
111. Mauersberger W (1985) Correlation between grade of malignancy of gliomas and their computer tomographic density values. In: Voth D, Krauseneck P (eds) Chemotherapy of gliomas. De Gruyter, Berlin New York, pp 95–99
112. Maurer K, Rochel M (1984) Early auditory evoked potentials (EAEP) in children with neoplastic lesions in the brain stem. In: Voth D, Gutjahr P, Langmaid C (eds) Tumours of the central nervous system in infancy and childhood. Springer, Berlin Heidelberg New York, pp 99–104
113. Maurer K, Rochel M, Gutjahr P, Voth D (1983) Early auditory evoked potentials (EAEP) in neurosurgery—A new method for diagnosis and location of posterior fossa tumors in childhood. Adv Neurosurg 11: 238–244
114. Merrem B (1970) Die Ventrikeldrainage. Zbl Neurochir 31: 127–148
115. Merrem G, Goldhahn W-E (1982) Neurochirurgische Operationen, 2nd edn. Springer, Berlin Heidelberg New York
116. Mindermann Th, Gruber UF (1984) Bei welchen Operationen wird eine Antibiotika-Prophylaxe mit nur einer Dosis durchgeführt? Fortschr Med 10: 253–259
117. Münch F, van Deyk K, Rinker D, Epple E, Junger H (1982) Clinical application of computer assisted continuous monitoring of intracranial pressure. Adv Neurosurg 10: 378–381
118. Müntener J (1984) Surgical operating microscopes. Series M 600 from WILD Heerbrugg Ltd. Neurosurg Rev 7: 103–107
119. Mundinger F (1982) CT-stereotactic biopsy of brain tumours. In: Voth D, Gutjahr P, Langmaid C (eds) Tumours of the central nervous system in infancy and childhood. Springer, Berlin Heidelberg New York, pp 234–246
120. Mundinger F, Weigel K (1985) CT-stereotactic interstitial irradiation therapy of nonresectable and recurrent intracranial tumour in children and adolescents. In: Voth D, Krauseneck P (eds) Chemotherapy of gliomas. De Gruyter, Berlin New York, pp 241–259

121. Nadjmi M, Piepgras U, Vogelsang H (1981) Kranielle Computertomographie. G Thieme, New York

122. Neuwelt EA, Glasberg M, Frenkel E, Clark WK (1979) Malignant pineal region tumors. J Neurosurg 51: 597–607

123. Norlen G (1949) Contribution to the surgical treatment of inoperable tumors, causing obstruction of the Sylvian aqueduct. Acta Psychiatr (København) 24: 629–637

124. Obrador S, Soto M, Gutierrez-Diaz JA (1976) Surgical management of the tumors of the pineal region. Acta Neurochir (Wien) 34: 159–170

125. Olivecrona H (1967) The surgical treatment of intracranial tumours. In: Olivecrona H, Tönnis W (eds) Handbuch der Neurochirurgie, vol IV. Springer, Berlin Heidelberg New York, pp 1–301

126. Ommaya AK (1963) Subcutaneous reservoir and pump for sterile access to ventricular cerebrospinal fluid. Lancet ii: 983–984

127. Oppenheim H (1902) Die Geschwülste des Gehirns, 2. Aufl. A Hölder, Wien

128. Oppenheim H, Krause F (1913) Operativer Erfolg bei Geschwülsten der Sehhügel- und Vierhügelgegend. Berl Klin Wschr 50: 2316–2321

129. Page LK (1977) The infratentorial-supracerebellar exposure of tumors in the pineal area. Neurosurgery 1: 36–43

130. Pampus F (1953) Zur Technik der Ventrikeldrainage. Zbl Neurochir 13: 219–223

131. Pecker J, Scarabin JM, Brücher JM, Vallée B (1979) Démarche stéréotaxique en neurochirurgie tumorale. Rennes

132. Pecker J, Scarabin JM, Dekkiche M, et al (1981) Place de la chirurgie dans le traitment des gliomes malins supratentoriels. Neurochir (Paris) 27: 287–293

133. Pendl G, Koos WTh (1983) Infratentorial-supracerebellar approach to the pineal and mesencephalic region in children. Adv Neurosurg 11: 263–269

134. Pobloth A, Jörg J, Kass W (1985) EEG, SEP, VEP examinations during the treatment of malignant gliomas. In: Voth D, Krauseneck P (eds) Chemotherapy of gliomas. De Gruyter, Berlin New York, pp 135–137

135. Pöll W, v Waldhausen W, Brock M (1980) Infection rate of continuous monitoring of ventricular fluid pressure with and without open cerebro-spinal fluid drainage. Adv Neurosurg 9: 363–366

136. Poppen JL (1943) Ventricular drainage as a valuable procedure in neurosurgery. Report of a satisfactory method. Arch Neurol Psychiat 50: 587–589

137. Raimondi AJ, Gutierrez FA (1975) Diagnosis and surgical treatment of choroid plexus papillomas. Childs Brain 1: 81–115

138. Rand RW (1978) Microneurosurgery, 2nd edn. Mosby, St Louis

139. Ransohoff J, Lieberman A (1978) Surgical therapy of primary malignant brain tumors. Clin Neurosurg 25: 403–411

140. Ratcheson RA, Ommaya AK (1968) Experience with the subcutaneous CSF reservoir. New Engl J Med 279: 1025–1031

141. Raudzens PA, Shetter AG (1981) Intraoperative monitoring of brain stem auditory evoked potentials. J Neurosurg 57: 341–348

142. Ray BS (1964) Surgery of recurrent intracranial tumors. Clin Neurosurg 10: 1–30

143. Regan D (1972) Evoked potentials in psychology, sensory physiology and clinical medicine. Chapman Hall, London

144. Richard KE (1977) Liquorventrikeldruckmessung mit Mikrokatheter und druck-kontrollierte externe Liquordrainage. Acta Neurochir (Wien) 38: 73–87

145. Richard KE (1978) Long-term measuring of ventricular CSF pressure with tumours of the posterior fossa. Adv Neurosurg 5: 179–183

146. Richard KE, Heller R, Frowein RA (1982) Internal shunt of perioperative pressure-controlled ventricular fluid drainage (C-VFD) in children and juveniles with in-

fratentorial tumours. In: Voth D, Gutjahr P, Langmaid (eds) Tumours of the central nervous system in infancy and childhood. Springer, Berlin Heidelberg New York, pp 257–264

147. Richard KE, Günther H, Eickschen M, Hahn G (1983) Externe Liquor-Langzeitdrainage beim posthämorrhagischen Hydrozephalus des Frühgeborenen. In: Voth D (Hrsg) Hydrocephalus im frühen Kindesalter. Enke, Stuttgart, S 181–186

148. Richard KE, Rabebold K (1985) Intracranial pressure monitoring in postoperative treatment of supratentorial and infratentorial gliomas (brief communication). In: Voth P, Krauseneck P (eds) Chemotherapy of gliomas. De Gruyter, Berlin New York, pp 133–134

149. Roosen K, Havers W, Schaaf J (1982) Indications and experiences with the Ommaya-reservoir for treatment of CNS neoplasms in childhood. In: Voth D, Gutjahr P, Langmaid C (eds) Tumours of the central nervous system in infancy and childhood. Springer, Berlin Heidelberg New York, pp 265–269

150. Rout, D, Sharma A, Radhakrishnan VV, Rao VR (1984) Exploration of the pineal region: observations and results. Surg Neurol 21: 135–140

151. Sano K, Matsutani M (1983) Microsurgery of teratoma and germinoma involving the diencephalon and the brain stem. Neurosurg Rev 6: 51–55

152. Schaltenbrand G, Walker AE (1982) Stereotaxy of the human brain, 2nd edn. G Thieme, Stuttgart New York

153. Schürmann K, Voth D (1975) Neurochirurgie. In: Baumgartl F, Kremer K, Schreiber HW (Hrsg) Spezielle Chirurgie für die Praxis, Bd I/2. G Thieme, Stuttgart, S 831–1019

154. Schwarz M, Voth D (1982) Palliative operations: internal shunt, ventricular fluid drainage, ventriculo-cisternostomy (Torkildsen) and interventriculostomy (Leksell). In: Voth D, Gutjahr P, Langmaid C (eds) Tumours of the central nervous system in infancy and childhood. Springer, Berlin Heidelberg New York, pp 214–217

155. Schwarz M, Keßel G, Voth D (1983) Über die Bedeutung der intraventrikulären Druckmessung im Rahmen der Diagnostik des Hydrocephalus internus. In: Voth D, Gutjahr P, Glees P (Hrsg) Hydrocephalus im frühen Kindesalter. Enke, Stuttgart New York, S 105–111

156. Schwarz M, Keßel G, Mahlmann E, Voth D (1985) Measurement of intracranial pressure. Techniques and indications. In: Voth D, Krauseneck P (eds) Chemotherapy of gliomas. De Gruyter, Berlin New York, pp 124–132

157. Seeger W (1980) Microsurgery of the brain, vol 1 and 2. Springer, Wien New York

158. Siesjo BK (1984) Cerebral circulation and metabolism. J Neurosurg 60: 883–908

159. Stein BM (1979) The infratentorial supracerebellar approach to pineal lesions. J Neurosurg 35: 197–203

160. Stockard JJ, Rossiter US (1977) Clinical and pathological correlates of brain stem auditory response abnormalities. Neurology 27: 316–325

161. Symon L, Wang AD, Costa e Silva IE, Gentili F (1984) Perioperative use of somatosensory evoked responses in aneurysm surgery. J Neurosurg 60: 269–275

162. Takeuchi K (1984) Natural history of gliomas. Neurochir (Stuttg) 26: 42–46

163. Takizawa T (1984) The carbon dioxide laser surgical unit as an instrument for surgery of brain tumours—its advantages and disadvantages. Neurosurg Rev 7: 135–144

164. Thomas DGT, Graham DI (1980) Brain tumours—scientific basis, clinical investigation and current therapy. Butterworths, London

165. Torkildsen A (1939) A new palliative procedure in cases of inoperable occlusion of the Sylvian ductus. Acta Chir Scand 82: 177–185

166. Vällfors B, Bergdahl B (1984) Automatically controlled bipolar electrocoagulation—"COA-COMP". Neurosurg Rev 7: 187–190

167. Virchow R (1863–1867) Die krankhaften Geschwülste, Bd 3. Hirschwald, Berlin

168. Voth D (1974) Antibiotika in der Praxis—Neurochirurgie. In: Frey R (Hrsg) Antibiotika in der Praxis. Aesopus, Lugano München, S 213–222

169. Voth D, Nakayama N (1976) Ein neues ventilgesteuertes System für die präliminare Ventrikeldrainage (technische Beschreibung und klinische Erfahrungen). Neurochir (Stuttg) 19: 196–201

170. Voth D, Hey O, Nakayama N, Emmrich P (1977) Die kontinuierliche Registrierung des intrakraniellen Druckes (intraventrikuläre Messung) im Rahmen der pädiatrischen Intensivmedizin. In: Emmrich P (Hrsg) Pädiatrische Intensivmedizin. G Thieme, Stuttgart, S 104–109

171. Voth D (1981) New aspects on antibiotic therapy in neurological surgery. In: Dietz H, Metzel E, Langmaid C (eds) Neurological surgery. G Thieme, Stuttgart New York, pp 326–330

172. Voth D, Gutjahr P, Langmaid C (1982) Tumours of the central nervous system in infancy and childhood. Springer, Berlin Heidelberg New York

173. Voth D, Schürmann K, Schwarz M (1982) Ventriculocisternostomy by the method of Leksell—indications, technique and results. In: Voth D, Gutjahr P, Langmaid C (eds) Tumours of the central nervous system in infancy and childhood. Springer, Berlin Heidelberg New York, pp 283–288

174. Voth D, Schwarz M, Hüwel N, Mahlmann E (1982) Shunt therapy in medulloblastoma? Adv Neurosurg 10: 348–356

175. Voth D, Schwarz M (1982) New light on the technique and indication for ventriculocisternal drainage according to Leksell (interventriculostomy). Neurosurg Rev 4: 179–184

176. Voth D (1982) Standard methods and microneurosurgery: The operative treatment of supra- and infratentorial tumours. In: Voth D, Gutjahr P, Langmaid C (eds) Tumours of the central nervous system in infancy and childhood. Springer, Berlin Heidelberg New York, pp 199–213

177. Voth D (1983) Perioperative prevention of infection with antibiotics in neurosurgery. In: Proc 13. Internat Congr Chemotherapy, part 9. Wien

178. Voth D, Gutjahr P, Glees P (1983) Hydrocephalus im frühen Kindesalter. Enke, Stuttgart

179. Voth D, Krauseneck P (1985) Chemotherapy of gliomas. De Gruyter, Berlin New York

180. Voth D (1985) Perioperative prevention of infection in neurosurgery. In: Antibiotics and chemotherapy, vol 33. Karger, Basel, pp 1–19

181. Wackenheim A, Jeanmart L, Baert AL (1980) Craniocerebral computer tomography. Springer, Berlin Heidelberg New York

182. Wende S, Aulich A, Kretzschmar K, Grumme Th, Meese W, et al. (1977) Die Computertomographie der Hirngeschwülste. Eine Sammelstudie über 1658 Tumoren. Radiologie 17: 149–156

183. Wernicke C, Hahn R (1982) Idiopathischer Abszeß des Occipitallappens, durch Operation entleert. Virchows Arch Path Anat 87: 335–344

184. Wolf AP (1981) Special characteristics and potential for radiopharmaceuticals for positron emission tomography. Sem Nuclear Med 2: 2–12

185. Yaşargil MG (1969) Microsurgery. G Thieme, Stuttgart

186. Youmans JR (1973) Neurological surgery. Saunders, Philadelphia London Toronto

187. Young B (1981) Reoperation for glioblastoma. J Neurosurg 55: 917–921

188. Zeitler E (1985) Kernspintomographie. Deutscher Ärzte-Verlag, Köln

Author's address: Prof. Dr. D. Voth, Neurochirurgische Universitätsklinik, Langenbeckstrasse 1, D-6500 Mainz, Federal Republic of Germany.

3

Neurosurgical Interventions for Intracranial Metastases

D. Voth

Department of Neurosurgery, University of Mainz School of Medicine,
Mainz, Federal Republic of Germany

Introduction

In any neurosurgical material among the space-occupying neoplastic lesions in the brain there is an average frequency between 3 and 5% of deposits from malignant tumors of extracranial origin, *i.e.* metastases[1, 2, 7]. Definite regularities exist as regards the frequency with which particular tumors give rise to cerebral metastases and likewise as regards the incidence of solitary metastases (about 50% of cases), while in about a half of these patients we find several metastases. These lesions can involve the cerebral hemispheres, as well as the cerebellum and the brain stem[26, 28].

Data on the Morbidity

In the large series of cases, for instance those of Bushe[3, 4], Penzholz[16, 17], Vieth and Odom[27], as well as from Simionescu[23] opinions are fairly uniform about the absence of any sex predominance and of an incidence predominantly between the ages of 50 and 60 years[10–12]. In all the large series analysed the most frequent primary tumor was *bronchial carcinoma*[14, 15] with an incidence of between 27.5 and 40%; only in the paper of Störtebecker[24] are renal and adrenal tumors said to be the most frequent. The second most frequent are metastases from *carcinoma of the breast* (10–22.6%), followed by deposits from *hypernephroma* (7.0–8.5%). All other lesions are definitely less frequent, including the whole spectrum from carcinomas of the gastro-intestinal tract to skin tumors, especially the melanomas[6], and the not insignificant group with an unrecognized or not detectable, primary tumor (11.8–14%) (see Jellinger, this volume).

The *clinical symptoms* correspond to those of a rapidly progressive cerebral lesion, without however showing any specific features[5, 18]. As regards the *diagnosis*, the relevant chapter of this book may be referred to.

Indications for Operation

Corresponding to the opinions of other authors we only consider there is a definite indication for the removal of the metastasis: 1st, if it is a solitary lesion, 2nd, if the primary tumor is accessible to treatment, or 3rdly, if the above is not or is only conditionally the case, if the cerebral metastasis is limiting the expectation of life.

While multiple metastases provide a clear contraindication to any operative treatment, it can, for instance, be approved in the case of a solitary metastasis when there is an unrecognized or not detectable primary tumor, if the cerebral symptoms compel some urgency. If the primary tumor is recognized and is accessible to treatment the indication for a cerebral operation can likewise be approved. If the primary tumor is recognized but is untreatable the neurosurgeon must decide what is the life-expectation from the point of view of the primary lesion. If this time is definitely and seriously reduced by the solitary metastasis, one should, in general decide to operate on the intracranial space-occupying lesion.

In some cases the decision about operating is by no means easy and should be given very careful consideration.

Operative Technique

Special descriptions are not necessary here, as basically the same procedures are employed as for intrinsic brain tumors[20]. Nevertheless one must frequently be satisfied with an excision of the metastasis with the aid of the ultrasound unit (CUSA). The discovery of smaller metastases can from time to time be facilitated by means of intraoperative sonography (Fig. 1). It is also necessary to take not of other

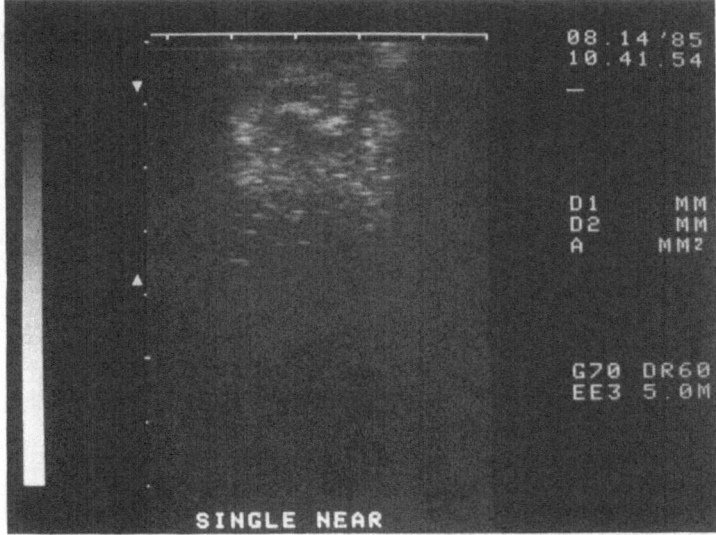

Fig. 1. Discovery of a small metastasis with central necrosis by means of intraoperative sonography

criteria, in respect of functionally important areas and their protection, and finally, also the endeavor to do as radical a removal of the metastasis as possible, with an adequate margin of safety into healthy tissue.

Results of Operation

Essentially the prognosis is less favorable, on the one hand because of the basic condition and, on the other, through the possibility of intracerebral recurrences and the possible appearance after an operation of further deposits, not previously apparent[8, 9, 13, 19].

In spite of this, in large series the patients survive longer in general, than without an operation[21, 22, 25, 29, 30].

Furthermore, in the paper by Vieth and Odom[27], for instance, 13.5% of the patients are still living after one year and a good 3% survive for up to ten years.

Against the background of the absolutely hopeless prognosis in the absence of any intracranial intervention, these figures should encourage an active policy, especially with improved treatment of the primary tumor, and even in the longer term more favorable results seem possible to achieve.

References

1. Black P (1979) Brain metastasis: Current status and recommended guide-lines for management. Neurosurgery 5: 617–631
2. Bremer AM, West CR, Didolkar MS (1978) An evaluation of the surgical management of melanoma of the brain. J Surg Oncol 10: 211–219
3. Bushe K-A (1972) Intrakranielle Metastasen. Langenbecks Arch Chir 332: 369–375
4. Bushe K-A (1983) Operative Therape. In: Krauseneck P, Mertens HG (Hrsg) Therapie maligner Neoplasien des Gehirns. Perimed, Erlangen, S 29–33
5. Capon A, Hildebrand J, Verbist J, Frühling J, Baleriaux D (1976) Changes in regional blood flow produced by dexamethasone in patients with brain metastases. Acta Neurol Belg 76: 325–330
6. Fell DA, Leavens ME, McBride ChM (1980) Surgical versus non-surgical management of metastatic melanoma of the brain. Neurosurgery 7: 238–242
7. French LA, Ausman JI (1977) Metastatic neoplasma to the brain. Clin Neurosurg 24: 41–46
8. Galicich JH, Sundaresan N, Arbit E, Passe S (1980) Surgical treatment of single brain metastases: factors associated with survival. Cancer 45: 381–386
9. Haar F, Patterson RH jr (1972) Surgery for metastatic intracranial neoplasms. Cancer 30: 1241–1245
10. Heimpel H, Herfarth C, Schreml W (eds) (1980) Metastasen. Huber, Bern Stuttgart Wien
11. Jänisch W, Günthert H, Schreiber D (1976) Pathologie der Tumoren des Zentralnervensystems. Fischer, Jena
12. Karrer K, Fleischmann E, Hochpöchler F (1984) Site of the primary in intracranial metastases. Adv Neurosurg 12: 10–14
13. Lang EF, Slater J (1964) Metastatic brain tumors. Results of surgical and nonsurgical treatment. Surg Clin North Amer 44: 865–872

14. MacGee EE (1971) Surgical treatment of cerebral metastases from lung cancer. J Neurosurg 35: 416–420

15. Magilligan DJ Jr, Rogers JS, Knighton RS, Davila JC (1976) Pulmonary neoplasm with solitary cerebral metastasis. J Thorac Cardiovasc Surg 72: 690–696

16. Penzholz H (1968) Die metastatischen Erkrankungen des Zentralnervensystems bei bösartigen Tumoren. Acta Neurochir (Wien) [suppl] 16

17. Penzholz H (1984) Surgical management of metastatic brain tumors. Adv Neurosurg 12: 3–9

18. Posner JB (1974) Diagnosis and treatment of brain metastases. Clin Bull 4: 47–57

19. Potthoff PC, Keim H (1984) Comparison of radiotherapy alone compared with surgery plus irradiation in two groups of patients with brain metastases. Adv Neurosurg 12: 79–86

20. Ransohoff J (1975) Surgical management of metastatic tumors. Sem Oncol 4: 21–27

21. Raskind R, Weiss SR, Manning JJ, Wermuth RE (1971) Survival after surgical excision of single metastatic brain tumors. Amer J Roentgenol 111: 323–328

22. Schnaberth G, Brunner G (1982) Zerebrale Metastasen als klinische Erstmanifestation eines Karzinoms. Wien Klin Wschr 94: 83–86

23. Simionescu MD (1960) Metastatic tumors of the brain. A follow-up study of 195 patients with neurosurgical considerations. J Neurosurg 17: 361–373

24. Störtebecker TP (1954) Metastatic tumors of the brain from a neurosurgical point of view. A. Follow-up study of 158 cases. J Neurosurg 11: 84–111

25. Tarnoff JF, Calinog TA, Byla JG (1976) Prolonged survival following cerebral metastasis from pulmonary cancer. J Thoracic Cardiovasc Surg 72: 933–937

26. Tornow K, Voigt M (1984) Computer tomographic diagnosis of intracranial metastases. Adv Neurosurg 12: 15–18

27. Vieth RG, Odom GL (1965) Intracranial metastases and their neurosurgical treatment. J Neurosurg 23: 375–383

28. Weiss LG, Gilbert HA, Posner JB (1980) Brain metastasis. G K Hall, Boston

29. Winston KR, Walsh JW, Fischer EG (1980) Results of operative treatment of intracranial metastatic tumors. Cancer 45: 2639–2645

30. Zimm S, Wampler GL, Stablein D, Hazra T, Young HF (1981) Intracerebral metastases in solid-tumor patients: natural history and result of treatment. Cancer 48: 384–394

Author's address: Prof. Dr. D. Voth, Neurochirurgische Universitätsklinik, Langenbeckstrasse 1, D-6500 Mainz, Federal Republic of Germany.

4

Stereotactic Biopsy and Technique of Implantation (Instillation) of Radionuclids

F. Mundinger

Abteilung Stereotaxie und Neuronuklearmedizin, Neurochirurgische Universitätsklinik, Freiburg, Federal Republic of Germany

Since the early 1950's, the effect of Curie (Brachy-Curie) therapy* of intracranial tumors by direct interstitial or intracavitary implanting of radioactive isotopes could first be demonstrated only in small volume tumors or cysts; in some cases the effect was even curative[4, 8, 17, 25, 49, 70, 74—76, 84, 98, 99, 102, 113, 116, 129, 132, 137, 145, 148, 152]. This therapy has only become possible by using stereotaxic operation methods. With a stereotactic device attached to the patient's head, the tumor is aimed at with a cannula, precalculated to the exact millimeter. Only after the biopsy, which in any case should be carried out first, the radioactive isotopes are interstitially implanted into the tumor, or the cysts are instilled, if indicated.

In the following, the stereotactic biopsy technique and the results, the technique of Curie (Brachy-Curie) therapy (CiT, BCiT) and the results and indications are reported:

1. Biopsy for Differentiation of Intracranial Processes and Optimization of Therapy

The nature of every unverified, progressive intracranial lesion should be histologically confirmed to determine whether it is a neoplasm or other. This applies

---

* The term "brachytherapy" is, in the English scientific literature, understood as "therapy at short range". According to the expert opinion of Priv.-Doz. Dr. K. Hackl, of the Ancient History Seminar, University of Bale, Switzerland, presumably this is a false ethymological interpretation, since the ancient Greek adjective "βραχύς" is, in combination with a noun, mainly used to characterize lapses of time, *e.g.* in the sense of "short-time therapy". We proposed the term "Curie therapy" as early as in the 1950's to define "low-dose rate interstitial irradiation with radioisotopes" as a permanent implantation and the term "Brachy-Curie therapy" for the "interstitial after-loading techniques with "high-dose rates".

whatever its location, and whether or not there are solitary or multiple lesions. This is essential before the planning of any conservative or radiation treatment. The exception to this is when an open exploratory operation is primarily indicated, during the performance of which adequate biopsy material can be obtained for conventional histological examination. This holds true even today, when modern CT or MRI devices have improved differential diagnosis. However, even with CT and MRI as a result of misinterpretation diagnostic errors can occur and, as a result of this, the wrong treatment may be selected and no cure may be achieved[85, 86, 93, 156].

The clinician cannot but be dismayed when, for example, he sends a patient for percutaneous radiation with the diagnosis of a "ring" glioblastoma, on the CT basis of a solitary deep-seated round focus with a ring structure, and later on the autopsy shows an abscess which could have been drained and rinsed out by stereotactic puncture and treated successfully with antibiotics. On the other hand, in lesions of the brain stem, pons, basal ganglia or the cerebral white matter close to the midline, there is a considerable risk of causing severe functional deficits when obtaining biopsy material by means of an open operation, the so-called exploratory craniotomy.

Today stereotactic biopsy is the method of choice as it avoids the above-mentioned risks, and rules out the danger of uncertainty, as for example in the mistaking small foci. Furthermore it eliminates the possibility of error inherent in freehand puncture.

With this method, tissue can be obtained with 1 mm precision from foci larger than 3 mm in diameter and can be histologically compared with the surrounding tissue. Treatment can be decided upon immediately, even if the intraoperative examination of a smear preparation has still to be completed. This method was introduced into stereotactic technique, in the early 1960's[97]. In cases of inflammatory, hemorrhagic, necrotic focal or systemic disease conservative treatment can be initiated. In other cases, as soon as the localized low grade astrocytoma of the brain stem, pons or the basal ganglia is confirmed, interstitial CiT can be performed immediately, or, when there is a cyst, a catheter for drainage can be implanted.

For a deep-seated intraventricular, dysontogenetic tumor, ependymoma or meningioma, microsurgical total resection can subsequently be aimed for. In such cases, percutaneous irradiation, which affects the tumor itself far less than the rest of the brain, is not indicated. Particularly in cases of deep-seated, nonresectable processes, the evaluation of the cases treated exclusively with conventional irradiation suffers from the lack of histological confirmation, so that benign cysts, hematomas, low-grade gliomas, dermoids, teratomas, etc., cannot be recognized among expanding and displacing lesions which are radiated as tumors.

Naturally they show good long-term results, although they could have and should have been either treated by operation or local radiotherapy with good palliative or recurative results or would have also cured themselves without any therapy at all. In cases of nonresectable tumors, e.g. malignant gliomas, the grading can be established intraoperatively. A decision can also be made whether the combination of CiT or BCiT with percutaneous irradiation is indicated or the latter alone in combination with or without chemotherapy.

One of the advantages of the stereotactic biopsy of intracranial lesions is that the focus to be punctured can be reached exactly, to the nearest millimeter using a thin needle or a biopsy probe. With our stereotactic device any previously selected point or focus, whether intracranial, intracerebral, or intracerebellar, can be punctured from any point on the surface of the skull. Careful selection of the angle of puncture and its adjustment to the location of the focus to be punctured ensures the protection of functionally important areas and larger vessels. The risk of functional damage is thus reduced to a minimum.

The biopsy material is usually taken along the puncture tract. Specimens are taken continuously, beginning in the healthy tissue, through the pathological tissue to the other side, into reactively changed or healthy tissue. A morphological profile can thus be provided at the same time. This procedure has a further advantage in that it includes the infiltration zone of tumors which escapes every other diagnostic method. Stereotactic biopsy, particularly of multiple foci, was developed together with Birg, using a modification of the stereotactic device of Riechert and Mundinger[9, 10, 12, 80, 127, 128].

Multiple biopsy specimens can be obtained through a small burr hole (6 mm in diameter) with various approach angles, all being calculated beforehand by computer. For lesions in both hemispheres, a bilateral burr hole is necessary.

Previously, target points for stereotactic biopsy used to be localized with the aid of invasive neuroradiological techniques such as pneumo-encephalography, ventriculography, arteriography, plain X-ray (because of calcification). Radionuclide-scintigraphy, in particular, made it possible to localize to the exact millimeter nuclid-storing foci and determine their size, as do confirm our numerous biopsy controls.

Today, CT and MRI improved decisively the stereotactic technique of biopsy and CiT.

a) Technique of CT (MRI) Stereotaxy for Biopsy and Implantation of Radioisotopes

As a rule the whole procedure is performed under local anesthesia. General anesthesia is used only in cases with transcerebellar approach and in children under 6 years of age.

The decisive breakthrough was the direct integration of CT and MRI into the computer-stereotaxy method. A simplification of the method was then achieved, with the target precision being 1 mm. This technique which the author developed in collaboration with Birg[11, 13, 14, 89—91, 101] and which has been named "CT stereotaxy" or "MRI stereotaxy" will be briefly described.

Essentially three possibilities of combining CT, MRI and stereotaxy (ST) can be distinguished:
   1. The indirect methods[1, 7, 32, 40, 48, 51, 52, 59, 62, 120, 125, 130, 134].
   2. The direct methods[10, 14, 22, 23, 31, 58, 82, 83, 85, 91].
   3. The expost methods[13, 134].

Using the indirect methods, the position of the ST device in relation to the CT sections is determined by means of wire or synthetic glass structures scanned simultaneously. The use of this method is recommended if the size of the ST device

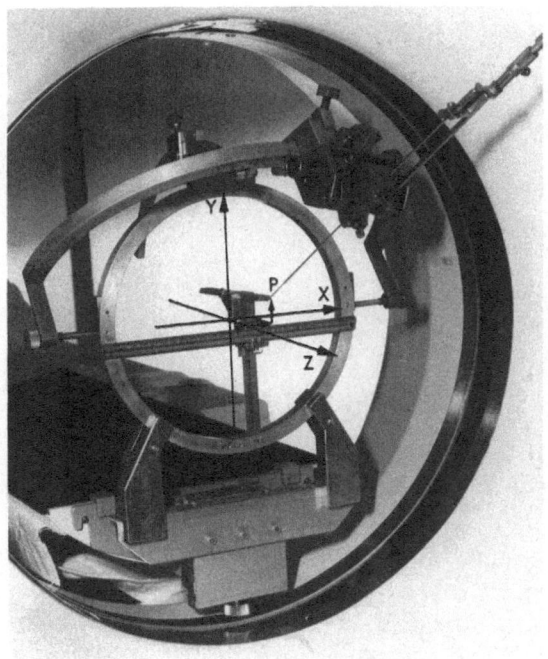

Fig. 1. Presentation of the CT scanner gantry with the stereotaxic device developed by Riechert and Mundinger in the computer compatible modification by Mundinger and Birg. The cartesian target point coordinates of the stereotactic device are identical with the coordinates of the CT, the zero-point of the stereotactic device being located in the origin of the CT scanner

is larger than the gantry of the CT scanner or if the spatial synchronization of the two coordinate systems cannot be achieved for other reasons.

Using the direct methods which we have introduced, the CT or MRI scans are produced while the ST device is attached to the patient's head. After the correct adjustment of both systems, the target coordinates can be measured directly (Fig. 1).

Using the expost method, the projected CT or MRI sections scaled according to the X-ray distortion are plotted onto a transparent sheet and transposed to the corresponding X-rays. This is done manually or by means of a computer program. Thus, the shape of the tumors, of the ventricles or other brain structures taken from the CT or MRI sections coincide automatically with the corresponding structures shown on the X-rays.

The direct method is the most exact and of primary importance for the future. This technique requires that the patient be scanned with the stereotactic base ring attached to his head.

Stereotactic device (STD): In this case, any stereotactic device can be used. However, the following conditions should be met: the base ring or polygonal frame of the device must fit into the CT scanner or MRI gantry and it must be adjustable

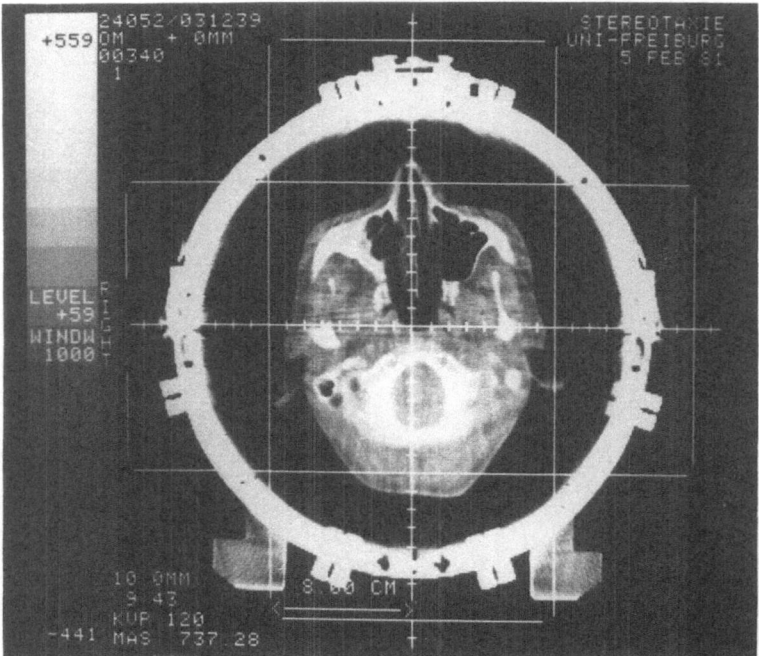

Fig. 2. The stereotactic operation show the following figures: After fixing the ST ring to the patient's head, the patient is laid on the CT table and the ST base ring is fixed to the adjustable holder (see Fig. 1). The coordinates of the stereotactic base ring are brought to coincidence with the coordinates of the CT gantry. The zero-plane of the base ring is thus in coincidence with the zero-plane of the CT layer, and also the zero-points

so that the origin of the device coincides exactly with the center of the CT scanner or the center of the magnetic field. During the scanning process, none or only few artifacts are permitted to originate in the operation area. Therefore, we use our own STD[127, 128] in the computer compatible version of Mundinger and Birg[9, 80] (Fig. 5)*.

Attachment to the head: The ST base ring may be fixed to the patient's head by acrylic holders and screws which produce few or no artifacts on the X-rays or magnetic field (Fig. 5). According to our CT experiences, metal holders and screws may also be used without any problems if the base ring is fixed to the skull at such a level that the area to be scanned is either above or below the ring. For MRI stereotaxy, nonmagnetic alloys or synthetic material are obligatory for the base ring.

The further procedure of targeting are shown in one case in Figs. 2–8.

The operation takes place in the operating room. Into the holder of the base ring an additional full size radiograph is built for AP and lateral views. The parameters (angles, depths of probe) for the stereotactic device can be calculated

---

* Producer of our STD: F. L. Fischer MET GmbH, D-7800 Freiburg/Federal Republic of Germany.

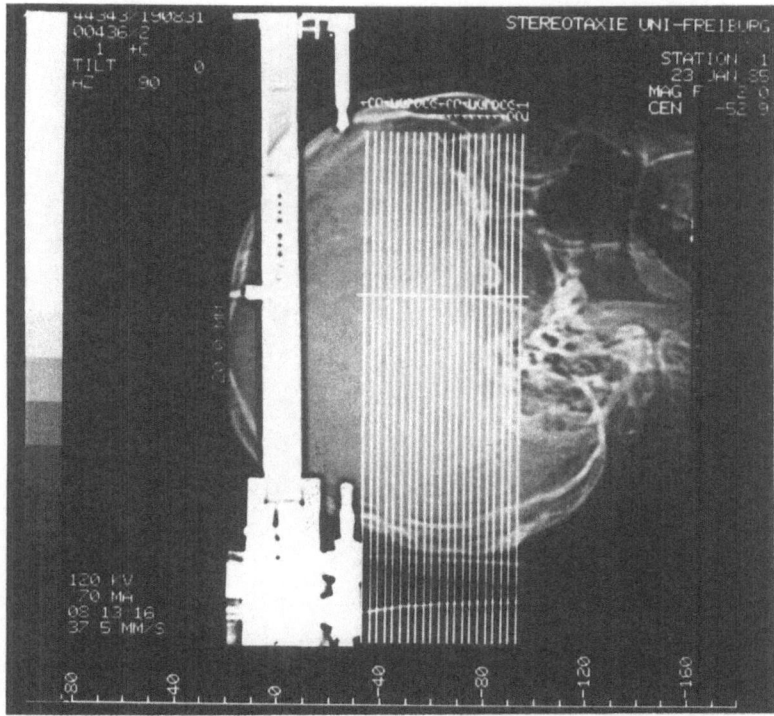

Fig. 3. CT sections are produced parallel to the stereotactic base ring (middle of the ring = zero-plane) with distances of 5 mm or 1.5 mm in the case of smaller processes (*e.g.* brain stem processes). The scanning area is determined using the so-called Scout-view-feature. In this case the base ring is fixed in a high head position. According to the Scout-view image and the axial CT section on the level of the stereotactic base ring, the coincidence of the origin of the CT scanner and that of the stereotactic device (STD) as well as the parallelism of the CT sections to the ST base ring is adapted. Then the coordinates of the CT scanner coincide with those of the STD, and no further calculations of the target point is required; all the coordinate values taken from the CT sections also apply to the STD. The same is true for MR stereotaxy when the center of the magnetic field coincides with the point of origin of the stereotactic coordinate system. After producing the CT scans, the axial images are determined for that section where the target structure (*e.g.* tumour shape) has reached its largest extension. The size and volume of the target structure is measured with the aid of the distance-measure feature. Next, the cross-hairs are moved to the center of the target structure and the resulting coordinates are reorded[83]

using the coordinate information. While these calculations are done on-line or off-line, the patient is brought into the operating room and is prepared for surgery in the usual manner. This procedure applies to all tumors in the hemispheres, in the mesencephalon, diencephalon, brain stem and pons area, and for all approaches, whether transcerebral, transcerebellar, or transnasal-transsphenoidal, transmeatal or transorbital. The accuracy of the described method has been tested. The deviation result was that none of the coordinates revealed on the CT images differed

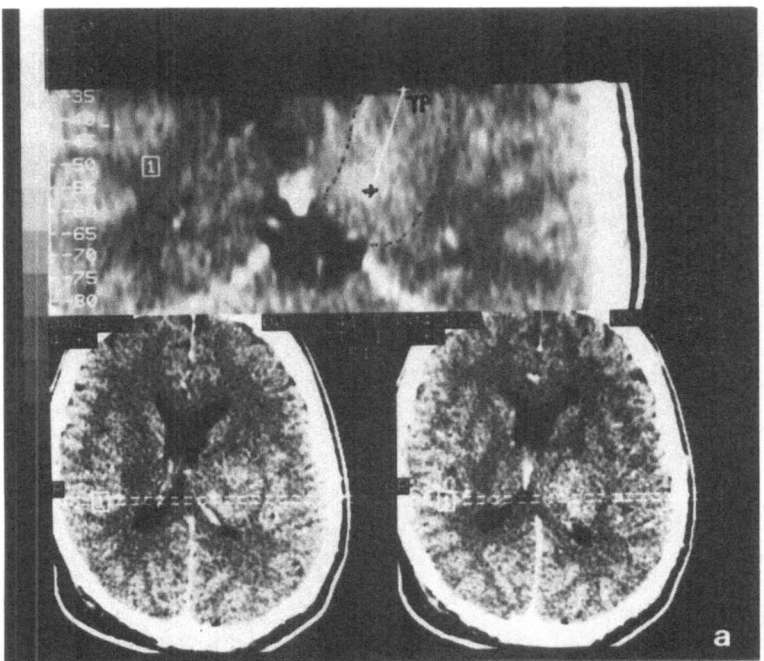

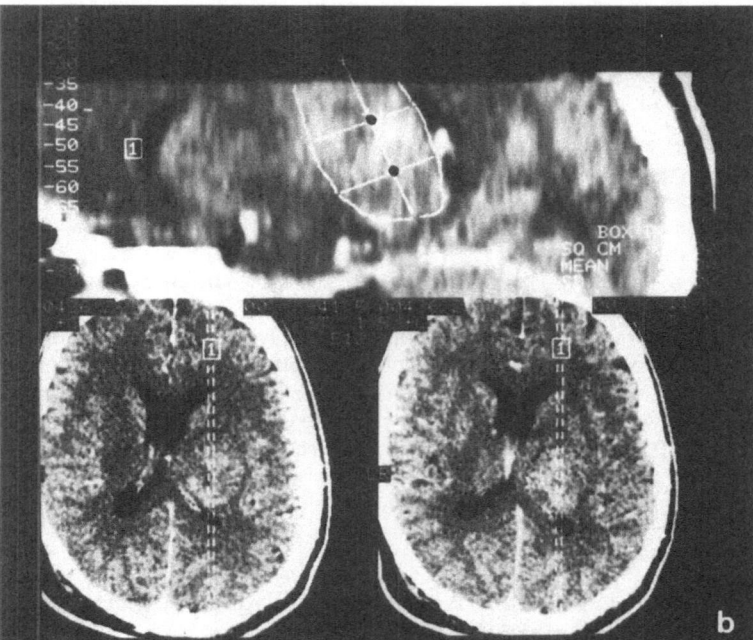

Figs. 4a and **b.** More precisely is the evaluation of tumor extension in the sagittal (*a*) and coronal (*b*) reconstructions. In this case of an anaplastic astrocytoma of the left basal ganglia the angle of puncture is selected in such a way that, in case of spherical lesions, the biopsy forceps can be introduced into the center, in cylindrical lesions along the axis of the cylinder. In cases of geometrically more complicated lesions (also in terms of a later distribution of the radionuclides for therapy) the forceps can be put into the various areas at different angles of puncture. After that, the cannula track and thus the trephination point are determined; the corresponding coordinate values are taken from the sagittal and coronal reconstruction images

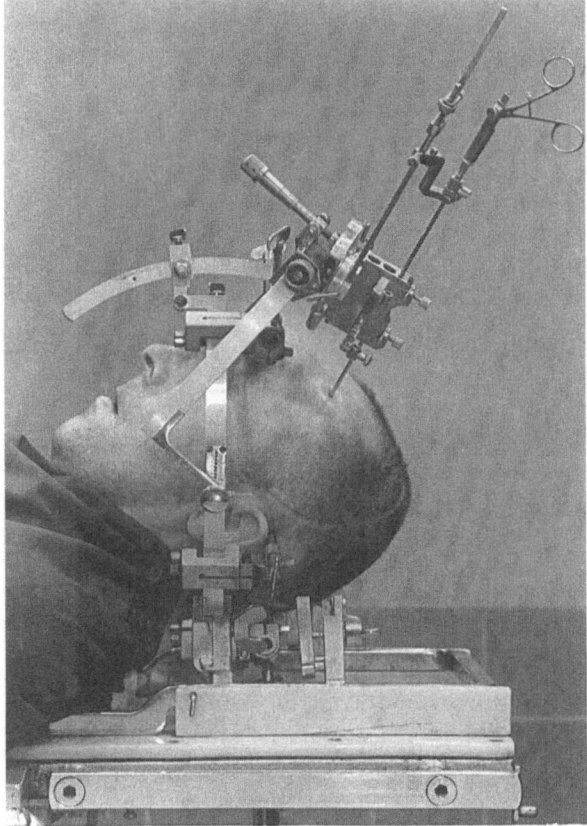

Fig. 5. The trephination hole is made at the site that has been previously determined in the CT (MRI); subsequently, the combined set of cannulas is introduced in order to perform the biopsy and implantation of nuclides. The figure shows the lateral view of our stereotactic device. For reasons of better presentation, the sterile cover has been omitted. The biopsy cannula is placed *in situ*

by more than 0.6 mm. At this time, in MRI stereotaxy the deviation of the coordinates amounts to less than 2 mm. This proves that the degree of accuracy of the method is so high that it is most suitable for stereotactc biopsy and the treatment of intracranial or scull base tumors (Table 1).

b) Technique of Biopsy

With a 2.5 cm incision, a burr hole 6 mm in diameter is made in the direction of the first target point. After coagulation of the dura, the outer cannula with the biopsy probe (or implantation probe) is led to the target point, step by step (Figs. 5 and 6).

The first biopsies are taken, before the tumor surface is reached, mainly from the perifocal edema or reactive gliosis. The next biopsies are taken at distances of 1

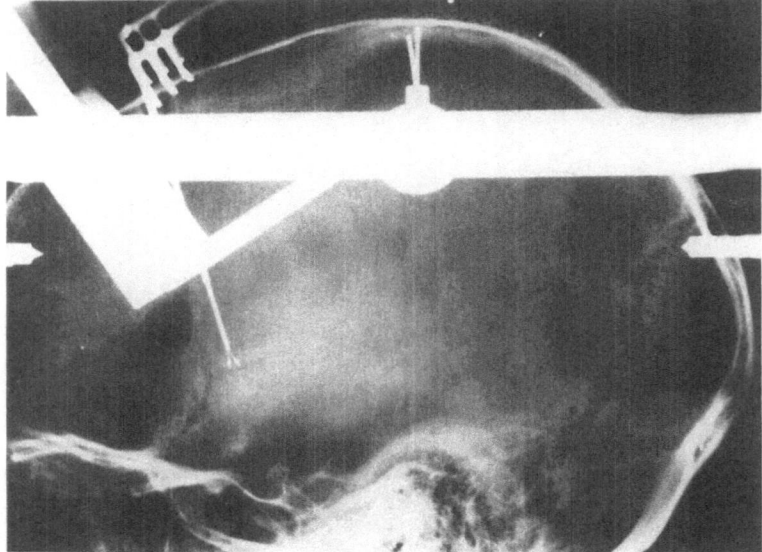

Fig. 6. For biopsy we use a set of cannulas, each of which consists of two cannulas with one having a smaller diameter so that it can be slid into the other. The cannula used for the brain midline area has a diameter of only 1.1 mm. The biopsy forceps, which are 0.8 mm in diameter, are introduced through the inside cannula (see Fig. 5). Two claw-like jaws of the forceps take hold of the tissue and snip it off. The amount of tissue is 1–3 mm³. The forceps have a head piece with millimeter intervals (up to 30 mm) to prolong the desired length of the clamps without having to be followed by the outer cannula, which is secured in the guide rail of the stereotaxic device

Table 1. Advantages of CT and MRI stereotaxy

Advantages of CT and MRI stereotaxy
Direct anatomo-morphologic visualization of the structures
Direct determination of target points
Less need of indirect invasive neuroradiological methods, *e.g.* ventriculography (intraarterial angiography)
Fewer complications
Increased range of indications with regard to age contraindications
Better results

or 2 mm up to the target point, sometimes up to the opposite side of the lesion and again into the perifocal tissue. A number of 5 up to 20 samples are submitted to the neuropathology department for paraffin embedding and special staining[31, 56, 57, 119, 124, 125]. Other smear preparations stained with methylene blue are immediately examined intraoperatively.

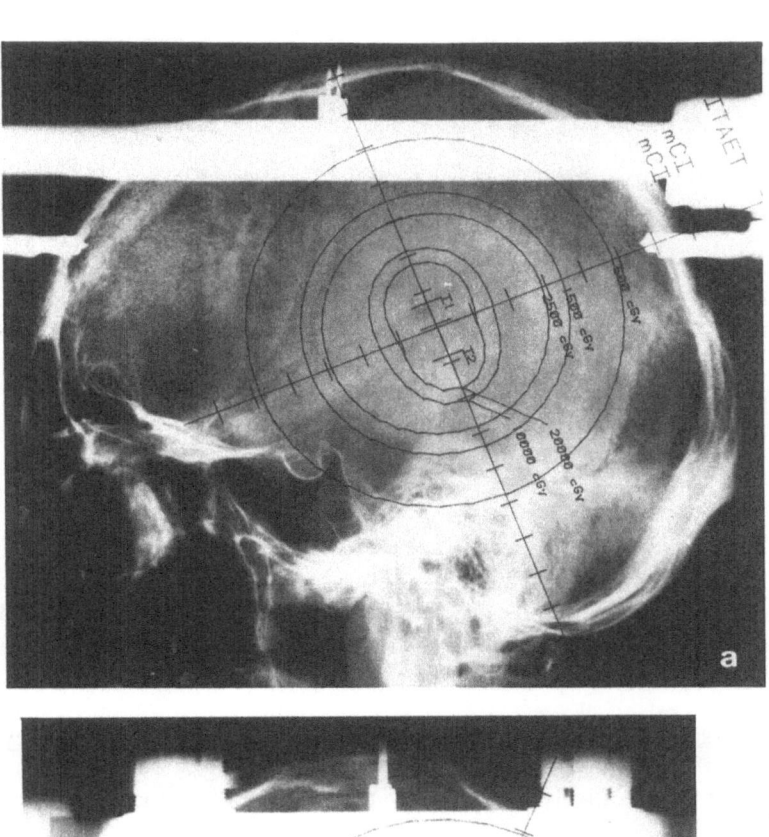

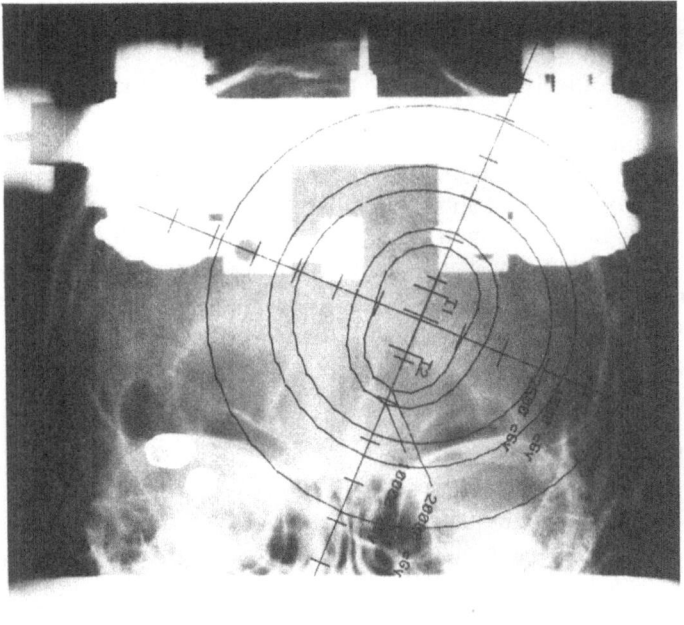

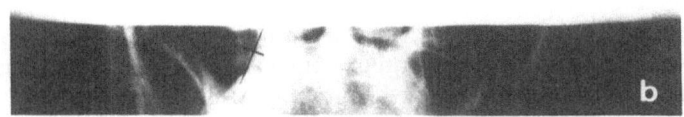

Figs. 7a and **b.** After biopsy, in this case of an anaplastic astrocytoma (WHO III) of the left basal ganglia, CiT with two I-125-seeds was performed. The lateral (**a**) and a.p. (**b**) X-ray films show the isodose distribution. The 2nd inner ring covers the tumor surface (peripheral tumor dose). Implanted total activity 18.4 mCi, 100 Gy on the tumor border

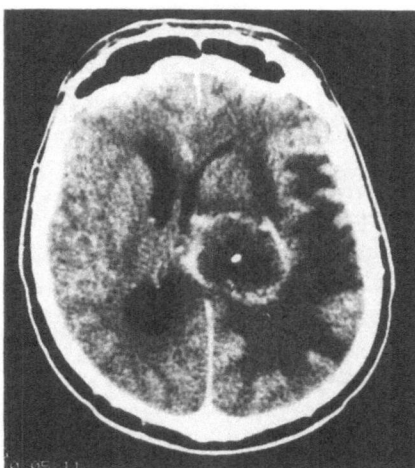

Fig. 8. F. J., 54 years. Anaplastic astrocytoma of the left basal ganglia. 7 months after [125]J CiT (seed centrally implanted), the anaplastic astrocytoma is centrally necrotized. The CT with enhancement shows a hyperdense ring structure as well as a perifocal edematous reaction

The classification and the grading of the tumor, *e.g.* low grade astrocytomas (WHO grade I or II) or anaplastic astrocytoma (WHO grade III and IV) can be established intraoperatively in the smear preparation. This makes it possible to decide immediately on further radiotherapeutic procedures. The bioptic confirmation of the tumor localization, in particular the determination of infiltration and the exact extent of the tumor, also enables us to correct the dosimetry.

Stereotactic biopsy is done in the peripheral areas of the focus in a recurrent tumor or where progressive growth of the focus has been established in the CT or MRI (*e.g.,* after operation, interstitial radiotherapy (RT) or percutaneous irradiation), in order to examine the residue of tumors left after operation or parts of a recurrent tumor, as well as for the purpose of making a distinction between tumors and radiation necroses.

c) Clinical Results of Biopsy

Among more than 2,500 stereotactic biopsies since 1965, from January 1981 to December 31, 1984, 893 CT stereotactic interventions have been performed. Table 2 shows a list of the CT stereotactic biopsies and the diagnoses.

In most cases, a CT stereotactic biopsy was performed in order to classify the tumors and administer the CiT, or to exclude inflammations, abscesses, necroses, hemorrhage, infarcts, etc.

The evaluation of the bioptic material from 600 patients gave the following results: Combined cytological (smear preparations) and histological examination of paraffin-embedded samples revealed the tumor type and approximate grading in 492 (82%) cases. In 66 patients (11%), a clinically suspected neoplasm was

Table 2. Diagnosis of 893 CT stereotactic biopsies (January 1981–December 31, 1984)

Histology of glial tumors	Number of cases
Astrocytoma I	87
Astrocytoma II	247
Astrocytoma III	149
Glioblastoma IV	88
Oligodendroglioma	30
Total	601

Histology of nonglial tumors	Number of cases
Ependymoma	9
Choroid papilloma	4
Medulloblastoma	5
PNET	23
Meningioma	9
Germinoma	20
Teratoma	8
Epidermoid	4
Craniopharyngioma	28
Colloid cyst	6
Metastases	68
Unclassified tumors	6
Total	190

Histology of nontumorous processes (mostly in CT and MRI displayed as tumor)	Number of cases
Hemorrhage	32
Glioses	55
Abscesses	15
Total	102

excluded. In the remaining 42 cases (7%), the presence of a tumor was confirmed but the available samples did not allow an unequivocal classification of the neoplasm. In our series we had a 95% agreement between the results of the smear preparations and those of the paraffin sections[57, 119].

The indications and advantages of the CT and MRI stereotaxy are given in Table 3.

d) Consecutive Procedures After Biopsy

Since the classification and the nature of the lesion is usually established intraoperatively by the smear preparation, it can be decided right away whether CiT

Table 3. Advantages of CT-guided stereotactic biopsy

I	To obtain reliable specimens from different parts of unilocular and multilocular, even small foci (no "free-hand" puncture)	
II	To avoid diagnostic errors (tumor/no tumor) To avoid wrong (failed) therapy (operation, irradiation, conservative treatment) As a lower-risk replacement of the so-called "test" craniotomia (such as posterior fossa region)	
III	Localization of the tumor	intracerebral, extra-cerebral, cerebellar, brain stem/pons region
IV	Classification and grading (I–IV, WHO)	with different therapeutic consequences, *e.g.* sensitive to ionizing irradiation, cytostatics
V	Tumor size and reaction of the surrounding structures (demarcation against edema, gliosis), dosimetry for local CiT.	

Table 4. Type of treatment after stereotactic diagnostic biopsy of 1,413 cases (1965–December 31, 1984)

Type of procedure		Number of cases
Permanent interstitial CiT	^{192}Ir	256
	^{125}J	287
(+ external irradiation)		86
Temporary interstitial 13 CiT		79
External irradiation		257
Cyst drainage (catheter implantation)		93
Tumor resection		91
No subsequent therapy		443

should be started immediately during the same operation (Figs. 7 and 8) or whether the lesion should be resected by open operation. A stereotactic biopsy has no limiting effect on the subsequent microsurgical resection of benign tumors (*e.g.*, intraventricular tumors, ependymomas). The histologically confirmed indication is an advantage for the surgical procedure (Table 4).

The same applies to anaplastic gliomas and glioblastomas of the hemispheres which, as a result of their size and localization, are no longer appropriate for an operative intervention or CiT. It also applies to patients who, due to their poor general condition or their advanced age, cannot be further burdened with an operation. In any case, having the results from a biopsy facilitate the decision as to whether or not an operative intervention is advisable at all (*e.g.*, it would not be sensible any more in case of an extended butterfly glioblastoma) and if preference should be given to percutaneous RT. The percutaneous RT of malignant tumors is also carried out after the indication has been histologically confirmed, whereby benign cysts, necroses, low-grade gliomas, or inflammatory foci, etc, can be excluded.

Abscesses and cysts are punctured immediately following the biopsy and, if necessary, drained with stereotactically implanted catheters[100]. Inflammatory for degenerative diseases are diagnosed and are given conservative treatment. Aneurysms and vascular deformities are contraindications, which is another reason why angiography, apart from its role in reducing the risk of puncture, is absolutely indispensable before the stereotactic biopsy is performed.

In cystic tumors (astrocytomas, glioblastomas, craniopharyngiomas), the interstitial or intracavitary radiation is combined within the same session with a stereotactic puncture and a drainage of the cyst, using a catheter. In cystic craniopharyngiomas the catheter is directed in such a way so that it drains the contents of the cyst via the ventricular system. In addition, it is equipped with a metallic reservoir (Rickham reservoir) which is fixed into the trephination point so that later on the reservoir may be percutaneously punctured and thus the cyst pressure may be relieved.

If an occlusive hydrocephalus is already present due to the obstruction of the interventricular foramen (Monro) or the Sylvian aqueduct caused by the tumor, an additional ventricular catheter is stereotactically introduced uni- or bilaterally after the implantation of the nuclides. At a later date, this ventricular catheter can be extended without another brain operation to a ventricular-atrial or ventricular-peritoneal shunt in order to drain the increased CSF pressure.

2. Curie (Brachy-Curie) Therapy (BCiT)

The CT-guided stereotaxic biopsy and interstitial or intracavitary CiT-BCiT for intracranial processes or the skull base are principally neurosurgical operations. However, the cooperation of the radiotherapist is mandatory. We differentiate (Table 5).

Table 5. Stereotactic CiT

		Time for dose accumulation
BCiT (high-dose rate irradiation)	a) after loading contact-irradiation device (*e.g.* GammaMed, ^{192}Ir, ^{137}C, ^{60}Co	0.1–1 hour
	b) temporary implantation of catheter systems (^{125}J, ^{192}Ir)	5–50 hours
CiT (continuous low-dose rate irradiation)	a) permanent implantation (^{32}P, ^{90}Y, ^{109}Pd, ^{186}Re, ^{198}Au)	8 days
	b) for protracted long-term irradiation (^{125}J, ^{182}Ta, ^{192}Ir)	150–200 days

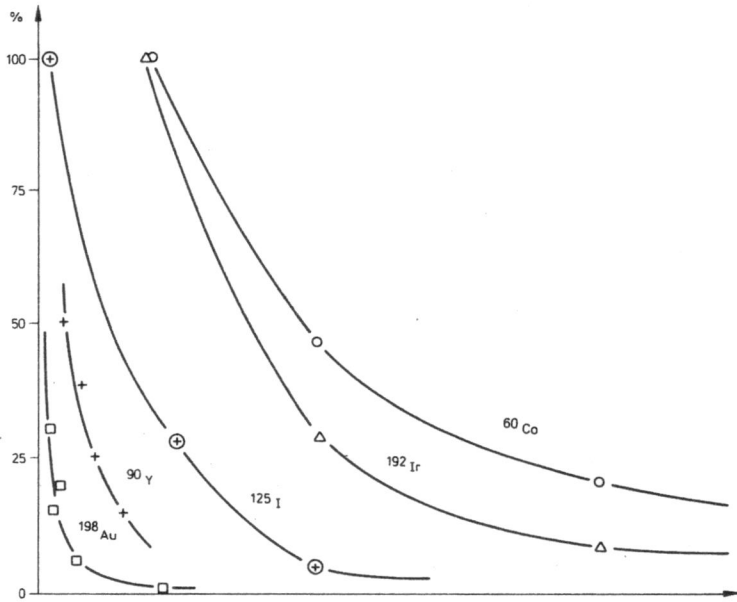

Fig. 9. Decrease of dosis with different radiopharmaceuticals

1. Brachy-Curie therapy (BCiT): an emitter with high Curie activities is inserted into the tumor for a short time, giving the tumor dose within minutes or a few days.

2. Curie therapy (CiT), the permanent implantation of radioactive emitters. The emitter is "lost" and administers the dose to the tumor within a few days to months.

The radiobiological differences between high-dose rate BCiT using an afterloading contact irradiation device for ^{192}Ir (GammaMed) (p. 18), *i.e.,* with the dose administered within minutes, and temporary implantation over a period of several days are only minor. This is because the tumor necrosis is replaced by a glial scar or it melts into cyst.

With low-dose CiT, especially using ^{192}Ir, the perifocal edema, in particular, is kept to a minimum, thus providing a better tolerance for this form of therapy than for BCiT. However, it is indicated only for certain morphological malignancies. There is not enough time for protected long-term irradiation in cases of anaplastic gliomas or other malignant tumors. In such cases, BCiT must be chosen, if necessary in combination with long-term irradiation or percutaneous irradiation. This combination is frequently employed by us.

In Table 6 the most common radiopharmaceuticals are compiled with a description of their physical characteristics. The decision as to which emitters are to be utilized is based upon the size of the tumor volume to be radiated. The variation with which the dosis decreases, *i.e.,* how sharply it drops off, measured from the emitter surface, must also be taken into consideration when making this decision (Fig. 9). The tumor volume also determines whether one or more radiation sources

Table 6. Principal physical properties of the nuclides used in interstitial radiation therapy of brain tumors

Nuclide	$T_{1/2}$	E_γ	E_β	K
$^{32}_{15}$P	14.3 days	—	1.71 (~ 100%)	—
$^{60}_{27}$Co	5.27 years	1.17 (100%) / 1.13 (100%)	0.31 / 1.48 (0.15%)	13.2
$^{90}_{39}$Y	2.7 days	1.75 (< 0.005%)	2.27 (~ 100%)	—
$^{109}_{46}$Pd	13.8 hours	0.31–0.77 (< 0.005%)	1.02 (100%)	—
$^{125}_{53}$I	60.2 days	0.0275 (73.8%) / 0.0272 (37.8%) / 0.031 (19.9%)		1.4
$^{134}_{55}$Cs	2.15 days	0.61 (100†) / 0.80 (72†)	0.66 (76%)	3.4
$^{182}_{73}$Ta	115 days	1.12 (100†) / 1.19 (60†)	0.51 (100†) / 0.44 (60†)	6.1
$^{186}_{75}$Re	3.7 days	0.137 (100†)	1.07 (71%) / 0.93 (21%)	0.062
$^{192}_{77}$Ir	74.6 days	0.31 (100†) / 0.47 (164†) / 0.1–1.06	0.67 (44%) / 0.54 (40%)	5.0
$^{198}_{79}$Au	2.7 days	0.41 / 0.68 (0.5%) / 1.09	0.96 (98.6%) / 0.29 (1%)	2.3

Legend

$T_{1/2}$: Physical half-life

E_γ: maximum intensity of radiation in MeV

E_β: maximum intensity of β radiation in MeV

(%): intensity of quants per 100 decays

(†): relative frequency of decays

K: point source dose rate constant in $\dfrac{r \cdot cm^2}{h \cdot mCi}$ for gamma radiation

must be implanted and according to which planted and accogeometrical scheme the implantation must be carried out, so that the dose distribution within the tumor region is sufficiently high and as homogeneous as possible.

A first approximation is carried out with the CT or MRI software. Subsequently, the number and localizations of the implants are with their coordinates defined (even for geometrically complicated tumor volumes), as well as the activities to be implanted in order to adapt the peripheric tumor isodose lines to the tumor surface. This is done with the help of our interactive dosimetry program system[15]. Other programs have been described by several authors[20, 21, 43, 51, 118, 121–123, 138, 146].

a) Radiobiology of the Low-Dose Rate CiT

The biological effect is defined by the dose rate. The lower the dose rate, the more reduced is the biological effect within a given radiation dose. This is why the exposure time has to be extended and the dosage raised. Proceeding from the radiobiological effect of the different examined systems, the dose rate must not be too low since in such cases the "critical dose rate" is reached and mitoses are therefore no longer prevented. The dose rate varies from cell system to cell system, depending upon the cell cycle period (720–900 rads per cell cycle of an inhibiting mitosis)[38, 126].

The dose rate effect is in normal tissue more pronounced than in tumor tissue. By applying the continuous low dose rate exposure for the interstitial intratumoral placement of the emitter, the surrounding normal tissue is spared better relative to the tumor tissue. For the above-mentioned reasons, our CiT as permanent implantation of emitters of a long half-life (^{192}Ir and ^{125}J) is radiobiologically indicated above all for tumors with longer cell cycle periods[44, 45, 72, 74, 77, 79, 81, 87, 92, 94].

This is one of the advantages of the "protracted long-term irradiation with low-dose rates", the CiT as introduced by the author, above all in cases of low-grade brain tumors. Conventional teletherapy techniques, in comparison with CiT techniques, do not allow a sufficiently high-dose to be absorbed in the tumor without considerably affecting the brain situated within the area of the cone of rays. With the doses which are applied *lege artis,* the low-grade brain tumors must therefore be considered as radioresistant. This also accounts for the low effectiveness of external radiation techniques in low-grade tumors.

The dose rate effect is the result of the "repair of sublethal damage" (SLD), redistribution in the cell cycle, reoxygenation of cells and repopulation of the tumor. These well-known facts need no elaboration here, but it should be briefly pointed out that decades of our experience with the continuous low dose rate irradiation have shown that the cell is affected lethally in the critical target site (assumed to be desoxyribonucleic acid; ionizing events occur at all critical target sites) when using the permanent implantation of ^{192}Ir (peripheral tumor dose 120 Gy) as well as ^{125}J (peripheral tumor dose 100 Gy).

The sharp dose drop-off of the intratumorally implanted emitter towards to the periphery also accounts for the demonstrated tendency that the repair SLD is more efficient in normal tissue than in tumor tissue, even if the SLD has been reached in the direct surroundings of the tumor.

This corresponds to our clinical experience obtained in the CT follow-up[158]; the reaction in the tumor periphery, accompanied by a bioptically confirmed edema or a gliosis, recedes within the period of several months up to 2 years. The varying ionization densities are a further factor in that the perifocal reaction is greater after applying the [125]J CiT than after the [192]Ir. In terms of "strength of reaction", [125]J can apparently be characterized as being situated between the gamma radiation and the particle radiation (α and β particles, fast neutrons) which are known to have a high linear energy transfer (LET) radiation and to produce cell damage without any possibility of repair. The X-ray photons of the [125]J have a higher total energy on the one hand but a lower linear transfer energy on the other and therefore cause less damage to the tissue per unit length of trajectory than the particle radiation. Hypoxic cells which are localized in the partly necrotizing parts, also of the low-grade glioma, repair the SLD less efficiently than the euoxic cells (see p. 152). This tendency is found much more distinctly in the anaplastic tumors and glioblastomas which are often centrally necrotized.

From the radiobiological viewpoint, the continuous low-dose rate irradiation of the interstitial CiT has the above-mentioned advantages. Nonresectable low-grade tumors, localized in deeply-seated structures, e.g. of the midline, but also nonresectable parts or recurrencies of hemispherical tumors, can be destroyed depending on the dosage given. In order to achieve this end, however, a knowledge of the dignity of the tumor is by all means required as well as a complete mastery of a precise implantation technique. The surrounding, functionally important normal brain tissue, neuronal systems or nuclei areas are either not affected by the killing of the cells or they have the possibility of a better repair mechanism.

Morphologically, the investigation has, for the ^{192}Ir and [125]J CiT, shown a tumor necrosis which is marked sharply towards the periphery[18, 19, 29, 56, 65, 72, 76, 144]. In the higher linear transfer energy of the ^{192}Ir, the necrosis is slightly less sharp than with [125]J. The decision as to which emitter is of more advantage must be made based on the infiltration size.

If, for example, in the surrounding healthy tissue of astrocytomas which demonstrate an unsharpe transitory zone in the CT, MRI and in the biopsy, which is carried out step by step from the periphery to the tumor, an unsharp transitory zone with the rests of tumor cells within the reactive gliosis, and therefore an extended infiltration zone is found, the radiation of ^{192}Ir is rather indicated due to its higher energy than the reaction of [125]J.

As we clearly must avoid lesions of functionally important structures which are localized in the immediate surroundings of the tumor, for example in tumors of the hypothalamus, thalamus, midbrain/brain stem region, a sharply defined tumor necrosis should be aimed at. In such cases the [125]J CiT is indicated. Morphologically, both emitters lead to a radionecrosis. The partly cystic liquefaction of the tumor which is in most cases localized in the white substance area only, has then the advantage that using the CT-stereotactic procedure the cyst may be punctured and drained, thus obtaining inner decompression of the brain. It is still unclear why with the same physical characteristics and dosage the radiobiological mechanisms are different in some tumors, as for example, in tumors which are localized in the grey substance area, and why involution instead of cyst formation occurs, with the tumors healing with a glial scar. Such questions call for further investigation and observation.

b) Radiobiology of High-Dose Rate Brachy-Curie Therapy (BCiT)

The afterloading techniques of interstitial radiation with ^{192}Ir or ^{137}C contact radiation devices with high-dose rates allow us within minutes to intraoperatively administer the ionization dose which as required for the cell death.

The larger doses in the immediate vicinity of the emitter (a legitimate objection) are not a problem. On the contrary, the center of malignant tumors is usually badly vascularized and thus hypoxemic, as our biopsy examinations confirm over and over again. Oxygen deficiency, however, leads to greater radioresistance, so that a 30–100% higher dose is necessary in these areas in order to achieve the same radiation effect as in tissue with normal oxygen content[26, 36, 76, 117].

In the marginal zone of the tumor, on the other hand, the cells with a shorter premitotic resting stage are predominant. These, however, show greater radiosensitivity. In the peripheral infiltrating zone a lower dose is therefore sufficient for inactivation. We can deal with these radiobiological factors with interstitial implantation. We can therefore also avoid the difficulties involved in percutaneous radiation of body tumor such as the spherical shape of the skull, varying tissue radiosensitivity, unintentional overdosage with the danger of concommitant peak formation in healthy tissue and underdosage in the area of the tumor.

The relative sharp dose drop off makes it possible to keep the radiation necrosis largely limited to the tumor and to protect the surrounding healthy brain tissue. In the BCiT we administer the tumor dosage within a few minutes or hours. This is an advantage in view of the close correlations between the dose distribution over a period of time and the varying speed of recovery, depending on the activity of the cell distribution. With the BCiT we block the recovery process of the tumor which is dependent on the oxygen supply.

By means of the short-lived dose accumulation with the high dose rate irradiation devices (e.g. GammaMed®) the so-called "active centers" become quickly concentrated within a minimal amount of time. These active centers are based on direct ionization and on chemically effective intermediate products which live for an extremely short time. The strong concentration and the addition of these "active centers" (Hug) within a minimum amount of time by means of a single radiation with a high dose rate is also favorable for tumors having a slow cycle time, where fractionation reduces the radiation effect. This means that interstitial BCiT can also destroy low grade astrocytomas (rich in fibers and cells), spongioblastomas and oligodendrogliomas, and other tumors which respond disappointingly to conventional external radiation methods[3, 5, 24, 27, 28, 30, 55, 64–67, 83, 88, 95, 102, 104, 135, 140, 141, 143, 154].

According to our experimental and clinical experiences[78] BCiT is significantly reinforced by thymine, analogous to radiosensitizers and antimetabolites; this may be demonstrated by our experiments on DS carcinoma-sarcomas of rats. In comparison to the control series, the tumor stops growing temporarily for 14 days after GammaMed BCiT after the administration of 5-brom-2-deoxycytidin for several days previously. The combination with 5-fluorine-uracil (5-FU), which inhibits the thymine synthesis, enhances this effect[37]. Much more effective is pretreatment with 5-bromo-2-deoxyuridine (BUDR), which is incorporated into the deoxyribonucleic acid as a substitute for thymine. This BUDR incorporation is strengthened much more with methotrexate (MTX) than with 5-FU.

The folic acid-reductase inhibitor MTX blocks the thymidilate-synthetase. This is the enzyme that effects the methylization to thymine. With a 6-day pretreatment with the combination BUDR and antimetabolites, followed by GammaMed irradiation, we were able to eliminate five sixths of the tumors in the animals. The results can still be improved if small doses of MTX are administered daily over a period of 4 weeks after irradiation. Apparently, with BCiT the blood-brain barrier in the area of the tumor is broken down making it possible for the MTX, and other cytostatic agents which otherwise do no pass the blood-brain or blood-tumor barrier, to work their way into the tumor. After we had incorporated the mitosis-inhibiting radiosensitizing substance Synkavit® (sodium salt of 2-methyl-1,4-naphtohydrochinon-diphosphate)[68] as an electron acceptor, and actinomycine D which blocks the transcription of genetic information from the DNA, we were able to increase the biological radiation effect by 1½ times, thereby reducing the dosage by 40%.

In order to obtain a reinforcement of the local cell-killing effect, further investigation is needed to find out to which extent, by applying the low dose rate CiT, the conditions may also be improved which would better locally concentrate the cytostatic agents applied during the absorption of the radiation dose. According to our experimental investigations with radiosensitizers such as MTX which we applied in addition to BCiT[104], this effect can be expected.

In future, even more importance may be attached to this kind of treatment, where RT is combined with radiosensitizers[33, 131, 142, 144, 147].

Such clinical investigation regarding the low dose rate irradiation is unknown to us.

BCiT is contraindicated for tumors of the midline, regardless of their dignity, since the very high concentration of "active centers" with the subsequently occurring radioactive and radioregressive changes happen too suddenly and are not tolerated by the midline structures. The decompensations cannot even be compensated with highest doses of dexamethasone or cortisone, nor with the sedation of the central nervous system, through the use of a "lytic cocktail".

According to our experience, the intraoperative BCiT should therefore be limited to either nonresectable or remaining or recurrent tumors of the white substance of the hemispheres or the corpus callosum. In other regions it should only be applied in fractions of 2–3 boosts of 8–10 Gy and in combination with CiT or external radiation. The dose level depends on how far away from the midline structures the tumor is localized. The more peripheric, the higher the single dose can be (between 35 and 45 Gy of the peripheral tumor dosage).

The physical and radiobiological advantages of CT-(MRI-)guided stereotactic interstitial BCiT are summarized as follows:

The oxygen-enhancement rate (OER) is lower than 1, and the relative biological efficacy (RBE) higher than 1. Above the critical dose rate, the repopulation of proliferate cells is faster in the normal brain tissue than in the tumor, and the redistribution of cell fractions tends to the more radiosensitive M (also G_2) phase.

Thus, the chances of removing the tumor are greater than 80%. When compared to chemotherapy, the local biological effect on the tumor is a 100 times greater. When compared to the percutaneous fractionated radiation, the tolerance by the healthy brain tissue is better, thus increasing the probability of sparing the surrounding brain tissue.

The attenuation of the energetic γ rays in the brain tissue is the same for photoenergies between 25 and 643 keV and thus for the majority of interstitially utilized radionuclides as in the brain gliomas themselves (with a scattering of value of only 1%). Therefore, an especially important advantage is the dose drop off of the interstitially implanted radionuclide to the periphery. For these reasons, interstitial CiT can be applied even in cases of recurrencies in which by a previous application of external (percutaneous) radiation the threshold of tolerance by the healthy brain tissue has been reached. Moreover, the volume determination in the CT and MRI is improved, thus giving the advantage of a more precise peripheral tumor isodose distribution.

Increased doses may occur in the immediate surroundings of the emitter, possibly followed by a cystic liquefaction. The cysts may be stereotactically punctured and drained without any risk at all. In cases of brain tumors, as opposed to other organ tumors, the formation of a radionecrosis is insignificant.

Hence, sufficiently high local doses may be administered and factors such as radiosensitivity or radioresistance may be disregarded, since by the application of an emitter with the appropriate physical characteristics, in combination with an optimum dosimetry, the destruction will be limited essentially to the tumors.

When compared to open surgery[39, 60, 64, 153, 160], stereotactically implanted emitters are better tolerated. The brain tumor is, as a rule, solitary and with the CT-guided stereotactic puncture technique accessible in any localization, even in midline areas. It is a precise method which is almost entirely without risk. The exception to this is the case of multiple metastases in which, if there are more than three knots, the stereotactic technique is not indicated. The same applies to the centers of the motor system and language in which, due to the mutilation effect, open surgery is in most cases naturally not an option.

The fact that the patient is only hospitalized for a few days, is another psychologically important factor.

3. Techniques of Implantation of Radionuclides

a) Curie Therapy

In cases where interstitial CiT is indicated, the radionuclide (^{125}J, ^{192}Ir) is implanted into the precalculated target points, directly following the biopsy and using the same hollow sound. The seeds are enclosed in a radiation-protected magazine. The magazine is then put into an intermediate piece which is again put into the cannular cone. The seeds are ejected from the magazine at the target site with the aid of a

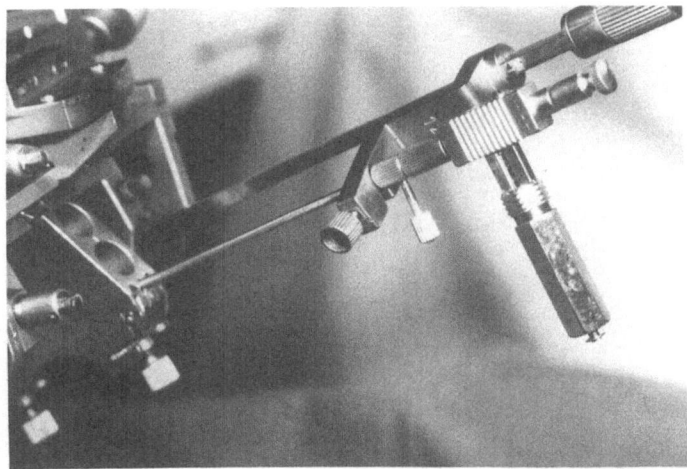

Fig. 10. The number and activity of the radiation-protected ^{192}Ir-^{125}J seeds, calculated by means of a specialized program (developed together with Birg), are distributed within the tumor using a special applicator (modified "Mick-applicator")

mandrin (Fig. 10). If the radionuclide must be distributed at several different targets within the tumor, the precalculated angles for the probe are adjusted one after the other, and the point of the hollow sound is led to these targets, thus implanting the calculated radio-activities. The emitters must be distributed within the tumor in such a way that on the "low lines" within the tumor, as well as on the tumor surface itself, sufficiently high doses of cell inactivation are absorbed[76, 146]. With the aid of CT-guided computer stereotaxy, the exact distribution within the tumor, using one and the same 7 mm small bony burr hole, is without any problem (see Figs. 1–3).

Whether a central implant (Fig. 11) or multiple implants should be interstitially inserted and geometrically distributed depends on the size and shape of the tumor (Fig. 12).

Smaller cerebral tumors or metastases situated cortically or subcortically are stereotaxically resected as completely as possible through the small bony opening with a cortical incision of only 5–6 mm. Later, intracavitary radiation of the resection wall can be performed either intraoperatively by means of a contact radiation device, (*e.g.* ^{192}Ir GammaMed) or using ^{125}J in an after loading catheter implantation.

Cysts or cystic tumors are first drained and then irradiated intracavitary. We puncture craniopharyngioma cysts through the anterior horn and insert the catheter in such a way that the cholesteremic cystic fluid can be drained via the ventricular system and the shunt system, if there is one.

As our long-term results have proved, this procedure is sufficient in most cases[72, 157]. For cystic craniopharyngiomas, intracavitary β radiation, *e.g.*, with ^{90}Y glucose, ^{198}Au or ^{186}Re colloid, is helpful[4, 16, 86, 88, 114, 115, 133, 148, 159].

Unfortunately, due to the various national radiation protection laws, not all radionuclides are presently allowed to be used despite their very favorable physical characteristics, for example, and the demonstrated clinical success obtained with

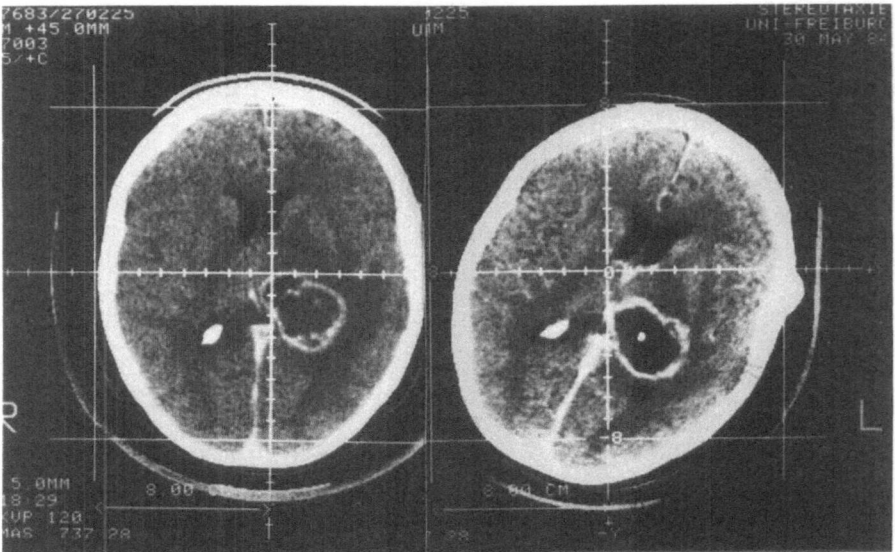

Fig. 11. H. U., 58 years. Anaplastic glioma (WHO grade III-IV) of the left basal ganglial block, including the internal capsule. **Left:** Before CiT (peripheral tumor dosage 100 Gy, radius 17 mm, activity 17.5 mCi). **Right:** 8 months after ^{125}J CiT only (additional external RT was rejected. Without tumor growth, a central necrosis has occurred. In the center, the ^{125}J seed can be recognized. Survival time after CiT: 12 months

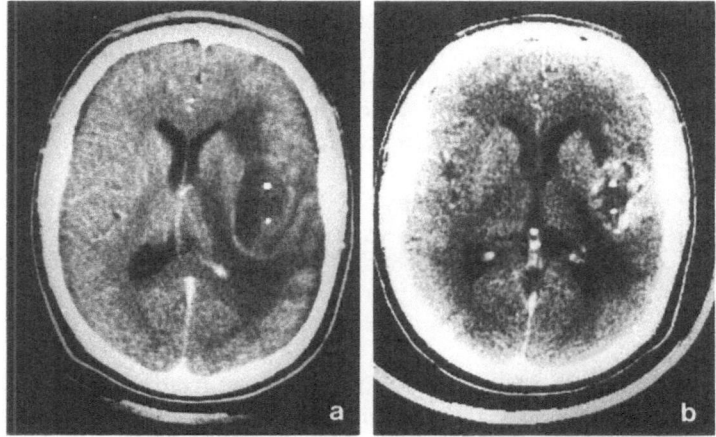

Fig. 12. K. A., 50 years. Fibrillary astrocytoma with suspected anaplastic component (WHO grade II–III) temporal, on the left side. *a* 1 month after ^{125}J CiT (2 seeds, total activity 36 mCi, peripheral tumor dosage 120 Gy). Midline shift of the ventricular system, accompanied by a perifocal edema around the tumor which shows a narrow hyperdense halo. *b* 2½ years later. Shrinkage and devitalization of the tumor. The ventricular system is developed again and is central in position. The hypodense perifocal areas probably correspond to a gliosis. The patient is, in the meantime, back to work as a highschool teacher of languages and sports

them[71, 72, 76]. They may not be applied in spite of the existence of, in part large-scale, radiation protection installations which were constructed in the 1950's and 1960's. For these reasons we had to give up the intraoperative permanent implantation of large tumor volumes with ^{192}Au seeds[69] and ^{182}Ta seeds[70], as well as the ^{60}Co afterloading BCiT[72] and the infiltration of macromolecular suspensions of gold (graphite adsorbate), even though the clinical results with these radionuclides were excellent. The stereotactic implantation of ^{198}Au seeds—radiated according to the β radiation dose—or that of ^{90}Y seeds can be limited to small tumor volumes only. In cases of large volumes, the exact adherence to the seed distances, marked in the form of a grid[146], is too time-consuming. There would always remain underdoses areas from which the existing tumor grows or begins anew. In addition, the risk of hemorrhages is provoked.

For the above reasons, the author introduced the ^{192}Ir into brain tumor therapy in 1959 and ^{125}J seeds in 1979, for very low dose rate irradiation as a permanent implantation method ("protracted long-term irradiation").

^{125}J seeds may also be distributed in larger tumor volumes without any conflicts with the radiation protection laws. Restrictions, however, do exist for the usage of ^{192}Ir in larger tumor volumes. (In such cases, ^{192}Ir after-loading BCiT is the "way out".)

These two nuclides are indicated for permanent implantation which is the method of choice in cases of low-grade tumors such as pilocytic and fibrillar astrocytomas, and here, above all in the brain midline area and at the base of the skull. In numerous publications we have reported on the techniques and long-term results[71–103, 105–112]. In cases of so-called maligne intracranial tumors, the radioisotope therapy is mainly indicated as BCiT therapeutical application.

b) Technique of Brachy-Curie Therapy (BCiT)

The method which we are using at present is carried out by means of the after-loading technique which is as follows: ^{192}Ir or ^{125}J, predominant among other radionuclides, are encapsulated in hollow needles or threaded in synthetic catheters and thus administered to the tumor temporarily a) for 4–10 days or b) for minutes or hours.

In method a), either one or more implants are inserted, depending on the size of the tumor, forming points, or catheter systems with seeds are led through the tumors[6, 22, 23, 32, 34, 35, 41, 42, 46, 47, 53, 54, 61, 72, 76, 127, 139, 155]. When compared to permanent implantation, the dose rate of BCiT is higher, e.g. in the first case amounting to a peripheral tumor dosage of 60 Gy, in 6 days 0.4 cGy/h[136]. Papers summarizing these techniques, the dosimetry and the results, have been published[22, 43, 72, 76, 82, 86, 88, 151].

However, the BCiT with ^{192}Ir, applied in the course of several days, requires considerable radiation protection measures, above all for the nursing staff. Therefore we early abandoned this technique, giving preference to intraoperative BCiT using the ^{192}Ir GammaMed contact radiation device, 1963 constructed by us[73, 103], or the after-loading ^{125}J catheter system.

The after-loading ^{125}J BCiT is, according to our own method, applied as follows: The stiff silicone outer catheter is first stereotactically introduced; by means of a small plastic fixation with a centrally drilled hole through which the catheter is guided, the intracerebral catheter is fixed in such a way that the platelet is fixed subgaleally at the outer edge of the bone (Fig. 13).

For radiation protection reasons subsequently the inner catheter, filled with ^{125}J seeds, is inserted into the outer catheter. Immediately above the fixation platelet, both catheters are squeezed together with the aid of a hemoclip, thus being

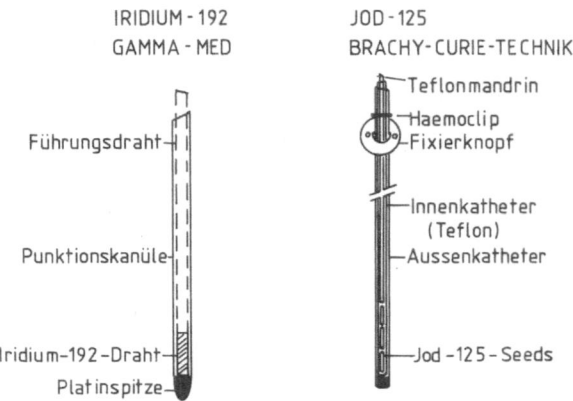

Fig. 13. Afterloading

fixed. The catheters are cut off directly above the clip and the incision subsequently closed completely with a few sutures (Fig. 14).

We attribute the fact that we have not had a single case of a wound infection to the practise of suturing. No wound infection occurred even in cases where the catheter remained *in situ* over a period of 5–7 days until the calculated dose had been administered. At the end of the radiation, one or two stitches are removed, the catheter is taken out together with the platelet and additional suturing is carried out. In some cases we removed the inner catheter only and exchanged it again at a later time with a inner catheter filled again with ^{125}J (fractionation) dependent on the clinical course.

In such cases, as well, no complication has ever occurred, as the follow-ups, carried out over a period of several years, have shown. In our opinion, the introduction of various catheters filled with ^{192}Ir seeds in the form of a grid[130, 139] in order to obtain a better homogeneous dose distribution within the tumor, is not necessary, since a necrosis with possible cystic liquefaction is a desired reaction and the inner decompression is obtained by puncture of the cyst.

c) Contact Radiation Devices

Contact radiation devices are for use with high dose rates. There exists a variety of different devices and application systems but we use our own ^{192}Ir contact radiation

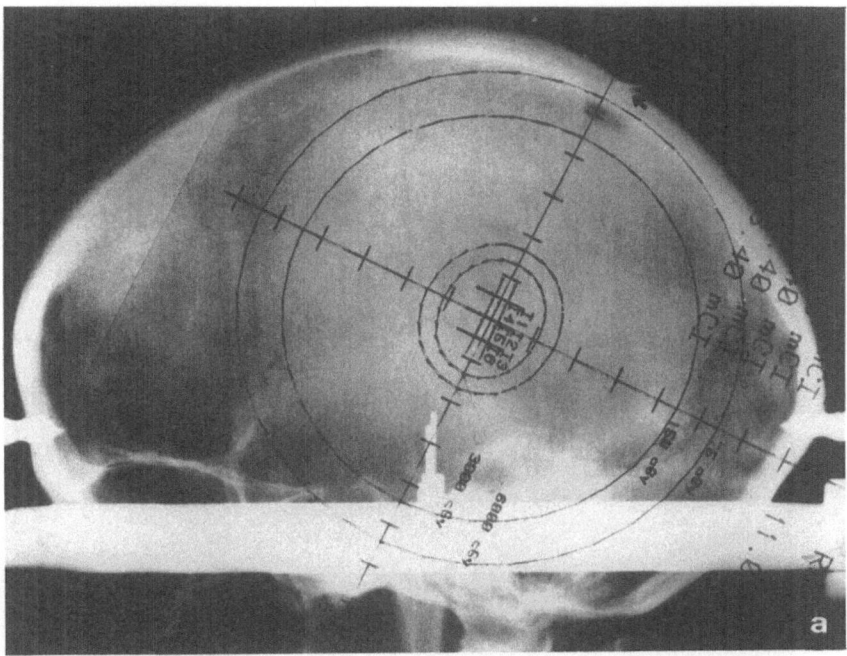

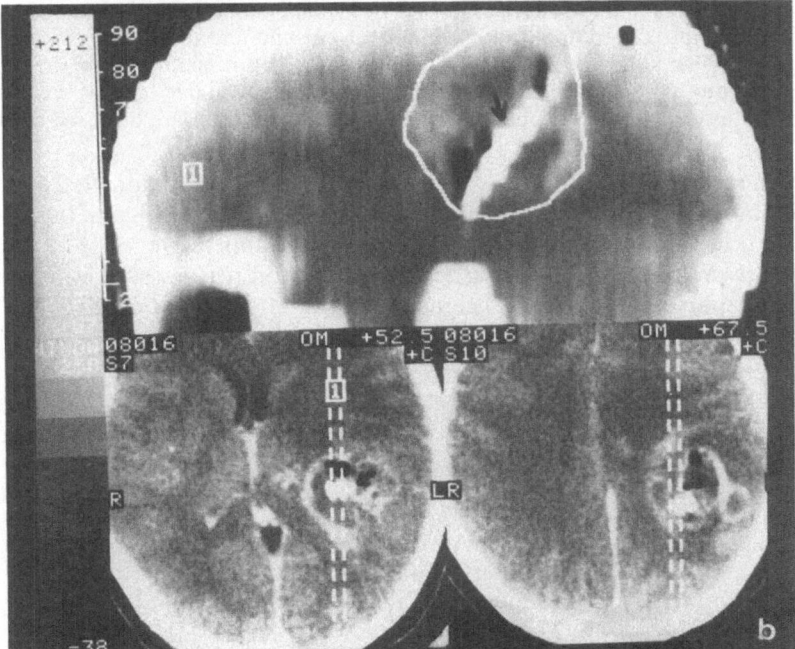

Fig. 14. R. M., 53 years. Anaplastic astrocytoma, in the left parietal region, extending to the basal ganglia. BCiT with ^{125}J. If no seeds with high activities are available, 2 catheters can be placed parallelly side by side, each of them filled with 3 seeds of ^{125}J. It was done in this case. For the period of the administration of the dosis (156 hours), the catheters are fixed by means of a metal-clip above the tubular collar, as has been described. *a* The lateral X-ray picture shows the arrangement of the seeds and the isodose distribution. The outer ring corresponds to the peripheral tumor dosage (30 Gy). (arrow: fixing of the catheter with metal-clip). *b* CT in the sagittal reconstruction through the double catheter (arrow). The punctiform dark spots are small air bubbles which have been pressed into the tumor during the biopsy

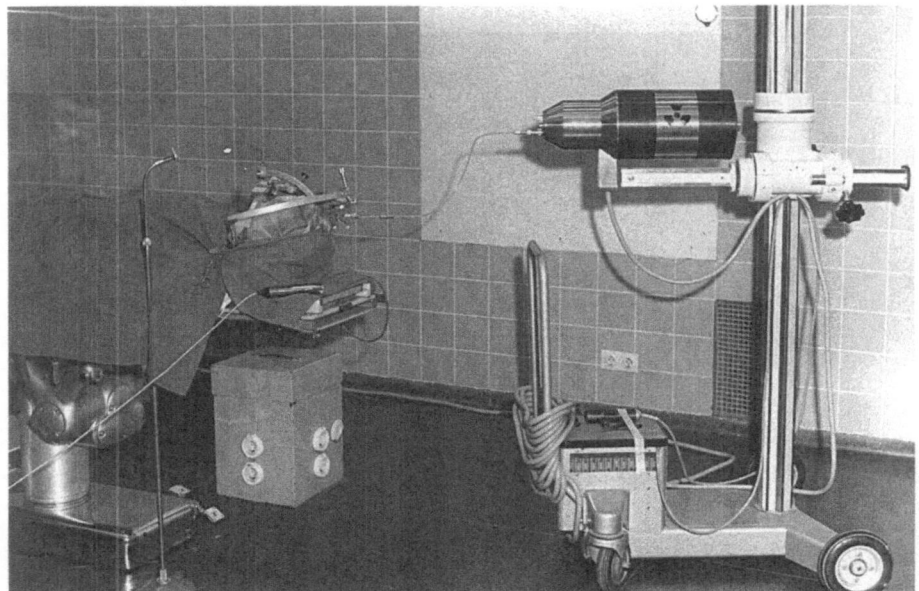

Fig. 15. ^{192}Ir-contact radiation device GammaMed [103] The connecting tube is attached to the stereotactically introduced application cannula at one end and to the exit channel of the shielding container at the other. With the aid of the remote automatic control the emitter is introduced into the intertumorally inserted application cannula and is automaticlly withdrawn into the shielding container after the calculated exposure has been completed

device. In collaboration with Sauerwein [103], we developed an automated apparatus for radiation with ^{192}Ir called "GammaMed"* (Fig. 15). The design of this device is such that it fulfills all requirements for an intraoperative or postoperative application. With the aid of the afterloading method it is possible to reach high activities capable of producing necroses in the tumor within a period of a few

---

Fig. 16. H. N., 36 years. *a* anaplastic astrocytoma (WHO grade III). State after two open operations and external irradiation (50 Gy). Lateral X-ray picture with two positions of the GammaMed cannula and isodose distribution. The outer ring corresponds with the surface of the astrocytoma recurrence. The peripheral tumor dosage is 25 Gy with an exposure period of 5 minutes, 12 seconds. *b* Row on the **left:** Immediately before BCiT with the ^{192}Ir contact radiation device GammaMed. Row on the **right:** 4 months later. The shift of the ventricular structures in the front parts towards the right has clearly receded. The tumor parts of the frontal corpus callosum can no longer be demonstrated. Both anterior horns have again developed rostrally. The cella media parts are also developed again. The ring-shaped hypodense structure does not point at a cyst but at necrotic tissue, as was shown in the biopsy. Survival time after GammaMed irradiation: 10 months. Total survival time: 58 months

---

* Producer of "GammaMed": Isotopen-Technik Dr. Sauerwein, D-5657 Haan/Rheinland 1, Federal Republic of Germany.

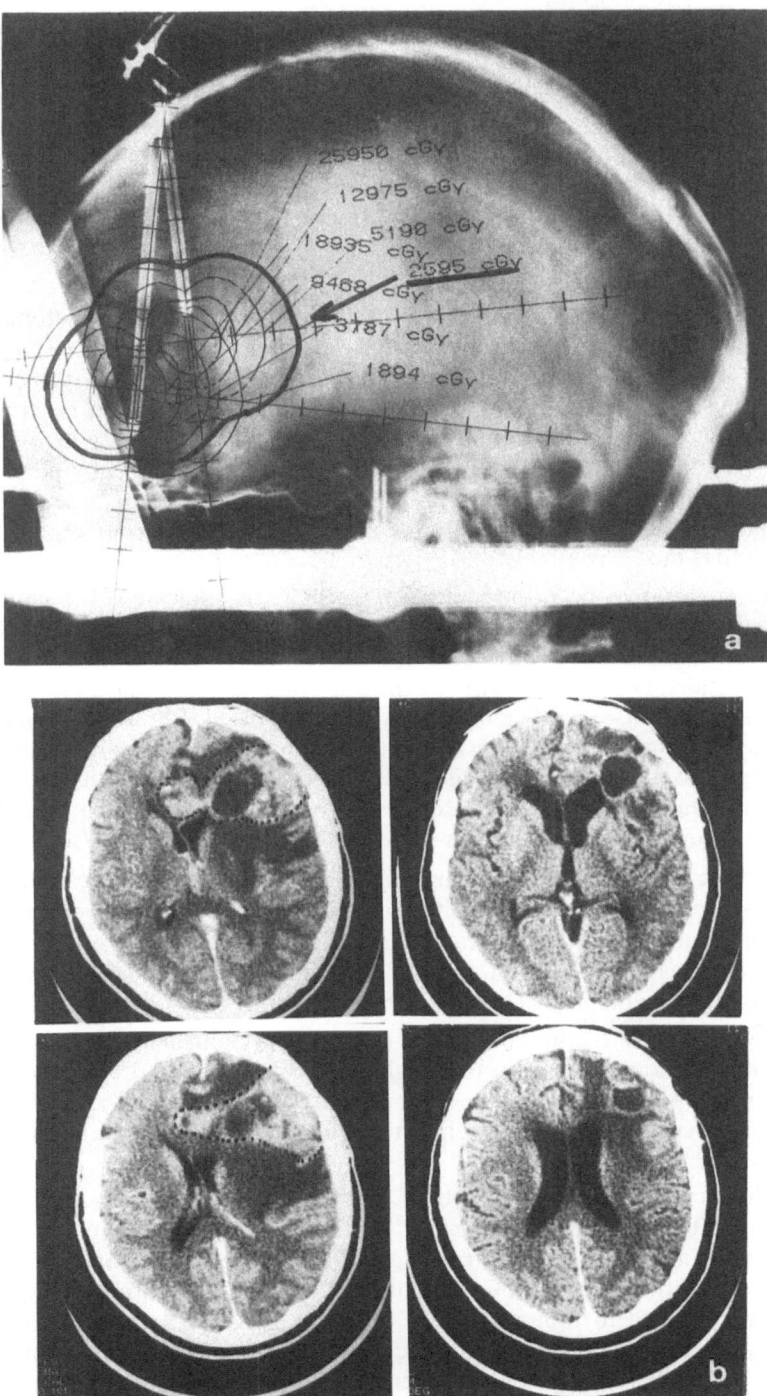

minutes. The ^{192}Ir emitter up to 120 Ci strength, is manufactured by Philips-Duphar, Amsterdam, the Netherlands, in the form of a cylinder, 1 mm in diameter and of variable length. It is contained in a Monel metal shell 1.8 mm in diameter and of appropriate length, usually of 10 mm. When not in use, the emitter is placed into the center of a heavy metal container of ellipsoid shape which eliminates all environmental radiation. This shielding device weighs 30 kg and has a shielding capacity for maximally 150 Ci of ^{192}Ir. The shielding device is placed in a protective container which hangs on a mobile stand or support and can be moved automatically.

The ^{192}Ir emitter is attached to a flexible cable or tube and can be automatically moved from the shielding container through a channel equipped with a shutter and guided by a sterilizable extension of the cable or tube which is then attached to the cannula used for the radiation. Following delivery the desired dose of radiation and with the aid of a time program, the emitter is automatically withdrawn towards its original position within the device which is, in turn, automatically closed by a shutter. A radiation detector incorporated into the protective container, monitors and safeguards the correct return of the emitter into the shielding device. We are still using the first model routinely.

If intraoperative or postoperative ^{192}Ir BCiT is indicated, the cannula is stereotactically introduced to the target point for the intraoperative afterloading contact irradiation which is carried out after the cannula position has been checked radiographically. Depending on the size and geometry of the volume to be radiated (e.g. square shaped), several cannulas may be introduced (Fig. 16) through which the emitter is successively introduced. By shifting one cannula in the tumor axis to different positions, radiation periods of various lengths can be programmed in such a way that the peripheral tumor dose may even be adapted to complicated geometrical tumor shapes (e.g. bear- or dump-bell-shaped) (Fig. 17).

The more recently developed GammaMed II has an emitter drive which may be programmed. In addition, several different activity levels may be programmed so that an optimum interstitial or intracavitary irradiation is carried out more easily on even complicated geometrical tumor forms. The dose for the tumor surface is, depending on the volume, 40–45 Gy in one sitting.

In cases where a fractionation into 2–3 sessions is planned in combination with fractionated external radiation, the single dose can be reduced correspondingly. The additional peripheral tumor dose should not exceed 100–120 Gy. One radiation session lasts, depending on the present activity loading, from a few minutes to about half an hour.

Radionecrosis takes place in about one third of the cases, along with cystic liquefaction at a later time ("radioknife"). After 2–5 weeks, an increased perifocal edema occurs in many cases, requiring higher doses of dexamethason. According to our clinical experiences, the application of the ^{192}Ir contact radiation of high dosage is, however, limited to tumor volumes of under 125 cm^3 (5 cm in diameter). In applying the full dosage, this "radiosection" is only tolerated in tumors of the cerebral and cerebellar hemispheres (edema). For lager hemisphere gliomas (grade IV), however, the combination with percutaneous radiation is in any case advisable and indicated. In tumors which infiltrate into the gray substance (basal ganglia), the

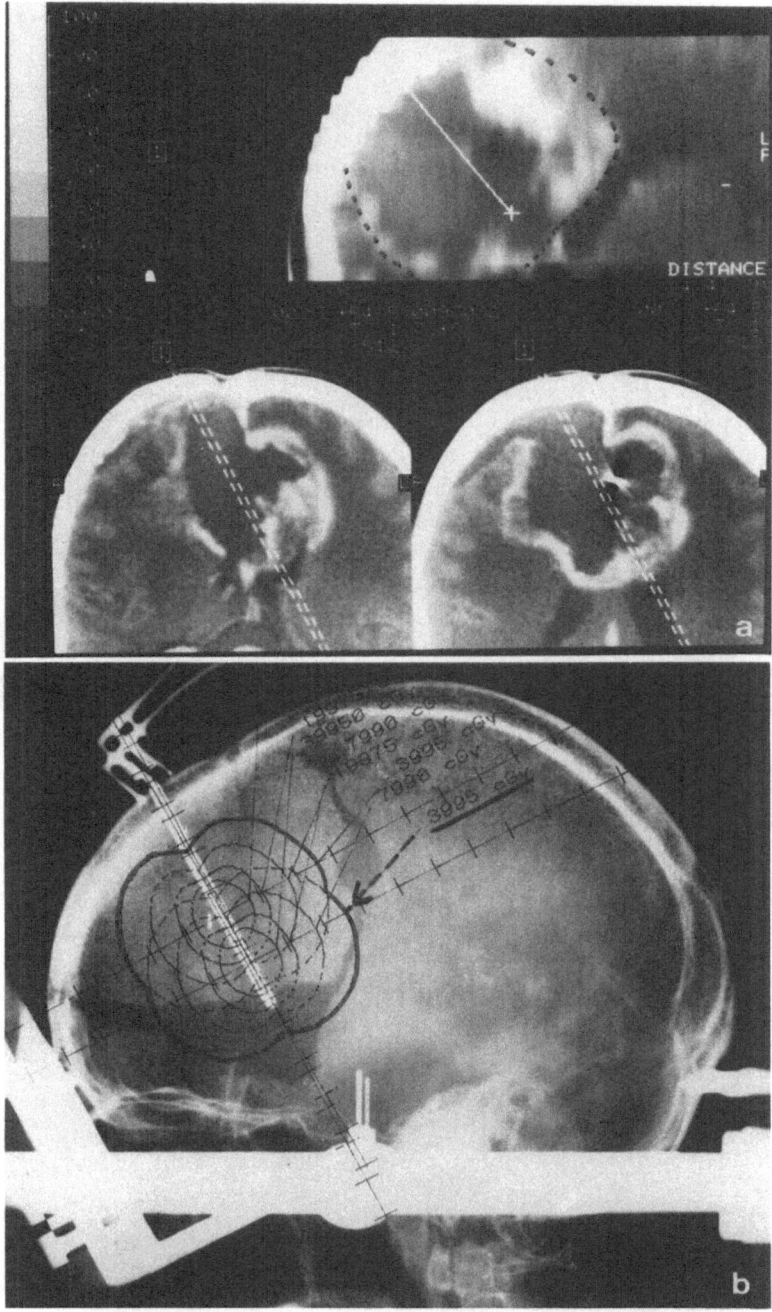

Fig. 17. N. M., 46 years. Glioblastoma multiforme (WHO grade IV). Two open operations and external irradiation. Centrally necrotizing recurrence. [192]Ir BCiT with GammaMed. *a* Oblique CT reconstruction through the plane which corresponds the way of approach, with representation of the tumor extension. *b* The lateral X-ray picture shows the GammaMed cannula *in situ*, as well as the isodose distribution. The peripheral tumor dosage (30 Gy) corresponds to the outer ring (2 positions). *c* Corresponding oblique CT reconstruction (90° to Fig. 17a). *d* The a. p. X-ray picture shows the GammaMed application cannula *in situ*. The peripheral tumor dosage is marked (radius 25 mm, 40 Gy). By shifting the emitter within the cannula, or by using several different cannula positions, the required peripheral tumor dosages can be implanted even in geometrically complicated radiation volumes

(Figs. 17c and d: see next page)

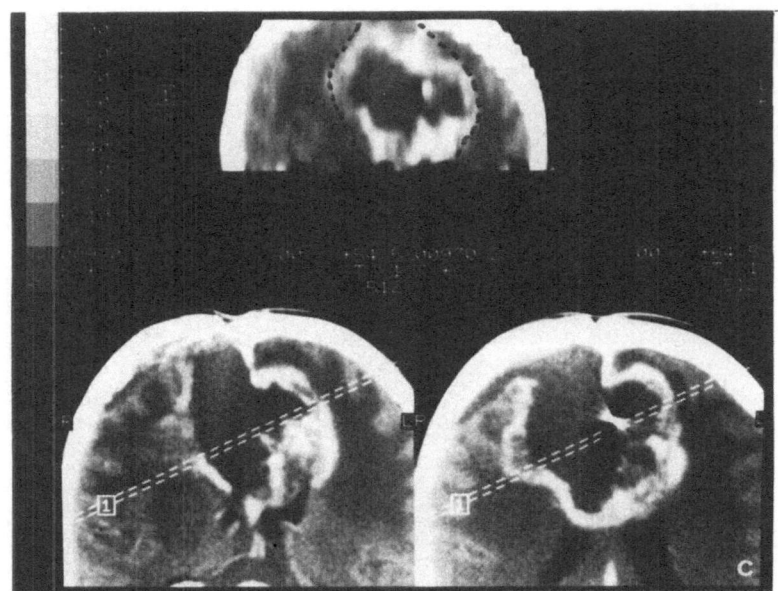

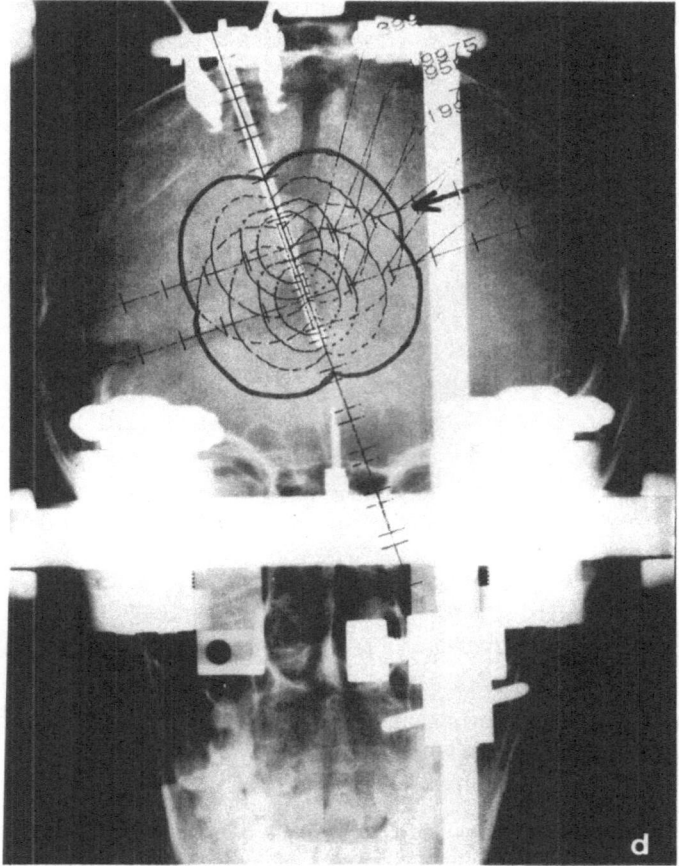

Figs. 17c and *d*

tumor surface dose should not exceed 12 Gy per session. In such cases, a combination with permanent implantation is indicated for tumors of smaller volumes whereas for larger volumes of grades III and IV percutaneous radiation is advisable. In recurrances after percutaneous irradiation or insufficient regression of the tumor volume a BCiT is additionally indicated for smaller volumes.

4. Results of BCiT

We have interstitially and stereotactically treated a total of 1,709 patients. Tables 7 and 8 show the radionuclides which were used in 1.587 patients, as well as the histological diagnoses. From 1951 to 1969 we treated the first series of 534 patients

Table 7. Radionuclides and number of stereotactic interstitial irradiation procedures (1952–December 31, 1984)

^{32}P	6
^{60}Co	179
^{90}Y	44
^{182}Ta	21
^{198}Au	129
^{125}J	331
^{125}J Brachy Curie Therapy	35
^{192}Ir GammaMed	284
^{192}Ir	558
Total	1,587

Table 8. Bioptically confirmed histology and number of interstitial irradiation (1952–December 31, 1984)

Glioblastoma	244
Astrocytoma	618
Oligodendroglioma	112
Ependymoma	38
PNET	39
Meningioma	21
Metastases	47
Sarcoma	11
Pituitary adenomas	254
Craniopharyngioma	40
Other lesions	85
Hypophysectomy	57
Pallidotomy	21
Total	1,587

Table 9. Postoperative survival times of patients with brain tumors following radiation with interstitially permanent implanted radioisotopes and combinations

Tumor Classification	Radioisotope	$t_{\bar{x}} \pm s$ (months)	t max (months)	t min (months)	Surviving patients (months)
Glioblastoma	198Au + roentgen	8.5 ± 4.9	12.0	5.0	
	182Ta		6.4		
	182Ta + 60Co	14.3 ± 2.0	15.8	12.7	
Astrocytoma (dedifferentiated)	198Au	6.5 ± 3.0	13.0		
	198Au + 60Co		45.9		
	182Ta	26.7 ± 19.1	14.8	7.5	
	182Ta + 60Co		30.1		
	182Ta + 60Co + roentgen				
Oligodendroglioma (dedifferentiated)	198Au + roentgen	17.4 ± 2.0	28.7	16.0	
	198Au + 182Ta		43.8		
	198Au + 60Co		33.0		
	182Ta		6.9		
Ependymoma	198Au		17.7		
Malignant meningioma	182Ta				85.9
	182Ta + 60Co		30.5		
	182Ta + roentgen		56.5		

intraoperatively and postoperatively. Among these patients, 305 were suffering from tumors. The postoperative mean survival times of the patients where radioactive sources had been implanted which were in part combined (Table 9) indicated clearly that even in 1970 our results were satisfying.

Table 10 shows the survival times of the deceased patients, subdivided into groups according to the types of neoplasms, and those who were still alive on the cut-off day (December 31, 1967). At that time 70.3% of our patients treated with the ^{192}Ir "GammaMed" irradiation were still alive, a figure which surpasses the results obtained in our ^{60}Co series. In spite of the partly good results using other nuclides we had to discontinue their application for the above reasons, especially that of the ^{60}Co BCiT.

^{192}Ir GammaMed irradiation, on the other hand, has a wider application and a simpler, more manageable technique than other methods. It can be used stereotactically in all tumors of the cerebrum and cerebellum either primarily or during craniotomy or in the postoperative phase or in recurrencies.

Meanwhile we have treated 284 patients (Table 7) in this way. Survival time with a useful life has increased with better tolerance of the radiation. A second term evaluation of 179 patients covered a period of 11 years (1968–1979). We compared open surgery alone with additional percutaneous radiation, applying additional interstitial ^{60}Co BCiT, with the interstitial ^{192}Ir GammaMed BCiT, with or without radiosensitizing substances[92]. Our results demonstrated that in glioblastomas and oligodendrogliomas, the survival times of patients who had undergone surgical therapy alone were significantly shorter than those of the ^{192}Ir GammaMed group (p < 0.005), although the differences between the individual radiation therapy methods were not significant. However, interstitial BCiT showed the longest mean survival times for all types of tumors, with the exception of astrocytomas. In comparison to the earlier ^{60}Co BCiT, the ^{192}Ir GammaMed BCiT method has proven better results (Table 11).

According to our experience, the biological radiation effect is raised by 60%[78, 95, 104] by applying for several days the intravasal pretreatment with thymine analogous radiosensitizers and antimetabolites (5-bromine-2-deoxyuridin, 5-fluoruracil, methotrexat as well as with the mitosis-inhibiting radiosensitizing substance Synkavit® (natrium salt of 2-methyl-14-naphto-hydrochinon-diphosphate) introduced by Mitchel[68] as an electron acceptor, and with the actinomycin D which blocks the transcription of genetic information of the DNS.

Obviously the BBB is destroyed in the tumor area so that subsequently MTX, CCNU or BCNU can be accumulated to a greater extent (see page 12). It is possible that the oxygen donator Metronidazol[142] plays a role in this therapy method. In combination with these radiosensitizers and metabolites, the average survival times in patients with glioblastomas and oligodendrogliomas are better than with the postoperative ^{192}Ir GammaMed therapy alone. The death curves show a more favorable effect with radiosensitizing and higher survival quotas in cases of astrocytomas and oligodendrogliomas. Only patients from the radiosensitized group were alive on the target day (Table 12).

The type of tumor also has a significant influence on the survival time (p < 0.001); astrocytomas and oligodendrogliomas are known to have a better prognosis in comparison with the other tumors. The same holds true for the polar

Table 10. Postoperative survival times of malignant brain tumor patients following radiation with interstitially ^{192}Ir GammaMed Brachy Curie therapy [76]

Classification	Dead patients			Surviving patients		
	Months	Localization	Histology at reoperation	Months	Localization	Reoperation
Glioblastoma	23.7*	f	no tumor	49.4	p-t	no tumor
	9.6	f	tumor + necrosis	39.6	f	tumor
	9.0	c-p-t	—	37.7	f-c	no tumor
	8.7	t-o	—	24.8	t-o	—
	6.0	f-c-t	tumor + necrosis	21.9	t	—
	3.1	c	—	17.2	f-c	no tumor
	2.7	t-o	—	16.4		—
	0.8*	f	—	14.9	f	—
				13.7	c-p	—
Astrocytoma (dedifferentiated)	26.7	c-p	tumor	38.5	f-t	—
	18.7	t l	tumor + necrosis	30.7	f	tumor
	17.4	c-p	tumor + necrosis	21.0	f	—
	2.9	t-p-o l	—	14.7	t l	—
				12.1	f	—
Ependymoma (dedifferentiated)	5.7**	p-o l	no tumor	13.8	f l	—
Oligodendroglioma (dedifferentiated)	61.2	f	tumor	26.2	f-c	no tumor
	18.7	f	tumor	23.2	f	no tumor
	14.0	p-o	tumor + necrosis	24.3		tumor + necrosis
Melanoblastoma	30.3	p-o	no tumor	16.2	f	—
Malignant glioma	8.4	c-t l	—	24.0	t-o	—
Sarcoma	3.7	f	—	37.0	f-t	—
Malignant meningioma				30.9	c	no tumor
				20.7	c	—

* Dead by complication after reoperation.

** Dead by emboli after radiation.

f = frontal, c = central, p = parietal, t = temporal, o = occipital localization, l = left hemisphere. Surviving patients are listed only when irradiated more than one year ago.

Table 11. Comparison of various methods of treatment in 305 patients[92]

	Surgery		Surgery + percutaneous irradiation		Surgery + interstitial ^{60}Co irrad		Surgery + ^{192}Ir GammaMed irradiation	
	n	t_s	n	t_s	n	t_s	n	t_s
Glioblastoma multiforme	10	125 ± 110	23	250 ± 235	31	290 ± 208	71	283 ± 206
Astrocytoma	7	692 ± 619	10	744 ± 427	29	512 ± 565	47	669 ± 502
Oligodendroglioma	7	314 ± 131	4	537 ± 528	7	650 ± 578	32	1,070 ± 919
Ependymoma	5	290 ± 70	5	363 ± 71	9	647 ± 1,013	8	912 ± 948

n = number of cases.
t_s = survival time in days.

Table 12. Survival after interstitial Ir-192-GammaMed BCiT with/without radiosensitization (179 patients)[92]

	n +	n −	t_s +	t_s −	$t_{max.}$ +	$t_{max.}$ −
Glioblastoma	62	9	9.6 ± 6.9	8.3 ± 6.8	35.3*	23.6
Astrocytoma	43	4	22.1 ± 16.9	24.1 ± 16.7	65.3*	47.5
Oligodendroglioma	25	7	37.2 ± 33.4	30.1 ± 18.5	111.5*	63.3
Metastasis	6	2	24.4 ± 35.2	9.1 ± 0.8	95.5*	9.6
Ependymoma	6	2	24.1 ± 22.1	49.3 ± 59.9	55.8*	93.1
Undifferentiated meningioma	2	1	16.7 ± 16.5	28.8	28.4	28.8
Other tumors	7	3	10.1 ± 10.9	28.3 ± 19.2	32.5	46.1
Total	151	28				

* = still living.
n = number of cases.
t_s = survival (months).
$t_{max.}$ = maximum survival (months).
+/− = with/without sensitization.

location of the tumor and for the average target dose (40 Gy), but not for the sex of the patient, except for the tendency among female patients towards glioblastomas. What is significant, however, is the age of the patient; patients under 40 years of age show a better prognosis for glioblastomas and a more favorable tendency for the other types of tumors. The catamnestic evaluations reveal that 77% of the patients who are still alive at that time show a satisfactory to very good state of health (see also Fig. 18). In the light of the evidence, one can justifiably ask the question whether the combination of a prior treatment with radiosensitizers and a follow-up treatment with cytostatic agents would not yet further improve the BCiT results (see Krauseneck, this volume).

The following results were revealed by the latest, and third series of 79 patients which was evaluated recently[96], with special emphasis on anamnesis, pretreatment in cases of recurrences of high-grade tumors and quality of life (according to the Karnofsky scale):

5. New Results of BCiT

Tables 13 and 14 show the pretreatment and median survival time, being the harder evaluation criterion than the mean survival time which was used in the past. It is evident that even in cases of recurrences of the hemispheric tumor, e.g. in glioblastomas, an additional 5–7 months of life can be gained for the patient, especially after ^{192}Ir GammaMed irradiation but also after ^{125}J afterloading BCiT. For interstitial RT, the patient must only be hospitalized for a few days. What is even more important than the survival time itself, is the survival quality, as determined according to the Karnofsky scale (Fig. 18). It is improved after the radiotherapeutic intervention and then remains constant at the preoperative level, only sinking during the final weeks before death. This tendency has already been demonstrated in all of our previous cases.

Parietal tumors have better median survival times (Table 15). This experience has also been confirmed by other therapeutical centers. Leibel et al.[61] reported a series of 53 patients with malignant gliomas, recurrent after surgery and conventional RT who underwent implantation with removable high activity ^{125}J sources between January 1980 and September 1984. In all patients, tumor

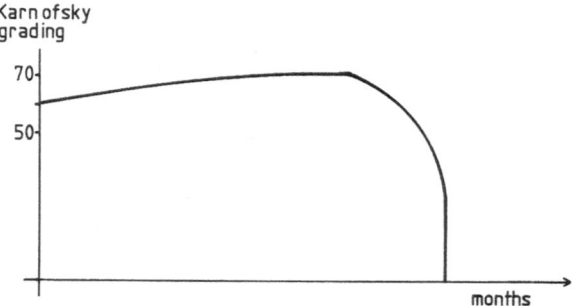

Fig. 18. Clinical trend of 69 patients with intracranial tumors treated with BCiT

Table 13. Previous treatment of 14 stereotactically biopsied nonglial intracranial tumors before BCiT (1975–1984)

Histology	"Open" biopsy	Partial resection	External irradiation	Without confirmed histology	Number of cases
Meningioma	0	1	0	0	1
Metastases	0	2	3	0	10
Unclassified tumor	0	1	1	1	1

Median time of anamnesis, pretreatment and median survival time after ^{192}Ir GammaMed and ^{125}J afterloading BCiT

		Number of cases	Median time of anamnesis months (min./max.)	Pretreatment resection/irradiation Number of cases	Median survival time after BCiT (months) +	Median survival time after BCiT (months) *
Papilloma	^{192}Ir	1	1		58 (1)	
	^{125}J	0	0			
PNET	^{192}Ir	1	1		2	
	^{125}J	0	0			
Meningioma	^{192}Ir	0	0	1		
	^{125}J	1	15	0	19	
Metastases	^{192}Ir	4	2(2–7)	2	9	8 (1)
	^{125}J	6	2	3	13	9 (1)
Unclassified tumor	^{192}Ir	0	0			
	^{125}J	1	24		5	

(Continuation of Table 13: see next page)

* = still living.
+ = dead (number of cases).

(Table 13 continued)

Additive external irradiation after ^{192}Ir GammaMed and ^{125}J afterloading BCiT

		Number of cases	BCiT therapy	Additive external irradiation	Median survival time (months)
Papilloma	^{192}Ir	1	1	0	58
	^{125}J	0	0	0	0
PNET	^{192}Ir	1	1	0	2
	^{125}J	0	0	0	0
Meningioma	^{192}Ir	0	0	0	0
	^{125}J	1	1	0	19
Metastases	^{192}Ir	10	4	1	9.5
	^{125}J		6	2	14
Unclassified tumor	^{192}Ir	0	0	0	0
	^{125}J	1	1	0	5

Table 14. Previous treatment of 65 stereotactically biopsied cerebral gliomas before BCiT (1975–1984)

Histology	"Open" biopsy	Partial resection	External irradiation	Without confirmed histology	Number of cases
Astrocytome II	3	5	4	1	8
Astrocytome III	0	10	9	3	26
Oligodendroglioma III	0	3	0	0	3
Glioblastoma IV	1	6	3	0	28

Median time of anamnesis, pretreatment and median survival time after ^{192}Ir and ^{125}J afterloading BCiT

		Number of cases	Median time of anamnesis months (min./max.)	Pretreatment resection/irradiation Number of cases	Median survival time after BCiT (months) +	*
Astrocytoma II	^{192}Ir	6	16 (10–114)	5	13	40 (4)
	^{125}J	2	8/58	4	12	7 (1)
Astrocytoma III	^{192}Ir	15	6 (1–50)	10	7	7 (3)
	^{125}J	11	4 (1–24)	9	4	26 (2)
Oligodendroglioma III	^{192}Ir	2	85/7	3	5	0
	^{125}J	1	27	0	7	0
Glioblastoma IV	^{192}Ir	17	2 (1–8)	6	4	6 (4)
	^{125}J	11	2 (1–22)	3	5	3 (1)

* = still living.
+ = dead (number of cases).

Additive external irradiation after ^{192}Ir GammaMed and ^{125}J afterloading BCiT of 65 cerebral gliomas (1975–1984)

		Number of cases	BCiT therapy	Additive external irradiation	Median survival time (months)
Astrocytoma II	^{192}Ir	8	6	1	26
	^{125}J		2	0	9
Astrocytoma III	^{192}Ir	26	15	5	7
	^{125}J		11	7	5
Oligodendroglioma III	^{192}Ir	3	2	0	5
	^{125}J		1	0	7
Glioblastoma IV	^{192}Ir	28	17	9	10
	^{125}J		11	6	5

Table 15. Regional distribution and median survival of intracranial tumors treated by BCiT
(1975–1984)

Regional distribution	Number of cases	^{192}Ir	^{125}J	Median survival rate (months)
Frontal	21	13	8	7
Temporal	20	14	6	6
Parietal	30	14	16	8
Hypothalamus	2	2	0	4
Thalamus	5	2	3	3
Midbrain, pons	1	1	0	8

progression had been documented after previous external RT; many of them had been also treated chemotherapeutically (usually nitrosoureas), either as part of the primary treatment or because of recurrences. Patients were considered evaluable if they were alive and available for the first evaluation 9 weeks after implantation. Twenty-three of the implantations into recurrent malignant gliomas resulted in responses of 2 to 17 months' duration. Stabilization of disease was achieved in 9 patients for 3 to 15 months whereas continued progression occurred in 13 cases.

The median survival time of the 42 patients treated for recurrent malignant gliomas with ^{125}J afterloading BCiT is 18 months with 50% of the patients remaining alive. Patients with glioblastomas had a median survival of 9 months while in patients with anaplastic astrocytomas the median survival has not been reached, with 78% alive after 2 years. The quality of life of these patients has been varying. The minority are unable to care for themselves, whereas many return to work, school, or houshold activities.

Of the 7 patients of the Szikla series[149] with grade III gliomas, 86% were still alive after 3 years and 55% after 5 years. Of the 9 patients with grade IV gliomas, 44% were alive after one and 19% after two years. They were treated either exclusively with ^{192}Ir BCiT or in combination with external radiation. Szikla et al.[150] reported also a combined experience made in various neurosurgical centers in France. A median survival rate of 12.7 months was described in 11 patients whose tumors were found to measure greater than 5 cm. Their analysis also comprised a group of 28 patients with grade II–III gliomas measuring between 3 and 5 cm. 70% of this group showed stabilization of their disease for as long as three years after implantation.

Among others, Dyck[22, 23] applied our technique. Out of a total of 31 patients who underwent CT-guided stereotactic biopsy and insertion of an afterloaded removable ^{192}Ir interstitial implant, 25 patients showed a definite tumor regression for 4 to 18 months from the time of implantation. 3 patients showed evidence of tumor stabilization for 4 to 14 months. 3 patients showed evidence of tumor progression.

In cases of malignant growth, we often combine CiT with ^{192}Ir or ^{125}J, mostly applicated in tumors around the midline, with external radiation or, above all in

Table 16. Stereotactic biopsy, histology, CiT (^{192}Ir, ^{125}J) and external beam irradiation of 277 intracranial nonglial tumors (1965–1984)

Histology	Number of cases	Biopsy only	External irradiation only	CiT with ^{192}Ir	CiT with ^{125}J	Additive external irradiation
Ependymoma	20	5	2	6	9	1
Papilloma	8	3	0	4	1	0
Medulloblastoma	6	4	4	0	2	0
PNET	24	12	8	4	8	0
Meningioma	14	8	0	2	4	0
Germinoma	35	18	16	7	10	13
Teratoma	13	9	1	3	1	0
Craniopharyngioma	59	43	0	8	8	1
Epidermoid	9	6	0	3	0	0
Colloid cyst	10	9	0	1	0	0
Metastases	69	56	35	2	11	2
Unclassified tumor	10	6	2	3	1	0

Stereotactic biopsy, histology, CiT (^{192}Ir, ^{125}J) and external beam irradiation of 924 cerebral gliomas (1965–1984)

Histology	Number of cases	Biopsy only	External irradiation only	CiT with ^{192}Ir	CiT with ^{125}J	Additive external irradiation
Astrocytoma I	196	75	4	60	61	2
Astrocytoma II	363	182	32	83	98	14
Astrocytoma III	174	112	79	21	41	25
Oligodendroglioma II	52	20	1	21	11	0
Oligodendroglioma III	12	5	2	6	1	1
Glioblastoma IV	127	96	88	13	18	23

Table 17. 3 and 5 years survival expectancy in maligne gliomas after stereotactic interstitial ^{192}Ir and ^{125}J CiT (1965–1980)

	Number of cases	3 years	5 years
Astrocytoma III	62	66%	43%
Oligodendroglioma II + III	36	61%	22%
Glioblastoma IV	50	17% (2 years)	

recurrences, with a "boost", using the ^{192}Ir GammaMed. A survey of our cases is shown in Table 16. Our partial results of earlier series, dealing with tumors which are commonly characterized as malignant, have been published elsewhere[71, 72, 76, 82, 88, 109].

In Table 17, one of the partial evaluations is shown[88].

The results of CiT of malignant brain tumors classified according to the different cerebral regions, are listed in Figs. 19 and 20 for the hypothalamic region and in Figs. 21 and 22 for the pineal region. The results for the thalamic region are listed in Table 18.

The median survival times for the tumors treated with CiT, as compared to tumors which were solely biopsied, above all in the thalamic region, are much longer.

The fundamentally better results of CiT in cases of low-grade gliomas have been published elsewhere[108–110].

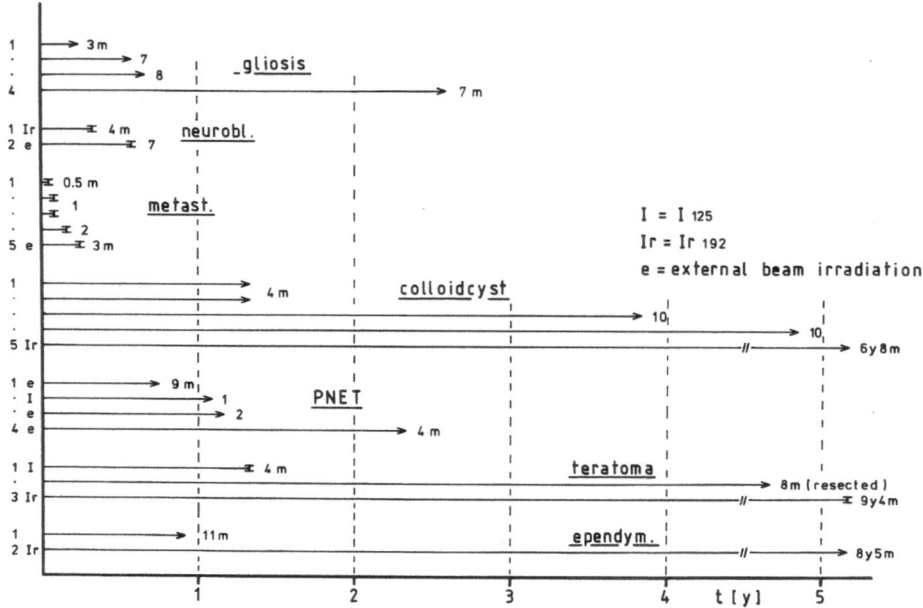

Fig. 19. Survival time of *diverse tumors* of the hypothalamic region after stereotactic CiT[107]

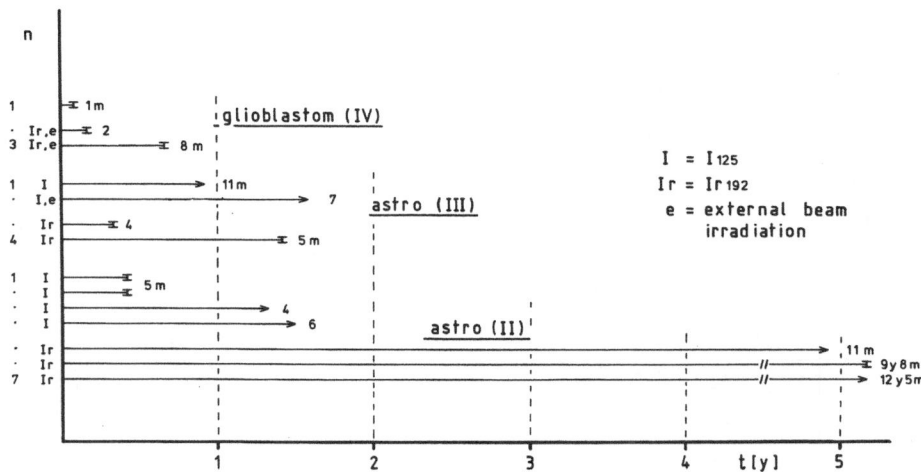

Fig. 20. Survival time of *gliomas* (grades II–IV) of the hypothalamic region after stereotactic CiT[107]

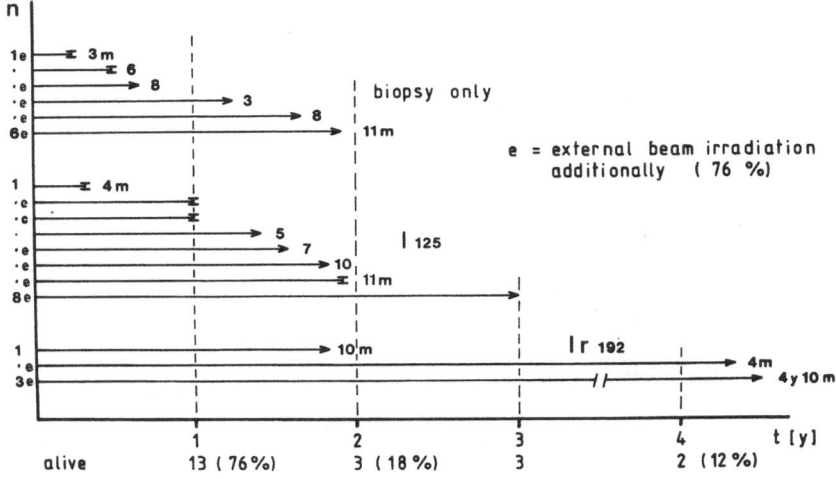

Fig. 21. Survival time of *germinomas* (WHO grade IV) of the pineal region after stereotactic CiT[106]

6. The Place of BCiT in the Treatment Plan

High dose rate BCiT is not indicated for tumors of the midline except in anaplastic tumors, when the dose is fractionated and administered in "boosts", possibly in combination with external radiotherapy and cytostatic agents. Interstitial irradiation is indicated for midline tumors and applied as CiT, using ^{125}J and ^{192}Ir for permanent implantation, even in cases of malign tumors of grades III and IV

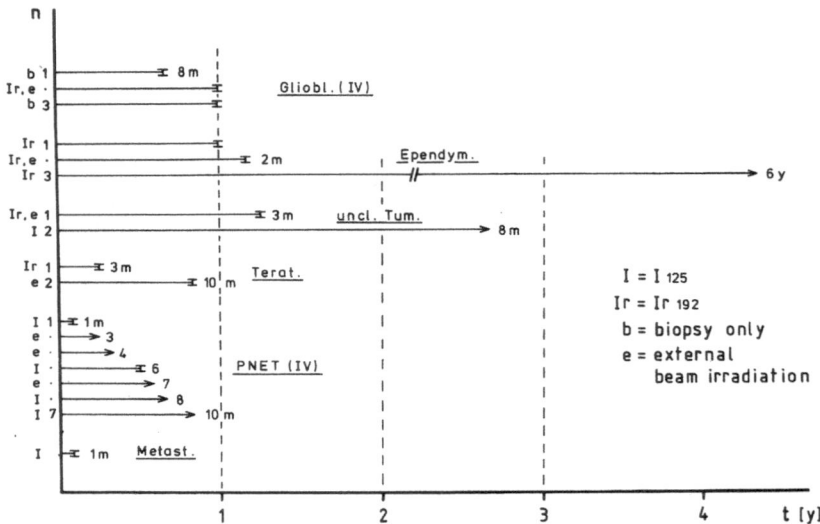

Fig. 22. Survival time of *diverse tumors* of the pineal region after stereotactic CiT[106]

Table 18. Median survival time of patients with anaplastic thalamic gliomas (n = 84)

Tumortype	^{192}Ir	^{125}J	Biopsy only
		Months	
Astrocytoma III	5	16	3
Astrocytoma IV	8	6	3

Median survival time of 23 metastases of the thalamic region

	Number of cases	Months
^{192}Ir permanent implantation	1	6
^{125}J permanent implantation	2	6 + 17
^{125}J BCiT	2	12 + 13
Biopsy only	18	1–7

(Fig. 23). For low-grade tumors of the midline, low dose rate CiT is, according to our experience and long-term results in more than 25 years, the method of choice. The details of low dose rate CiT of low-grade tumors of the midline are not discussed. This has been published elsewhere[92, 94, 97, 102, 105–111].

However, we cannot agree with the opinion of Gutin and Bernstein[32] that in low-grade tumors of the midline area, preference should be given to external RT

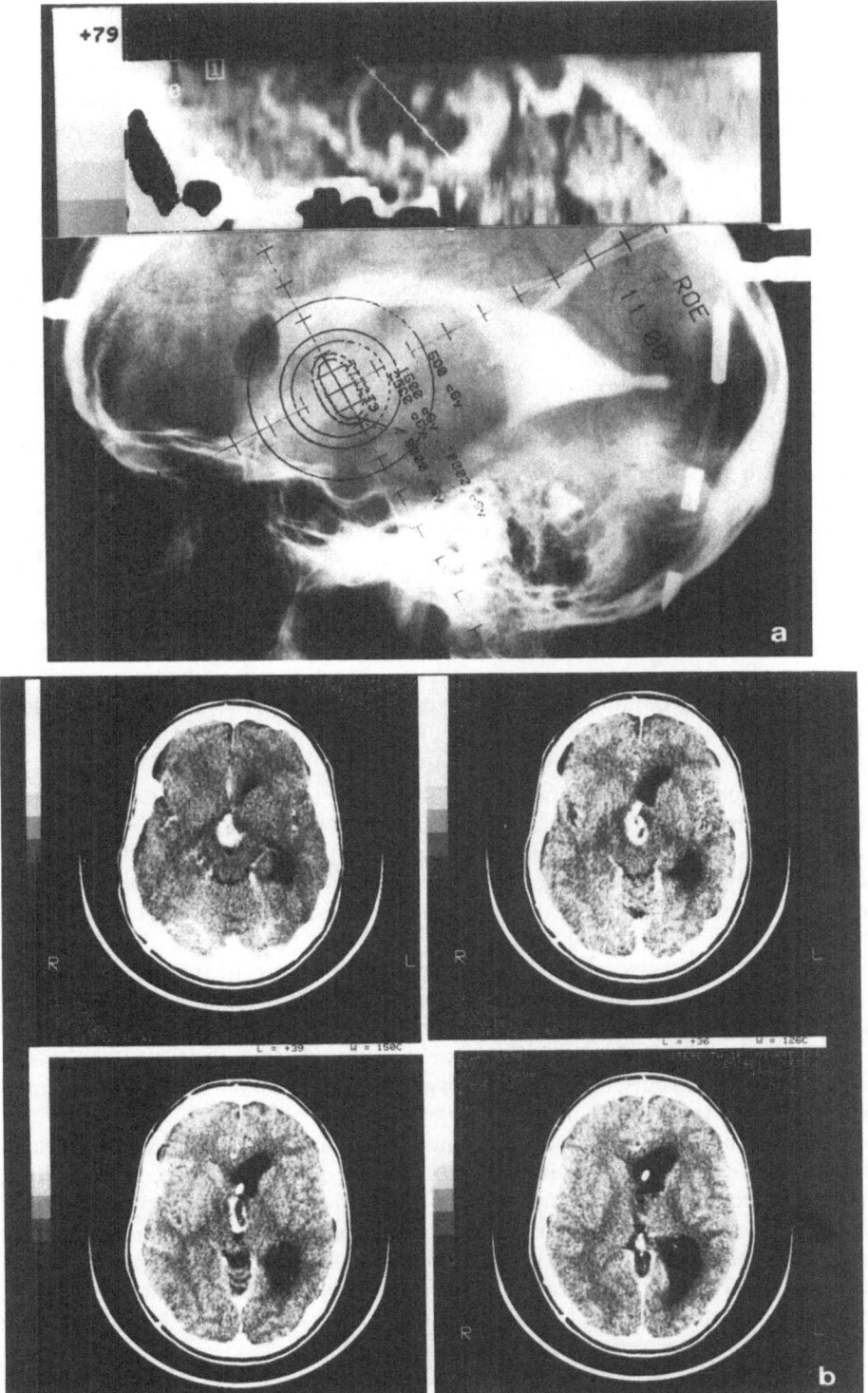

Fig. 23. E.G., 27 years. Anaplastic astrocytoma of the diencephalon (WHO grade III).
a Above: Sagittal reconstruction of the centrally necrotic astrocytoma. **b** 17 months after [125]J
CiT. The CT with enhancement presents scarred and in parts necrotic changes. The tumor
has clearly shrunk. For reasons of insufficient drainage by the left atrioventricular shunt, the
valve had to be exchanged. Survival time: Since onset: 24 months. Since [125]J CiT: 19 months

and not to CiT. The histological, radiobiological and clinical follow-up data hold against the primary external RT of low-grade tumors. Even more so, these tumors which are histologically classified as benign or semi-benign, show high radioresistance for doses of 55–65 Gy, to be absorbed at the focus by means of external RT methods "lege artis".

The low-grade tumor itself shows in the gray matter of the midline, as well as in the brain stem/pons area, histologically either hardly any or very small radioregressive changes, without any reduction of the tumor volume. This has been repeatedly proved by biopsy. Clinical effects of improvement on the one hand interfere with the affection of the surrounding normal brain tissue on the other hand, mainly the white matter in the radiation cylinder. In the sense of an inner decompression, this region either shrinks by microcystic necroses or glial volume reduction and glial scars, or the ventricular plexus secretion is reduced.

High dose rate BCiT should therefore be limited to tumors which are in a narrow sense also histologically malignant, as far as they are localized in the hemispheres. According to our own experience, based on the comparison of long-term results, BCiT is indicated as follows: In cases of nonresectable tumors of functionally important regions, with special emphasis on medial hemisphere regions.

Craniotomy with open resection should be carried out in such cases where the tumor is accessible without severe functional deficits being caused and where a good palliative effect can be expected. In cases of malignant tumors or metastases, the craniotomy should be immediately followed by external (percutaneous) irradiation. Depending on the morphology and dignity, these measures can be additionally supported by an appropriate cytostatic therapy.

If the short-term CiT control reveals that either the tumor does not sufficiently react to the external RT, or grows further or a new, interstitial BCiT is indicated in cases where small-volume conditions are still given (Fig. 24). The MRI follow-up of the externally irradiated cases seems to be a problem today, since even with irradiation doses of 20 Gy, extended signal foci are shown which blur the tumor itself[93].

If the basal ganglia are already affected by the tumor, the further therapeutic steps should depend upon the patient's general state, the existing functional deficits and the speed of growth; depending on these factors, the treatment will be either limited to applying corticoids or possibly continuing the combination of chemostatic and cytostatic agents, if an active therapy appears advisable and promising at all with regard to the quality of life.

Depending on the further clinical course, BCiT may again immediately follow, possibly after another operative resection of the necroses has been carried out, causing clinical improvement. It appears to be important that also the re-BCiT therapy is carried out in cases of tumor rests or recurrences consistently and at an early stage and that we should not wait until, on the one hand, the tumor volume has also for this type of therapy grown hopelessly big and, on the other hand, percutaneous radiation, which has previously been carried out to an optimum degree, cannot be repeated any more.

In some cases we have carried out a combination of BCiT (25–40 Gy) with additional permanent implantation of ^{192}Ir or ^{125}J (70–90 Gy). Here we consider the

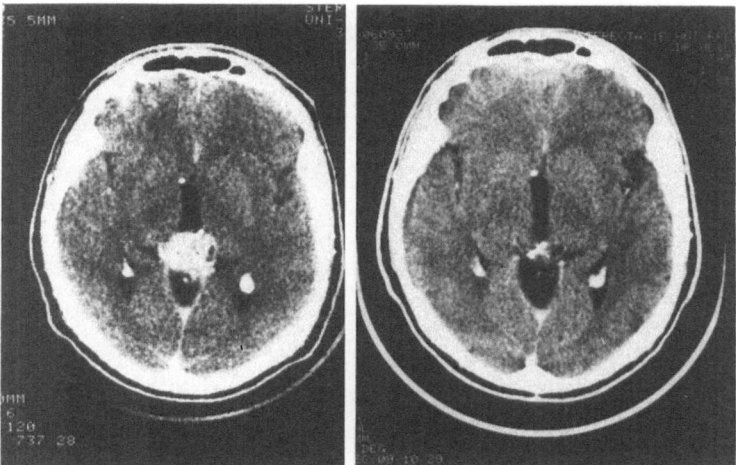

Fig. 24. H. H. P., 47 years. Recurrence of a primitive neuroectodermal tumor (PNET) with a caudally adjacent cyst, after open surgery and external irradiation. The illustration on the *left* shows the recurrence before the ^{125}J CiT (8.7 mCi, peripheral tumor dosage 80 Gy). Illustration on the *right:* 1 year later. The patient is fully able to work in his profession. The neurological, above all the ophthalmological findings have completely receded. Survival time: 24 months

advantage to be in the fact that the applied dose can be administered gradually over a period of time which results in a less severe reactive perifocal edema and makes the therapy more tolerable. This combination is indicated for malignant tumors in the commissural systems and in the white matter near the third ventricle, *e.g.*, the corpus callosum, posterior ventricle triangle, mediotemporal and frontocaudal parts of the hemisphere, etc.

BCiT with ^{125}J or ^{192}Ir may be applied in the hemispheres in cases of morphologically low-grade brain tumors, if they are well demarcated[22, 23, 35, 81–88, 149–151]. According to our experience with large numbers of patients, however, the protracted long-term radiation with very low dose rate permanent implantation of ^{125}J and ^{192}Ir has proved to be the better therapy method in these cases.

Due to radiation protection laws, the permanent implantation of *larger* tumor volumes using ^{192}Ir or other γ-ray emitters such as ^{182}Ta, is unfortunately no longer permitted in most countries, although their effectiveness has been demonstrated[70, 72, 76]. The use of these emitters is therefore limited to the implantation of smaller tumor volumes. Due to the radiation protection laws of the different countries, including West Germany, also the permanent implantation of higher activities of ^{192}Ir, or ^{182}Ta, etc which were formerly used by us is today impossible.

Therefore we have made a virtue of necessity in such cases by carrying out a combinaton of permanently implanted ^{192}Ir and ^{125}J in order not to exceed the permitted γ-ray doses of ^{192}Ir. This was done because, according to long-term examinations, the ^{192}Ir has proved superior to the ^{125}J in cases of low-grade tumors, as is shown by the evaluations of the life expectance (see p. 22 and Fig. 25).

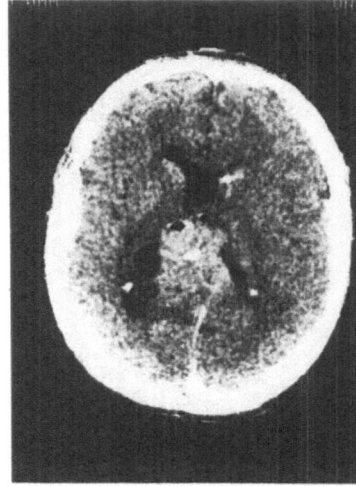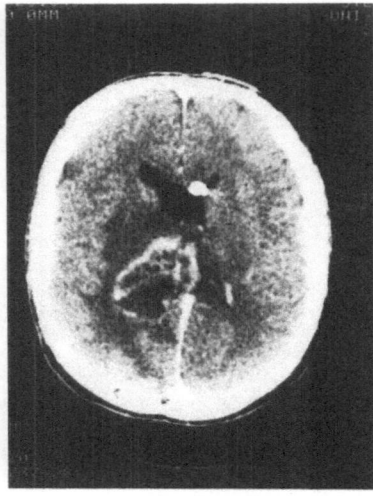

Fig. 25. L. U., 35 years. Recurrent pinealoblastoma. A shunt had been implated in 1980, followed by percutaneous RT and partial resection in December 1983. Now, recurrence 6 months after open surgery. **Left:** 2 days after implantation of a [125]J seed on June 26, 1984 (activity 15.8 mCi, peripheral tumor dosage 90 Gy, radius 17 mm). **Right:** 5 months later. The malign tumor is to a large extent necrotized and has, as a whole, not grown. The perifocal edema has increased. Survival time: 11 months after CiT

If the growth of the focus is revealed in the further clinical course and a tumor recurrence can be demonstrated by the CT stereotactic biopsy, an [125]J re-implantation is in cases of midline tumors exlusively indicated if, from the functional point of view, it is still advisable at all; (Fig. 26) in some cases it may be combined with an external "boost", added to the focal dose. Tests using ^{32}P capsules, ^{90}Y seeds and [198]Au seeds are, according to our own experience, not very promising, since the exact distribution of the nuclides in a close-mashed grid is technically almost impossible and the recurrences start to grow faster from the low-dose lines of the underdosed areas[69–72, 146].

7. Indications for Curie (Brachy-Curie) Therapy and Combined Radiotherapy

The decision on which method to use and which radioactive sources to apply depends on the histological diagnosis, the grading of the tumor, the localization within the brain, the tumor volume and the infiltration direction.

According to our experience, the following clinical indications, possibly in combination with external radiation and cytostaticas well as chemotherapy, have proved to be advisable in cases of nonresectable tumors (Table 19).

The local (focal) interstitial and intracavitary application of the radionuclides in intracranial tumors has effectively expanded the therapy, or has even become the treatment method of choice, as for example in cases of nonresectable low-grade midline tumors.

Based on our 33 years' experience with more than 1,900 interstitial radiation interventions using radioisotopes, among them 1,587 (December 31, 1984) carried out by means of the stereotactic operation method, the following clinical indications have become obvious:

It should be taken into account that, in larger brain tumors of the hemispheres, open surgery with, if possible, total or subtotal removal of tumor should be tried. Should, however, the removal or partial resection of a tumor prove impossible because of anticipated severe functional deficits, or should for other reasons open

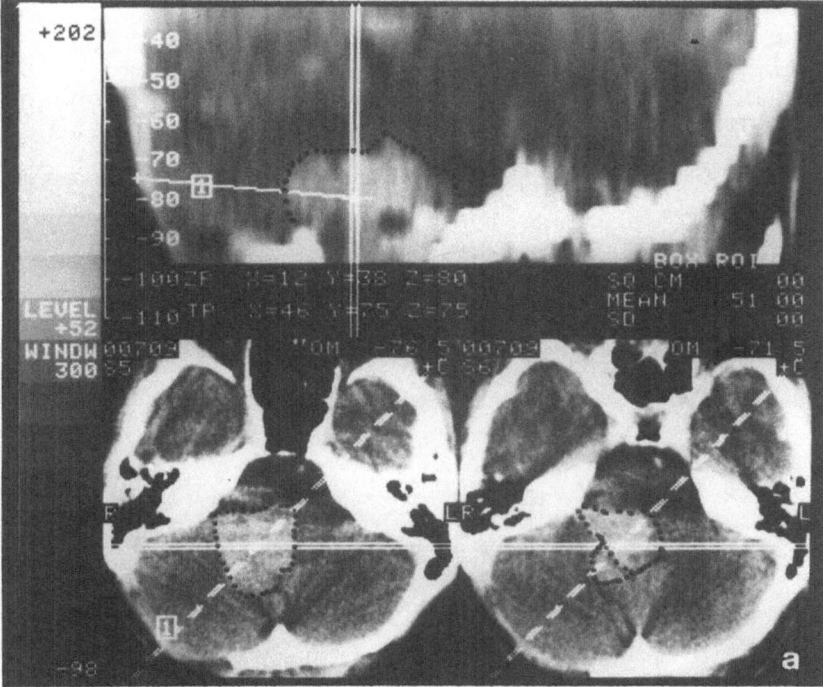

Fig. 26. O. T., 33 years. Malignant recurrent ependymoma (WHO grade II-III) in the right medial cerebellar hemisphere and vermis, infiltrating the brain stem, after open surgery. Clinically: abasia, astasia, very serious vertigo and vomiting, so that an anti-emetic had to be injected every 30 minutes. CiT stereotaxic approach: transcerebellar, on the right side. *a* The oblique CT reconstruction above shows the extension of the ependymoma, with enhancement represented hyperdensely. The figures below show, in two planes, the oblique approach through the osteoclastic craniotomy site. The tumor outlines are marked. The coordinates for the target point and the trephination point are displayed below the reformated picture. *b* On the radiograph, the cannula in the target point. Implantation of [125]J seed (activity 3.5 mCi, peripheral tumor dosage 70 Gy). The isodoses are superposed. 6 months later, an additional ^{192}Ir implantation was carried out (activity 1.0 mCi, peripheral tumor dosage 100 Gy). *c* The ^{192}Ir seed is easily distinguishable. Proof of a tumor is no longer possible. Clinical improvement with complete disappearance of neurological symptoms and signs. The patient can work as a teacher again

(Figs. 26 b and c: see next page)

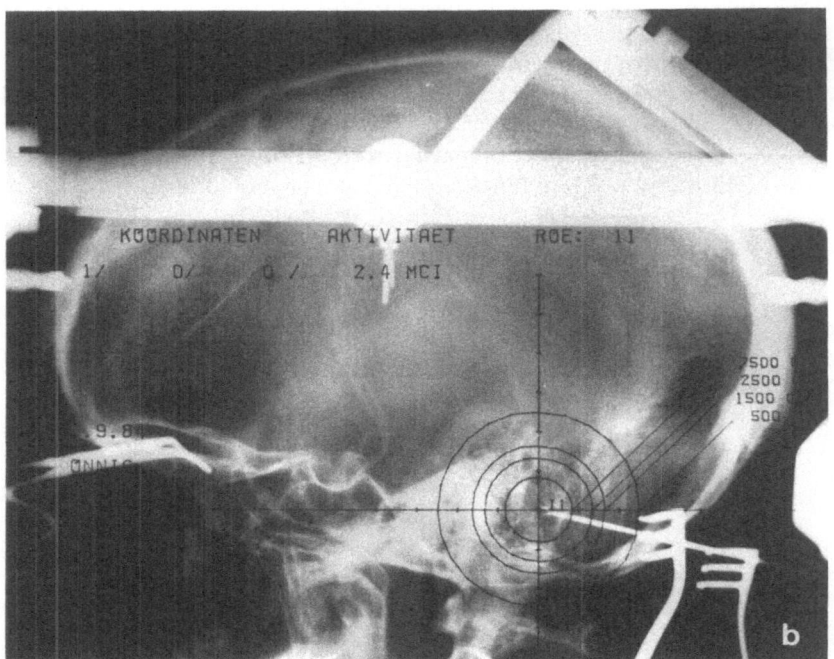

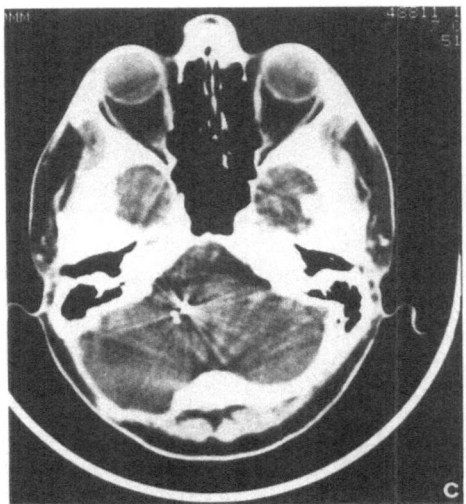

Figs. 26 b and *c*

Table 19. Indications for CiT stereotactic high-dose rate ^{192}Ir or [125]J BCiT (temporary implantation) of intracranial malign tumors

	Biopsy obligatory
Primary BCiT	small volume hemispheric tumors tumors in functional important region (central, temporal, parietal) nonresectable deep-seated tumors
Secondary BCiT	after operation and external irradiation recurrances after external irradiation

Not indicated in processes around midline structures

Table 20. Clinical indications

1. BCiT plus external irradiation (evt. Chemotherapy)	(a + b) Anaplastic glioma (grade III, IV) glioblastoma, malignant ependymoma; melanoma; medulloblastoma; sarcoma; metastasis
2. BCiT alone	Small-volume malignant tumors as recurrent malignant tumors after external irradiation (also CiT)
3. CiT alone	(a) Cysts; small-volume glioma; glial, nonglial and extracerebral tumors; hypophysis-adenoma and recurrences
	(b) Glioma (grades I, II); ependymoma; dysontogenetic tumors; extracerebral benign and semibenign tumors or recurrences even of malignant midline tumors
4. CiT plus external irradiation	Anaplastic glioma (grade II–III); germinoma; pineoblastoma-cytoma
5. External irradiation (including neuroaxis)	Inoperable large-volume anaplastic glioma; multiple metastases; medulloblastoma; germinoma (PNET); malignant extracerebral tumors

surgery be contraindicated, then stereotactic CiT-BCiT therapy is indicated (Table 20).

1. In anaplastic tumors (grade III or IV) of the hemispheres, the combination of interstitial BCiT and percutaneous RT allows an effectiv increase in the local dosage, thus improving the palliative result (Fig. 27). If the anaplastic tumor is detected at an early stage and if it fulfills the conditions for small-volume irradiation, BCiT alone is indicated first.

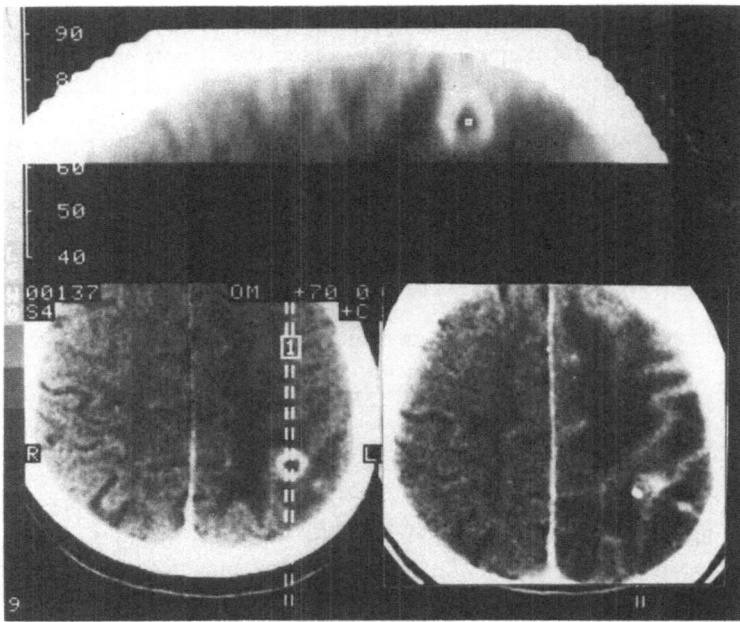

Fig. 27. V. B., 42 years. Leukemic infiltrate, on the left, parietal, 2 months after external radiation. BCiT with [125]J, tumor dosage 40 Gy. 13 months later, ring structure with a growth tendency. **Upper** and **bottom left:** Before the [125]J permanent implantation (radius 12 mm, activity 7.5 mCi, tumor dosage 100 Gy). **Bottom right:** 5 months later, no evidence of a recurrence. The implanted [125]J seed is easily recognizable

2. Regular CT control is used to decide whether re-implantation or additional percutaneous irradiation is indicated. After fully combined treatment, recurrent tumors can again be treated with BCiT.

3. Experience has shown that tumors of grades I and II do not react satisfactorily to the external irradiation technique. If the boundaries of the tumor can be easily demarcated, CiT, combined with additional therapeutic measures such as cyst puncture, catheter systems etc, is indicated, and long-term, palliative and curative results can be achieved.

For extended nondelimited hemisphere gliomas of grades I and II, corticoid therapy alone should be applied. A surprisingly long palliative effect can sometimes be achieved with this treatment.

4. For the transition to anaplastic tumors (grade II and III), CiT is preferred in combination with percutaneous RT.

5. External RT may be indicated[2, 50, 66, 67], if necessary in combination with radiosensitizers and cytostatic agents[63] whenever the anaplastic tumor (grades III or IV) is already infiltrating extensively and whenever the patient's general condition and functional deficits, as well as any spread into the brainstem and basal ganglia do not any longer justify CiT-BCiT[63]. In such cases, priority must be given to enabling the patient to live a purposeful and worthwile life rather than forcing a statistically longest-possible palliative result.

References

1. Apuzzo MLJ, Sabshin JK (1983) Computed tomographic guidance stereotaxis in the management of intracranial mass lesions. Neurosurgery 12: 277–284
2. Atac MS, Blaauw G (1979) Radiotherapy in brain-stem gliomas in children. Clin Neurol Neurosurg 81: 281–290
3. Atkinson AB, Allen IV, Gordon DS (1979) Progressive visual failure in acromegaly following external pituitary irradiation. Clin Endocrinol (Oxf) 10/5: 469–479
4. Backlund EO (1973) Studies on craniopharyngiomas. III. Stereotaxic treatment with intracystic yttrium 90. Acta Chir Scand 139: 237–247
5. Bataini JP, Ennuyer A, Dhermain P, Jaulerry C, Diaz de Bedoya LV (1975) Radiothérapie des tumeurs cérébrales de l'adulte à exclusion des gliomes hémi-spheriques. Neurochir (Paris) 21: 391–399
6. Bell AG (1903) Letter to the editor. Arch Roent Ray 8: 64
7. Bergstroem M, Greitz T, Steiner I (1980) An approach to stereotaxic radiography. Acta Neurochir (Wien) 54: 157–165
8. Bernstein M, Gutin PhH (1981) Interstitial irradiation of brain tumors: a review. Neurosurgery 9: 741–750
9. Birg W, Mundinger F (1973) Computer calculations of target parameters for a stereotactic apparatus. Acta Neurochir (Wien) 29: 123–129
10. Birg W, Mundinger F (1982) Direct target point determination for stereotactic brain operations from CT data and the calculation of setting parameters for polar-coordinate stereotactic devices. Appl Neurophysiol 45: 387–395
11. Birg W, Mundinger F (1984) CT-guided stereotaxy with the Riechert/Mundinger apparatus for biopsy and interstitial curietherapy of intracranial processes. J Neuro-Oncol 2: 280
12. Birg W, Mundinger F, Klar M (1977) Computer assistance for stereotactic brain operations. Adv Neurosurg 4: 287–291
13. Birg W, Krebber L, Mundinger F (1979) Ein einfaches Verfahren für die Übertragung von Tomographie-Scan-Schichten auf das Röntgenbild, insbesondere für die funktionelle Neurochirurgie. Fortschr Neurol Psychiat 47: 637–640
14. Birg W, Mundinger F, Mohadjer M, Weigel K, Fürmaier R (1985) X-ray and MR-stereotaxy for the functional and nonfunctional neurosurgery. Appl Neurophys 48: 22–29
15. Birg W, Schneider J, Bauer S, Mundinger F (1979) An interactice program system for the stereotactic interstitial implantation of radionuclids in brain tumors. In: Szikla G (ed) Stereotactic cerebral irradiation. Biomed Press Elsevier/North-Holland, pp 77–80 (INSERM symposium no 12)
16. Bond WH, Richards D, Turner E (1965) Experiences with radioactive gold in the treatment of craniopharyngioma. J Neurol Neurosurg Psych 28: 30–38
17. Danlos H (1905) Quelques considérationes sur le traitement des dermatoses par le radium. J Physiother (Paris) 3: 98–106
18. Davis RL, Barger GR, Gutin PhH, Philips ThL (1984) Response of human malignant gliomas and CNS tissue to I-125-brachytherapy: A study of seven autopsy cases. Acta Neurochir [suppl] 33: 301–305
19. Davis RL, Gutin PhH, da Silva V, Hattner R, Wara W (1984) The effect of I-125 brachytherapy on the radionuclide and CT scans in malignant gliomas with pathologic correlations. J Neuro-Oncol 2: 284–287
20. Dutreix A, Marinello G, Wambersie A (1982) Dosimétrie en curiethérapie. Masson, Paris
21. Dutreix A, et al. (1976) Développement actues du système de Paris — deuxième partie. J Radiol 60: 319–325

22. Dyck P (1983) Stereotactic biopsy and brachytherapy of brain tumors. University Park Press, Baltimore
23. Dyck P, Bouzaglou A, Solti-Bohman LG, Gruskin Ph (1983) Computer-aided, CT-guided biopsy and brachytherapy of brain tumors. Bull Clin Neurosci 48: 122–138
24. Franke HD (1980) Two years of experience with fast neutrons (DT, 14 MeV) in clinical tumor therapy at Hamburg-Eppendorf. In: Kärcher K-H, Kogelnik HD, Mayer H-J (eds) Progress in radio-oncology. G Thieme, Stuttgart New York
25. Frazier CH (1920) The effects of radium emanations upon brain tumors. Surg Gynecol Obstet 31: 236–239
26. Fritz-Niggli M (1959) Strahlenbiologie. G Thieme, Stuttgart
27. Galassi E, Tognetti F, Frank F, Gaist G (1984) Extraneural metastases from primary pineal tumors. Review of the literature. Surg Neurol 21: 497–504
28. Godwin JT, Farr LE, Sweet WH, Robertson JS, Stikkley EE, Locksley HB (1955) Pathological studies of eight cases of glioblastoma multiforme treated by thermal neutron capture by 13-10. Cancer 8: 601–615
29. Groothuis D, Ostertag Ch, Vick N (1984) Changes in brain capillary permeability caused by I-125 interstitial radiation. J Neuro-Oncol 2: 283–284
30. Greenberger J, Cassady JR, Levene MG (1977) Radiation therapy of thalamic, midbrain and brain stem gliomas. Radiology 122: 463–468
31. Gruskin P, Saeger KL, Carberry JN (1983) Neuropathology of stereotactic biopsies. In: Dyck P (ed) Stereotactic biopsy and brachytherapy on brain tumors. University Park Press, Baltimore, pp 63–78
32. Gutin PhH, Bernstein M (1984) Stereotactic interstitial brachytherapy for malignant brain tumors. Prog Exp Tumor Res 28: 166–182
33. Gutin PhH, Bernstein M, Sano Y, Deen DF (1984) Combination therapy with 1,3-bis(2-chloroethyl)-1-nitrosourea and low dose rate radiation in the 9 L rat brain tumor and spheroid models: Implications for brain tumor brachytherapy. Neurosurgery 15: 781–786
34. Gutin PhH, Phillips ThL, Hosobuchy Y, Wara WM, Mackay AR, Weaver KA, Lamb S, Hurst S (1981) Permanent and removable implants for the brachytherapy of brain tumors. Int J Radiat Oncol Biol Phys 7: 1371–1381
35. Gutin PhH, Philips ThL, Wara WM, Leibel SA, Hosobuchi Y, Levin VA, Weaver KA, Lamb S (1984) Brachytherapy with removable iodine-125 sources for the treatment of recurrent malignant brain tumors. Acta Neurochir [suppl] 33: 363–366
36. Gutin PhH, Wara WM, Philipps ThL, Wilson CB (1980) Hypoxic cell radiosensitizers in the treatment of malignant brain tumors. Neurosurgery 6: 567–576
37. Habers E, Chandhuri NK (1959) MTX, FU and BUDR in nucleic acid metabolism. J Biol Chem 234: 1255–1262
38. Hall EJ, LAM Y-M (1978) The renaissance in low dose-rate interstitial implants. Front Radiat Ther Oncol 12: 21–34
39. Hardy J (1975) Transsphenoidal microsurgical removal of pituitary microadenomas. Prog Neurol Surg 6: 200–216
40. Heilburn MP, Robert TS, Apuzzo MLJ, Wells TH, Sabshin JK (1983) Preliminary experience with Brown-Roberts-Wells (BRW) computerized tomography stereotaxic guidance system. J Neurosurg 59: 217–222
41. Henschke UK (1958) Artificial radioisotopes in nylon ribbons for implantation in neoplasms. Proc Int Conf Peaceful Uses Atomic Energy 10: 48–53
42. Hilaris BS (1978) Techniques for interstitial and intracavitary radiation. Cancer 22: 745–751
43. Hilaris BS (ed) (1975) Handbook of interstitial brachytherapy. Mass Publ Sci Group, Acton

44. Hilaris BS, Henschke UK, Holt JG (1968) Clinical experience with long half-life and low-energy encapsulated radioactive sources in cancer radiation therapy. Radiology 91: 1163–1167

45. Hilaris BS, Kim JA, Tokita N (1976) Low energy radionuclides for permanent interstitial implantation. AJR 126: 171–178

46. Hochberg GH, Pruitt A (1980) Assumptions in the radiotherapy of glioblastoma. Neurology (NY) 30: 907–911

47. Holt G, Hilaris BS, Balter S, Ragazzoni GD, Philips RF, Laughlin JS (1968) Experience with computerized implant dosimetry. AJR 102: 688–693

48. Huk W, Baer U (1980) A new targeting device for stereotaxic procedures within the CT scanner. Neuroradiology 19: 13–17

49. Imm W, Fürste O, Ostertag Ch, Mundinger F, Wehinger H (1978) Intralumbale Radiogoldapplikation (^{198}Au) zur Prophylaxe zentral nervöser Leukämie-Rezidive. Dtsch Hämatologenkongreß, Göttingen, Oktober 1978

50. Jellinger K, Volc D, Podreka I, Grisold W, Flament H, Vollmer R, Weiss R (1981) Ergebnisse der Kombinationsbehandlung maligner Gliome. Nervenarzt 52: 41–50

51. Kelly PJ, Kall BA, Goerss SG (1984) Computer simulation for the stereotactic placement of interstitial radionuclide sources into computer tomography-defined tumor volumes. Neurosurgery 14: 442–448

52. Kelly PJ, Kall BA, Goerss SG (1984) Computer assisted stereotactic biopsies utilizing CT and digitized arteriographic data. Acta Neurochir [suppl] 33: 233–235

53. Kelly PJ, Olson MH, Wright AG (1978) Stereotactic implantation of iridium-192 into CNS neoplasms. Surg Neurol 10: 349–354

54. Kelly PJ, Olson MH, Wright AE, Giorgi C (1979) CT localization and stereotactic implantation of Ir-192 into CNS neoplasms. In: Szikla G (ed) Stereotactic cerebral irradiation. Elsevier/North-Holland Biomedical Press, Amsterdam, pp 123–128 (INSERM symposium no 12)

55. Kjellberg RN (1979) Stereotactic Bragg peak proton radiosurgery results. In: Szikla G (ed) Stereotactic cerebral irradiation. Elsevier/North-Holland Biomedical Press, pp 233–240 (INSERM symposium no 12)

56. Kiessling M, Kleihues P, Gessaga E, Mundinger F, Ostertag ChB, Weigel K (1984) Morphology of intracranial tumours and adjacent brain structures following interstitial iodine-125-radiotherapy. Acta Neurochir [suppl] 33: 281–289

57. Kleihues P, Volk B, Anagnostopoulos, J, Kiessling M (1984) Morphologic evaluation of stereotactic brain tumors biopsies. Acta Neurochir [suppl] 33: 171–181

58. Koslow M, Abele MD, Griffith RC, et al. (1981) Stereotactic surgical system controlled by computed tomography. Neurosurgery 8: 72–82

59. Laitinen LV, Liliequist B, Fagerlund M, Eriksson AT (1985) An adapter for computed tomography-guided stereotaxis. Surg Neurol 23: 559–566

60. Laws ER, Taylor WF, Clifton MB, Okazaki H (1984) Neurosurgical management of low-grade astrocytoma of the cerebral hemispheres. J Neurosurg 61: 665–673

61. Leibel StA, Gutin PhH (1985) Stereotaxic interstitial implantation for the treatment of malignant brain tumors. Int Congress Radiology, XVIth Hawaii, July 1985

62. Leksell L (1971) Stereotaxis and radiosurgery. An operative system. Charles C Thomas, Springfield, Ill

63. Levin VA, Wara WM, Davis RL, et al. (1985) Phase III comparison of BCNU and the combination of procarbazine, CCNU, and vincristine administered. J Neurosurg 63: 218–223

64. Levy LF, Elvidge AR (1956) Astrocytomas of the brain and spinal cord. A review of 176 cases, 1940–1949. J Neurosurg 13: 413–443

65. Liwnicz BH, Berger TS, Liwnicz RG, Aron BS (1985) Radiation-associated gliomas: A report of four cases and analysis of postradiation tumors of the central nervous system. Neurosurgery 17: 436–445

66. Lütolf UM, Glanzmann CH, Aberle HG, Horst W (1978) Ergebnisse der Radiotherapie bei 68 inoperablen Hirntumoren (1950–1975). Strahlentherapie 154: 8–10

67. Marsa GW, Probert JC, Rubinstein LJ, Bagshaw MA (1973) Radiation therapy in the treatment of childhood astrocytic gliomas. Cancer 32: 646–655

68. Mitchell JS (1953) Acta Radiolog 116: 431

69. Mundinger F (1956) Eine einfache Methode der lokalisierten Bestrahlung von Großhirngeschwülsten mit radioaktivem Gold. Münch Med Wschr 98: 23–25

70. Mundinger F (1958) Beitrag zur Dosimetrie und Applikation von Radio-Tantal (Ta^{182}) zur Langzeitbestrahlung von Hirngeschwülsten. Fortschr Röntgenstr 89: 86–91

71. Mundinger F (1963) Die interstitielle Radio-Isotopen-Bestrahlung von Hirntumoren mit vergleichenden Langzeitergebnissen zur Röntgentiefentherapie. Acta Neurochir (Wien) 9: 89–109

72. Mundinger F (1966) Treatment of brain tumors with radioisotopes. In: Krayenbühl H, Maspes M, Sweet C (eds) Progress of neurological surgery, vol I. Karger, Basel, pp 202–257

73. Mundinger F (1969) Erfahrungen mit der stereotaktischen interstitiellen Brachytherapie mit Ir^{192}-"GammaMed" bei infiltrierenden Hirntumoren. Fortschr Röntgenstr 110, 254–261

74. Mundinger F (1969) Die intraselläre protrahierte Langzeitbestrahlung von Hypophysenadenomen mittels stereotaktischer Implantation von Iridium^{192}. Acta Radiol 8: 55–62

75. Mundinger F (1970) Intraselläre Iridium^{192}-Permanent-Implantation bei Hypophysenadenomen. In: Bushe K-A (Hrsg) Fortschritte auf dem Gebiet der Neurochirurgie. Hippokrates, Stuttgart, S 83–87

76. Mundinger F (1970) The treatment of brain tumors with interstitially applied radioactive isotopes. In: Wang Y, Paoletti P (eds) Radionuclide applications in neurology and neurosurgery. Charles C Thomas, Springfield, Ill, pp 199–265

77. Mundinger F (1970) Interstitial radioisotope therapy of intractable diencephalic tumors by the stereotaxic permanent implantation of iridium-192, including bioptic control. Conf Neurol 32: 195–203

78. Mundinger F (1972) Combined treatment of experimental DS-tumors and infiltrating cerebral gliomas with interstitial Curie-therapie and radiosensitizing drugs. In: Proceed fourth europ congr neurosurgery. Present limits of neurosurgery. Avicenum, Prag, p 77

79. Mundinger F (1975) Interstitial Curie-therapy in the treatment of pituitary adenomas and for hypophysectomy. Progr neurol Surg 6: 326–379

80. Mundinger F (1975) Stereotaktische Operationen am Gehirn. Grundlagen — Indikationen — Resultate. Hippokrates, Stuttgart

81. Mundinger F (1979) Rationale and methods of interstitial iridium-192-Brachy-Curie-therapy and iridium-192 or iodine-125 protracted long term irradiation. In: Szikla G (ed) Stereotactic cerebral irradiation. Elsevier/North-Holland Biomedical Press, pp 101–116 (INSERM symposium no 12)

82. Mundinger F (1981) Die stereotaktische interstitielle Therapie nicht resezierbarer intracranieller Tumoren mit Ir-192 und Jod-125. In: Wannenmacher M, Schreiber HW, Gauwerky F (Hrsg) Kombinierte chirurgische und radiologische Behandlung maligner Tumoren. Urban & Schwarzenberg, München, S 90–112

83. Mundinger F (1982) Implantation of radioisotopes (Curietherapy). In: Schaltenbrand G, Walker AE (eds) Textbook of stereotaxy of the human brain. Thieme, Stuttgart, pp 410–435

84. Mundinger F (1982) Stereotactic interstitial therapy of non-resectable intracranial tumours with iridium-192 and iodine-125. In: Kärcher KH, *et al.* (eds) Progress in radio-oncology II. Raven Press, New York, pp 371–380

85. Mundinger F (1984) CT-stereotactic biopsy of brain tumours. In: Voth D, Gutjahr P, Langmaid C (eds) Tumours of the central nervous system in infancy and childhood. Springer, Berlin Heidelberg New York, pp 234–246

86. Mundinger F (1984) Stereotaktische intrakranielle Bestrahlung von Tumoren mit Radioisotopen (Curie-Therapie). In: Dietz H, Umbach W, Wüllenweber R (Hrsg) Klinische Neurochirurgie, II: Klinik und Therapie. G Thieme, Stuttgart New York, S 519–565

87. Mundinger F (1984) Langzeitbestrahlung nicht resezierbarer intrakranieller Hirntumoren. Die CT-stereotaktische interstitielle Curie-Therapie mit Jod-125-Seeds. Münch Med Wschr 126: 126: 1176–1179

88. Mundinger F (1985) Technik und Ergebnisse der interstitiellen Hirntumorbestrahlung. In: Heilmann HP (Hrsg) Handbuch der medizinischen Radiologie, Bd XIX/4: Spezielle Strahlentherapie maligner Tumoren. Springer, Berlin Heidelberg New York, S 179–214

89. Mundinger F, Birg W (1981) CT-aided stereotaxy for functional neurosurgery and deep brain implants. Acta Neurochir (Wien) 56: 245

90. Mundinger F, Birg W (1984) Stereotactic biopsy of intracranial processes. Acta Neurochir [suppl] 33: 219–224

91. Mundinger F, Birg W (1984) CT stereotaxy in the clinical routine. Neurosurg Rev 7, 219–224

92. Mundinger F, Busam B, Birg W, Schildge J (1979) Results of interstitial iridium-192-Brachy-Curie therapy and iridium-192 protracted long term irradiation. In: Szikla G (ed) Stereotactic cerebral irradiation. Elsevier/North-Holland Biomedical Press, pp 303–320 (INSERM symposium no 12)

93. Mundinger F, Weigel K, Fürmaier R, Volk B (1986) CT, MRI and stereotactic biopsy. In: Poeck K, Freund HJ, Gänshirt H (eds) Neurology. Springer, Berlin Heidelberg New York, pp 469–476

94. Mundinger F, Hoefer T (1974) Protracted long-term irradiation of inoperable midbrain tumors by stereotactic Curie-therapy using iridium-192. Acta Neurochir (Wien) 21: 93–100

95. Mundinger F, Jobski Ch, Vogt P, Fischer HU (1970) The interstitial Curie-therapy (GammaMed) after radiosensibilizing using bromdesoxyuridine/bromdesoxycytidine and antimetabolites on DS-carcinosarcoma of rats (preliminary report). Atomkernenergie (ATKE) 15: 157

96. Mundinger F, Kratz FG, Weigel K (1985) Stereotactic after-loading Brachy-Curie-Therapy with iridium-192 and iodine-125 in non-resectable intracranial or recurrent Tumours. XVIth international congress of radiology, Hawaii, July 1985

97. Mundinger F, Metzel E (1970) Interstitial radioisotope therapy of intractable diencephalic tumours by the stereotaxic permanent implantation of iridium-192, including bioptic control. Confin Neurol 32: 195–203

98. Mundinger F, Noetzel H (1958) Morphologie, Diagnostik und Therapie der malignen Hirngeschwülste. Zbl Neurochir 18: 19–27

99. Mundinger F, Noetzel H, Riechert T (1959) Erfahrungen mit der lokalisierten Bestrahlung von malignen Hirngeschwülsten mit Radio-Isotopen. Acta Neurochir (Wien) [suppl] 6: 171–182

100. Mundinger F, Ostertag ChB, Birg W, Weigel K (1980) Stereotactic treatment of brain lesions: biopsy, interstitial radiotherapy (iridium-192 and iodine-125) and drainage procedures. Appl Neurophysiol 43: 198–204

101. Mundinger F, Reinke M-A, Hoefer Th, Birg W (1975) Determination of intracerebral structures using osseous reference points for computer-aided stereotactic operations. Appl Neurophysiol 38: 3–22

102. Mundinger F, Riechert T (1967) Hypophysentumoren — Hypophysektomie. Klinik — Therapie — Ergebnisse. G Thieme, Stuttgart

103. Mundinger F, Sauerwein K (1966) "GammaMed", ein neues Gerät zur interstitiellen, nur einige Minuten dauernden Bestrahlung von Hirngeschwülsten mit Radioisotopen, auch intraoperativ anwendbar. Acta Radiol (Stockh) 5: 48–52

104. Mundinger F, Vogt P, Jobski Ch, Fischer H-U, Ostertag Ch (1972) Klinische und experimentelle Ergebnisse der interstitiellen Brachy-Curietherapie in Kombination mit Radiosensibilisatoren bei infiltrierenden Hirntumoren. Strahlentherapie 143: 318–328

105. Mundinger F, Weigel K (1984) Stereotactic Curietherapy of thalamic tumours. J Neuro-Oncol 2: 278

106. Mundinger F, Weigel K (1983) CT-stereotactic biopsy and interstitial radiotherapy of pineal region tumors. VIII. Mexican congress of neurological surgery, Acapulco, Mexico, July 1983

107. Mundinger F, Weigel K (1984) Indication and results of stereotactic Curietherapy with iridium-192 and iodine-125 for non-resectable tumors of the hypothalamic region. Acta Neurochir [suppl] 33: 323–330

108. Mundinger F, Weigel K (1984) Long-term results of stereotactic interstitial Curietherapy. Acta Neurochir [suppl] 33: 367–371

109. Mundinger F, Weigel K (1985) Long-term results of stereotactic Curietherapy (permanent-implantation) with iridium-192 and iodine-125 in non-resectable cerebral gliomas or recurrent tumours. International congress of radiology, Hawaii July 1985

110. Mundinger F, Weigel K (1985) CT-stereotactic interstitial irradiation therapy of non resectable and recurrant intracranial tumour in children and adolescents. In: Voth D, Krauseneck P (eds) Chemotherapy of gliomas. Basic research, experiences and results. De Gruyter, Berlin New York, pp 241–259

111. Mundinger F, Weigel K (1985) Results of CT-guided stereotactic Curie-therapy of midline tumors of the brain. Third international meeting on progress in radio-oncology, Wien, March 1985

112. Mundinger F, Weigel K, Mohadjer M (1984) CT-stereotaktische Biopsie und/oder interstitiell-extern kombinierter Strahlenbehandlung von Hirnmetastasen. In: Hirnmetastasen. Pathophysiologie, Diagnostik und Therapie. Akt Onkol 13: 128–143

113. Murray KJ, Blumberg A, Strubler K, Sirota R, Altman J (1984) Permanent radioactive iodine seed implants following radical resection in recurrent human malignant high grad astrocytomas. J Neuro-Oncol 2: 282

114. Musolino A, Munari C, Blond S, Betti O, Lajat Y, Schaub C, Askienazy S, Chodkiewicz JP (1985) Traitement stéréotaxique des kystes expansifs de craniopharyngiomes par irradiation endocavitaire beta (Re 186, Au 198, Y 90). Neurochir (Paris) 31: 169–178

115. Netzeband G, Sturm V, Georgi P, et al. (1984) Results of stereotactic intracavitary irradiation of cystic craniopharyngiomas. Comparison of the effects of yttrium-90 and rhenium-198. Acta Neurochir [suppl] 33: 341–344

116. Notter G (1959) A technique for destruction of the hypophysis using Y^{90}-spheres. Acta Radiol (Stockh) [suppl] 184: 1–128

117. Oehlert W (1967) Zur Histo-Pathologie des Strahlenschadens. Strahlenschaden in Forschung und Praxis 7: 201

118. Orton CG, Webber BM (1977) Time-dose factor (TDF) analysis of dose rate effects in permanent implant dosimetry. Int J Radiat Oncol Biol Phys 2: 55–60

119. Ostertag ChB, Mundinger F, Weigel K (1981) Biopsie stéréotactique et radiothérapie interstitielle des tumeurs cérébrales. Méd Hyg 39: 1994–2008

120. Perry JH, Rosenbaum AE, Lunsford, *et al.* (1980) Computed tomography-guided stereotactic surgery: conception and development of a new stereotactic methodology. Neurosurgery 7: 376–381

121. Pierquien B (1964) Précis de Curiethérapie. Masson, Paris

122. Pierquin B (1976) The destiny of brachytherapy in oncology. AJR 127: 495–499

123. Pierquin B, *et al* (1978) The Paris system in interstitial radiation therapy. Acta Radiol Oncol 17: 33–48

124. Pecker J, Scarabin JM, Brucher JM, Vallee B (1979) Démarche stéréotaxique en neurochirurgie tumorale. Pierre Fabre, Paris

125. Powell M, Olney J, Darling J, Thomas DGT (1984) Correlation of target site with histology and cell culture in CT-directed stereotactic biopsy. J Neuro-Oncol 2: 275

126. Van Putten LM, Kallman RF (1968) Oxygenation status of a transplantable tumor during fractionated radiation therapy. J Natl Cancer Inst 40: 441–451

127. Riechert T, Mundinger F (1956) Beschreibung und Anwendung eines Zielgerätes für stereotaktische Hirnoperationen (2. Modell). Acta Neurochir (Wien) 3: 308–337

128. Riechert T, Mundinger F (1959) Stereotaktische Geräte. In: Schaltenbrand G, Bailey P (Hrsg) Einführung in die stereotaktischen Operationen mit einem Atlas des menschlichen Gehirns. G Thieme, Stuttgart

129. Rougier A, Pigneux J, Cohadon F (1984) Combined interstitial and external irradiation of gliomas. Acta Neurochir [suppl] 33: 345–353

130. Salcman M, Sewchand W, Amin P, Bellis E (1984) CT-guided stereotactic surgery and interstitial irradiation for glial tumors. J Neuro-Oncol 2: 282

131. Sano K (1977) Chemo-radiotherapy of malignant brain tumors. In: Carrera R (ed) Neurological surgery, proceedings of the sixth international congress of neurological surgery, São Paulo ICRS no 433. Excerpta Medica, Amsterdam Oxford, pp 79–87

132. Sachs E, Moore S, Furlow LT (1937) Direct roentgen radiation of brain tumors during operation. Ann Surg 105: 658–661

133. Schaub C, Bluet-Pajot MT, Videau-Lornet C, Askienazy S, Szikla G (1979) Endocavitary beta irradiation of glioma cysts with colloidal 186-rhenium. In: Szikla G (ed) Stereotactic cerebral irradiation. Elsevier/North-Holland Biomedical Press, pp 293–302 (INSERM symposium no 12)

134. Schlegel WH, Scharfenberg J, Doll O, *et al.* (1982) CT-images as the basis of operating planning in stereotactical neurosurgery. Proceedings of the 1st international symposium on medical imaging and imaging interpretation ISMIII October 1982

135. Schulz MD, Wang CC, Zinninger GF, *et al.* (1968) Radic‑herapy of intracranial neoplasms, with a special section on the radiotherapeutic management of central nervous system tumors in children. Prog Neurol Surg 2: 318–370

136. Scott WP (1972) Permanent interstitial implantation technique using absorbable spacers. Am J Roentgenol 114: 620–622

137. Scott WP (1975) Interstitial therapy using nonabsorbable Ir-192 nylon ribbon and absorbable J-125 vicryl suturing techniques. Amer J Roentgenol 124: 560–564

138. Selker R, Eddy M, Anderson L (1984) A method of dosimetry planning and implantation of interstitial irradiation in glioma patients utilizing I-125. J Neuro-Oncol 2: 281

139. Sewchand W, Amin PP, Drzymala RE, Salazar OM, Salcman M, Samaras GM, Botero E (1984) Removable high intensity iridium-192 brain implants. J Neuro-Oncol 2: 177–185

140. Shaw CM, Sumi SM, Alvord EC Jr, Gerdes AJ, Spence A, Parker RG (1978) Fast-neutron irradiation of glioblastoma multiforme: Neuropathological analysis. J Neurosurg 49: 1–12

141. Sheline GE (1975) Radiation therapy of primary tumors. Semin Oncol 2: 29–42

142. Sheline GE, Wassermann ThH, Phillips TL (1979) The role of radiosensitizers in therapy of brain tumors. International symposium on multidisciplinary aspects of brain tumor therapy, Gardone Riviera, June 1979 (abstract book, p 59)
143. Shewmon DA, Masdeu JC (1980) Delayed radiation necrosis of the brain contralateral to original tumor. Arch Neurol 37: 592–594
144. Da Silva V, Gutin PhH, Bernstein M, Weaver K, Deen DF (1984) An animal tumor model for the study of radiation biology of I-125 interstitial brachytherapy. Acta Neurochir [suppl] 33: 311–315
146. Simon N, Silverstone SM, Roach LC, Warner RRP, Baron MG, Rudavsky AZ (1971) Intra-arterial irradiation of tumors, a safe procedure. AJR 112: 732–739
146. Sommermeyer K, Mittermaier L (1957) Untersuchungen über die Dosisverteilung in der Umgebung reiner Gammapräparate mit dem Fluoreszenzdosimeter. Strahlentherapie 102: 78–87
147. Walker MD (1975) Chemotherapy: adjuvant to surgery and radiation therapy. Semin Oncol 2: 69–72
148. Wycis HT, Robbins R, Spiegel-Adolf M, Meszaros J, Spiegel EA (1954) Studies in stereoencephalotomy III: Treatment of a cystic craniopharyngioma by injection of radioactive P-32. Confin Neurol 14: 193–202
149. Szikla G, et al. (1984) Interstitial and combined interstitial and external irradiation of supratentorial gliomas. Results in 61 cases treated 1973–1981. Acta Neurochir [suppl] 33: 355–362
150. Szikla G, Betti O, Szenthe L, Schlienger M (1981) L'expérience actuelle des irradiations stéréotaxiques dans le traitement des gliomas hémisphériques. Neurochir (Paris) 27: 295–298
151. Szikla G, Peragut JC (1975) Irradiation interstitielle des gliomes. Neurochir (Paris) [suppl] 2: 187–228
152. Talairach J, Bonis G, Szikla G, Schaub G, Bencaud J, Covello L, Bordas-Ferrer F (1970) Stereotaxic implantation of radioactive isotopes in functional pituitary surgery. Techniques and results. In: Wang Y, Paoletti P (eds) Radionuclide applications in neurology and neurosurgery. Charles C Thomas, Springfield, Ill, pp 267–325

Author's address: Prof. Dr. F. Mundinger, Abteilung Stereotaxie und Neuronuklearmedizin, Neurochirurgische Universitätsklinik, Hugstetter Strasse 55, D-7800 Freiburg i. Br., Federal Republic of Germany.

5

Radiation Therapy of Brain Tumors

R. Sauer

Strahlentherapeutische Klinik und Poliklinik der Universität Erlangen-Nürnberg, Federal Republic of Germany

1. Introduction

Radiation therapy (RT) is the most important treatment modality following surgery in brain tumors. Most of them respond to radiation administered either in the form of an external beam, or as interstitial implants. Usually, postoperative RT considerably prolongs the recurrence-free survival of the patients, and ameliorates their symptoms when tumors reoccur. RT as the sole therapeutic measure is indicated in only a few exceptional cases. Most frequently, it is an unsatisfactory therapeutic alternative, and remains a stopgap. At the very least, the surgeon must provide a biopsy specimen so that the diagnosis of a tumor, including grading, can be reliably established. This applies also, and in particular, to the diagnosis of recurrence after prior irradiation, in order not to confuse a recurrent tumor with radiation-associated late effects.

Indications for Radiotherapy

For most brain tumors, the results obtainable with RT are not satisfactory not even when used in combination with surgery. In particular, megavoltage irradiation is ineffective in arresting the further growth of glioblastoma multiforme, despite very high doses and large treatment volumes. In palliative RT, the indications are more or less open to discussion. The radiotherapist should be allowed wide powers of discretion, and he must take account of the consequences of the current tumor situation, the short- and middle-term prognosis, and the situation of the patient.

Principally, the following indications for *primary RT* of brain tumors apply:

— The tumor is central in location. A surgical intervention would increase the tumor-related symptoms.

— The tumor involves vital structures, *e.g.* the basal ganglia, brain stem, third ventricle, midbrain. In such cases, surgery would be associated with a high mortality risk.

— The tumor is highly radiosensitive, *e.g.* medulloblastomas, germinomas, or malignant lymphomas and, after biopsy and, possibly, decompression of elevated intracranial pressure, can be controlled by irradiation alone in a high percentage of the cases.

— In optic glioma, RT alone, applied after cautious biopsy, can bring about long-term freedom from symptoms without surgery-related side effects.

— The tumor lesion is recognized as a metastatic deposit of an extracranial malignancy. Although, clinically, only one site may be suspected, multiple tumor sites are usual. Rare exceptions are solitary brain metastases that occur as a differential diagnostic problem, or a long-term controlled primary site that is radioresistant, *e.g.* kidney or colon cancer.

Postoperative irradiation is generally advocated for the following tumor types: astrocytoma grade III—IV, ependymoma, medulloblastoma, pinealoma, sarcoma, hemangioblastoma, and malignant lymphomas.

In the following types of tumor, postoperative irradiation is indicated only if tumor removal has been incomplete:
astrocytoma grade II, oligodendroglioma, meningioma, pituitary adenomas, craniopharyngioma, chordoma, neurinoma.

2. Fundamentals of Radiotherapy

The tumors of the central nervous system (CNS) are of particular interest for local therapy, since, irrespective of whether they are benign or malignant, and unlike most other malignant tumors, they very rarely spread via the bloodstream. The therapeutic concept can concentrate on mastering a local problem, namely, eradication of the primary lesions without having to struggle with the overwhelming problem of distant metastases—so often the cause of failure and death in patients with other types of cancer[30].

Despite the noninvasive growth of benign tumors, (*e.g.* pituitary adenoma, meningioma, craniopharyngioma, optic glioma, cerebellar astrocytoma), they often present problems if resection is attempted, owing to their proximity to critical structures.

Malignant tumors (*e.g.* high-grade astrocytoma, dysgerminoma, and medulloblastoma) infiltrate adjacent nervous tissue and frequently spread beyond the primary site through the parenchyma, corpus callosum or subarachnoidal space (SAS). Malignant tumors in contact with the ventricular system of SAS may disseminate via the cerebrospinal fluid (CSF) pathways. This is particularly seen in medulloblastomas, high-grade ependymomas, germ cell tumors and malignant gliomas of the posterior fossa[29, 43, 274, 278]. Effective local treatment relatively diminishes the appearance of primary recurrence and often controls or eradicates the seeding in the SAS and ventricles, if it is directed primarily to the entire craniospinal axis.

2.1. Radiation Sensitivity and Radioresistance

The effectiveness of ionizing radiation in the treatment of tumors is based upon sensitivity differences between tumor tissue and healthy tissue. Although the physical laws of energy absorption, and the subsequent physico-chemical or biochemical processes, are qualitatively similar in all cells, tumor cells and normal cells usually differ both in the extent of the lethal and sublethal radiation injury, and also in their capacity for initiating repair. The degree of this quantitative difference represents the therapeutic gain. This means that radiotherapy can injure, or possibly even destroy, and tumor tissue that is more vulnerable to radiation than the immediately adjacent healthy brain tissue. Tumors are considered radioresistant when their capacity for repair or cell replacement equals that of the surrounding brain tissue.

Thus, the radiation sensitivity of the whole brain or neural tissue sets a limit to our radiotherapeutic efforts. In addition, the capacity of the brain tissue for effecting repair is low and, decreases with age[199]. The brain stem, spinal cord, and the infantile brain are considered to be particularly vulnerable to radiation. But the capacity of the various parts of the brain to compensate possible late radiation sequelae also differs. Thus, late radionecrosis in the midline region or in the spinal cord has a more serious effect than in the frontal and temporal lobes or on the surface of the cerebral hemisphere where it can be surgically removed.

The *sensitivity of brain tumors* varies over a wide range. Certain germ cell tumors are considered to be highly sensitive to radiation. These are followed by malignant lymphomas and medulloblastomas. In contrast, the glioblastoma is one of the most malignant and most treatment-resistant human malignancies.

Age is a major factor in the treatment of gliomas. Although they may be more radiosensitive in young children, the tolerance levels are lower. Thus, the therapeutic ratio is the same as in adults, although smaller doses are required. Young children with malignant gliomas appear to have a higher survival rate than older patients[30, 213].

The mechanisms responsible for *radioresistance,* can be listed in simplified form as follows:

— *Genuine radioresistance* of the tumor cells. As a result of summation, even small differences can have a large effect.

— The *number of tumor stem cells* and the volume of the tumor are now recognized as the most important prognostic factors with respect to radiation sensitivity. It may thus make good sense to diminish the tumor cell mass prior to initiating radiotherapy.

— The *tumor cell proliferation* varies considerably among the various tumors. It may be so high that the tumor can recover completely in the interval between the individual fractions (repopulation).

— Poor *supply of oxygen* to a tumor can make it radioresistant, since the tumor cells surviving a radiation insult cannot reoxygenate during the treatment-free interval.

The radioresistance of certain tumors, in particular of the high-grade astrocytomas, remains one of the major unresolved problems in the field of oncology. Numerous attempts have been, and are being made, to overcome this resistance: higher radiation doses, modifications of fractioning patterns and the dose per fraction, the use of chemical radiosensitizers and hypoxic cell radiosensitizers, heavy particle beam radiation, hyperthermia, and brachytherapy.

2.2. Types of Radiation

RT uses a variety of types of radiation which produce ionization damage in the cells, tissues, or organs irradiated. The radiation involved here is either electromagnetic radiation, the so-called photon radiation (X- and gamma-rays), or corpuscular radiation (electron, neutron, proton, deuteron and alpha radiation).

Electromagnetic radiation involves the transport of energy through space as a combination of electric and magnetic fields, both of which undergo a change in magnitude with time. The quantity of energy involved may be termed a photon. Photons are classified in accordance with their mode of origin. The photon radiation produced by a telecobalt machine peaks at energies of 1.17 and 1.33 millions of volts (MV). The energy produced by a betatron or linear accelerator varies between 4 and about 40 MV.

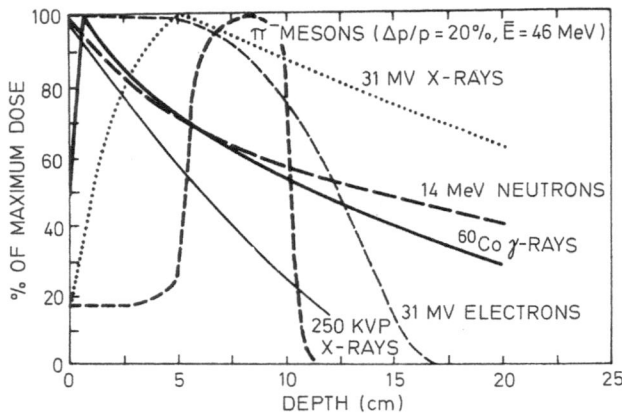

Fig. 1. The absorption of radiation in water as a function of the depth in cm. A number of different types of therapeutic radiation beams are represented. Note the steep decrease in dose of the various corpuscular radiations, electrons, neutrons and pi-mesons (courtesy of Horst, W., Conrad, B. (1966), Fortschr. Röntgenstr. 105: 299–321)

Corpuscular radiation comprises moving particles of matter. For clinical applications, electron radiation is employed, in a few centers also neutrons, and in 4 to 5 centers throughout the world, Pi-mesons. The energy of corpuscular radiation is expressed in millions of electron volts (MeV), and in the case of clinically employed electron radiation varies between 3 and 25 MeV, in the betatron up to 45 MeV.

The depth dose distribution increases with increasing energy. The character of the curve differs, in particular, between corpuscular radiation and electromagnetic radiation (Fig. 1). Thus, with electron irradiation, the depth of penetration of the radiation can be accurately determined by setting the most suitable radiation energy—with electromagnetic radiation, this cannot be done in the same manner.

2.3. Radiation Dose

2.3.1. Definitions

The dose defines the amount of radiation emitted by a source of radiation or absorbed by the body. Of biological importance is the dose absorbed within the body. The physical unit used is the rad or the Gray (Gy). 100 rad correspond to 1 Gy, which corresponds to 1 joule/kg.

The tumor dose is defined as the radiation dose within the target volume. It is expressed as isodose lines "enclosing" the target volume. Isodose lines connect together all the points at which the dose applied is identical. The highest (maximum) dose is delivered only to a point. It is usually made equal to 100%, and the isodose lines are expressed as percentages of the maximum dose.

2.3.2. The Effect of the Dose on Tumor Control

The radiation dose is determined by the histological type of tumor presenting, radioresponsiveness, anatomic site, and the level of tolerance of the surrounding normal structures. Total tumor doses range from 50 to 70 Gy/6–8 weeks, with daily fractions of 1.5–2.0 Gy each. Doses higher than 70 Gy have been shown not to result in a cure of grade IV tumors. Coned-down fields are recommended when doses to the whole brain reaches 35–40 Gy in the cases of children, 50 Gy in young adults, and 50–60 Gy in adults.

In *glioblastomas* (grade IV gliomas), a further increase in the total dose to 80 Gy, sometimes applied to very large volumes, has been able to improve only the 2-year survival rate[280], while no improvement in survival rates beyond 4 years was achieved in patients with grade III astrocytomas. On the other hand, the incidence of severe late radiation sequelae increased. For this reason, Salazar *et al.*[280] recommend that the total tumor dose be reduced again to 60 Gy.

In *medulloblastomas,* a dose-effect relation has been demonstrated in the ± 50 Gy range[24, 58, 63, 124]. A statistically significant correlation was found with the radiation dose delivered to the posterior cranial fossa: 12, 17, 35, and 50% survival rates, respectively, after < 50 Gy, as compared with 45–48, 71, 73, and 80%, respectively, after > 50 Gy (Table 1). No such relationship was found with respect to doses in the supratentorial or spinal regions under cerebrospinal irradiation (CSI).

Table 1. Dose-effect relationship in medulloblastomas. Posterior fossa dose and survival (from 182)

Author	No. of patients evaluated	5-year survival	
		< 50 Gy	≥ 50 Gy
Berry *et al.* (1981)	119	50%	73%
Chin and Maruyama (1981)	20	12%	80%
Cumberlin *et al.* (1979)	19	17%	71%
Harisiadis and Chang (1977)	55	35%	45–48%

Table 2. Dose-effect relationship in ependymomas. Dose to primary tumor volume and survival (from 182)

Author	No. of patients evaluated	5-year survival	
		< 45 Gy	⩾ 45 Gy
Kim and Fayos (1977)	32	20%	46%
Marks and Adler (1982) (4th ventricle tumors only)	25	33%	70%
Phillips *et al.* (1964)	25	0%	87%
Salazar *et al.* (1975)	28	10%	56%

Table 3. Dose-effect relationship in pineal-suprasellar tumors. Dose to primary tumor volume and failure rate (from 182)

Author	No. of failures/Total treated patients	
	< 45 Gy– < 50Gy	⩾ 50 Gy–55 Gy
Abay *et al.* (1981)	2/19	1/8
Bradfield and Perez (1972)	3/7	1/6
Jenkin *et al.* (1978)	0/9	2/22
Sung *et al.* (1978)	15/32	4/40
Total failure rate	25/67 (37%)	8/76 (11%)

In *ependymomas*, available dose-response data are limited. An improvement in the five-year survival rate was reported in patients who had been irradiated with ⩾ 45 Gy to the primary tumor (0, 10, 20, 33%, respectively, as compared with 46, 56, 70, 87%)[164, 210, 250, 279]. Recommendations for dose levels of approximately 50 Gy/5–6 weeks are easily confirmed (Table 2).

A dose-effect relationship has also been found for the tumors of the *pineal* and *suprasellar regions*[1, 43, 157, 277, 318]. The dose levels compared were < 45–50 Gy versus ⩾ 50–55 Gy (Table 3). Salazar *et al.*[277] reported tumor recurrences in 57% of patients receiving ⩽ 50 Gy, and in 31% of those given higher doses.

2.4. Treatment Volume

The treatment volume, particularly for glioblastoma multiforme, medulloblastoma, ependymoma, and the pineal-suprasellar tumors, is a matter of discussion.

2.4.1. Glioblastoma multiforme

A major argument advanced for the use of whole-brain irradiation is the infiltrative growth pattern of the high-grade astrocytomas in the ipsilateral hemisphere, across the corpus callosum or between the thalami[138, 204, 357]. The implications of such infiltrative growth for the treatment volume were discussed by Concannon *et al.*[62]. On the other hand, the pattern of failure after treatment, which alone is of clinical significance, is local recurrence. True multicentric tumors seen in 3–6% of the cases, are less common than once assumed[138, 269]. With the aid of CT and MRI, tumor localization can be improved to the extent that the parts of the brain invaded by the tumor can be identified, and true multicentricity detected. For this reason, we reject the routine use of whole-brain irradiation, and recommend that, in glioblastoma multiforme, the treatment volume should be restricted—albeit with a generous margin—to the region of the tumor alone.

2.4.2. Medulloblastoma

The biology of the medulloblastoma is well documented. In 10 to 15% of the cases, subarachnoidal and ependymal infiltration are identified at presentation in the meninges overlying the cerebellum or within the supratentorial ventricular system[239]. Metastases are detected along the cerebrospinal axis outside of the posterior cranial fossa in one third of the cases when treatment is restricted to the region of the primary tumor[218]. Seeding to the spinal cord has been found by myelography at the time of the diagnosis in 10 to 35%[72]. For this reason, together with the primary tumor region, the entire neurocranium and spinal axis should also be irradiated, with 30 to 35 Gy[30].

2.4.3. Ependymoma

The incidence of CSF metastases of intracranial ependymomas ranges from 0 to 28%[182]. Bloom[30] reviewed 598 cases from the literature, and established an overall incidence of CSF seeding of 12%. A significantly higher incidence of CSF seeding was seen for high-grade ependymomas than for low-grade tumors[30, 164]. The highest occurrence was found in high-grade lesions located in the posterior fossa. Hence, in this subgroup, the routine use of craniospinal irradiation is well founded. Using CSI, improved disease-free survival in ependymoma patients has been reported[30, 210, 279]. However, statistically significant data that support the routine use of CSI are still lacking.

2.4.4. Pineal Tumors and Suprasellar Germinomas

In pineal tumors and suprasellar germinomas, the reported incidence of sub-arachnoidal seeding through the ventricular system is between 0 and 50%[30, 45, 69, 157, 277, 318]. Sung *et al.*[318] reported an incidence of risk of such metastases in 10% of all tumors of the pineal region, and in 42% of the suprasellar germinomas, after five years. This indicates a possible role for cerebro-axis irradiation in these tumors[30, 318]. So far, however, all attempts to correlate the irradiated volumes with recurrence-free survival have failed. Nevertheless, very small fields ($< 10 \times 10 \, cm^2$) are associated with a greater risk of recurrent disease[110, 157, 318]; than is the irradiation of large volumes.

2.5. Dose per Fraction

The total radiation dose is usually applied in daily fractions of $\leqslant 2$ Gy. Any increase in the fraction size is associated with the danger of late injury to the normal brain tissue. For this reason, only in patients with a very short life expectancy individual doses of > 2.0–2.5 Gy per day should be given, that is, in patients who will die before brain necrosis develops (glioblastoma multiforme and brain metastases).

2.5.1. Hyperfractionation

In RT of brain tumors, hyperfractionation (superfractionation) is attempted in the largely radiation-resistant glioblastoma multiforme. This technique is defined as an increased number of fractions, a decrease in the fraction size (< 2 Gy), and a classical overall treatment time. In theory, the total dose should either remain unchanged, or increase. The rationale for this form of treatment is not well known, but the following points are conceivable:

— Using smaller doses per fraction may approximate to a situation similar to that achieved with continuous low-dose radiation techniques[305].

— It is assumed that hyperfractionation can improve local tumor control if the tumor response is dominated by hypoxic cells, or if the tumor cells are slower to repair sublethal insults than normal tissue[76].

— The oxygen enhancement ratio decreases with decreasing dose per fraction when the dose is applied in several fractions per day[221]. This results in a reduced influence of hypoxia, and produces the advantageous features of brachytherapy.

— The tolerance of the normal tissue increases, since repair processes are concluded already after 4 to 6 hours, while taking much longer in tumor tissue.

2.5.2. Accelerated Fractionation

Accelerated fractionation (rapid fractionation) means a shortening of the overall treatment time with higher dose per fraction and unchanged or reduced total dose. In accordance with our present-day knowledge of radiobiology, it is indicated in rapidly proliferating tumors. A disadvantage, however, is the greater injurious effect on the normal tissue.

Therefore, in cases of *glioblastoma multiforme,* the total tumor dose should be reduced to 35–38.5 Gy by increasing the dose per fraction from 2 to 3.5 Gy, while still achieving the same effect as > 50 Gy administered in a conventional fractionation pattern[136]. However, this procedure did not lead to an improvement in survival rate. It is possible, indeed, that an increase in total dose to > 35 Gy with this rapid fractionation pattern, might even reduce survival.

Between 1971 and 1976, the Radiation Therapy Oncology Group (RTOG) carried out a study in 1,902 patients with *brain metastases,* to establish the suitable dose per fraction[39, 40]. The response of patients receiving ultrarapid treatment, which means 10 Gy/1 fraction or 12 Gy/2 fractions, as assessed by improvement in neurological function was comparable to that of patients receiving the longer schedules (20 Gy, 30 Gy or 40 Gy/1–4 weeks). The rate of improvement in neurological function, treatment-associated morbidity and median survival were also comparable with those of patients receiving 20–40 Gy in 1–4 weeks. However, the duration of the improvement, the time elapse to progression of the neurological deficits, and the rate of complete healing of the neurological symptoms, were generally reduced as compared with patients who had received 10 or 12 Gy administered in 1 and 2 days, respectively. On the basis of this study, the application of 10–12 times 3 Gy (30–36 Gy total dose)/2–2½ weeks, has found general acceptance as a suitable fractionation pattern for the RT of brain metastases.

2.5.3. Acceleration by Hyperfraction

More recent clinical concepts combine hyperfractionation with acceleration. Multiple daily fractions of less than 2 Gy are applied up to a total daily dose of more than 2 Gy. In this manner, the same total dose can be given as with customary fractionation in a shorter period of time, but with excellent tolerance by the healthy tissue. It is possible that the higher dose applied over a shorter period, increases tumor reoxygenation[160], and reduces the extent of the repopulation of tumor cells during the radiation series[70].

Unfortunately, these new therapeutic approaches have failed to improve treatment of high-grade astrocytoma[145, 249, 307]. Shin et al.[305] investigated the effect of three fractions per day in a prospective, randomized clinical trial of patients with malignant astrocytomas. 35 patients were randomized to 40 Gy/45 fractions/3 weeks whole-brain irradiation with a subsequent local boost of 10 Gy/5 fractions/1 week (SF); 34 other patients were treated with conventional fractionation patterns, receiving 34 Gy/17 fractions applied to the whole brain over 3½ weeks, with a subsequent local boost of 16 Gy/8 fractions/1.5 weeks (CF). In both treatment groups, additional CCNU was administered. The one- and two-year survival was 54 and 21% in the group with superfractionation, and 32 and 10%, respectively, in the group with conventional fractionation. The median survival for the CF and SF groups were 9 months and 13 months, respectively. The difference in survival was not statistically significant. The other advantages of SF include a shorter mean duration of steroid administration, and improved performance status following RT. Although the superiority of SF RT in the protocol published by Shin et al.[305] may be explained by factors other than the radiation mode, further continuing studies are required to determine the role of SF radiation therapy in the management of malignant astrocytomas.

2.6. Chemical Radiosensitizers

The use of chemotherapy to treat tumors of the brain should be considered, in the first instance, fort the rapidly progressive malignant gliomas, i.e. astrocytomas and oligodendrogliomas, grade III and IV. The blood-brain barrier (BBB) is a major limiting factor for the effectiveness of chemotherapy. Although the BBB is no longer existent in the necrotic center of a malignant glioma, it is still effective in the proliferating marginal areas. Thus, only substances that can penetrate the CSF spaces are effective[128, 195, 225]. An effect on malignant gliomas is exhibited by the nitrosoureas BCNU, CCNU and methyl-CCNU, by procarbazine, possibly also

VM 26, VP 16 and vincristine[179]. Administered either alone or in combination, these agents achieve remissions in up to 30% of the cases[30, 135, 154].

Thus, although chemotherapy alone is ineffective in the treatment of malignant gliomas, in certain cases, the combination of BCNU and RT does appear to accomplish the longest median survival times, and is, therefore, considered the standard treatment in clinical trials. In 30 or 40% of the patients, however, the increase in median survival is achieved at the cost of hematological toxicity and depression of the bone marrow function[135, 154, 321, 338, 340, 341]. This information has been established by the BTSG in a number of phase III protocols[340, 341]. The administration of BCNU prolongs the median survival in comparison with patients receiving surgery alone, by eight weeks. Here, postoperative RT is considerably more effective, adding 20 weeks to median survival. The combination of surgery, irradiation and BCNU, however, does not prolong median survival but increases the number of long-term survivors. Krauseneck et al.[180] reported a median survival of 16–17 months in patients with high-grade astrocytomas after surgery, postoperative irradiation and BCNU ± VM 26. The more powerful lipophilic nitrosourea derivative Semustine (methyl-CCNU) did no prove superior to BCNU[341]. The combination of BCNU and radiotherapy resulted in the best median survival—52 weeks—and the best long-term results. To date, it has, unfortunately, not been possible to improve the results of the combination surgery + RT + BCNU by the addition of other drugs or by other combinations, e.g. CCNU, vincristine, methotrexate, procarbazine or prednisone (COMP protocol[154]). Orally administered CCNU is significantly inferior to BCNU[246].

In summary, not all patients benefit from the combination of RT + BCNU. This is clearly the case in about 30% who die within the first 6 weeks. A further third of the patients have a survival gain of several months, while the remaining third— the long-term survivors—have a chance of surviving, symptom-free, for a number of years.

2.7. Hypoxic Cell Radiosensitizers

Thanks to their electron-affinic properties, hypoxic cell radiosensitizers have a similar radiochemical effect to oxygen, but are metabolized more slowly. For this reason, they are expected to reach deeply seated hypoxic areas by diffusion (Fig. 2). In addition, they have a cytotoxic effect on hypoxic cells, and may enhance the effect of other chemotherapeutic agents[44, 161, 326].

Among the electron-affinic agents, the derivatives of nitroimidazole (metronidazole and misonidazole) have been tested both experimentally[4, 97] and clinically. In particular misonidazole was expected to be effective in the treatment of malignant brain tumors[114, 325, 338, 342]. Ash et al.[11] showed that oral misonidazole reached peak blood levels after about 2 hours. After 4 to 6 hours, 80 to 90% of the maximum blood level was measured in the CSF, and up to 90% of the blood level in the central, necrotic tumor tissue, and in cystic fluid.

Misonidazole was used as a single agent, and in combination with BCNU. The predicted enhancement ratio is between 1.3 and 1.7, which implies that, for a given

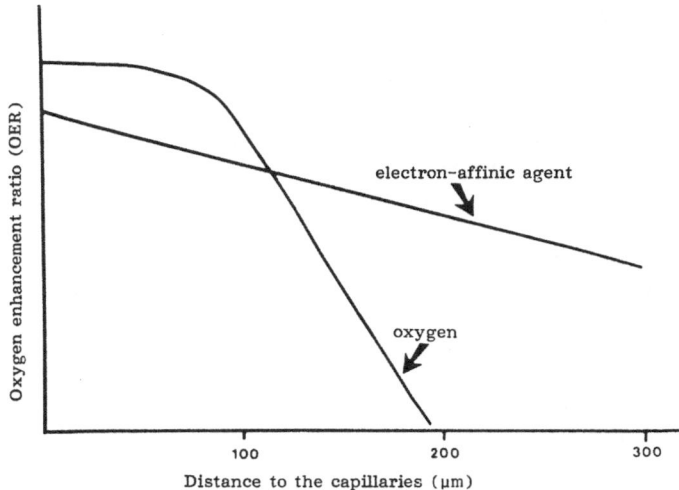

Fig. 2. Electronaffinic substances (radiosensitizers) have, in comparison with oxygen, a longer diffusion pathway, and penetrate more deeply into the tissue (courtesy of Bamberg M, *et al.* (1984) Verh Dtsch Krebsges 5: 221–227)

dose of irradiation, misonidazole will increase its effectiveness by about 30 to 70%[338].

In the first controlled study in patients with supratentorial glioblastomas treated with posteroperative irradiation and metronidazole, there was an initial increase in survival as compared with RT alone, but only within the first 12 months[338]. As for misonidazole, the considerable neurotoxic side effects limit the size of the fraction and the overall dose, so that, in humans, the sensitizing effect found in animal experiments, cannot be fully utilized (see[30, 325]). The following national studies revealed no advantage of adding misonidazole to RT, despite variations in dose and fractionation[26, 52, 120, 145, 273, 297]. This suggests that it is doubtful whether, in malignant gliomas, hypoxia does in fact have any radiobiological significance with respect to therapy resistance.

2.8. Heavy Particle Beam Irradiation

In an attempt to overcome the resistance to therapy of malignant gliomas, neutrons, pi-mesons and heavy ions have been used, too (see[77]). Heavy particle beam irradiation is available at a few centers in Europe and North America. As compared with the photon radiation common employed at the radiotherapeutic centers, these beams cause a more dense ionization per unit length of their path within tissues. This has a greater effectiveness in killing tumor cells and in rendering possible cell survival less capable of sublethal repair. The effect of heavy particle beams is less dependent upon tissue oxygen than that of photon radiation, and also less dependent on the phase of the cell cycle. These biological properties gave reason to hope that greater local control of the more radioresistant tumors might be achieved.

Recent studies were disappointing. In the London neutron therapy trial involving high-grade astrocytomas, pathological evidence of total or near-total tumor destruction was found in 69% of the cases after 13–15.60 Gy tumor dose delivered with 7.5 MeV neutrons[54]. In contrast, after 6 MV photon irradiation at doses of 50–55 Gy, such evidence was found at autopsy in only 14% of the cases. Despite the clearly greater biological effect of the neutrons, however, particle beam therapy resulted in no prolongation of survival. Furthermore, it was associated with more marked radiation-induced changes in the cerebral white matter leading to progressive dementia. A similar experience was reported from Seattle, where 8 MeV neutron radiation was employed to treat patients with glioblastoma multiforme, and compared with a historical series treated with megavoltage irradiation[247]. In order to reduce the powerful side effects of treatment on healthy brain, attempts at combining photon and neutron treatment have been undertaken. Unfortunately, no improvement in survival rates as compared with neutron therapy alone was observed. Owing to the high level of morbidity, mixed-beam RT cannot at present be recommended for treating brain tumors[21, 188].

2.9. Hyperthermia

Hyperthermia, *i.e.* local heating to 41–43 °C is directed against therapy-resistant parts of the tumor in which, both in combination with ionizing radiation and also with cytotoxic chemotherapeutics, it results in greater cell damage than can be produced by one of the modalities used alone[117, 118]. There is evidence that during hyperthermia, the temperature in the tumor tissue might be higher than that in the adjacent healthy tissue. Hyperthermia lowers the tissue pH, at > 41 °C inhibits the repair of subtotal cell damage and, at > 42.5 °C, has cytotoxic effect. In contrast to other fields of cancer therapy, hyperthermia has hardly been tried in the treatment of brain tumors. Occasional case reports on external local hyperthermia[25, 134, 284, 287] do not seem particularly hopeful. However, it may be possible that treatment with a combination of hyperthermia and radiotherapy can enhance the response of malignant gliomas. In our experience, however, the tumors started growing again rapidly after treatment.

At present, the prerequisites for hyperthermia of tumors of the brain, in terms of hardware and technical application, including methods of recording the temperature in the brain tissue, are not yet available. Before clinical trials can be initiated, the effects of hyperthermia, either alone or in combination with cytotoxic drugs and RT, on healthy brain tissue must be investigated. For if the thermal enhancement ratio turns out to be identical for tumor tissue and healthy brain tissue, no therapeutic gain can be expected.

2.10. Brachytherapy
(Permanent and Removable Radioactive Implants)

In view of the results of the BTSG[343] which revealed a statistically significant increase in median survival of glioblastoma patients when a high radiation dose was applied (difference between 50 and 60 Gy significant at p = 0.004), it may be expected in other tumors, too, that, application of higher doses of radiation might improve local tumor control. However, the delivery of doses of external irradiation in excess of 60 Gy is accompanied by brain necrosis[303]. Brachytherapy employing radioactive implants permits a very high radiation dose to be applied to an exactly defined tumor volume, without burdening the surrounding healthy brain tissue to above the tolerance threshold. Interstitial implantations can be employed either alone or to augment the dose delivered by external beam irradiation in the treatment of primary brain tumors, and would also permit the radical retreatment of recurrent malignant gliomas. Depending upon the therapeutic concept and the histology of the tumor, a suitable dose rate can be selected. This is done by making a choice between permanent and temporary application, and in favor of a given radioactive isotope from among the variety of radioactive materials available, or by selecting a given specific activity[113, 233, 323, 329].

2.11. Focal Radiosurgery

Focal radiosurgery is the name given to an irradiation technique in which narrow, highly collimated radiation beams produced by a cobalt 60 unit, an ultrahard photon beam of a linear accelerator, or a high-energy proton beam of a cyclotron, is focused, stereotactically, to a target within the brain, to produce there a high, locally delimited dose[14, 192]. If the dose gradient at the margins of the irradiated volume is very steep, a necrosis dose can be applied in a single session, while, at the same time, exposing the surrounding healthy brain tissue to a negligible dose of radiation.

At present, there are three types of radiation facilities that have been specially adapted for use in focal radiosurgery:
— the gamma unit[14, 193],
— Bragg-peak irradiation[166] and
— moving-field irradiation using a linear accelerator[130, 317].

A prerequisite for this technique of radiosurgery is its combination with a stereotactic localization system. The technique has been used in particular to treat intracranial arteriovenous malformations.

3. Radiotherapeutic Technique

3.1. Radiation Treatment Planning

Treatment planning is a medical and physico-technical procedure that is undertaken in the following steps: Case history and physical examination, special examinations, definition of the tumor volume, and of the target volume, isodose planning, and choice of the treatment technique, simulation and localization of the radiation fields.

3.1.1. Typing and Grading

A knowledge of the nature, histology and degree of malignancy, and also of the primary or metastatic nature of a tumor of the brain are the basis for any decision as to treatment, and also for treatment planning. RT is indicated only if it can be expected to improve survival or the quality of survival.

3.1.2. Tumor Volume (Fig. 3 a)

A second precondition for deciding on treatment, is an accurate knowledge of the pretherapeutic extent of the tumor. If the patient has been submitted to surgery, the radicality of the intervention must be known, as also the geography of possible postoperative histologically suspected or macroscopically detectable residual tumor. For this purpose, the radiotherapist requires

a detailed surgical report,

a histological report (as far as possible with histological workup of the margins) and

the complete diagnostic workup.

The latter comprises physical and neurological examinations, visual field and fundoscopic examination. CT scanning of the brain has become one of the most important procedures for diagnosing and localizing tumors. Occasionally, the CT scan can be supplemented by MRI, that permits a better differentiation between tumor, perifocal edema and normal brain or bone tissue. It also permits the representation of the brain and spinal cord in the sagittal plane, and is superior to CT in the assessment of the base of the skull and the posterior cranial fossa.

Skull roentgenograms can be useful for RT planning, since they show the surgical defect, the position of the surgically introduced catheters, clips or other markers of the surgical cavity. In primary tumors metastasizing to the CSF, CSF cytology should be a routine procedure in order to exclude carcinomatous meningiosis.

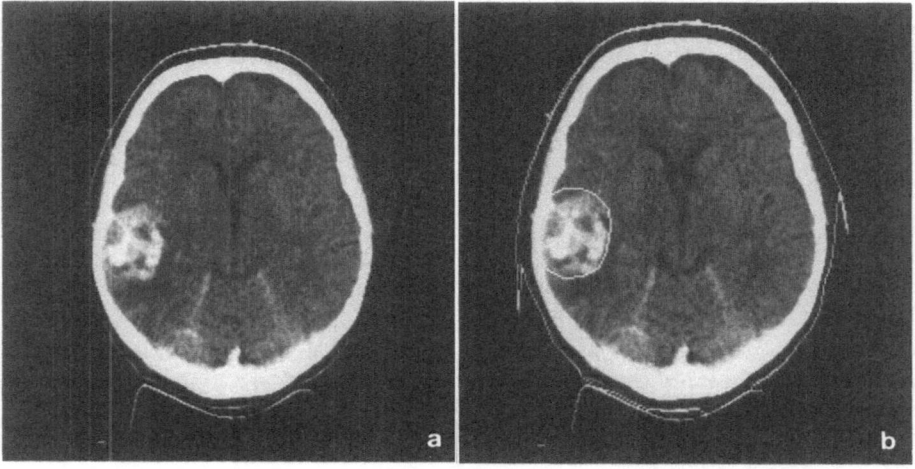

Fig. 3. Treatment planning in the case of glioblastoma with the aid of CT. *a* The CT reveals the extent of the tumor (tumor volume). *b* Demarcated tumor volume. *c* Target volume. *d* Three treatment portals. *e* Isodose distribution

3.1.3. Target Volume (Fig. 3 b)

On the basis of a knowledge of the localization, volume and histology of the tumor, and a consideration of the dose-limiting vital structures, *e.g.*, the eyes, hypophysis, hypothalamus, brain stem and spinal cord, the radiotherapist determines the target volume. The dose should be delivered uniformly to the target volume, avoiding hot spots. Critical tissue and organs should be spared as far as possible. The maximum dose must always lie within the tumor volume.

3.1.4. Dosimetry (Fig. 3 c)

The planning of the isodose distribution is done on the basis of representative CT cross-sections, usually with a computer-aided treatment planning system. The entire process of treatment planning can be followed on a video screen. Various arrangements of isodose curves can be calculated and displayed on the video screen within a matter of minutes.

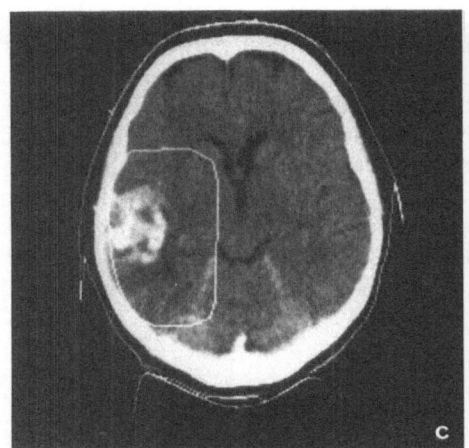
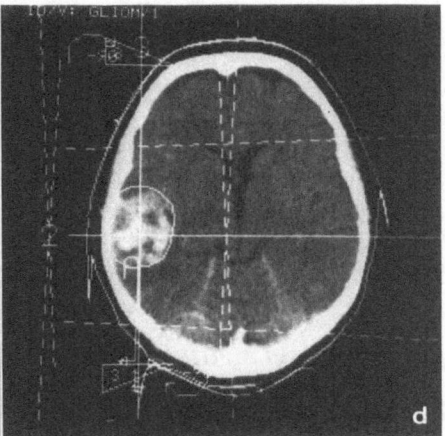
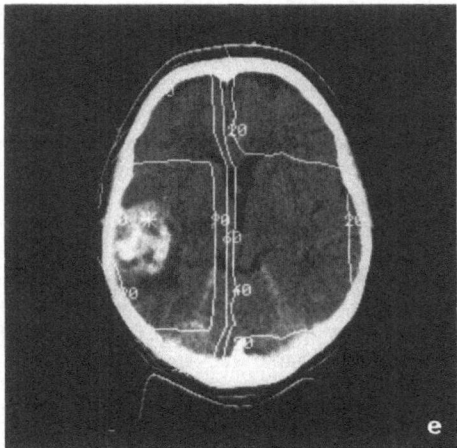

It must first be decided whether fixed beams or the rotation technique is to be employed. Then, the fields, their size, and possible wedges are decided upon. The most suitable isodose plan is determined, individually, by the radiophysicist and the radiotherapist working together. In general, field arrangements as shown schematically in Fig. 4 for different tumor sites and extension, have proved useful.

3.1.5. Simulation and Localization of the Treatment Portals (Fig. 4)

The simulation (localization) of the radiation fields is effected on a radiographic unit, the so-called therapy simulator, on which the radiation fields can also be documented on localization films. The geometrical features of the simulator are identical with those of the megavoltage treatment machine.

The patient is placed in the treatment position. His head is accurately positioned with immobilization aids (see section 3.2.). In some cases, it may be necessary to immobilize the entire body of patient. The radiation portals are marked on the radiation mask, and individual shielding is carried out to protect vital structures. In Erlangen, the portals, shieldings, laser marks, and the configuration of the individual absorbers are identified on polyethylene masks (Fig. 5).

Films obtained on the treatment machine confirm and document correct field settings for the radiotherapy proper. During the course of treatment, a number of repeat verification films are obtained. It is our practice to prepare portal films every two weeks. Localization films, the portal films and isodose printouts from the treatment planning computer, have to be stored for 30 years. In addition, the field arrangements, their marking on the patient's skin or the treatment masks, are documented with polaroid photographs, which are kept in the treatment file.

3.2. Technical Setting Devices

Treatment masks made of polyethylene fix the patient's head in reproducible treatment position. These masks bear the marked-in radiation fields, absorbers and laser coordinates, etc. Since the radiation fields no longer need to be marked on the skin, the patients can be treated on an outpatient basis (Figs. 6 and 7).

Fig. 4. Arrangement of treatment fields in tumors of various locations. *a* Frontal midline tumor with infiltration of both cerebral hemispheres: here, narrow laterally opposed open fields are indicated. *b* Large tumor with involvement of both hemispheres, *e.g.* high-grade astrocytoma. Initially, whole-brain irradiation via laterally opposed open fields are applied, followed by a local boost applied to a reduced treatment volume. *c* Frontal tumor on the right, *e.g.* a low-grade astrocytoma. The radiation technique of choice is two fields arranged at an angle of 90 degrees to each other, with wedge filters. *d* Parietal tumor on the right. Small-volume irradiation via three fields employing the cross-field technique and wedge filters. *e* Narrow frontal tumor in the midline, *e.g.* a meningioma of the sphenoid bone. Irradiation is effected via a narrow ventral open field and two lateral fields with wedge filters. *f* Tumor in the region of the sella, *e.g.* a pituitary adenoma or a craniopharyngioma. Here, the rotation beam technique is indicated

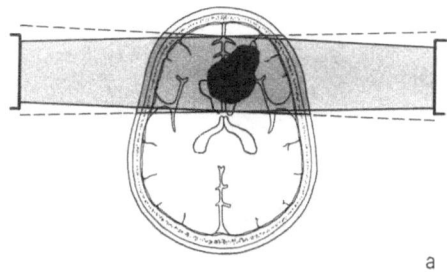

a

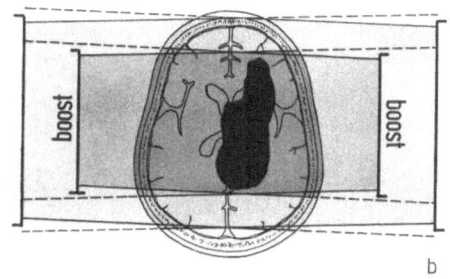

b

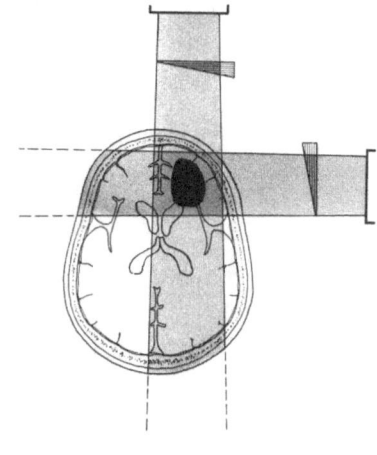

c

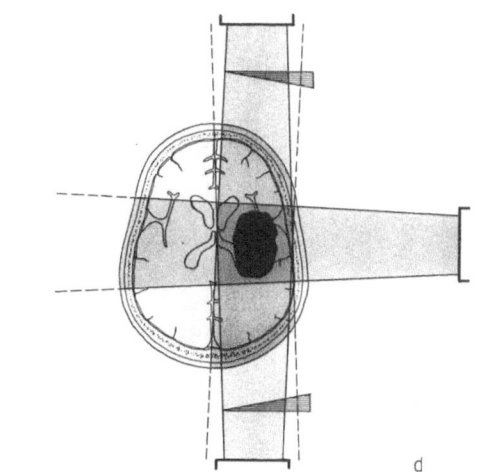

d

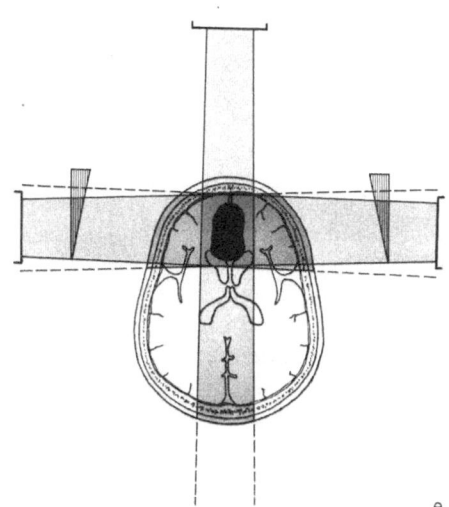

e

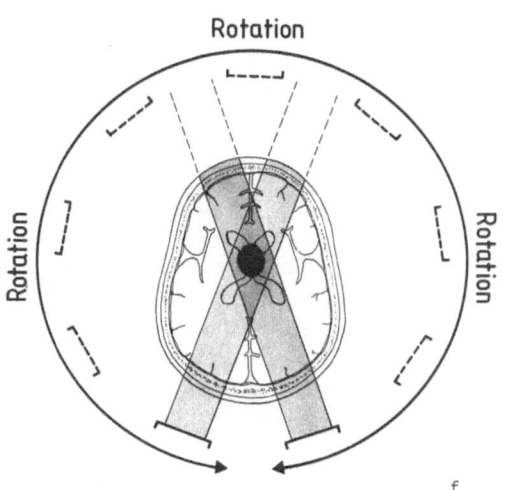

f

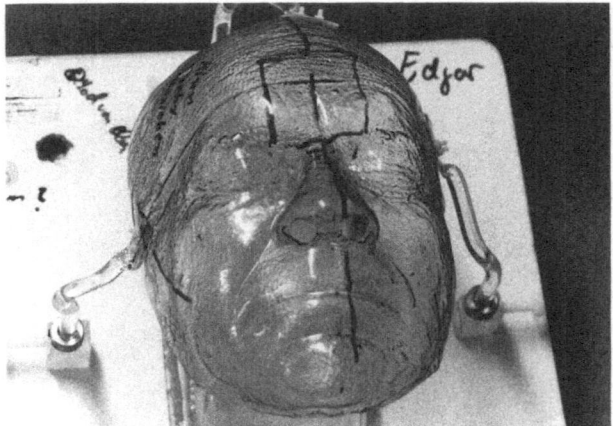

Fig. 5. Individually prepared treatment masks bearing the laser coordinates and setting field for rotation radiotherapy

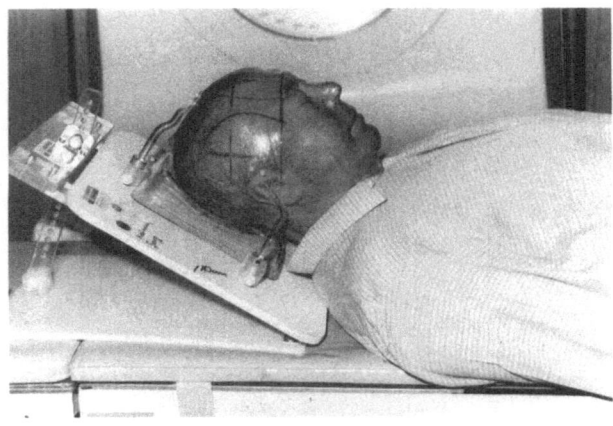

Fig. 6. Patient wearing the treatment mask and positioned for irradiation treatment. The transparent, closely fitting mask can hardly be recognized on the patient

Casts made of plaster of Paris, polyurethane, expanded polystyrene, etc., are also employed to ensure reproducible patient positioning.

Bite blocks are also made for each patient individually. The geometry of the bite block is defined during simulation, and remains unchanged throughout the entire course of treatment. By biting firmly on the block, the patient keeps his head in the reproducible treatment position (Fig. 8).

Laser coordinates are necessary to ensure the geometrically accurate and "tilt-free" positioning of the patient's body and head for the daily treatment sessions (Fig. 9).

Individual absorbers make possible an individually-shaped treatment volume, and considerably reduce radiogenic complications in the healthy tissue (Fig. 10).

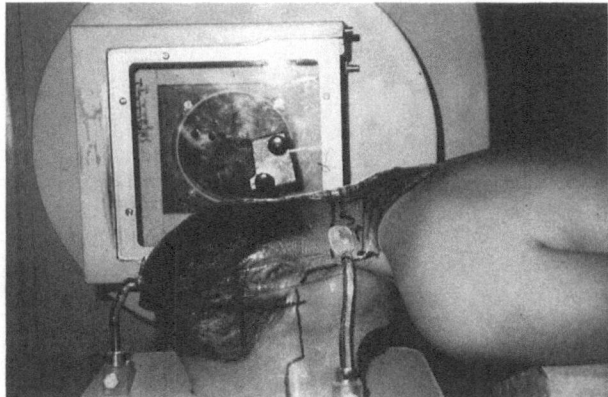

Fig. 7. Patient in treatment position for irradiation of a medulloblastoma. The laser coordinates, the field delimitations and the configuration of the individual absorber are marked on the mask. The individual absorber is mounted on a plexiglas plate and inserted into the radiation head of a linear accelerator

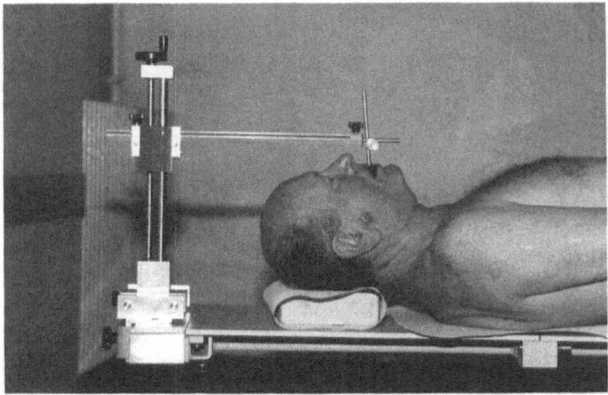

Fig. 8. Individually made bite block. Its position is determined in the simulator during the establishment of the radiation fields. By firmly biting on the block, the patient keeps his head, reproducibly, in the treatment position (Prof. Bohndorf system, Würzburg)

3.3. Interstitial Brachytherapy Technique

The interstitial brachytherapy of brain tumors has received new impetus as a result of the introduction of CT, various stereotactic devices [149, 192, 233, 324], computer-aided treatment planning, the afterloading principle, iodine-125, and new forms of applying iridium-192.

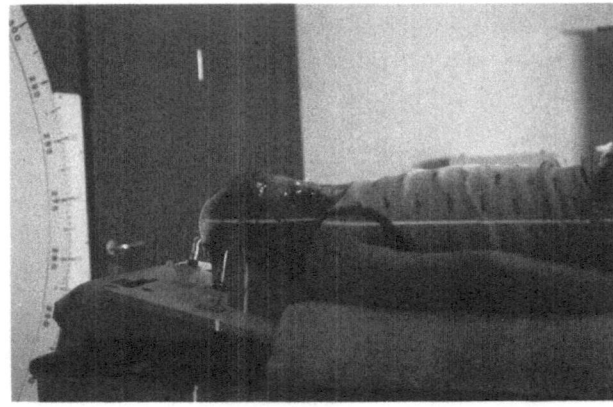

Fig. 9. Laser coordinates facilitate the accurate geometrical positioning of the patient, who is in the prone position for treatment of a medulloblastoma

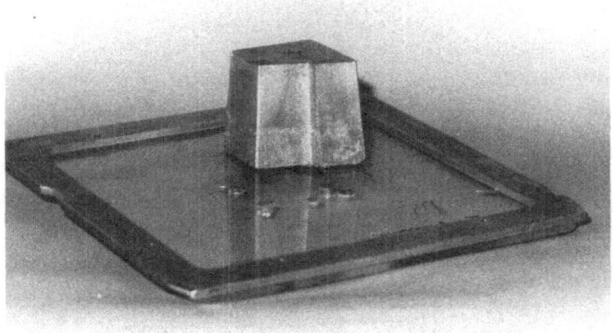

Fig. 10. Individual absorber as used to protect the facial part of head in the treatment of acute lymphatic leukemia. To facilitate the daily setting-up procedure, the absorber is firmly mounted on a plexiglas plate, which is inserted into the accessory holder at the radiation head of the linear accelerator

3.3.1. Erlangen Implantation Technique

We apply the permanent or removable iodine-125 implants with the aid of the CT-controlled stereotactic device[149] (Figs. 11 and 12). It comprises a head support and a phantom with three rings (targeting ring with targeting device, burrhole ring, tumor ring with target point) movable along a single axis. With the aid of CT measurements, we establish the reference point for the hollow needle. From the projection of this reference point onto the CT image of the target point, and or the

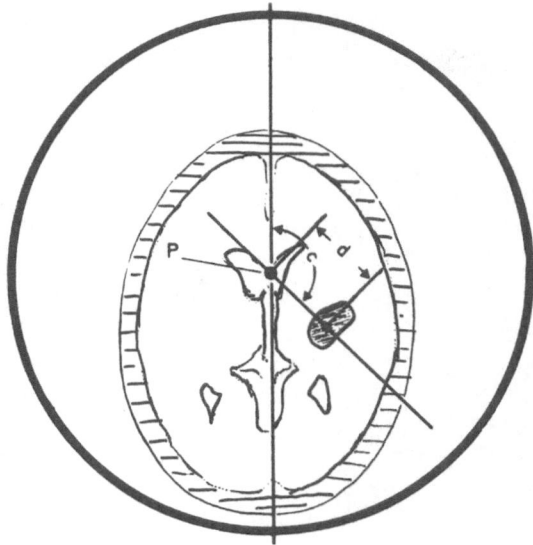

Fig. 11. Erlangen implantation technique for iodine-125 seeds. The reference point for the hollow needle is defined with the aid of CT measurements. From the projection of this reference point onto the CT image of the target point and of the burrhole, the polar coordinates and angle, are obtained

burrhole, the polar coordinates, distance and angle are obtained (Fig. 11). On the basis of these parameters, with the aid of a phantom or a computer program, the coordinates for the probe can be derived. The procedure is carried out under general anesthesia. We use iodine-125 seeds with an activity of 30–50 mCi each, which are kept in place by an afterloading coaxial silicone catheter that is closed at the cranium side with a Rickham reservoir[330] (Fig. 12).

3.3.2. Temporary Implantation

In temporary implantation, we employ a total activity of roughly 200 mCi iodine-125, corresponding to 0.25–1.0 Gy/hour at the surface of the tumor. This modality is to be recommended in high-grade gliomas for local boosting, either prior to or after external beam therapy, or for treating recurrent lesions.

3.3.3. Permanent Implantation

The permanent, centrally placed implantation makes use of an activity of 10–60 mCi iodine-125, resulting in a dose rate of 0.06–0.1 Gy/hour at the surface of the tumor. In agreement with Mundinger, we use this technique for the primary treatment of low-grade astrocytomas. An additional, small-volume external boost may sometimes be necessary.

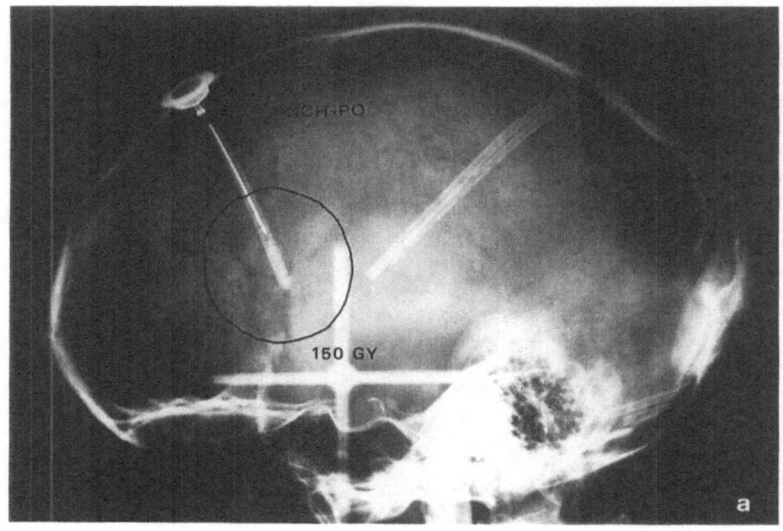

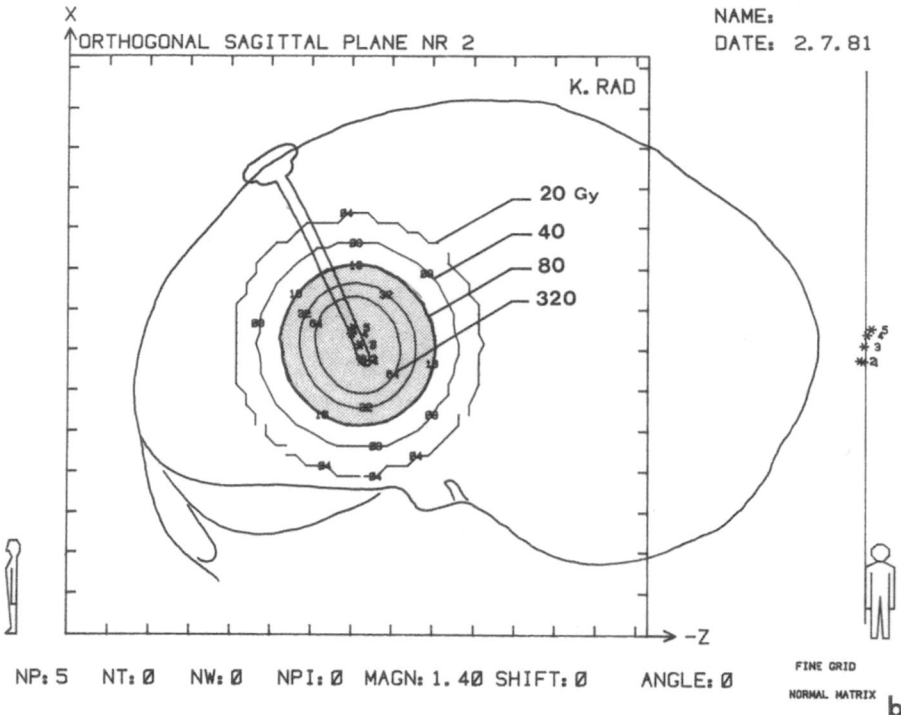

Fig. 12. The iodine-125 seeds are located within a silicone catheter, which is connected to a Rickham reservoir. **a** Catheter with seeds *in situ*. **b** Isodose distribution

4. Special Radiotherapy of Brain Tumors

4.1. Low-Grade Astrocytomas

Grade I and II astrocytomas[162, 163] are readily delimitable and, very slow-growing tumors. In supratentorial astrocytomas, a permanent cure can only rarely be achieved. Recurrent lesions following surgical removal appear late, usually after several years. About two thirds of all patients with low- and intermediate grade cerebral astrocytomas show a malignant transformation of the tumor, so that the recurrence-free interval is shortened[189]. Müller et al.[231] reported that 56% of the recurrent tumors of 72 patients with primary grade I astrocytomas became grade II, and a further 30% grades III and IV. Laws et al.[189] saw transformation into high-grade astrocytomas in 49%.

Recommended therapy: The primary treatment of choice is surgical excision. Any residual tumor should be treated by postoperative small-volume irradiation.

The assumption that low-grade astrocytomas are radioresistant is not correct[30]. Several studies indicate that postoperative RT results in an improvement in survival as compared with surgery alone[41, 42, 96, 101, 189, 190]. The five-year survival rate was 25% for grade I astrocytomas and 0% for grade II patients treated by surgery alone[190]. With postoperative RT the five-year survival rates were 58% and 25%, respectively. The survival rates of 80 patients with diffusely invasive astrocytomas were significantly better after postoperative RT than after surgery alone (median survival 5 versus 2.2 years; five-year survival 50% versus 21%[101].

Radiation technique: Partial brain irradiation with a safety margin around the area of resection is recommended. The arrangement of fields is dictated by the localization of the tumor (Fig. 4).

Radiation dose: 55–60 Gy/6–8 weeks. Since the life expectancy is relatively favorable, the tolerance limits of the affected parts of the brain should not be exceeded.

Prognosis: 20–50% of the patients with grade I astrocytomas, and 0–25% of those with grade II astrocytomas survive for 5 years after surgery, 10–15 and 0–6%, respectively, survive for 10 years[35]. Postoperative RT that meets the present-day technical requirements, can improve the 5-year survival rate of all patients with low-grade astrocytomas to 30–40%.

4.2. High-Grade Astrocytomas (Glioblastomas)

Grade III astrocytomas should be differentiated from grade IV astrocytomas (synonym for glioblastoma multiforme) on account of the better prognosis of the former[176, 212, 271, 278, 280, 291, 300].

Glioblastoma multiforme, which accounts for 30% of all gliomas, is the most common and most malignant of all the brain tumors. It is almost never radically operable, rapidly recurs, and is one of the most radioresistant and chemotherapy-resistant tumors in man. A risk of tumor dissemination into the ventricular system and the subarachnoidal space, has been reported[84, 275, 278]. However, this fact is of little relevance as long as effective local treatment of glioblastoma remains unavailable.

Recommended therapy: Surgical decompression and excision of the tumor are the primary treatment of choice. In this way, the main tumor mass, including the necrotic part of the tumor, is removed, the intracranial pressure decreased and the tumor volume greatly reduced. This reduction in tumor mass is one of the major prerequisites if RT is to have its maximum effect. In any case, high-dose radiation is applied postoperatively. It is considered to be proven that combination treatment of surgery and postoperative RT improves survival as compared with surgery alone[28, 41, 280, 291, 300, 332, 341, 343]. In a review of the literature covering 450 patients treated with surgery alone, and 619 patients receiving combination therapy, Bloom[28] showed that this positive effect of postoperative RT persists for only 2 years. In the third year, the results of the treatment are equally poor.

If there is any doubt as to the resectability of a glioblastoma, and if surgery would be associated with a high risk of complications, we recommend RT without prior surgery—in combination with chemotherapy. The results are presumably better than after surgery alone. This applies for tumors in the dominant cerebral hemisphere, and those invading the opposite side, the basal ganglia, midbrain, brain stem or third ventricle. Tönnis and Walther[332] achieved a mean survival of 7 months with RT alone, and in Bouchard's[41] series 44% of the patients survived for one year.

In patients with glioblastoma, the best survival rates seem to be achieved with a combination of surgery, postoperative RT and BCNU (see section 2.6.). In the studies of the BTSG[341] the median survival after combination treatment was 52 weeks. We prefer BCNU to CCNU, and administer 80 mg BCNU/m^2 body surface as intravenous infusion in the first 3 days of RT, and again for 3 days at intervals of 6 weeks, as long as tolerance remains good, in some cases continuing for the rest of the patient's life.

High-grade astrocytomas are not curable, and the additional life span gained by treatment is only small. For this reason, the question frequently raised, as to whether treatment of high-grade astrocytomas is indicated at all, is justified, in particular when the associated period of hospitalization is long. It should be remembered that treatment gives patients with grade III astrocytoma a 20% chance of surviving for five years (see Mundinger). Moreover, a study conducted by the RMH (Royal Marsden Hospital) showed that 34% of patients with high-grade astrocytoma submitted to surgery and postoperative RT, were enabled to return to work and lead a normal, active life. A further 24% were in a moderately good, functional state, while in 42%, function remained poor. This means that almost 60% gained something from treatment[32].

Radiation technique: For the irradiation of high-grade astrocytomas, whole-brain irradiation has always been considered necessary. The rationale was the occasionally diffuse or multicentric growth, the frequent involvement of the contralateral hemisphere, and the occasional occurrence of metastases in the ventricular system and cerebrospinal canal[278]. Today, when CT scanning permits an accurate macroscopic localization of the tumor, and largely excludes a multicentric origin, whole-brain treatment is no longer justifiable. Glioblastoma

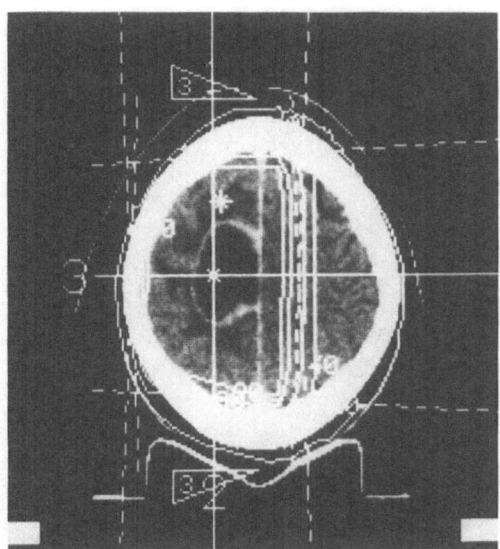

Fig. 13. Half-brain irradiation in the case of a glioblastoma multiforme located near the midline. Three-field cross-beam wedge technique

multiforme is a unifocal disease in more than 90% of the cases. Following RT, 80% and more of tumor recurrences occur within 2 cm of the original primary site[138]. For this reason, we irradiate a large volume that includes a generous margin of clearance around the primary tumor. In very large gliomas that cross the midline, this might represent nothing less than whole-brain irradiation. Usually, even in the most unfavorable case, a half-brain irradiation is sufficient (Figs. 13 and 14).

Radiation dose: For whole-brain irradiation, 50 Gy should not be exceeded. Also in large-volume irradiation, after 50 Gy, the volume is reduced and a local boost of 10–20 Gy applied. Doses of > 70 Gy are, we believe, not justified. The dose per fractions is $\leq$ 2 Gy/five times a week. If dose fractions of 3.5 Gy per day are applied, a total dose of 35–38.5 Gy/2–2½ weeks should not be exceeded[136]. This fractionation has the advantage of shortening hospitalization. By and large, the nature of dose fractioning in the case of glioblastoma appears to be irrelevant for the prognosis or—expressed differently—the optimal fractionation pattern for high-grade astrocytomas has not yet been established[49, 145, 249, 307].

As for the assumption that an increase in the radiation dose with external beam radiotherapy is capable of improving the tumor control rate, the opinions in the literature are divided. Salazar *et al.*[280], using a whole-brain dose of up to 75–80 Gy, were able to improve the survival of patients with grade IV astrocytomas in the first 2 years, and within the first four years in the patients with grade III lesions. Most patients to benefit were those aged under 45. In a dose-response analysis of the BTSG involving 621 patients[343], a stepwise improvement in the survival was observed in patients who had received 50, 55, or 60 Gy. The median survival was 28, 36, and 42 weeks, respectively. The difference between 50 and 60 Gy was statistically significant with p = 0.004 (Fig. 15).

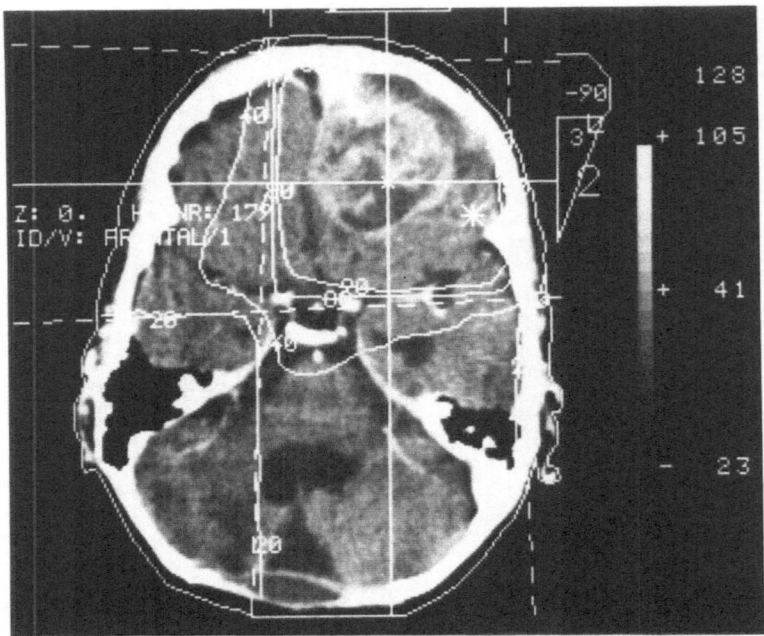

Fig. 14. Glioblastoma multiforme located frontally on the right; large-volume irradiation applied via a 2-field cross-beam wedge technique

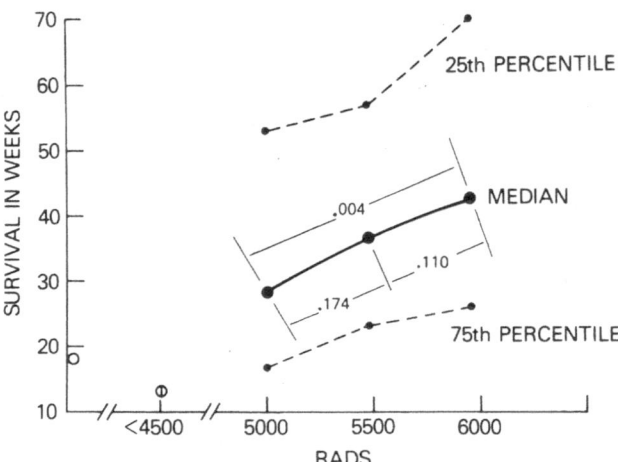

Fig. 15. The median survival of patients receiving no radiotherapy (0), less than 4,500 rads (∅), and 5,000, 5,500, or 6,000 rads (●), and survival at the 25th and 75th percentile and the Gehan-Wilcoxon-test p value for significance (courtesy of Walker *et al.* (1979), Int J Radiat Oncol Biol Phys 5: 1725–1731

Shryver *et al.* (1976) irradiating only a small volume, applying 50 Gy/6 weeks, achieved the best therapeutic results. The one-year survival rate was 64%, 43% of the patients survived two years, and 33% three years, while Catteral *et al.*[54] found that an increase in dose from 50 Gy to 55 Gy decreased survival.

Prognosis: The mean life expectancy of untreated patients with glioblastoma multiforme is 2–3 months. After surgery alone, 50% of the patients die within the first 4–6 months, and almost all have died within 2 years[15, 341]. Postoperative RT prolongs the median survival to 8 to 9 months. After radical surgery and postoperative RT the median survival can be 12 months[277, 291, 300, 332, 341–343].

In patients with grade III lesions, survival is better, and a number of series report survival rates of 20 to 30% at five years[47, 281, 291].

The problem of radioresistance of the high-grade astrocytomas has not yet been resolved. Further clinical investigations are necessary in order to establish the suitable dose, the suitable fractionation pattern, and the suitable irradiation mode. Further, it must also be determined whether chemical radiosensitizers, hypoxic-cell radiosensitizers, heavy particle beam irradiation or hyperthermia under conditions other than those so far investigated are capable of improving local control.

4.3. Oligodendrogliomas

Oligodendrogliomas are slowly growing, relatively benign tumors with a long pretherapeutic and postoperative evolution. Owing to the fact that they are usually highly invasive, they can rarely be completely extirpated. Recurrences occur late, so that the five-year survival figure says little about the overall performance[228].

Recommended therapy: The primary aim is to achieve as complete a surgical excision as possible. On account of the slow growth and the relative rarity of the tumors the value of additional postoperative RT is difficult to assess. In recent series[30, 226, 243, 302, 304] a favorable effect of RT on inoperable or recurrent tumors was found. The authors noted a clinical improvement, and Bloom[30] also reported an objective regression of the tumor in the CT scan. Postoperative irradiation is recommended whenever there are any doubts as to the radicality of surgery. Already in the historical series treated by Harvey Cushing, patients receiving postoperative irradiation did better than those submitted to surgery alone[266].

Radiation technique: We recommend small-volume irradiation with an adequate margin of clearance in accordance with Fig. 4, and a dose of 50–60 Gy/6–7 weeks.

Prognosis: The five-year survival rate after surgery and postoperative RT is up to 80%. The ten-year survival rate drops to 25–30%[302, 304, 347], the 15-year survival rate to 15–20%[30].

4.4. Unbiopsied Tumors (Deep-seated Unverified Tumors)

Tumors in the basal ganglia, brain stem, midbrain, and third ventricle, are usually sent to RT without prior histological verification. With the introduction of the operating microscope and more modern stereotaxic techniques, however, the percentage of unbiopsied patients is constantly decreasing[260].

Surgical series of midline intraaxial (nuclear) tumors show that the majority of such lesions are astrocytomas, which respond well to irradiation. They are followed by high-grade gliomas (about 15%) and hamartomas (5–10%)[6]. These tumors invade and destroy the healthy nuclei and fiber tracts, with the result that the symptoms progressively worsen. The prognosis of children with bilateral tumors of the hypothalamus is better than that of children with unilateral tumors of the thalamus, and equally as good in tumors with cysts and calcifications and < 5 cm in diameter[6].

Recommended therapy: Tovi et al.[334] showed that the best treatment for unbiopsied deep-seated tumors was radical RT without prior surgery. Surgical measures should be restricted to a shunt procedure or, at most, a biopsy[57, 220].

Radiation technique: Depending upon the localization of the tumor, either a rotation beam technique or small-volume irradiation with crossed beams (Fig. 4) is usually employed. The dose to be delivered should be 50–60 Gy/5–6 weeks.

Prognosis: In the series reported by Tovi et al.[334], 33% of the patients receiving RT alone, survived for 5 years, and 26% for 10–23 years. In contrast, 6 out of 10 patients in whom surgery was attempted died in hospital, only one subject survived for 5 years.

4.5. Tumors of the Brain Stem

Most brain stem tumors are found in children, are usually not excisable, and are not always accessible to bipsy. In view of this, the therapeutic aspects concerning these tumor localizations might also have been discussed in section 4.4.

The majority of these tumors are diffusely invasive astrocytomas with a high tendency to transform into glioblastomas. A minority (approximately 20%) are juvenile pilocytic astrocytomas which are more circumscribed, grow more slowly, and have a protracted evolution[208, 213, 299]. The cervicomedullary tumors are much more frequently low-grade astrocytomas than the more rostrally, antero- or posterolaterally situated lesions[88]. Twenty-five per cent of the brain stem tumors disseminate via the CSF. The pontine tumors are invasive and often spread rostrally into the midbrain, caudally into the medulla, and also in the direction of the cerebellum.

Recommended therapy: In many cases, treatment can merely be palliative. Here, RT has a good and objectifiable effect in 65–80% of the patients[109, 213, 299, 337].

Radiation technique: With respect to field size and beam localization, it should be remembered that tumor invasion takes place not in a vertical direction, but rostrally, caudally and laterally. Most expediently, two adequately long lateral fields and a dorsal field are set. The posterior part of the third ventricle, hypothalamus, and the supra- and infratentorial parts of the posterior brain (pedunculi cerebri et cerebelli) must be covered by the target volume.

Radiation dose: The required dose is 50–60 Gy/5–6 weeks. Kim et al.[165] observed that the results of treatment were dependent upon the dose administered. The overall five-year survival rate was 20%, the 10-year survival rate 10%, while the relevant figures for patients who had received > 50 Gy tumor dose were 32 and 18%, respectively.

Prognosis: The decisive prognostic criterion is not so much the histopathological type, but the location of the tumor (with the exception of glioblastoma multiforme). Thus, the prognosis of tumors of the pons and the medulla, is better than that of tumors located in the thalamus, hypothalamus or midbrain[299]. Following RT, the recurrence rate is high. The 5-year survival rate is between 13 and 30%[3, 30, 41, 132, 165, 202, 240, 245, 294, 315], but 5-year survival rates of 30–50% have been reported, too[109, 300, 351].

4.6. Pineal Tumors and Suprasellar Germinomas

Pineal tumors are space-occupying lesions of the pineal body. Accounting for only 1% of all brain tumors, they represent a rare group. Histologically, the pineal tumors are classified in accordance with their tissue of origin[45]:

1. Germ cell tumors
Germinoma (highly radiosensitive),
teratoma (benign teratoma, embryonal cell carcinoma, choriocarcinoma, endodermal sinus tumor (varying radiosensitivity, in some cases low).

2. Pineal cell tumors
Pineocytoma (low radiosensitivity),
pineoblastoma (highly radiosensitive).

3. Glial tumors
e.g., astrocytoma, glioblastoma.

4. Miscellaneous
Ependymoma, meningioma, choroid plexus papilloma, benign cysts, etc.

Up to 30% of the various tumors of the pineal body tend to disseminate into the cerebro-spinal SAS[45, 69, 157, 277, 318]. These are germinomas, malignant teratomas, pineoblastomas and high-grade astrocytomas.

Not infrequently, the early symptoms that lead to the diagnosis of an intracranial germ cell tumor, are neuroendocrine disorders[254]. The diagnosis can be made, in a nonstressful manner, on the basis of raised tumor marker in the CSF, a positive CSF cytology, or by means of a stereotactic biopsy.

Recommended therapy: Up until recently, primary RT was considered to be the treatment of first choice. A surgical approach to pineal tumors, and even the taking of biopsies from the tumor, was considered too risky, on account of the position of the lesion (30–60% surgical mortality). Recently, however, Bruce and Allen[45] have reported acceptable results with surgical biopsy, subtotal or macroscopically total resection of tumors in the area of the pineal body. These authors chose a posterior approach. An indisputable advantage of this procedure is that it provides knowledge of the histology of the tumor, which can be determinative for the further therapeutic procedure: If benign or radioresistant lesions are present, postoperative RT is not necessary.

Torkildsen[33] proposed the placement of a shunt where necessary, and then applying only radiotherapy. In order to avoid biopsy-taking, Bloom[30] proposed starting treatment with local RT of the pineal body region. After applying a dose of about 20 Gy/2.5 weeks, a repeat CT scan is done in order to establish the response of the tumor. If there has clearly been regression, it may be assumed that the tumor was either a germinoma or, perhaps, a pineoblastoma. In this case, the volume treated is extended to include the entire CSF compartment. A surgical attack on the tumor is not necessary.

Chemotherapy of pineal tumors and suprasellar germinomas is still in the cradle. In cases of the radiosensitive tumors, and in view of the low side effects of RT, we see no indication for primary chemotherapy. However, an attempt at

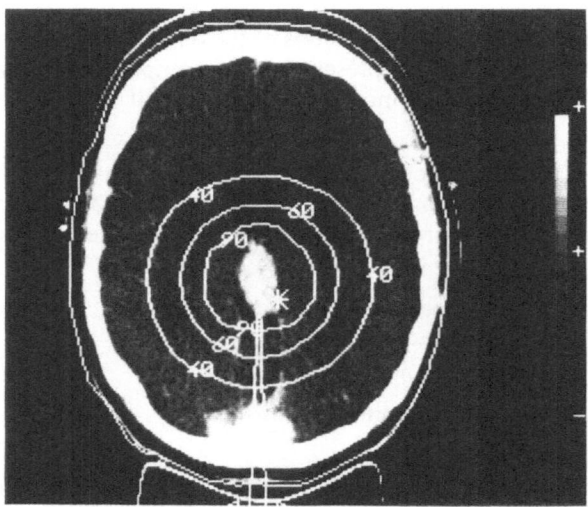

Fig. 16. Histologically confirmed pinealoma. Small-volume 360°-rotation technique as the first stage of percutaneous radiation therapy. After 20 Gy/2.5 weeks, irradiation of the entire craniospinal fluid space is followed

chemotherapy might be useful in residual or recurrent suprasellar or pineal tumors[335]. In patients with ventriculo-peritoneal, or ventriculo-atrial shunt, chemotherapy may protect against metastasization through the shunt[184].

Radiation technique: Both in histologically verified and in unbiopsied tumors, we begin with local RT of the primary tumor region. We give preference to the rotation-beam technique and employ a generous margin of safety that includes the third ventricle and the aqueduct (Figs. 4 and 16). 20 Gy are administered in 2–2.5 weeks.

Routine cerebrospinal axis irradiation with 30 Gy/3.5–4 weeks is justified in all patients with confirmed or suspected germinomas or pineoblastomas[30, 261]. In unbiopsied patients in whom no response can be detected after the administration of 20 Gy, and in all other tumor types, irradiation is restricted to the region of the primary tumor.

The patient is treated in the prone position. The technical details are described in section 4.8.

Radiation dose: In cases of highly radiosensitive tumors, a dose of 45–55 Gy/5–7 weeks applied to the region of the primary tumor is indicated, and 30 Gy/3.5–4 weeks applied to the cerebrospinal axis. In all tumor which, treated in accordance with the concept of Bloom[30], show a poor response to primary RT, 55–60 Gy applied to the pineal body region is indicated.

Table 3 shows a collection of reports from the literature[182], which reveals that with increasing radiation dose (< 50 Gy versus $\geqslant 50$ Gy) the local control rate increases, while the recurrence rate diminishes.

Prognosis: The prognosis of pineal tumors and suprasellar germ cell tumors depends upon the histological picture. It is relatively good in the case of germinomas and astrocytomas, with 5-year survival rates of up to 80%[157] and poorer in pineal cell tumors, malignant teratomas and high-grade astrocytomas. The 5-year survival rate for all pineal tumors and suprasellar germ cell tumors is 50–80%[7, 43, 45, 64, 224, 241, 259, 261, 268, 277, 318, 345]. Postradiotherapy recurrences occur in the region of the primary tumor (16%), elsewhere in the brain (10%), and in the spinal canal (14%)[43, 157, 277, 318].

4.7. Cerebral and Cerebellar Astrocytomas in Children

These lesions are low-grade astrocytomas with a characteristic histological picture, referred to as spongioblastomas[357] or pilocytic astrocytomas of the juvenile type[270]. The tumors are very slow-growing, so that a long period of symptom-free survival does not necessarily mean a cure. Some patients with only partial tumor resection do just as well over a long period as those whose tumors have been, macroscopically, totally excised[47, 65, 103]. Recurrent lesions have been observed after a symptom-free interval of more than 40 years[168].

In benign cerebellar astrocytomas, local invasion of the leptomeninges is relatively common[171, 264, 275]. The picture of benign juvenile astrocytoma usually persists over many years, even in the case of a recurrence; malignant transformation is rare[23, 168, 264]. High-grade astrocytomas of the cerebellum are rare in children[23, 100, 275].

In contrast to the cerebellar astrocytomas, the juvenile cerebral astrocytomas are more rarely benign, have a tendency toward malignant degeneration, and are often so unfavorably sited that radical surgery is not possible[30, 171, 213]. Nevertheless, they have a much better prognosis than in adults (Table 4).

Recommended therapy: In children with infratentorial, *i.e.*, cerebellar astrocytomas, total macroscopic excision should be the aim of primary treatment. But even partial removal makes good sense. Whether postoperative RT is indicated in low-grade cerebellar astrocytomas has not yet been definitively decided. However, postoperative radiation after subtotal removal of the tumor does seem to make the long-term results identical with those achieved by radical tumor removal[111, 290].

After complete excision of the tumor, postoperative RT is given only in high-grade astrocytomas.

Primary RT is indicated in inoperable situations, *e.g.*, cerebral astrocytomas or brain stem tumors which are not radioresistant. Long-term remissions over five years of 45% have been reported[30, 213, 290]. Whenever accessible, the space-

R. Sauer:

Table 4. Treatment results in cerebral astrocytomas and unverified tumors in children and adults (South Thames Cancer Registry, 1958–1974[30])

| | 5-year survival rate | | | |
| | Children (< 15 years) | | Adults (> 15 years) | |
	No. pts.	%	No. pts.	%
Astrocytomas All grades of malignancy	106	45%	2067	5%
Unverified tumors	144	27%	1363	13%

occupying lesions should be biopsied prior to RT since treatment decisions are oriented to the type of tumor presenting. In cerebellar tumors, biopsy prior to RT is obligatory.

Radiating technique: Small-volume irradiation in accordance with the recommendations shown in Fig. 4 is indicated. In infratentorial glioblastomas, there are good reasons that militate in favor of cerebrospinal irradiation[275].

Radiation dose: The dose applied depends upon the histology of the tumor: in low-grade astrocytomas, 40–45 Gy/5–6 weeks (children < 1 year), 45–50 Gy/5–7 weeks (children aged > 1 year), and 50–60 Gy/6–7 weeks (children aged > 3 years, and young adults) are applied. For high-grade astrocytomas, we recommend a dose of between 50 and 60 Gy/6–7 weeks, depending upon the age of the child involved.

Prognosis: Patients with cerebellar low-grade astrocytomas have the best prognosis. The curability at 5 years is about 90%, and at 10 years up to 85%[30, 47, 61, 66, 103, 111, 213, 299]. Even after subtotal tumor excision and recurrent disease, symptom-free survival rates extending from years to decades have been reported[37, 74, 171, 196, 214].

The prognosis of the cerebral astrocytomas is appreciably poorer. Nevertheless, with a five-year survival rate of about 45%, it is still considerably better than in adults, where the corresponding figure is only 5% (Table 4).

In the RMH series comprising 88 children under 16 years of age with intrinsic cerebral gliomas, the prognosis of thalamus tumors was worst, while that of tumors of the cerebral hemispheres, third ventricle and hypothalamus, was more favorable (Table 5). In the Erlangen case material of juvenile astrocytomas of the cerebellum, the brain stem and the cerebrum (1978–1983), a five-year survival of 75 ± 16%, and a ten-year survival of 67 ± 20% was calculated. The children with cerebellar astrocytomas had the best prognosis[290].

4.8. Medulloblastoma

This malignant tumor arising in the vermis of the cerebellum above the roof of the fourth ventricle, occurs largely in childhood and, with an incidence of 20–25%, is the most common of the brain tumors found in children[29, 234, 236]. It is rare in adults[172].

The medulloblastoma is markedly invasive, and has a great tendency ($> 30\%$) to throw off "seedings" via the CSF into the SAS and the ventricles[72, 218, 239]. In roughly 5% of the cases, metastases are also found outside of the CSF, mainly in the skeleton, lungs, and in the lymph nodes[172, 235]. Berry *et al.*[24] found that at the first relapse, 35% of the patients had systemic metastatic disease.

Recommended therapy: Only exceptionally can the medulloblastoma be cured by surgery alone[65]. The extent of the excision, in combination with RT, may have a positive effect on the prognosis[24, 238, 258]. This statement is, however, at variance with the experience reported by Bouchard[41], according to which patients receiving needle biopsy and irradiation, had a better prognosis than did those submitted to surgery and postoperative RT.

Table 5. Cerebral hemisphere gliomas (excluding verified ependymoma). Survival in all children referred for radiotherapy (Royal Marsden Hospital 1952–1976[30])

Site	No. pts.	Survival		
		5 years %	10 years %	15 years %
Cerebral lobes	37	38	34	34
Third ventricle + hypothalamus	33	66	53	53
Thalamus	18	20	20	20
Total	88	45	38	38

The question as to whether an external CSF drainage increases the systemic metastasization rate or not has, so far, not been answered[112, 139, 258]. However, a factor that militates in favor of reducing elevated intracranial pressure by drainage prior to primary tumor surgery, is the resulting improvement in the patient's general condition.

Due to the appreciable radiosensitivity of the medulloblastoma, RT of the primary tumor region and the whole cerebrospinal axis represents the most effective of the therapeutic measures available[17, 29, 30, 35, 58, 124, 248, 306, 310]. Of particular importance is a homogeneous distribution of dose along the cerebro-spinal axis for recurrent lesions tend to occur most readily in underdosed areas[159, 306, 310].

The use of chemotherapy may bring about a further improvement in the results obtained with a combination of surgery and RT[22, 30, 234]. It is also still unclear whether chemotherapy develops a greater effect when administered immediately following surgery, that is, before RT. Points that militate in favor of giving chemotherapy before irradiation are the unimpaired bone marrow tolerance found at the time, the still intact BBB, and also the fact that the CNS has not yet been burdened by ionizing radiation. An aim of this procedure is to bring about some reduction in the radiation dose[236]. In this way, it is hoped to reduce the incidence of adverse effects of treatment.

An argument for placing chemotherapy *after* radiation treatment, is the fear that chemotherapy might delay the administration of RT, which is the most effective therapeutic measure available, thus possibly reducing its effectiveness. This would then reduce the patient's chances of being cured[30].

Radiation technique: Using the Manchester technique[248] radiation is, today, always applied to the region of the primary tumor, the whole cerebrospinal axis down to and including the second sacral vertebra, simultaneously. Treatment is to be started as soon as possible after surgery, with large-volume irradiation of the CSF compartment[144]. Only in exceptional cases is it permitted to start treatment with a boost to the posterior cranial fossa, that is, with small-volume irradiation. Such a procedure may be indicated after prior chemotherapy, particularly when the induced leukopenia has not yet "bottomed out".

By and large, the irradiation technique corresponds to that described by Bloom[28] and its variations (*e.g.*,[18]): the patient is placed in the prone position (Fig. 17). The head is positioned in a treatment mask (Fig. 7), the body immobilized, if necessary, in a plaster of Paris mold. The cerebro-spinal axis is irradiated from the intervertebral space C 2/3 or C 4/5 to S 2 inclusively, using a moving field technique, via one or several stationary fields from dorsal. The width of the field is 4–6 cm. Electron beams have the advantage of lower hematological and gastrointestinal toxicity. However, an energy of at least 18 MeV[209] is required.

The brain is irradiated isocentrically via two lateral opposing fields, shaped with individual absorbers. The caudal edge of the field is matched exactly to the edge of the light field of the dorsal spinal field, by rotating the collimator as shown in Fig. 17. In addition, the divergence of the caudal edge of the skull field can be compensated by appropriate cranial tilting of the central beam or by tilting the table appropriately. The junction between the skull fields and the spinal fields is daily shifted between C 2/3 and C 4/5 in order to avoid possible hot spots or underdosing.

Even when irradiation is carried out with the greatest care, dose peaks of up to 30% can occur in the region of the cervical spinal cord[18, 229, 279], when the X-radiation of a linear accelerator is employed. With telecobalt treatment, hot spots are observed in only 10% of the cases[18, 55, 229]. Therefore a gap of 5–10 mm is recommended between the skull fields and the dorsal spinal field.

Radiation dose: The radiation dose applied is 50–55 Gy/7–8 weeks to the posterior cranial fossa, 35–45 Gy/4–6 weeks to the whole brain, and 30–35 Gy/4.5–5 weeks to the spinal axis. In the case of children younger than 2 years, the dose to the posterior fossa should be reduced to 45 Gy/6–7 weeks[24, 34, 106, 151, 156, 175, 212, 218, 299]. With increasing dose, the local control rate and survival rates also increase[24, 58, 63, 124, 151, 175, 299, 306] (Table 1).

Prognosis: Today, using a combination of surgery and optimal RT, 2-year survival rates of 60–70%, five-year survival rates of 40–60%, and 10-year survival rates of 30–40% can be achieved[17, 24, 30, 105, 121, 124, 132, 144, 222, 294, 299, 306]. These figures relate to patients who had received complete RT. For all patients treated, therefore, the overall mortality rate will probably be 10–15% higher[30].

In medulloblastoma of the adult, the prognosis is better than in children, although, only in the first ten years following treatment[34]. 70% of the recurrences occur within two years, with a median of 18 months. Recurrent lesions are most

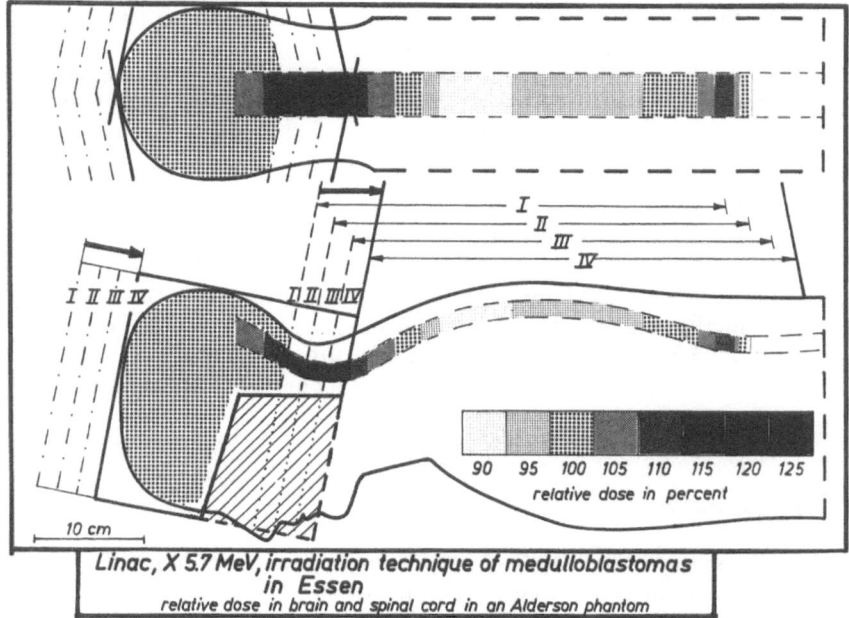

Fig. 17. Dose distribution with abutment of the lateral skull fields with the dorsal spinal field in radiation treatment of medulloblastoma, using 5.7 MV photon beams. Measurements on the Alderson phantom. Essen moving-field technique. The overdosage in the cervical part of the spinal cord of 25–30%, can be recognized (Bamberg M, *et al.* (1980) Strahlentherapie 156: 1–17)

frequently found in the posterior cranial fossa, followed by the subarachnoidal space[34, 124, 310].

National and International Protocols

1. In 1970, a pilot study was initiated at the RMH, in order to assess the feasibility and possible value of adjuvant chemotherapy (vincristine, CCNU, and, in some cases, intrathecal methotrexate) in children with medulloblastoma treated with radical surgery and cerebrospinal axis irradiation[28]. The 5-year survival of a group of 37 children treated with adjuvant chemotherapy was better than in an historical series without chemotherapy (71% versus 32%, p < 0.001)[30].

2. In 1975, a randomized multicenter cooperative trial was initiated by the International Society of Pediatric Oncology (SIOP). Forty-four centers, mainly in Europe, contributed 280 patients with medulloblastoma under 16 years of age to the study[33]. The treatment schedule was based on that of the RMH pilot study. The analysis done in 1982 showed that the overall disease-free survival of the patients receiving adjuvant chemotherapy was greater than that of those not receiving chemotherapy, but the difference was only nominally statistically significant (p = 0.046). However, significant results militating in favor of chemotherapy were obtained in certain high-risk subgroups, *i.e.* children aged less than 2 years

(p = 0.058), those in whom the tumor was only partially excised (p = 0.002), and those with brain stem involvement (p = 0.003).

3. The Children's Cancer Study Group (CCSG) and the Radiation Oncology Group (RTOG) initiated a trial with the same chemotherapy as applied in the SIOP study, but with the addition of prednisone as maintenance therapy. Here, no significant difference was found in the survival rate of the indicidual treatment groups[90, 91].

4. In 1980, the Gesellschaft für Pädiatrische Onkologie (GPO) started a trial with postoperative preradiotherapeutic ("sandwich") chemotherapy (procarbazine, vincristine, intermediate-dose methotrexate with citrovorum factor rescue, intrathecal methotrexate and dexamethasone). The study has not yet been concluded. In the first years, the results obtained are similar to those achieved in the SIOP and the CCSG/RTOG studies[234]. (See Jacobi and Kornhuber).

4.9. Ependymoma

Ependymomas constitute 8–10% of all pediatric intracranial tumors[60]. They arise from the ependymal cells anywhere along the ventricular system and—rather uncommonly—in the spinal canal[102, 105, 210, 250, 276, 348]. 15–25% of the tumors are classified as "ependymoblastomas" or—more correct—high-grade ependymomas. They proliferate faster than ependymomas, and contain cells of the embryonal type that show increased mitotic activity[30, 102, 276, 348, 359].

Ependymomas may spread along the cerebrospinal axis like medulloblastomas (for review of the literature see[30, 182, 348]). The incidence of seeding is reported to be between 12 and 20%.

The risk of CSF dissemination is about 20–35% in high-grade ependymomas located in the posterior fossa[30, 61, 164, 182, 252, 276, 300].

In low-graded posterior fossa ependymomas, the probability of CSF dissemination is only about 10%[30, 61, 252, 276].

In tumors with supratentorial location, the risk of CSF dissemination is still not known with any degree of accuracy. It appears to be moderate for high-grade tumors[102, 155, 203]—approximately 20%—and low for low-grade ependymomas[30, 164, 252].

Recommended therapy: An accurate decision with regard to therapy, can be made only after surgical exploration. The attempts should always be made surgically to remove as much of the tumor as is feasible. Nevertheless, the relationship between gross resectability and curability, remains an unanswered question[41, 348, 356]. On account of their invasive growth and localization, the tumors are usually not totally removable at surgery, and often recur without postoperative irradiation. The exceptions are a number of ependymomas arising, tongue-like from a narrow base in the fourth ventricle, that are possibly curably resectable[320].

There is general agreement that, irrespective of the extent of the tumor resection, postoperative RT should be given. Opinion as to the volume to be treated, however, remains controversial. In agreement with others[35, 164], we recommend the following strategy:

— Postoperative irradiation of the whole cerebrospinal axis in all patients with high-grade tumors, irrespective of their location, and in all those with posterior fossa lesions, irrespective of the malignancy grade.

— Irradiation exclusively of the primary tumor region with a generous margin of clearance in patients with low-grade supratentorial ependymomas.

In contrast to the experience with medulloblastomas, adjuvant chemotherapy for ependymomas merely postpones, but does not prevent, recurrence[30]. In the SIOP trial, this subgroup had no gain with respect to survival.

Radiation technique: The radiation technique is the same as the employed for medulloblastomas (see section 4.8.).

Radiation dose: The required dose to the region of the primary tumor is 50–60 Gy/6–8 weeks. In children younger than 2 years, the dose is reduced to 45 Gy/6–7 weeks. The rest of the brain and spinal cord receives 35–45 Gy/5–6 weeks[30, 102, 164, 210, 250, 276]. In collected results from the literature (see Table 2) the five-year survival rate improved in patients whose primary tumor had been irradiated with > 45 Gy. After the application of < 45 Gy, the five-year survival rate in the individual treatment groups was 0, 10, 20, and 33%, while, in the same groups after > 45 Gy, the respective figures were 46, 56, 70, and 87%[182].

Prognosis: With a combination of surgery and postoperative RT, five-year survival rates of between 40 and 90% are achieved[30, 42, 102, 106, 155, 164, 181, 210, 228, 250, 276, 279]. After surgery alone, the results are considerably less encouraging[228, 265].

The dominating prognostic factors are age and tumor grade. For low-grade ependymomas, the five-year survival rate is 60–100%, and for high-grade tumors, roughly 15%. Only Bloom[30] has reported better survival rates for high-grade ependymomas, but maintained for only 6 years posttreatment.

4.10. Pituitary Adenomas

Pituitary adenomas account for up to 10% of all the intracranial tumors[81, 122]. According to autopsy statistics, they are, indeed, found in 10–20% of the pituitaries previously unremarkable in appearance[80, 163]. As a rule, they arise in the anterior lobe, where they lead to an excessive production of hormones, or to anterior lobe insufficiency. Later, the tumors grow into the extrasellar space. When they extend to about 1.5 cm above the sella, they compress the optic chiasma, which leads to visual field defects, loss of sight, and atrophy of the optic nerve (chiasma syndrome). At the beginning of the nineteen-seventies, some 80% of patients with pituitary tumors first consulted an ophthalmologist for disturbances of vision. Today, only about 30% of the patients have such problems[93, 353]. The reason for the early detection is the advances made in endocrinological diagnosis.

Pituitary adenomas are classified according to their endocrine function. The percentage of hormonally inactive adenomas is constantly decreasing, since due to immunohistochemistry and cell culture explants, the production of hormone can now be demonstrated in the so-called hormonally inactive tumors[5]. Previously, RT had its permanent place in the treatment of pituitary adenomas. Impressive therapeutic results were reported after RT alone, or after surgery and adjuvant RT[173, 201, 253, 301].

The introduction and standardization of *microsurgery*, both for transsphenoidal and transcranial interventions, permits selective adenomectomy while preserving the remaining pituitary functions. These advances in surgery have been promoted by rapid developments in the field of neuroradiology: with the aid of thin-layer tomograms of the third CT generation, and representation of the tumor in three planes, and also MRI, not only can microadenomas in the anterior pituitary lobe be represented, but expansion of the tumor into the extrasellar régions can be better delimited. As a result, the morbidity and mortality of surgical interventions have been appreciably reduced. Together with new endocrinological techniques, the new radiological procedures permit a more accurate determination of the initial functional and morphological situation, and comparison of the effectiveness of various therapeutic procedures.

Unfortunately, it has, so far, not been possible with the modern diagnostic procedures, to objectify the *effect* of RT comprehensively and over a longer period of time. Most of the large case series are from the period prior to the introduction of CT and the endocrinological techniques. In the meantime, it has been seen that even in patients who became symptom-free after RT, the hormone levels first remained unchanged, and fell only after months (up to 10) years (see Sheline[301]). Studies comparing the control rates and complications of megavoltage irradiation with those of other therapy modalities are completely lacking. Accordingly, at present, the place of RT in the treatment concept for pituitary adenomas can hardly be defined or convincingly reasoned.

4.10.1. GH-secreting Adenomas (Acromegaly)

Pituitary adenomas leading to acromegaly can be removed via a transsphenoidal approach, and the growth hormon level is reduced to below the targeted threshold of 5 ng/ml in 70–80% of the patients. In adenomas developing within the sella, this can be achieved in up to 90%[20, 93–95]. If, as normalization criterion, not merely the basal growth hormone level, but also suppression by oral glucose to below 2 ng/ml is taken as parameter, these results worsen by about 10%. A further worsening of 10% results when the inadequate rise in growth hormone in response to TRH is taken into account. In addition, the preoperative basal level of growth hormone also plays a part. Thus, normalization of growth hormone levels above 50–100 ng/ml decreases appreciably as compared with lower levels[95]. These observations suggest that postoperative residual tumor is apparently more common than was first thought.

Conventional, externally applied *photon irradiation* is effective in the treatment of acromegaly (for a review see[82, 301]). The clinical control rate (the above-mentioned reservations should be noted) is between 80 and 90%, the effect being dose-dependent. In the few series in which the growth hormone level was measured prior to and after irradiation, it was shown that RT is capable of significantly lowering the growth hormone levels, provided that enough time is allowed to elapse before the determination is made[82, 104, 177]. Probably the best studied group of acromegaly patients treated with conventional megavoltage therapy, was reported by Eastman et al.[82]. A total of 47 patients were irradiated with a tumor dose of 40-50 Gy. The GH level dropped slowly but constantly over a period of up to 10 years (Table 6). Serum phosphate and plasma glucose normalized "analogously" to the

Table 6. The effect of radiotherapy on the growth hormone excess in cases of acromegaly (data from the literature)

Author	No. pts.	Radiation dose (Gy)	Follow-up period	GH* before RT** (ng/ml)	GH* after RT**	
					< 10 ng/ml	< 5 ng/ml
Eastman *et al.* (1979)	42	40–50	2 years	6–250	38%	17%
	33	40–50	5 years	6–250	73%	42%
	16	40–50	10 years	6–220	81%	69%
Giovanelli *et al.* (1980)	24	no data	1–6 years	6.5–110	66%	37%
Lawrence *et al.* (1977)	12	35–65	1–4 years	20–332	75%	58%
Erlangen (Buchfelder 1984)	11	50	4–24 months	11–380	9%	0%

  * Growth hormone.
 ** Radiotherapy.

growth hormone levels. No relationship was found to exist between the level of excess GH prior to irradiation, and the therapy response. However, other pituitary functions diminished progessively throughout the course of the observation period.

The biological effectiveness of alpha and photon radiation is virtually identical with that of proton radiation[201]. For practical concerns, this radiation plays no therapeutic role. However, it does appear that the pituitary deficits are more marked in patients treated with proton radiation than in those receiving megavoltage photon beam treatment[207].

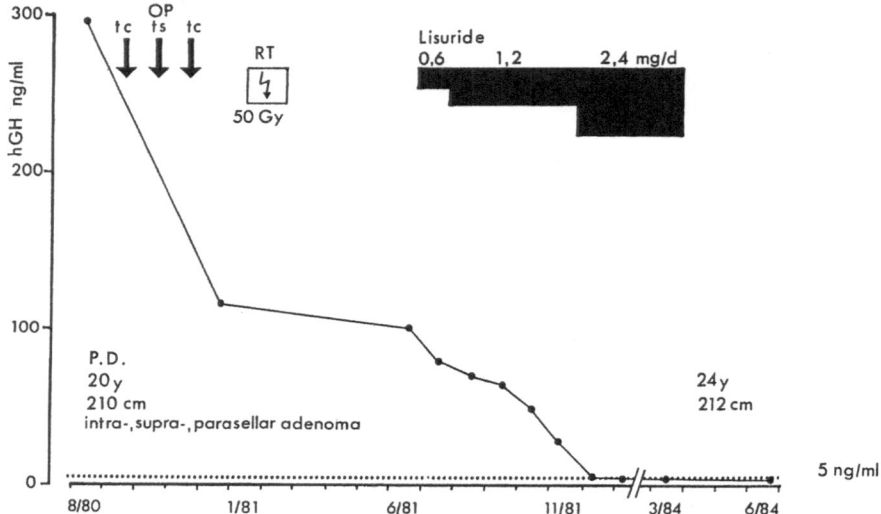

Fig. 18. Growth hormone level in a 20-year-old male patient with acromegaly caused by a giant adenoma. Three operations failed to normalize the excessive hormone level. In response to percutaneous radiotherapy with 50 Gy, the growth hormone level dropped again constantly. Additional dopamine agonists finally normalized the GH level to 5 ng/ml

These so far incomplete results appear to show that the control rates after transsphenoidal hypophysectomy and RT are similar. As compared with surgery, however, RT has the disadvantage of a slow onset of the therapy response and also the undesirable side effect of partial or total "hypophysectomy". For this reason, an attempt will be made to treat GH-producing adenomas with primary microsurgery. Primary RT is indicated only if rapid monitoring of the hormone level is not essential, the patient refuses surgery, or is in an inoperable state.

Postoperative RT is always indicated in suspected or proven incomplete removal of the adenoma, that is

— in patients with large tumors in whom the growth hormone levels do not normalize immediately after surgery (Fig. 18) and

— in all invasively proliferating tumors, even when the postoperative growth hormone levels have normalized.

4.10.2. ACTH-secreting Adenomas (Cushing's Syndrome)

In more than 90% of patients with Cushing's syndrome (CS), Fahlbusch et al.[95] detected microadenomas in the anterior lobe of the pituitary. On account of the fact that ACTH-secreting microadenomas are frequently diffuse, and sometimes expand beyond the gland, microsurgical treatment in Cs is one of the technically most difficult operations. Clinical and endocrinal biochemical remission is achieved in 75–90% of the patients[95, 123].

Conventional pituitary *irradiation* can control CS in 50–80% of the cases (for review see[301]). In the study by Orth and Liddle[242] a total of 51 patients were irradiated with 40–50 Gy, 44 of whom were followed up between 1 and 14 years. The criteria for the response to therapy were the excretion of 17-hydroxy-corticosterone in the urine, mean plasma cortisol concentration, and diurnal rhythms. On the basis of these criteria, 10/44 patients were cured, an additional 13 improved so that no further therapy was necessary. The remaining 21 patients were managed by secondary bilateral adrenalectomy.

The available data on the value of RT in CS are, at present, very incomplete. The effect of postoperative irradiation after primary microsurgical adenomectomy should be investigated.

4.10.3. Nelson's Syndrome (NS)

NS represents an ACTH-secreting pituitary adenoma following bilateral adrenalectomy (in hyperplasia of the adrenal cortices) to treat hypothalamo-hypophyseal CS, which is associated with progressive enlargement of the sella, hyperpigmentation and increasing ACTH levels. The results of treatment, whether by surgery, RT or a combination of both, are unsatisfactory. Normalization of the ACTH levels in response to surgery is observed in only a few cases[94, 122, 206, 353].

The role of RT in the treatment of NS is uncertain. Possibly, however, prophylactic irradiation of the region of the pituitary may lower the incidence of Nelson's syndrome, which occurs in about 10–15% of patients submitted to bilateral adrenalectomy[158, 242]. However, "Nelson's tumors" have been observed even despite high-dose prophylactic irradiation in patients with bilateral adrenalectomy[227, 301]. Conventional RT, with and without surgical resection, has also been used to treat NS. Moore et al.[227] reported that 6 out of 7 patients who received RT alone (the one death was not due to the underlying disease) are still alive and well after a mean observation period of 9.4 years.

A summary of the results of conventional irradiation is given in Table 7. Despite the paucity of data in the literature on RT of NS, in particular in the field of endocrinological documentation, we are of the opinion that present standard treatment comprises surgical removal of the tumor followed by routine postoperative RT.

4.10.4. Prolactin-secreting Adenomas (Prolactinomas)

The epidemiologically largest group of pituitary adenomas are the prolactinomas. Prior to the introduction of prolactin assay, these tumors were usually termed nonfunctional chromophobe or mixed adenomas. Treatment with resection alone, results in a return of the serum prolactin level to the normal range in only 33% of

Table 7. Nelson's syndrome: treatment results, modified after Sheline[301]

Author	No. of pts.	Treatment modality	Follow-up period	Treatment results
McKenzie and McIntosh (1965)	2	RT (48 Gy)	no data	NED
Moore et al. (1976)	5	RT (28–100 Gy)	9.4 years	NED (6 patients)
	2	RT (30–50 Gy)		TRD (1 patient)
Nelson et al. (1965)	1	OP + RT (30 Gy)	1 month	ACTH normal
	2	RT (30–40 Gy)	5 months	ACTH unchanged
Sheline (1981)	1	RT (50 Gy)	6 months	uncontrolled
	1	OP + RT (40 Gy)	5 years	under control
	1	OP + RT (50 Gy)	2 years	under control
Erlangen (Buchfelder 1984)	1	OP + RT (50 Gy)	2.5 years	TRD
	4	OP + RT (50 Gy)	3 years	alive without symptoms
				ACTH level elevated

NED = no evidence of disease, TRD = tumor related death, OP = operation, RT = radiotherapy.

the patients. In microadenomas, the situation is more favorable, with up to 80% normalization[95]. Despite postoperative normalization of excessive PRL, however, later recurrence occurs in 16%[92, 94] to 50%[123].

While there is a wealth of reports on the effectiveness of surgical measures in prolactinomas, in particular microadenomas, data on the effect of conventional RT on prolactin excess is very limited. The reason is that a reliable method for prolactin determination has been available only for about 15 years, and that while surgery is followed by a rapid drop in prolactin levels, hyperprolactinemia responds only slowly—over years—to radiation therapy. Table 8 shows a comparison of our own results[46] with data from the literature.

In 8 patients who received RT alone, and in 15 surgical patients, Kleinberg et al.[167] noted identical effectiveness of the two modalities. In the case material reported on by Gomez et al.[108], the prolactin levels dropped in 62% after RT, initially relatively rapidly within one month, but then slowly over a period of 3 to 4 years. This is in agreement with the Erlangen observations in 23 patients receiving postoperative RT[46]. The series of Autunes et al.[13] comprised 30 patients with mainly largish tumors. Here, there was a tendency to employ surgery alone for the lower grade lesions, and RT alone for higher-grade tumors. Although the pretreatment serum prolacin levels were even more elevated in the RT group, treatment resulted in a drop in prolactin similar to that observed after surgery alone. Sheline[301] deduced from this that the prospects for normalization of prolactin levels depends primarily on magnitude of the excess prolactin level, but not upon the nature of the treatment given—whether surgery or RT. Autunes et al.[13] found no normalization of hyperprolactinemia when the serum concentrations exceeded 125 µg/l. Nor did we see any normalization in our patients when serum prolactin levels were in excess of 4,000 µU/ml—admittedly over much too short an observation period. At the present time, the available data in the literature do not permit any definitive statement on RT in the treatment of prolactinomas. We are of the opinion that such lesions should be irradiated if they do not respond to prior surgical or medical treatment.

In contrast to the ACTH- and GH-secreting adenomas, we now have an alternative to primary surgical treatment in the dopamine agonists, bromocriptine, lisurid and pergolid. The dopaminergics are suitable for the treatment of the small adenomas measuring between 5 and 7 mm, for reducing the volume of macroadenomas prior to transsphenoidal surgery, and for the treatment of residual tumors, where the prolactin levels remain elevated after surgery or RT[95]. Surgery is, we believe, indicated when dopamine agonists are not tolerated, when they have an inadequate therapeutic effect, and also in suprasellar tumors, in particular when pregnancy is planned[94, 95].

4.10.5. Hormonally Inactive Adenomas and Giant Adenomas

These lead to a pituitary anterior lobe insufficiency only in the late stage of development. Thus, as a rule, these tumors are diagnosed only when they have already expanded intracranially, and have compressed the optic nerve and given rise to the symptoms of a space-occupying process. They can grow into the sinus cavernosus, into the brain tissue, and into the sphenoidal cavity.

Table 8. Radiotherapy effect on prolactin excess in prolactinomas (modified after[301])

Authors	No. of patients	Treatment modality	Prolactin levels (µg/l)			Decrease	Galac-torrhea ceased	Menses resumed	Follow-up period (months)
			Before treatment	Before RT	After treatment				
Autunes *et al.* (1977)	8	OP + RT	21–3,600	NDA	3–490	87%	1/3	0/3	3–39
	6	RT	110–10,000	NDA	32–560	93%	2/3	1/3	13–72
Gomez *et al.* (1977)	16	OP	27–900	NDA	6–361	79%	4/12	3/13	1–28
	8	RT	38–480		12–200	62%	2/8	4/?	6–57
Kleinberg *et al.* (1977)	15	OP	4–3,000.	NDA	0.5–170	84%	5/15	2/12	NDA
	8	RT	61–10,000		32–1,000	74%	3/8	2/6	NDA
Sheline (1981)	4	OP + RT	37–1,300	—	28–450	50%	1/2	0/3	1–16
Erlangen (Buchfelder 1984)	23	OP + RT	1,600–197,000 µE/ml	42,980 µE/ml	25,570 µE/ml (mean value)	64%	0/4	0/11	3–48

OP = operation, RT = radiotherapy, NDA = no data available.

Owing to their localization, they cannot be completely removed by surgery. For this reason, after surgery alone, most patients, if followed-up for long enough, will be seen to develop recurrent disease[46, 87, 89, 131, 253]. In general, these tumors grow very slowly. If, therefore, a permanent cure is to be proven, the observation period must be adequately long. In the case series reported by Sheline[301], the mean time to recurrence for patients who failed to respond to surgery alone, was 4 years, and 9 years for those who developed recurrent disease after a combination of surgery and postoperative RT. Erlichman et al.[89] found a median time to recurrence of 2.4 years for patients treated by surgery alone, and of 3.5 years for those treated by surgery and postoperative RT.

The Erlangen material included 34 patients with hormonally active tumors, of whom 27 had been operated on at least once prior to RT. In 31 patients regularly monitored by CT over a period of 1 to 5 years, the tumor was clearly diminished in size in 12 cases after RT, had remained unchanged in 15, or had undergone cystic transformation, but had enlarged in only 4 cases. This demonstrates the efficacy of RT in large pituitary tumors, too. In the UCSF patients[301], those who had been given RT alone, and those in whom only partial tumor resection had been followed with postoperative RT, recurrent-free survival was identical. In contrast, only 49% of the patients treated by surgery alone were still alive and recurrence-free after 2 years, while no patient survived for 15 years or longer. And in patients who had received postoperative RT of at least 45 Gy, recurrent lesions were extremely rare, and the control rate was estimated to be about 95%.

Sheline[301] reported that in patients with relatively minor visual field deficits affecting a quarter of the visual field or less, radiation alone and surgical decompression were equally effective: in about two thirds of the patients, the visual field returned to normal. When the pretherapeutic visual field deficit affected two quadrants, RT alone brought about a 60% improvement rate, but no deficit disappeared completely. Here, surgery, with normalization in 32%, was more effective. An improvement in vision can be achieved in up to 80% of patients with hormonally inactive pituitary tumors by the transsphenoidal procedure[94].

Other authors, too, have reported favorable results achieved with RT, either alone or in combination[87, 89, 131, 177, 253]. Emmanuel[87] and Sheline[301] compared freedom from recurrence after surgery alone and after combined therapy. After 4 years, they observed a recurrence-free survival rate of 30% in patients receiving surgery alone, 75% after RT alone, and in 93% after surgery combined with postoperative RT. Pistenma et al.[253] also showed that the percentage of recurrence-free survivors after 5 years was almost 90%, both after RT alone and after surgery supplemented by irradiation.

Large space-consuming pituitary tumors, in particular the hormonally inactive tumors, should receive postoperative conventional RT. Although RT alone, in particular in small tumors, is effective, in general, surgical debulking of the tumor mass should be undertaken. This rapidly relieves the pressure on the neighboring tissue. Total removal needs not always be the aim of surgery.

Radiation technique (see Fig. 4): Simple opposed bilateral coaxial fields are acceptable for large tumor volumes in which the rotation technique does not achieve an adequate dose distribution within the target volume. Here, admittedly, the temporal lobes are, unnecessarily, subjected to a high radiation dose. In the

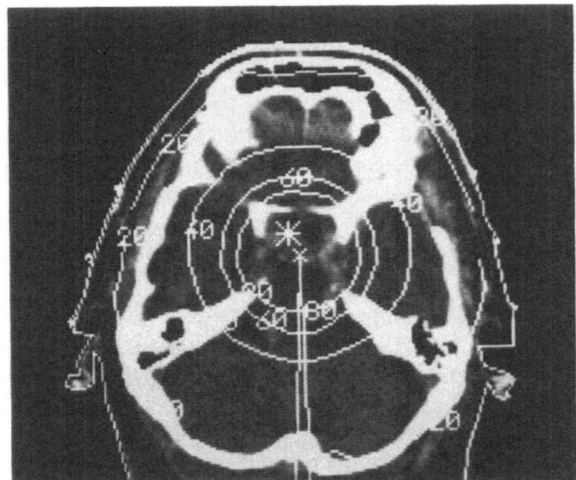

Fig. 19. Giant pituitary adenoma. The patient is in the supine position, and his head is fixed by means of a treatment mask. Full rotation through 360 degrees produces an ideal dose distribution

majority of cases, therefore, we give preference to the rotation beam technique. The full rotation through 360 degrees is, we feel, less subject to disturbances than the 220 degree rotation using wedges, described by Sheline[301] and produces an ideal dose distribution (Fig. 19).

Depending upon the extent of the tumor, the field size is $4 \times 4\,cm^2$ to $5 \times 6\,cm^2$, and includes the region of the primary lesion, the optic chiasma, and parts of the hypothalamus.

Radiation dose: We employ the conventional fractionation regimen of 1.8–2.0 Gy per day given five times a week to make a total dose of 45 Gy on the 90% isodose. This corresponds to a dose inhomogeneity of ± 5% (2.5 Gy) in the target volume. The results of the UCSF[301] showed that lower radiation doses result in a lower control rate. On the other hand, doses of > 50 Gy lead to complications affecting the hypothalamus and optic chiasma.

4.11. Craniopharyngioma

These benign, nonaggressive tumors originate in epithelial cell proliferations of the embryonal Rathke's pouch. Since such cell rests can spread into the transition zone between the neurohypophysis and adenohypophysis, the development of cranio-pharyngiomas is both intrasellar and suprasellar. Two thirds of the patients are children, in whom it is the most common nonglial intracranial tumor, accounting for about 9% of all intracranial neoplasms. 75% of the patients reveal calcifications in the skull X-ray. CT permits a distinction between cystic and solid tumor parts. The tumors give rise to dysfunction through their local "mass effect" and progressive expansion, and distortion of the surrounding tissue: headaches, visual impairment secondary to papilledema, visual field defects due to chiasmic and optic nerve involvement, hormonal defects such as growth retardation, diabetes insipidus and delayed or precocious puberty[140, 216].

Although they are histologically benign, craniopharyngiomas often develop a malignant effect, since they can invade neighboring structures such as the base of the skull, the carotid artery and hypothalamus. Therefore, they are rarely amenable to complete surgical extirpation—recent surgical statistics quote a figure of up to 30%. This is also confirmed by long-term CT follow-up over a period of years. In the Erlangen series[95], the tumors were amenable to surgical removal in 11/50 patients, complete removal being achieved in 16%. The surgical mortality rate is reported to be between 30 and 40% for transcranial operations. In a larger study[322] 10.5% of the patients died after the first radical tumor extirpation, 28.5% after a second radical procedure, but only 3% after less radical interventions. In the Erlangen series, one patient died postoperatively.

Recommended therapy: The primary aim of therapy is the complete surgical removal of the tumor, but without an excessive attendant risk. Recent reports indicate that percutaneous RT has an important, possibly even a curative role to play, and limited surgery with postoperative radical RT is, today, more than just a challenge to radical surgery.

Amacher[9] established that after so-called curative tumor resection, the recurrence rate is 19%, after subtotal resection 75%, but after subtotal resection followed by postoperative RT, "only" 30%. In the RMH[30, 31], 112 new patients received radical postoperative RT, 109 after limited excision. The 5- and 10-year survival rates in 46 children were 85 and 74%, respectively, and for 66 adults, 74 and 60%, respectively. No adverse effects of the RT were observed. According to the authors, the postoperative IQ levels, which tended to be low, but were still normal, must be directly related to the tumor disease, and not to the very often small-volume irradiation. Sung et al.[319] reported on 109 patients who had been treated surgically or with combined surgery and postoperative RT. Five- and 10-year survival rates were 62.9 and 48% in the 74 patients who received primary surgical treatment. The corresponding figures in 32 patients receiving combination therapy were 82.2 and 71%, respectively. The patients treated with surgery alone had a five-year and ten-year relapse-free survival of 31.5 and 17.4%, respectively, as compared with 76.3 and 43.8% following combined surgery and postoperative RT. The authors thus showed that combined treatment and total excision produce the same results. In another series[59] recurrent disease was observed in 44 to 67% of patients receiving subtotal resection, but in only 17% of those given postoperative RT. Danoff et al.[67] irradiated 19 children after either partial surgical resection, total gross resection or aspiration and biopsy. The five-year survival rate was 73%, the ten-year survival rate 64%. Their results are at least comparable, if not superior, to those of surgery. Other authors[50, 198, 263, 298, 331] confirmed the effectiveness of conservative surgery and postoperative RT in achieving long-term survival comparable with that of total excision in the treatment of childhood craniopharyngiomas.

Recently, results have been reported from Nijmwegen[143] on postoperative irradiation following subtotal resection of the tumor. The five-year relapse rate in the group without postoperative radiation therapy was 45%, and the five-year rate of death of disease was 27%. For the group that received postoperative RT, the five-year recurrence rate was only 11%, and no death of disease was observed in this group.

Radiation technique: We prefer a three-field technique with wedge filters in accordance with the scheme shown in Fig. 4, or a monaxial rotation technique. The target volume includes the sella, the suprasellar and parasellar structures. The patient is in the supine position, the base of the skull usually being vertical. Preferentially, it ought to be tilted a little more strongly in the direction of the chest.

Radiation dose: Following a proposal by Sung *et al.*[319], we recommend a dose of 50–55 Gy/6–6½ weeks after grossly total resection, but still present tumor rests in the postoperative CT scan. In patients with subtotal tumor removal or only minimal resection, we apply 55 Gy/6½ weeks in children, and 60–65 Gy/7–7½ weeks in adults.

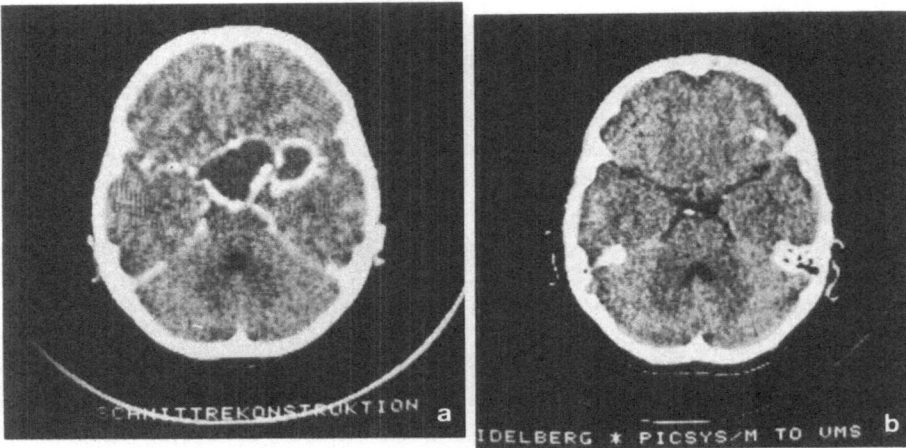

Fig. 20. *a* CT examination of an 8-year-old boy with a craniopharyngioma two ears after microsurgical tumor exstirpation. The picture shows two communicating cysts. *b* CT image of the same patient 5 years after intracavitary administration of yttrium-90. A tumor dose of 200 Gy to the inner surface of the cysts was calculated. The tumor disappeared completely. The boy is free of neurological symtoms. (The treatment was performed by Prof. V. Sturm, Heidelberg)

Palliative radiation by radioisotope therapy: Intracavitary radioisotope treatment of cystic craniopharyngiomas was introduced by Leksell *et al.*[194] in 1967. The stereotaxic puncture of the cyst is followed by radioisotope implantation using the following radioisotopes: phosphorus-32, gold-198, and yttrium-90[170, 316]. This treatment of a solitary cyst of a craniopharyngioma leads, in the majority of the cases, to shrinkage of the cyst, reduction of tumor mass, and thus, at least temporarily, to a good palliative result (Figs. 20 *a* and *b*).

4.12. Optic Gliomas

Gliomas of the optic nerve and optic chiasm are rare, accounting for only 1–2% of all the gliomas. 80% of such tumors manifest in childhood, usually within the first

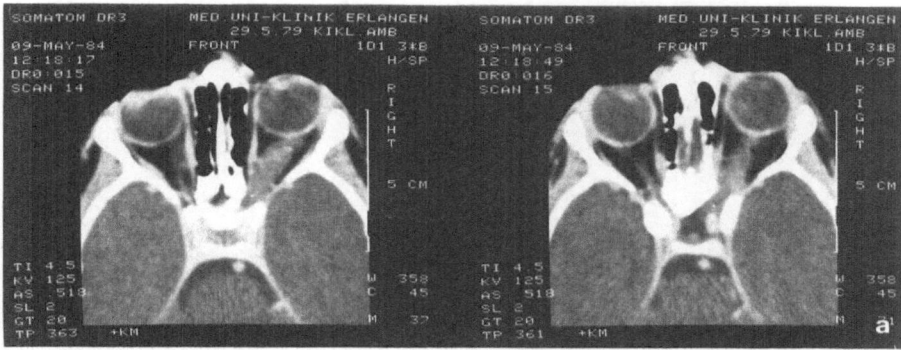

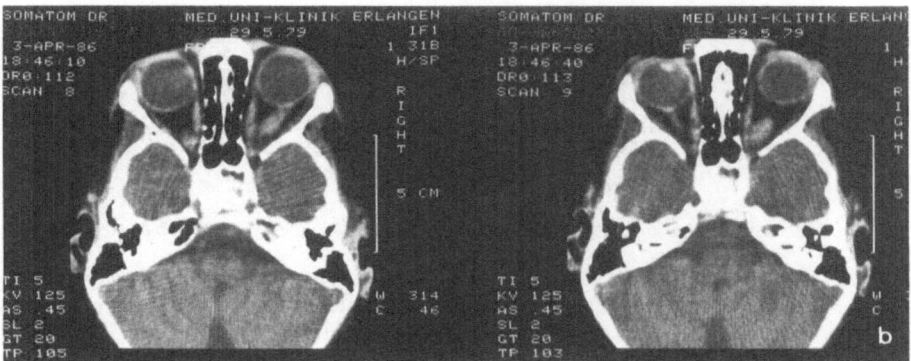

Fig. 21. Course of treatment of an optic glioma (astrocytoma grade 1) prior to (**a**), and 24 months after (**b**) radiation therapy. Radiotherapy led to a radiologically recognizable reduction in the size of the tumor

five years of life. The majority are low-grade astrocytomas of the so-called juvenile type [269, 270]. They are slow-growing and infiltrative, and, in particular in older patients, can transform into high-grade astrocytomas [68, 148, 205].

Tumors of the anterior portion of the optic nerve typically give rise to unilateral proptosis and reduced visual acuity. Chiasmal tumors cause bilateral restriction of vision and, under certain circumstances, hydrocephalus and hypothalamic functional deficits [75, 146, 147, 217, 223, 267, 328]. Although the tumors are indolent in their behavior, and grow slowly, they give rise to morbidity, and the larger and more dorsally located tumors lead to late mortality.

Recommended therapy: A pretreatment CT examination provides information on the localization and extent of the optic glioma. If, thereafter, there are any doubts as to the diagnosis, in particular in chiasmal tumors, surgical exploration is advised. By this means, craniopharyngiomas, meningiomas, suprasellar germinomas and hypothalamic gliomas may be excluded. Furthermore, a screening evaluation of the endocrine system is indicated [147, 223]. Only in unilaterally amaurotic patients should any attempt be made to achieve radical tumor excision.

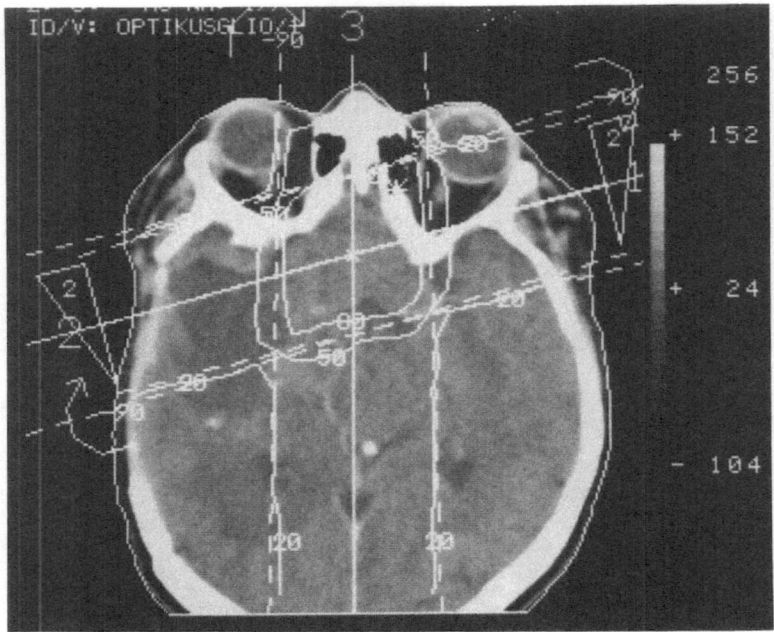

Fig. 22. Three-field cross-field technique with wedge filters, for the treatment of an optic glioma in the region of the chiasm and involving the anterior part of the right optic nerve. Two of the fields are lateral, the third frontal-oblique

Further indications for surgery are an increased intracranial pressure, progressive proptosis and pain[95, 217]. As a rule, the neurosurgeon will content himself with obtaining a biopsy to confirm the histological diagnosis, and then refers the patient for external conventional irradiation. We recommend RT for optic chiasmal glioma, for gliomas of the diffuse type, but also for unilateral tumors of the anterior portion of the optic nerve, provided that the affected eye has not gone blind.

Following RT, patients with progressive optic gliomas may have a favorable prognosis. Horwich and Bloom[146] observed an improvement in vision in 43%, stabilized vision in 48%, and a deterioration in vision in only 9% of the patients. In 18% of the cases, there was an increase in visual fields. 90% of the irradiated patients remained free from disease progression at a median follow-up period of 10 years. RT effected a reduction in exophthalmus, and in the radiologically demonstrable tumor bulk[68, 75, 78, 127, 267, 327] (Fig. 21).

Radiation technique: The target volume is determined on the basis of the CT findings. We employ two- or three-field techniques using wedge filters (Fig. 22).

Radiation dose: The total dose is 50–65 Gy/6–8 weeks with daily individual doses of 1.8–2.0 Gy. Montgomery *et al.*[226] discovered that a dose of < 50 Gy is inadequate. In their series, 4 out of 7 patients had tumor recurrence, while after > 50 Gy, none out of 9 patients showed any relapse. In accordance with Bloom[30], we reduce the dose to 45–50 Gy/5–6 weeks in children aged between 2 and 5 years, and to 40–45 Gy/4–5 weeks in children younger than 2 years.

Prognosis: Following combined treatment with limited surgery and radical irradiation, 75 to 90% of patients retain their vision. Between 75 and 100% are long-term survivors[30, 68, 146, 217].

4.13. Meningiomas

Meningiomas account for about 10% of all intracranial neoplasias. Most are histologically benign, grow slowly, and have a favorable natural history which, however, can vary widely. Anaplastic meningiomas are rare[269, 270].

The reported data on the value of RT for the postoperative treatment of incompletely resected or anaplastic meningiomas are controversial. The available data are sparse, but they militate against an often postulated radioresistance of meningiomas[30, 41, 53, 83, 191, 312, 346]. Radiation treatment given alone can ameliorate headaches in inoperable patients, improves visual impairment and ocular motor paresis, and reduces exophthalmus[30, 83]. Bloom[30] reported on 102 patients of whom 37 received RT either after limited surgery or as the sole form of treatment. The five-year recurrence-free survival rate was 73% as compared with 78% in 65 patients who had received postoperative RT after a grossly total or subtotal tumor excision. The corresponding ten-year recurrence-free survival rates were 60 and 61%, respectively. Thus, it appears that the radiation therapy had compensated the therapeutic shortcomings of incomplete tumor extirpation.

Recommended therapy: After complete tumor extirpation, RT is not indicated. We recommend postoperative RT in those meningioma patients who have a high risk of recurrent tumor, *i.e.* those

— with residual tumor,

— with infiltration of the tumor into the neighboring structures, and

— with unfavorable histological criteria suggesting potentially aggressive tumor behavior.

Wara *et al.*[346] reported from the UCSF on 92 patients following incomplete resection. Thirty-four of these patients had received postoperative irradiation, 58 had been treated solely by surgery. The recurrence rate without irradiation was 74% as compared with 29% after postoperative RT. The same differences were evident in those patients followed-up for 10 years or more. Carella *et al.*[53] and Solan and Kramer[312] confirmed that, when surgical excision is incomplete, postoperative RT seems to offer hope of long-term control, whether delivered in the immediate postoperative period or for salvage at the time of progression.

Radiation dose: 55–60 Gy/6–6½ weeks with 1.8–2.0 Gy per fraction.

4.14. Brain Metastases

8–9% of the patients with an invasive malignant growth develop brain metastases sometime during the course of the disease[153, 251, 255]. This makes brain metastases more common than primary brain tumors.

Malignant melanoma, small-cell lung carcinoma and germ cell tumors have a particularly marked tendency to metastasize to the brain. In absolute terms, among the patients with brain metastases, the most common primary tumors are lung and breast cancers, and are followed by unknown primaries[39, 40, 133, 153, 251, 255, 288, 289]. Apparently, over the last 20 years, the number of patients with diagnosed and therapy-requiring brain metastases has increased. The reasons for this are not known[251]. One reason might be that chemotherapy has prolonged the survival of patients with small-cell lung carcinoma, breast cancer, nonseminomatous tumors of the testes, etc., to such an extent that brain metastases can now appear clinically. This would seem a distinct possibility, since the commonly employed chemotherapeutic agents do not pass through the BBB, and thus have no therapeutic effect on the brain.

Metastatic cancer in the brain is more often multiple than single. The ratio varies, depending upon the histological type and nature of the primary tumor. In various treatment series, the incidence of solitary and multiple brain metastases differs. Neurosurgical series representing a positive selection, reveal solitary metastases in up to 85% of the cases[48, 73, 153, 187, 352, 354]. In radiotherapeutic and autopsy series, patients with multiple brain metastases predominate by far, accounting for about two thirds of the total[39, 153, 251, 255, 288, 289].

As the site of metastases, the cerebral hemispheres lead the cerebellum or brain stem by 2 to 1 to 3 to 1[153, 251].

Recommended therapy: Whole-brain irradiation is the primary treatment of choice. With this modality, the neurological symptoms can be improved to the extent that a neurosurgical intervention can be postponed or, in more favorable cases, be obviated altogether. This also applies to solitary metastases.

Primary neurosurgical intervention is indicated (see p. 131)

— in solitary metastases of a poorly radiosensitive tumor, *e.g.* hypernephroma, gastrointestinal tumor, malignant goitre, soft-tissue sarcoma, osteosarcoma,

— in unknown primary tumors, to permit histology, or in undecided differential diagnosis to primary brain tumor, and

— in suspected late metastasis of a long-term controlled primary tumor.

Postoperative cranial irradiation should follow grossly successful surgical extirpation of a solitary cerebral metastasis. Smalley *et al.*[309] were able to provide a rationale for this requirement. 51 postoperative patients were merely kept under observation, while 35 received adjuvant whole-brain irradiation. A comparison of the two groups revealed a marked difference in the failure pattern. Brain failure was seen as a component of eventual failure in 83 versus 30%, and was the sole site of eventual failure in 50 versus 3% of the observed and irradiated group, respectively. Survival from craniotomy was better in the irradiated group (median 23 months, mean 27.3 months) as compared with the observed group (median 12 months, mean 20.9 months). Eleven irradiated patients (31%) and 3 observed patients (6%) remained without any evidence of disease at the time of the last follow-up or intercurrent death. Similar results were obtained by Kreuser *et al.*[181a]. They concluded that patients treated by surgical excision and adjuvant RT may achieve long-lasting cerebral remission.

In principle, the treatment of brain metastases is indicated only when the remaining "tumor situation" is under control, and the patient can expect to survive, largely symptom-free, for a number of months.

Radiation technique: Whole-brain irradiation should always be given. Via laterally opposed fields, a midbrain dose of 30 Gy/2 weeks is applied.

Radiation dose: The national randomized Phase III trials of the RTOG[39, 40] showed that the following radiation doses or fractionation patterns are equal in their effect: 20 Gy/1 week, 30 Gy/2 weeks, and 40 Gy/3–4 weeks. This was also seen in the Erlangen protocol[289], < 30 Gy tumor dose/3 weeks does not suffice to control brain metastases (p > 0.05). The basic dose of 30 Gy/2 weeks can, in the presence of a good response and/or residual findings, be boosted by 10–15 Gy/1 weeks applied to a small volume.

In cases of recurrent brain metastases, it is possible to reirradiate the whole brain with 30–40 Gy/2–4 weeks[40, 185, 255].

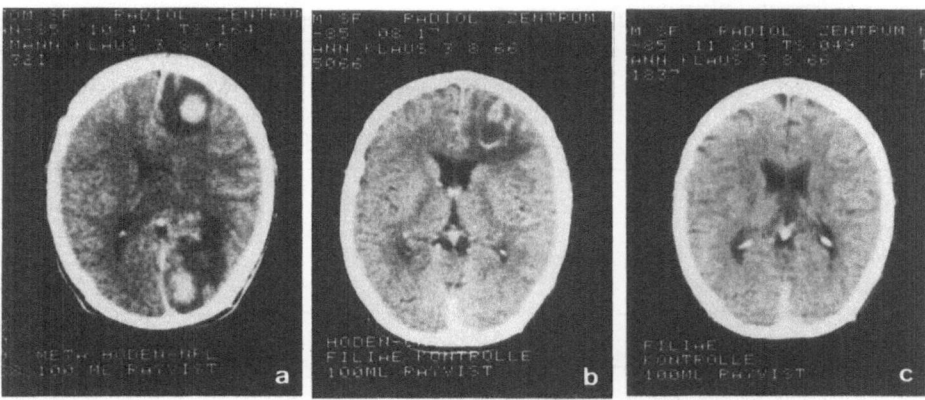

Fig. 23. Multiple brain metastases in a 19-year-old patient with a malignant teratoma of the testis. **a** Prior to radiotherapy. **b** After 36 Gy/2½ weeks whole-brain irradiation. **c** Nine months after termination of radiation therapy the brain metastases are no longer to be seen

Treatment results (Tables 9–11): After whole brain irradiation, 50–80% of the patients can expect partial or complete remission: improvement in neurological symptomatology, and regression or diminishment of the brain metastases (Fig. 23) observed in the CT scan[39, 56, 71, 133, 255, 288, 289, 336, 349]. Since, in the literature, the response to therapy is often expressed only in clinical terms, but not in terms of the CT scan, we propose not to differentiate between complete and incomplete remission.

The quality of the remission does not depend upon the nature and histology of the primary tumor[255, 289, 349]. Furthermore, it is of little importance whether solitary or multiple, supratentorial or infratentorial metastases present. There is, however, a clear correlation between the quality of remission and the radiation dose applied. In the Erlangen case material[289], only 11% of the patients had a remission after < 30 Gy/3 weeks, 56% after 30 Gy/2 weeks or 40 Gy/4 weeks, and as much as 80% of the patients who received > 40 Gy (Table 9). However, we do not wish to exclude the possibility that a positive selection occurred in that only those patients received a high radiation dose who showed a favorable course under treatment. There is agreement with RTOG observations to the effect that RT was more effective in

Table 9. Improvement of neurological symptoms following radiotherapy according to dose delivered. 252 patients with brain metastases

Dose (ret)	No. of patients	Overall remission	No change
< 1,100	75	8 (11%)	67 (89%)
1,101–1,300	57	32 (56%)	25 (44%)
1,301–1,500	77	64 (83%)	13 (17%)
> 1,500	43	37 (86%)	6 (14%)

Table 10. Survival of 252 patients with brain metastases following radiotherapy

	Mean (months)		Median (months)	
	1959–1974	1978–1983	1959–1974	1978–1983
Breast cancer	5.0	6.6	2	5
Lung cancer	7.8	5.7	2	3.5
Hypernephroma	0.6	7.4	0.5	6.5
Primary tumor unknown	7.7	5.4	5	5
Total	3.25	6.2	2	4

patients in a good general condition, that is, outpatients showed a better response than hospitalized patients[39].

Following RT alone, depending upon the composition of the case material and the nature of the treatment provided, between 5 and 40% of the patients survived for 1 year. The overall survival rate after one year is between 10 and 20%. The median survival is about 4–6 months[39, 56, 133, 255, 288, 336, 349].

Usually, brain metastases are an expression of advanced, always disseminated, tumor disease. For this reason, although RT can largely exclude brain metastasis as the immediate cause of death, it can improve the overall situation only marginally, and the survival rate merely within the immediately posttreatment months, perhaps within the course of a year (Table 10). In the Erlangen patient material 38% of the responders, were still alive after 1 year, of the nonresponders only < 5% (p < 0.05) (Fig. 24). The *one-year survival* also correlated with the radiation dose applied: after 1,100–1,300 ret*, 19% survived, after 1,300–1,500 ret 30%, and after > 1,500 42% of the patients[289]. The difference between these three dose ranges and that of < 1,100 ret is statistically significant (p < 0.05). It was found that the same parameters also had an influence on the median survival.

---

* The Nominal Standard Dose concept takes into account the total dose D in rad, the number of fractions N, and the overall treatment time T in days, thus: NSD (ret) = $D \times N^{-0.24} \times T^{-0.11}$.

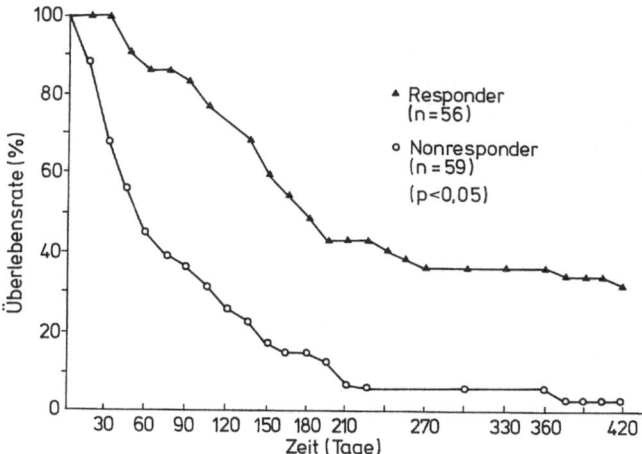

O Dose at site on necrosis
● Dose at tumor size
2, 4 or 6-multiple cases at some point

Fig. 24. Survival rate of 115 patients as a function of response to treatment. After one year, 38% of the responders are still alive, but only < 5% of the nonresponders

Table 11. Survival of 131 patients with brain metastases following radiotherapy. Prognostic factors

	Median survival (days)	
Age: < 65 years	115	
> 65 years	135	
Multicentricity:		
solitary	144	
multiple	126	
Dose delivered (ret):		
0–1,100	39	
1,101–1,300	123	
1,301–1,500	173	$p < 0.05$
> 1,500	173	
boost	208	
Treatment modality:		
radiotherapy	121	
surgery + radiotherapy	225	
Response to treatment:		
responders	178	$p < 0.05$
nonresponders	53	

In older patients (> 65 years), the median survival was, at 135 days, longer than in young patients, who survived for a median period of only 115 days (Table 11). Again, the nature of the primary tumor, and the number of brain metastases presenting, had no influence. Responders had a median survival of 178 days as compared with only 53 days in the case of the nonresponders. Eighteen patients, in whom a solitary metastasis had received a small-volume boost, had a median survival of 208 days. Versus patients who had received only the "basic dose", this was statistically significant (p < 0.05).

The results obtained by the Mayo Clinic with respect to postoperative RT after surgical resection of solitary metastasis, point into the same direction[309]: patients treated with the median dose of 39 Gy or more (n = 19) had a longer survival (median 27.5 months, mean 31 months) as compared to those treated with less than 39 Gy (median 13.5 months, mean 22.9 months). The survival advantage was associated with an improved local control rate in the brain.

5. Complications of Radiotherapy

RT of the primary and secondary tumors of the brain, as also adjuvant whole-brain irradiation employed in the treatment of leukemia, can induce brain injury. The CNS proves to be less radioresistant than it appeared to be some 30 years ago.

5.1. Definition

Radiation-induced brain injury is defined as injury to the healthy tissue which, following RT alone or in combination with other physical or chemical noxae with a deleterious effect on the nervous system, occur after a typical latency period. Such noxae are operations on the CNS, systemic or intrathecal chemotherapy, infections and injuries induced directly by the tumor itself. In these cases, then, we are talking about *combination injuries*. Radiation-induced complications are generally restricted to the irradiated volume, or arise within it.

A distinction of radiation-induced complications in accordance with their temporal course, is made between the acute reaction, early delayed reaction, and late reaction[36, 38, 79, 152, 186, 292].

5.1.1. Acute Reaction

An acute reaction can be observed within a matter of hours after the first irradiation treatment, or within the course of the first day of treatment (Table 12). Neuropathology shows intracellular and extracellular edema, inflammatory accompanying reactions, metabolic disorders of the glial and nerve cells and, rarely, even acute radionecrosis. These changes may regress completely, but, when they are marked, may also lead into a late reaction[199].

5.1.2. Early Delayed Reaction

Within a few weeks or months after RT, characteristic neurological symptoms can occur. In general, these are of a temporary nature and disappear again without

Table 12. Systematics of radiation injuries to the nervous system

	Latency	Course
1. *Acute reaction*		
Brain	hours	— reversible within hours
Spinal cord	hours	— often unrecognized; transverse lesion
Peripheral nerves	hours/days	— often unrecognized; completely reversible
2. *Early delayed reaction*		
Brain	2–8 weeks	— reversible within 6–8 weeks
Subform: Leukoencephalopathy	2–8 weeks	— in part reversible within 2–6 weeks in part becomes chronic
Spinal cord (Lhermitte's sign)	2–8 weeks	— reversible within 1–5 months — chronic form, rare
3. *Late delayed reaction* (late radionecrosis) Brain		— progression
Cerebral hemisphere	9 months– 7.5 years	relatively favorable prognosis
Midline region	1–36 months	poor prognosis, death within months
Subforms: — Pituitary-hypotha- lamus insufficiency	years	slow progression, good prognosis with substitution
— Psychomotoric deficiency sondrome	months– years	?
Spinal cord	4–25 months	— progression — when tetraplegia or paraplegia death within 18 months
Peripheral nerves	4 months– 10 years	— progression

treatment within a few weeks (Table 12). Most common is Lhermitte's sign in the region of the cervical and thoracic spinal cord. It can occur after large-volume irradiation of the upper section for malignant lymphoma, or after radiation of head and neck tumors. Neuropathology reveals focal areas of demyelinization of the white matter, perivascular lymphocyte and plasma cell infiltrates, vascular changes, disturbances of the BBB, edema, circumscribed hemorrhages, and necroses [152, 199].

Leukoencephalopathy is possibly a variety of early delayed reaction [303]. Radiologically, the ventricles are enlarged, and the subarachnoidal space widened, the CT scan of the brain contains hypodense areas, and there are intracerebral calcifications. These changes may be clinically asymptomatic, but they can also give rise to severe neurological deficits. Neuropathologically, the findings extend from a noninflammatory microangiopathy with surrounding necroses and microcalcifications, to a loss of the glia that may extend to severe, confluent, demyelinizing necroses of the white matter [256].

5.1.3. Late Reaction

The late CNS reaction can occur within months or years after treatment. It is usually progressive, irreversible, and finally leads to the death of the patient (Table 12). The white matter is more severely affected than the gray matter. The main neuropathological findings are vascular damage, necrosis and a perifocal edema. Sometimes, the late necrosis manifests clinically as a space-consuming lesion, and is often not distinguishable from a recurrent tumor in the CT scan (Fig. 25). Clinically, it has proven useful to differentiate the radiation injuries in accordance with their localization [142]. Radiation necroses of the cerebral hemispheres have a different morphology, a greater tolerance threshold, a longer latency period, and also a more favorable prognosis than those of the hypothalamus, brain stem or optic chiasma.

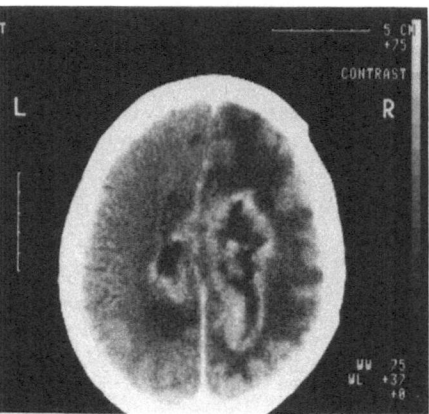

Fig. 25. Late necrosis in the right temporal lobe also involving the left hemisphere. The annular structures store contrast medium. Marked perifocal brain edema. On the basis of the CT scan alone, no differentiation can be made between tumor or recurrent tumor and late radionecrosis

5.2. Incidence of Radiation Injuries

The literature contains no adequately reliable information on the incidence of early and late radiation injuries, for four reasons:

— Most reports in the literature on early and late radiation reactions are anecdotal. They usually contain few details on the nature of the RT employed, such as single dose, total dose, tumor dose and maximum dose, nor do they provide information on the volume irradiated, the arrangement of the fields, radiation quality or dose-time relationship.

— In brain tumor patients, the follow-up period is usually short. In the high-grade astrocytomas, for example, it may be shorter than the latency period of the late reactions. Moreover, many patients are lost to follow-up in the special departments.

— The incidence of autopsies performed on brain tumor patients is low. But the differential diagnosis between a late and a recurrent tumor can only be clarified in biopsy or postmortem material.

— Information on the number of brain tumor patients receiving radiation therapy is completely lacking, and the actual number of diagnosed and histologically verified radiation reactions in the CNS is unknown.

5.3. Symptomatology

The patient's symptoms are dictated by the localization and extent of the lesion, together with the phase of the course of the radiation reaction (Table 12). For further details we refer to the review by Sauer[286].

5.3.1. Acute Reaction

During an acute radiation reaction, the tumor-induced symptoms are usually augmented.

Irradiation of the brain: uncharacteristic headache, such signs of increasing incranial pressure as nausea and vomiting, rarely, somnolence.

Irradiation of the spinal cord: Compression of the spinal cord caused by radiation edema can result in complete paraplegia.

Irradiation of the peripheral nerves: Lancinating pain and paresthesia in the area supplied by the nerve or nerve plexus.

Prophylaxis and therapy: Whenever RT involves high individual doses and large volumes, or when a space-consuming lesion with marked perifocal edema presents, and also whenever threatening or incomplete paraplegia symptomatology presents, we administer corticoids (1 mg cortisone/kg body weight) prophylactically. Occasionally, laminectomy may be indicated to relieve spinal cord compression.

5.3.2. Early Delayed Reaction

Commonly, the symptoms are uncharacteristic and transient.

Irradiation of the brain: lethargy, somnolence, enhancement of the tumor-related symptoms. Recurrence of neurological disturbances several weeks after termination of radiotherapy must not be misinterpreted as recurrent tumor.

Irradiation of the spinal cord: Lhermitte's sign is featured by electric-like shocks, paraesthesia, possibly also pain, in the shoulder girdle, back, buttocks and thighs when the spinal cord is stretched. It can be induced in the supine patient by flexion of the cervical spine, or by having the patient lift his straight legs.

Cortocoids accelerate the regression of early delayed reaction.

5.3.3. Late Delayed Reaction

5.3.3.1. Brain

The symptoms may be those of a space-consuming process: signs of elevated intracranial pressure, epileptic seizures, cranial nerve deficiencies, peripheral pareses, etc. The latency period for late necrosis in the region of the cerebral hemispheres is 9 months to 7.5 years, and in the midline region 1 to 36 months[142].

Dysfunctions of the *hypophysis-hypothalamus system* following irradiation treatment of pituitary adenomas, craniopharyngiomas, tumors of the roof of the pharynx, eyes, or inner ear, are more common than assumed by many radiotherapists until recently[46, 82, 107, 262, 272, 296, 301]. Older reports on a low incidence of radiation-induced pituitary functional disorders are not conclusive. For many of the patients described here received radiotherapy prior to the era of the assays for pituitary hormones. Already before RT, they also had tumor-related disturbances of some of the pituitary functions.

Samaan *et al.*[272] investigated the hypothalamic-hypophyseal function in 65 patients with irradiated tumors of the naso-pharynx, paranasal sinuses or orbits. The effective dose at the pituitary was 40 to 85 Gy. Three to 20 years after radiation therapy, the examined hormonal parameters indicated a disturbance in the function of the hypothalamus in 54/65 patients, and a primary pituitary insufficiency in 25/65 patients. Eastman *et al.*[82] investigated the function of the pituitary-thyroid axis, and the pituitary-adrenal axis in 47 patients with acromegaly. In patients who had received 40–50 Gy, they discovered secondary hypothyroidism and secondary adrenocortical insufficiency, whose incidence increased with time. The incidence of the hypothyroidism increased from 9% before treatment to 19% after 10 years, that of hypoadrenalism from 6% prior to irradiation to 30% after 5 and 39% after 10 years.

In our selected series of very large tumors[46], the incidence of disturbed pituitary function was already very high (67/75 patients) even before radiation therapy. In all functional deficiencies, the number of patients requiring substitution therapy increased with increasing observation time: 57 patients receiving hydrocortisone substitution versus 55 patients prior to radiotherapy; 57 patients receiving thyroxine replacement as compared with 49 prior to RT, and 38 patients receiving sexual hormone substitution as compared with 27 before irradiation. Since the incidence of diabetes insipidus did not increase, it may be concluded that the posterior lobe of the pituitary shows a greater radioresistance.

Intellectual Deficits

The long-term effects of irradiation of the brain on intelligence has been thoroughly investigated in children with leukemia[19, 85, 137, 183]. Since most of the patients had no primary CNS involvement, and had received cranial irradiation in accordance with various "prophylactic protocols", the effects of the treatment can readily be differentiated from tumor-induced effects. Significantly lower intelligence quotients were found in children receiving irradiation.

These early studies, however, were unable to stand up to a critical analysis. Walther and Gutjahr[344] established that the treatment of acute lymphatic leukemia (ALL) in childhood affected the basic psychomotoric processes rather than the cognitive processes. Harten et al.[126] discovered no intellectual deficiencies following chemotherapy and whole-brain irradiation. Whenever deficiencies did appear, they were related to the prior neurological findings or to the premorbid state of evolution. There were, however, discrete dysfunctions in the speed of psychomotoric process, which manifested in a general "slowing down". For the rest, the younger children did better than older children, thus discounting the supposed greater vulnerability of the brain in this group of children. Investigation carried out by Soni et al.[313] point in the same direction.

A high-dose whole-brain irradiation of children with 40–60 Gy does, however, results in clearly apparent functional disorders in long-term survivors (see[303]), Li et al.[197] observed moderate to severe intellectual deficiencies in 13/30 (43%) patients irradiated in childhood, after a latency period of 5–47 years. The most noticeable deficiencies, however, were seen in patients with large surgically inaccessible or particularly aggressive tumors. Such patients had been selected for radiation therapy, that is, they represent a negative selection. Sheline et al.[303] cite from the literature a number of statements to the same effect: patients with neurological injuries prior to irradiation show an impairment of intellectual abilities after treatment, too.

5.3.3.2. Spinal Cord

In late radiation necrosis of the spinal cord, the sensory nerve tracts are the first to be involved, and these are followed by the pyramidal tracts, then the motor tracts. The results are first sensory dissociation, then spastic pareses, possibly simultaneous or later flaccid pareses or a Brown-Séquard syndrome[79, 308]. Since demyelination can progress caudally, paraplegia or tetraplegia is also possible. Occasionally, late necroses of the spinal cord appear as space-consuming processes with myelographic stop, and elevation of the protein level in the CSF[79, 141, 215, 244]. Subsequently, atrophy gradually develops. The patients usually die as result of the paraplegic syndrome, of respiratory paralysis, pneumonia, pulmonary embolism or sepsis. In collective statistics reported by Franke and Lierse[99], 122/176 patients (69%) died of late necrosis of the spinal cord.

5.4. Radiation Tolerance of the Central Nervous System

The radiation tolerance of the nervous system varies. In the region of the cervical and thoracic spinal cord, but also in the midline structures, it is lower than in the cerebral hemispheres, and the peripheral nerves[36, 79, 98, 99, 129, 178, 244].

Table 13. Comparison of doses for various single doses and fractions per week. The tolerance thresholds in ret* do not correspond with those in neuret**

Fractions per week	10	5	5	5	4	4	5	4
Dose per fraction (Gy)	1.2	1.5	1.8	2.0	2.5	3.0	3.0	3.5

Total dose	NSD (ret) / NSD (neuret)							
30 Gy	1,010	1,010	1,070	1,110	1,170	1,250	1,280	1,310
	610	660	720	760	830	910	920	980
35 Gy	1,110	1,110	1,190	1,230	1,300	1,380	1,410	1,450
	660	710	780	820	900	*990*	*1,000*	*1,060*
40 Gy	1,220	1,220	1,300	1,340	1,420	1,510	1,540	1,590
	710	760	830	870	960	*1,050*	*1,070*	*1,140*
45 Gy	1,310	1,310	1,400	1,450	1,530	1,630	1,670	1,720
	750	800	880	930	*1,020*	*1,120*	*1,130*	*1,210*
50 Gy	1,410	1,410	1,500	1,560	1,640	1,750	1,790	1,840
	790	850	930	*980*	*1,080*	*1,180*	*1,200*	*1,270*
55 Gy	1,500	1,500	1,600	1,660	1,740	1,860	1,900	1,960
	830	890	*970*	*1,030*	*1,130*	*1,240*	*1,250*	*1,340*
60 Gy	1,580	1,590	1,690	1,750	1,850	1,970	2,020	2,070
	870	930	*1,020*	*1,070*	*1,180*	*1,290*	*1,310*	*1,400*
65 Gy	1,670	1,670	1,780	1,850	1,950	2,070	2,120	2,190
	900	*970*	*1,060*	*1,120*	*1,230*	*1,350*	*1,360*	*1,450*

  * NSD (ret) = D × N$^{-0.24}$ × T$^{-0.11}$.
 ** NSD (neuret) = D × N$^{-0.44}$ × T$^{-0.06}$.

5.4.1. Radiation Dose

5.4.1.1. Brain

The brain apparently tolerates 53 Gy and less administered with a conventional fractionation regimen (< 2 Gy) and with megavoltage beams. 60 Gy/30 fractions/6–7 weeks is considered a threshold dose for brain necroses[36, 42, 141, 200, 303, 355].

Lindgren[200] was the first to establish a relationship between dose and duration of treatment. He obtained, in the modified, double-logarithmic Strandquist diagram, a curve, a, having a slope of 0.26 to the X-axis. This curve defines a dose range with a high risk for brain necrosis. Values above this line represent an overdosage. The smallest dose that caused brain necrosis in the adult was, according to Lindgren[200], between 45 and 50 Gy/30 days. For the brain stem, Boden[36] calculated a regression line having a slope of 0.22, which pointed to a greater influence of treatment time.

Ellis[86] introduced into the dose-time relationship the number, and thus also the size, of the single fractions.

The Nominal Standard Dose concept applies to the healthy skin, and takes account of the total dose, D, in rad, the number of fractions, N, and the total treatment time, T, in days:

$$NSD \ (ret) = D \times N^{-0.24} \times T^{-0.11}$$

Table 13 shows the ret values for the fractionation regimens commonly employed today.

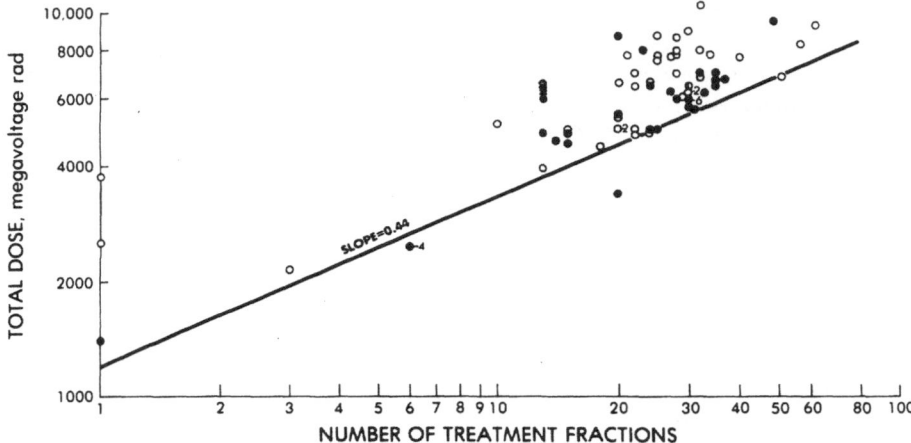

Fig. 26. Total dose in megavoltage ret equivalents in 40 patients with brain necroses reported in the literature, plotted against the number of single fractions. The regression line has a slope of 0.44. Most of the cases with brain necroses are located above this line (from Sheline *et al.* 1980)

In the meantime, it has been established that the Ellis formula is unsuitable for assessing the radiation risk, since the dose per fraction is much more important than the Ellis formula accounts for. Applied to the CNS, therefore, the Ellis formula would lead to overdosage. Sheline *et al.*[303] therefore modified the NSD (ret) concept, to provide an NSD (neuret) concept:

$$NSD \ (neuret) = D \times N^{0.44} \times T^{-0.06}$$

The indices for the number of fractions and radiation time were obtained in animal experiments on lumbar spinal cord (see[303]).

Sheline *et al.*[303] established that the total dose which can result in a brain necrosis, may be surprisingly small when the treatment time is short, the number of individual doses small, and the dose per fraction large. The regression line in Fig. 26 has a slope of 0.44. It marks the lowest dose at which a necrosis can occur. The highest incidence of necrosis was found between 1.000 and 1.100 neuret ($\cong$ 1.700 to 1.800 ret) corresponding to about 60 Gy/30 fractions/42 calender days. Only 4/80 patients with brain necroses had received < 1,000 neuret, corresponding to about 54 ± 2 Gy in 2 Gy/fraction.

Harris and Levene[125] discovered a similar situation following RT of pituitary adenomas and craniopharyngiomas. In 27 patients who had received daily individual doses of ≤ 2 Gy, no injury to the interbrain system occurred. 3/28 patients receiving individual doses of 2.5–3 Gy, however, developed injuries; two of them received a total dose of only 45 and 50 Gy, respectively. Similarly, Franke and Lierse[99], and Marks et al.[211] drew attention to the risks of applying high individual doses to the CNS.

5.4.1.2. Spinal Cord

Boden[36] indicated a tolerance threshold for the spinal cord of 35 Gy/17 days for large volumes, and 45 Gy/17 days for small volumes. Sinner[308] quoted 35–45 Gy/21 days or 37–48 Gy/28 days, or 41–52 Gy/43 days as the tolerance threshold. Abbatucci et al.[2] consider 50 Gy/25 fractions 35 days to be tolerable for the cervical cord, provided a volume of 3–5 vertebrae is not exceeded. For clinical purposes, it is generally assumed that 35–40 Gy/18–20 fractions/4 weeks represents the tolerance limit beyond which the spinal cord should not be irradiated.

5.4.2. Radiation Volume

For the spinal cord[2, 36, 244, 308] and the peripheral nerves[350], impressive data are available which show that with increasing treatment volumes, the radiation tolerance of the nervous system diminishes. It is to be assumed that this will also apply to the brain, although no experimental or unequivocal clinical data are available.

5.4.3. Interaction with Chemotherapeutics

Oncological chemotherapy given together with, or after radiotherapy, can sensitize the central nervous system for ionizing radiation and enhance radiation complications, respectively. And it is of no importance whether the drugs can pass the BBB or not, since it may be impaired in brain tumors, or even be nonexistent[339]. As a result, even such cytotoxic agents can interact with radiotherapy which, under normal circumstances, cannot pass the BBB. Of interest in this respect are methotrexate, vincristine, cytosine-arabinoside, L-asparaginase, presumably also leukerane, procarbazine, and the nitrosoureas BCNU and CCNU.

Best known is the situation in the case of methotrexate, the drug of choice in acute lymphatic leukemia in childhood. Even without whole-brain irradiation, this agent is capable of causing leukoencephalopathy, both after intravenous[8] and intrathecal[27] administration. In contrast, cranial irradiation with 18–24 Gy/2–3 weeks as sole prophylaxis in ALL, causes no leukoencephalopathy.

The risk of necrotizing leukoencephalopathy in children receiving ALL therapy is greatest when all three treatment modalities are employed: intrathecal MTX, intravenous MTX and whole-brain irradiation[27]. The risk may be 5– $> 50\%$ [12, 27, 115, 116, 257].

Price and Jamieson[257] differentiate the leukoencephalopathy risk, both with respect to the size of the radiation dose to the CNS, and the amount of MTX administered. For, leukoencephalopathy confirmed at autopsy, did not occur below a dose of 20 Gy, but was seen after 20–24 Gy in 9/51 patients (17%), in 2/16 patients after 25–30 Gy, and in 2/3 patients after > 30 Gy. Likewise, the behavior of the methotrexate dose: 3/29 patients (10%) developed leukoencephalopathy after 1–200 mg, 4/13 (30%) after 400–600 mg, and 5/16 patients (31%) after > 600 mg.

Habermalz et al.[116] pointed out that it is not known how wide the CSF spaces may normally be in childhood. In their study, the authors classified changes visible in the CT scan into 3 grades, and discovered posttreatment grade I and II abnormalities in 58% of the patients. As the authors suggest, grade I was probably a normal variant. Thus, a particularly critical eye must be cast on reports in the literature dealing with similarly high incidence rates of CT changes after CNS prophylaxis in ALL. A grade II abnormality was found by Habermalz et al.[116] in 27% of the patients. A grade III abnormality was never seen. A correlation between the duration of maintenance therapy and the size of the individual dose in whole-brain irradiation ($\gtrless$ 1.7 Gy) was apparent. In contrast, there was no dependence on the total RT, at least not in the range 8.5–24 Gy, or on the intensity of the induction phase of treatment.

5.5. Conclusions

In addition to the radiosensitivity of the tumor involved and the radiotolerance of the part of the brain affected, the life expectation of the patient should also be taken into account when deciding whether RT is indicated for brain tumors. In tumors with a favorable long-term prognosis, we recommend a cautious approach with respect to the size of the dose and dose per fraction, since the patients may well live long enough to develop brain necrosis. This also applies to RT in young patients and children. Here, it is generally assumed that the healthy tissue has a higher radiosensitivity, although clinical proof of this has not been clearly established.

Chemotherapy with cytostatic or cytotoxic agents given together with, prior to, or after, RT, can considerable enhance the radiogenic side effects in the CNS. If whole-brain irradiation has to be combined with intrathecal or intravenous methotrexate, the mildest side effects are seen after sequential application, the MTX being given preferentially prior to CNS irradiation.

References

1. Abay EO, Laws ER, Grado GI, Bruckman JE, Forbes GS, Gomez MR, Scot M (1981) Pineal tumors in children and adolescents. Treatment by CSF shunting and radiotherapy. J Neurosurg 55: 889–895
2. Abbatucci JS, Delozier T, Quint R, Roussel A, Brune D (1978) Radiation myelopathy of the cervical spinal cord: time, dose and volume factors. Int J Radiat Oncol Biol Phys 4: 239–248
3. Abramson N, Raben M, Cavanaugh PJ (1974) Brain tumors in children: analysis of 136 cases. Radiol. 112: 669–672
4. Adams GE, Dewey DL (1963) Hydrated electrons and radiobiological sensitization. Biochem Biophys Res Commun 12: 473–477
5. Adams AF, Mashiter K (1985) Role of cell and explant culture in the diagnosis and characterization of human pituitary tumours. Neurosurg Rev 8: 135–140

R. Sauer:

6. Albright AI, James HE (1985) Neurosurgical staging of midline intra-axial (nuclear) tumors. Cancer [Suppl] 56: 1786–1788
7. Allen JC, Nisselbaum J, Epstein F, Rosen G, Schwartz MK (1979) Alpha-fetoprotein and human chorionic gonadotropin determination in cerebrospinal fluid. J Neurosurg 51: 368–374
8. Allen JC, Rosen G, Metha BM, Horten B (1980) Leucoencephalopathy following high dose i.v. methotrexate chemotherapy with leucovorin rescue. Cancer Treat Rep 64: 1261–1773
9. Amacher AI (1980) Craniopharyngioma: the controversy regarding radiotherapy. Child's Brain 6: 57–64
10. Aronson SM, Garcia JH, Aronson BE (1964) Metastatic neoplasms of the brain: their frequency in relation to age. Cancer 17: 558–563
11. Ash, DV, Smith MR, Budgen RD (1979) Distribution of misonidazole in human tumors and normal tissues. Br J Cancer 39: 503–509
12. Aur, RJA, Simone JV, Verzosa MS, Hustu HO, Pinkel DP, Barker LF (1978) Leucoencefalopatia en ninos con leucemia linfocitica aguda sometido a terapeutica preventiva del sistema nervioso central. Sangre (Barc) 23: 1–12
13. Autunes JL, Housepian EM, Frantz AG, Holub DA, Hui RM, Carmel PW, Quest DO (1977) Prolactin secreting pituitary tumors. Ann Neurol 2: 148–158
14. Backlund EO (1971) A new instrument for stereotaxic brain tumor biopsy. Acta Chir Scand 137: 825–827
15. Bailey P (1945) Intracranial tumors, 2nd edn. Ch C Thomas, Springfield, Ill
16. Bailey P, Cushing H (1925) Medulloblastoma cerebelli. A common type of mid-cerebellar glioma of childhood. Arch Neurol Psychiat (Chic) 14: 192–223
17. Bamberg M, Sauerwein W, Scherer E (1982) Methoden und Ergebnisse der Strahlentherapie beim Medulloblastom. Strahlentherapie 158: 71–75
18. Bamberg M, Schmitt U, Quast EB, Bongartz H-E, Nau C, Bayindir V, Reichardt U (1980) Therapie und Prognose des Medulloblastoms. Fortschritte durch neuartige Bestrahlungstechniken. Strahlentherapie 156: 1–17
19. Bamford FN, Morris-Jones P, Pearson D, Ribeiro GG, Shalet SM, Beardwell CG (1976) Residual disabilities in children treated for intracranial space-occupying lesions. Cancer 37: 1149–1151
20. Baskin DS, Boggan JE, Wilson CB (1982) Transsphenoidal microsurgical removal of growth-hormone secreting pituitary adenomas (a review of 137 cases). J Neurosurg 56: 634–641
21. Battermann JJ (1980) Fast neutron therapy for advanced brain tumors. Int J Radiat Oncol Biol Phys 6: 333–335
22. Bellani FF, Gasparini M, Lombardi F, Zucali R, Luccarelli G, Migliavacca F, Moise S, Nicola G (1984) Medullablastoma. Results of a sequential combined treatment. Cancer 54: 1956–1961
23. Bernell WR, Kepes JJ, Seitz EP (1972) Late malignant recurrence of childhood cerebellar astrocytoma. Report of two cases. J Neurosurg 37: 470–474
24. Berry MP, Derek R, Jenkin T, Keen CW, Nair BD, Simpson WJ (1981) Radiation treatment for medulloblastoma. J Neurosurg 55: 43–51
25. Bicher HJ, Sandhu TS, Hetzel DW (1980) Hyperthermia and radiation in combination: a clinical fractionation regime. Int J Radiat Oncol Biol Phys 6, 861–866
26. Bleehen NM (1980) The Cambridge glioma trial of misonidazole and radiation therapy with associated pharmacokinetic studies. Cancer Clin Trials 3: 267–273
27. Bleyer WA, Griffin TW (1980) White matter necrosis, mineralizing microangiopathy, and intellectual abilities in survivors of childhood leukemia: associations with central nervous system irradiation and methotrexate therapy. In: Gilbert HA, Kagan AR (eds) Radiation damage to the nervous system. Raven Press, New York, pp 155–174

28. Bloom HJG (1975) Combined modality therapy for intracranial tumors. Cancer 35: 111–120
29. Bloom HJG (1979) Adjuvant therapy for residual disease in children with medulloblastoma. In: Methé G, Salmon SE (eds) Recent results in cancer research. Springer, Berlin Heidelberg New York, pp 412–422
30. Bloom HJG (1982) Intracranial tumors: response and resistance to therapeutic endeavors, 1970–1980. Int J Radiat Oncol Biol Phys 8: 1083–1113
31. Bloom HJG, Harmer CL (1976) Craniopharyngioma: General aspects and treatment. In: Bucalossi P, Veronesi U, Emanuelli H, Bellani F (eds) I tumori infantili. Casa Editrice Ambrosiana, Milano, pp 119–128
32. Bloom HJG, Peckham MJ, Richardson AE, Alexander PA, Payne PM (1973) Glioblastoma multiforme: a controlled trial to assess the value of specific active immunotherapy in patients treated by radical surgery and radiotherapy. Br J Cancer 27: 253–267
33. Bloom HJG, Thornton-Jones H (1983) Adjuvant chemotherapy for medulloblastoma: the multicentre controlled trial of the International Society of Pediatric Oncology (SIOP). In: Bloom HJG, Pichler E (eds) Chemotherapy of brain tumours in childhood. Proceedings 13th International Congress of Chemotherapy, Vienna, Wien Med Akad, pp 208/19-208/25
34. Bloom HJG, Wallace ENK, Henk JM (1969) The treatment of prognosis of medulloblastoma in children: a study of 82 verified cases. Am J Roentgenol 105: 43–62
35. Bloom HJG, Walsh L (1975) Tumors of the central nervous system. In: Bloom HJG, Lemerle J, Neidhardt MK, Voûte PA (eds) Cancer and children—clinical management. Springer, Berlin Heidelberg New York, pp 93–119
36. Boden G (1950) Radiation myelitis of the brain-stem. J Fac Radiol 2: 79–94
37. Bodian M, Lawson D (1953) The intracranial neoplastic diseases of childhood—a description of their natural history based on a clinicopathological study of 129 cases. Br J Surg 40: 368–392
38. Boellaard JW, Jacoby W (1962) Röntgenspätschäden des Gehirns. Acta Neurochir (Wien) 5: 533–564
39. Borgelt BB, Gelber R, Kramer S, Brady L, Chang C, Davis L, Perez C, Hendrickson F (1980) The palliation of brain metastases: final results of the first two studies by the Radiation Therapy Oncology Group. Int J Radiat Oncol Biol Phys 6: 1–9
40. Borgelt BB, Gelber R, Larson M, Hendrickson F, Griffin T, Roth R (1981) Ultra-rapid high dose irradiation schedules for the palliation of brain metastases: final results of the first two studies by the Radiation Therapy Oncology Group. Int J Radiat Oncol Biol Phys 7: 1633–1638
41. Bouchard J (1966) Radiation therapy of tumors and diseases of the nervous system. H. Kimpton, London
42. Bouchard J (1980) Central nervous system. In: Fletcher GH (ed) Textbook of radiotherapy. Lea & Febiger, Philadelphia, pp 444–498
43. Bradfield JS, Perez CA (1972) Pineal tumors and ectopic pinealomas. Radiology 103: 399–406
44. Brown JM (1982) Clinical perspectives for the use of new hypoxic cell sensitizers. Int J Radiat Oncol Biol Phys 8: 1491–1497
45. Bruce DA, Allen JC (1985) Tumor staging for pineal region tumors of childhood. Cancer [suppl] 56: 1792–1794
46. Buchfelder M (1984) Effekte der postoperativen Radiotherapie para- und suprasellärer Hypophysenadenome. Inaugural-Dissertation, Universität Erlangen-Nürnberg
47. Bucy PC, Thieman PW (1968) Astrocytomas of the cerebellum. A study of a series of patients operated upon over 28 years ago. Arch Neurol (Chic) 18: 14–19

48. Bushe KH (1984) Operative Behandlung der Hirnmetastasen. Akt Onkol 13: 151–156

49. Caldwell WL, Aristizabal SA (1975) Treatment of glioblastoma multiforme. Acta Radiol 14: 505–512

50. Calvo FA, Hornedo J, Arellano A, Sachetti A, de la Torre A, Aragon G, Otero J (1983) Radiation therapy in craniopharyngiomas. Int J Radiat Oncol Biol Phys 9: 493–496

51. Capra LG (1980) Radiotherapy of cerebral gliomas. In: Thomas DGT, Graham DI (eds) Brain tumours. Butterworth, London, pp 322–343

52. Carabell SC, Leonard AB, Weinstein AS, Richter MP, Chang CH, Weiler CB, Goodman RL (1984) Misonidazole and radiotherapy to treat malignant glioma: a phase II trial of the Radiation Therapy Oncology Group. Int J Radiat Oncol Biol Phys 7: 71–77

53. Carella R, Ransohoff J, Newall J (1982) Role of radiation therapy in the management of meningioma. Neurosurgery 10: 332–339

54. Catterall M, Bloom HJG, Ash DV, Walsh L, Richardson A, Uttley D, Gowing NFC, Lewis P, Chaucer B (1980) Fast neutrons compared with megavoltage X-rays in the treatment of patients with supratentorial glioblastoma: a controlled pilot study. Int J Radiat Oncol Biol Phys 6: 261–266

55. Chang CH, Housepian EM, Herbert C, jr (1969) An operative staging system and a megavoltage radiotherapeutic technic for cerebellar medulloblastomas. Radiology 93: 1351–1359

56. Chao JH, Phillips R, Nickson JJ (1954) Roentgentherapy of cerebral metastases. Cancer 7: 682–689

57. Cheek WR, Taveras JM (1966) Thalamic tumors. J Neurosurg 24: 505–513

58. Chin HW, Maruyama Y (1981) Results of radiation treatment of cerebellar medulloblastoma. Int J Radiat Oncol Biol Phys 7: 737–742

59. Chin HW, Maruyama Y, Young B (1983) The role of radiation treatment in craniopharyngioma. Strahlentherapie 159: 741–744

60. Cohen ME, Duffner PK (1984) Ependymomas. In: Cohen ME, Duffner PK (eds) Brain tumors in children: principles of diagnosis and treatment. Raven Press, New York, pp 136–155

61. Cohen ME, Duffner PK, Kun LE, D'Souza B (1985) The argument for a combined cancer consortium research data base. Cancer [suppl] 56: 1897–1901

62. Concannon JP, Kramer S, Berry R (1960) The extent of extracranial gliomas at autopsy and its relationship to techniques used in radiation therapy of brain tumors. Am J Roentgenol Radium Ther Nucl Med 84: 99–107

63. Cumberlin RL, Luk KH, Wara WM, Sheline GE, Wilson CB (1979) Medulloblastoma. Treatment results and effect on normal tissues. Cancer 43: 1014–1020

64. Cummings FM, Taveras JM, Schlesinger EB (1960) Treatment of gliomas of the third ventricle and pinealomas. Neurology 10: 1031–1036

65. Cushing H (1930) Experiences with cerebellar medulloblastoma: critical review. Acta Pathol Microbiol Scand 7: 1–86

66. Cushing H (1931) Experiences with cerebellar astrocytomas. A critical review of 76 cases. Surg Gynecol Obstet 52: 129–204

67. Danoff BF, Cowchock FS, Kramer S (1983) Childhood craniopharyngioma: survival, local control, endocrine and neurologic function following radiotherapy. Int J Radiat Oncol Biol Phys 9: 171–175

68. Danoff BF, Kramer S, Thompson N (1980) The radiotherapeutic management of optic nerve gliomas in children. Int J Radiat Oncol Biol Phys 6: 45–50

69. Dayan AD, Marshall AHE, Miller AA, Pick FJ, Rankin NE (1966) Atypical teratomas of the pineal and hypothalamus. J Path Bact 92: 1–28

70. Denekamp J, Harris SF (1976) Studies of the processes occurring between two sessions in experimental mouse tumors. Int J Radiat Oncol Biol Phys 1: 421–430
71. Deutsch M, Parson JA, Mercado R, jr (1974) Radiotherapy for intracranial metastases. Cancer 34: 1607–1611
72. Deutsch M, Reigel DH (1981) Myelography and cytology in the treatment of medulloblastoma. Int J Radiat Oncol Biol Phys 7: 721–725
73. Deviri E, Schachner A, Halevy A, Shalit M, Levy MJ (1983) Carcinoma of lung with a solitary cerebral metastasis—surgical management and review of the literature. Cancer 52: 1507–1509
74. Dewit L, van der Schueren E, Ang KK, van den Bergh R, Dom R, Brucher JM (1984) Low grade astrocytoma in children treated by surgery and radiation therapy. Acta Radiol (Oncol) 23: 1–8
75. Dosoretz DE, Blitzer PH, Wang CC, Linggood RM (1980) Management of glioma of the optic nerve and/or chiasm. Cancer 45: 1467–1471
76. Douglas BG (1982) Superfractionation: its rationale and anticipated benefits. Int J Radiat Oncol Biol Phys 8: 1143–1153
77. Douglas BG, Castro JR (1984) Novel fractionation schemes and high linear energy transfer. In: Rosenblum ML, Wilson CB (eds) Brain tumor therapy. Karger, Basel, pp 152–165 (Progr exp tumor res, vol 28)
78. Dunst J, Sauer R, Thiel HJ (1986) Zur Strahlentherapie der Optikusgliome. Strahlentherapie (im Druck)
79. Dynes JB, Smedal M (1960) Radiation myelitis. Am J Roentgenol 83: 78–87
80. Earl KM, Dillar SH (1973) Pathology of adenomas of the pituitary gland. In: Kohler PO, Ross GT (eds) Diagnosis and treatment of pituitary tumors. American Elsevier, New York, p 3
81. Earp HS, Ney RL (1982) Pituitary tumors. In: Holland JF, Frei E (eds) Cancer medicine. Lea & Febiger, Philadelphia, pp 1634–1647
82. Eastman RC, Gorden P, Roth J (1979) Conventional supervoltage irradiation is an effective treatment for acromegaly. J Clin Endocrin Met 48: 931–940
83. Effenterre RV, Bataini JP, Cabanis EA, Iba-Zizen MT (1979) High energy radiotherapy in the treatment of meningiomas of the cavernous sinus. Acta Neurochir (Wien) [suppl] 28: 464–467
84. Ehrlich SS, Davis RL (1978) Spinal subarachnoid metasis from primary intracranial glioblastoma multiforme. Cancer 42: 2854–2864
85. Eiser C (1981) Psychological sequelae of brain tumors in childhood: a retrospective study. Br J Clin Psychol 20: 35–38
86. Ellis F (1969) Dose, time and fractionation. A clinical hypothesis. Clin Radiol 20: 1–7
87. Emmanuel IG (1966) Symposium on pituitary tumors. 3. Historical aspects of radiotherapy, present treatment, techniques and results. Clin Radiol 17: 154–160
88. Epstein F (1985) A staging system for brain stem gliomas. Cancer [Suppl] 56: 1804–1806
89. Erlichman C, Meakin JW, Simpson WJ (1979) Review of 154 patients with nonfunctioning pituitary tumors. Int J Radiat Oncol Biol Phys 5: 1981–1986
90. Evans AE (1983) Therapeutic approaches to medulloblastoma and results: trial of the Children's Cancer Study Group (CCSG) and the Radiation Therapy Oncology Group (RTOG). Proc 13th Int Congr Chemother, Vienna (abstract) 208: 26–28
91. Evans AE, Anderson J, Jenkin RDT, Kramer S, Schoenfeld D, Wilson C (1979) Adjuvant chemotherapy for medulloblastoma and ependymoma. In: Paoletti P, Walker MD, Butti G, Knerich R (eds) Multidisciplinary aspects of brain tumor therapy. Elsevier/North-Holland Biomedical Press, New York Oxford, pp 219–222
92. Faglia G, Moriondo P, Travaglini P, Giovanelli MA (1983) Influence of previous bromocriptine therapy on surgery for prolactinoma. Lancet i: 133–134

93. Fahlbusch R (1981) Surgical treatment of pituitary adenomas. In: Beardwell C, Robertson GL (eds) The pituitary. Butterworth, London, pp 76–105
94. Fahlbusch R, Buchfelder M (1985) Present status of neurosurgery in the treatment of prolactinomas. Neurosurg Rev 8: 195–205
95. Fahlbusch R, Buchfelder M, Schrell U (1985) Neurochirurgische Therapie neuroendokrinologischer Störungen. Internist 26: 293–301
96. Fazekas JT (1977) Treatment of grades I and II brain astrocytomas: the role of radiotherapy. Int J Radiat Oncol Biol Phys 2: 661–666
97. Fowler JF, Adams GE, Denekamp J (1976) Radiosensitizers of hypoxic cells in solid tumors. Cancer Treat Rev 3: 227–256
98. Franke HD (1973) Die Strahlenempfindlichkeit des Nervensystems. In: Braun H, Henck F, Ladner H-A, Messerschmidt O, Musshoff K, Streffer Ch (Hrsg) Strahlenempfindlichkeit von Organen und Organsystemen der Säugetiere und des Menschen. Thieme, Stuttgart, S 172–194 (Strahlenschutz in Forschung und Praxis, vol XIII)
99. Franke HD, Lierse W (1978) Strahlenbedingte Reaktionen des Gehirns und des Rückenmarks. Strahlentherapie 154: 587–598
100. Fresh CB, Takei Y, O'Brien MS (1976) Cerebellar glioblastoma in childhood—case report. J Neurosurg 45: 705–708
101. Garcia DM, Fulling KH, Marks JE (1985) The value of radiation therapy in addition to surgery for astrocytomas of the adult cerebrum. Cancer 55: 919–927
102. Garrett PG, Simpson WJK (1983) Ependymomas: results of radiation treatment. Int J Radiat Oncol Biol Phys 9: 1121–1124
103. Geissinger JD, Bucy PC (1971) Astrocytomas of the cerebellum in children. Long term study. Arch Neurol (Chic) 24: 125–135
104. Giovanelli MA, Gaini SM, Tomei G, Motti EDF, Villani R (1980) Acromegaly: Surgical failures and recurrences. In: Derome PJ, Jedynac CP, Peillon F (eds) Second european workshop on pituitary adenomas. Asclepios, France, pp 253–262
105. Glanzmann C, Horst W, Schiess K, Friede R (1980) Consideration in the radiation treatment of intracranial ependymoma. Prognosis in 24 own cases and results in published series after different techniques of radiation treatment. Strahlentherapie 156: 97–101
106. Glanzmann C, Horst W, Seiffert H (1974) Radiotherapie in der Behandlung primärer Hirntumoren. Ergebnisse bei 208 Patienten und Literaturübersicht. Fortschr Röntgenstr 121: 644–652
107. Goldfine ID, Lawrence AM (1972) Hypopituitarism in acromegaly. Arch Int Med 130: 720–723
108. Gomez F, Reyes FI, Faiman C (1977) Nonpuerperal galactorrhea and hyperprolactinemia. Clinical findings, endocrine features and therapeutic responses in 56 cases. Am J Med 62: 648–660
109. Greenberger JS, Cassady JR, Levene MB (1977) Radiation therapy of thalamic, midbrain and brain stem gliomas. Radiology 122: 463–468
110. Griffin BR, Griffin TW, Tong, DYK, Russell AH, Kurtz J, Laramore GE, Groudine M (1981) Pineal region tumors: results of radiation therapy and indications for elective spinal irradiation. Int J Radiat Oncol Biol Phys 7: 605–608
111. Griffin TW, Beaufait D, Blasko JC (1979) Cystic cerebellar astrocytomas in childhood. Cancer 44: 276–280
112. Grote W, Nau HW, Lamers B (1982) Operatives Vorgehen beim Medulloblastom. Strahlentherapie 158: 63–70
113. Gutin PH, Chillips TL, Wara WM, Leibel SA, Hosobuchi Y, Levin VA, Weaver KA, Lamb S (1984) Brachytherapy of recurrent malignant brain tumors with removable high-activity iodine-125 sources. Neurosurgery 60: 61–68

114. Gutin PH, Wara WM, Phillips TL, Wilson CB (1980) Hypoxic cell radiosensitizers in the treatment of malignant brain tumors. Neurosurgery 6: 567–576

115. Gutjahr P, Kretzschmar K (1979) Akute lymphoblastische Leukämie und maligne Non-Hodgkin-Lymphome im Kindesalter. Dtsch Med Wschr 104: 1068–1071

116. Habermalz E, Habermalz HJ, Stephani U, Henze G, Riehm H, Hanefeld F (1983) Cranial computed tomography of 64 children in continuous complete remission of leukemia I: relations to therapy modalities. Neuropediatries 14: 144–148

117. Hahn GM (1979) Potential for therapy of drugs and hyperthermia. Cancer Res 39: 2264–2268

118. Hall EJ (1978) Hyperthermia. In: Hall EJ (ed) Radiobiology for the radiologist, 2nd edn. Harper and Row, New York London, pp 325–348

119. Hall R, Anderson J, Smart GA, Besser M (1980) Fundamentals of clinical endocrinology. Pitman Medical, London

120. Hatlevoll R, Lindegaard KF, Hagen S, et al. (1985) Combined modality treatment of operated astrocytomas grade 3 and 4. Cancer 56: 41–47

121. Hardy DG, Hope-Stone HF, McKenzie CG, Scholtz CI (1978) Recurrence of medulloblastoma after homogenous field radiotherapy. J Neurosurg 49: 434–440

122. Hardy J (1971) Trans-phenoidal hypophysectomy. J Neurosurg 34: 582–594

123. Hardy J (1982) Cushing's disease: 50 years later. Can J Neurol Sci 9: 375–380

124. Harisiadis L, Chang CH (1977) Medulloblastoma in children: a correlation between staging and results of treatment. Int J Radiat Oncol Biol Phys 2: 833–841

125. Harris JR, Levene MB (1976) Visual complications following irradiation for pituitary adenomas and craniopharyngiomas. Radiology 120: 167–171

126. Harten G, Stephani U, Henze G, Langermann HJ, Riehm H, Hanefeld F (1984) Impairment of psychomotor skills in children after treatment of acute lymphoblastic leukemia. Eur J Pediatr 142: 189–197

127. Harter DJ, Caderao JB, Leavens ME, Young SE (1978) Radiotherapy in the management of primary gliomas involving the intracranial optic nerves and chiasm. Int J Radiat Oncol Biol Phys 4: 681–686

128. Hazegawa H, Ushio Y, Hayakawa T, Yamada K, Mogami H (1983) Changes in the blood-brain barrier transport in experimental metastatic brain tumors. J Neurosurg 59: 304–312

129. Haymaker W, Lindgren M (1970) Nerve disturbances following exposure to ionizing radiation. In: Vinken PJ, Bruyn GE (eds) Handbook of clinical neurology, vol VII/14. North-Holland, Amsterdam, pp 388–401

130. Heifetz MD, Weseler M, Thompson R (1984) Single beam radiotherapy knife. J Neurosurg 60: 814–818

131. Henderson WR (1939) The pituitary adenomata: a follow-up study of the surgical results in 338 cases (Dr. Harvey Cushing's series). Br J Surg 26: 811–921

132. Hendrick EB, Hofmann HJ, Humphreys RP (1975) Treatment of infratentorial gliomas in childhood. In: Hekmatpanah J (ed) Gliomas: current concepts in biology, diagnosis and therapy. Springer, Berlin Heidelberg New York, pp 102–106

133. Hendrickson FR (1977) The optimum schedule for palliative radiotherapy for metastatic brain cancer. Int J Radiat Oncol Biol Phys 2: 165–168

134. Herbst M, Sauer R (1980) Zur Strahlentherapie in lokaler Hyperthermie — ein vorläufiger klinischer Erfahrungsbericht. Strahlentherapie 156: 331–335

135. Hildebrand J (1983) Chemotherapy of malignant supratentorial gliomas in adults: a ten-year experience of the EORTC brain tumor group. Proceedings of the 13th International Congress of Chemotherapy, Vienna (abstracts), p 249

136. Hinkelbein W, Bruggmoser G, Schmidt M, Wannenmacher M (1984) Die Kurzzeitbestrahlung des Glioblastoms mit hohen Einzelfraktionen. Strahlentherapie 160: 301–308

137. Hirsch JF, Pierre-Kahn A, Benveniste L, George B (1978) Les médulloblastomes de l'enfant. Survie et résultats fonctionels. Neurochirurgie (Paris) 24: 391–397

138. Hochberg FH, Pruitt A (1980) Assumptions in the radiotherapy of glioblastoma. Neurology 30: 907–911

139. Hoffmann HJ, Hendrick EB, Humphreys RP (1976) Metastasis via ventriculoperitoneal shunt in patients with medulloblastoma. J Neurosurg 44: 562–566

140. Hoffmann HJ, Hendrick EB, Humphreys RP, Buncic JR, Armstrong DL, Jenkin RDT (1977) Management of craniopharyngioma in children. J Neurosurg 47: 218–227

141. Holdorff B (1980) Der Unterschied zwischen zerebralen Hemisphären- und Mittellinien-Strahlenspätnekrosen und seine Bedeutung für die Strahlentherapie. Strahlentherapie 156: 530–537

142. Holdorff B (1983) Strahlenschäden des Gehirns und des Rückenmarks. In: Seitz D, Vogel P (Hrsg) Hämoblastosen, Zentrale Motorik, Iatrogene Schäden, Myositiden. Springer, Berlin Heidelberg New York Tokyo, S 158–170 (Verhandlungen der Deutschen Gesellschaft für Neurologie, vol II)

143. Hoogenhout J, Otten BJ, Kazem I, Stoelinga GBA, Walder SHD (1984) Surgery and radiation therapy in the management of craniopharyngiomas. Int J Radiat Oncol Biol Phys 10: 2293–2297

144. Hope-Stone HF (1976) Radiotherapy in modern clinical practice. Crosby Lockwood Stables, London

145. Horiot JC, van den Bogaert W, Ang KK, Chaplain G, van den Schueren E, Nabid, A, Vessiere M (1982) EORTC Experience with misonidazole combined with a multiple daily fractionated (MDF) radiotherapy. Inaugural meeting of the Europ Soc for Therap Rad and Oncol, London (meeting abstract)

146. Horwich A, Bloom HJG (1985) Optic gliomas: radiation therapy and prognosis. Int J Radiat Oncol Biol Phys 11: 1067–1079

147. Hoyte WF, Baghdassarian SA (1969) Optic glioma of childhood: natural history and rationale for conservative management. Br J Ophthalmol 53: 793–798

148. Hoyte WF, Meshel LG, Lessell S, Schatz NJ, Suckling RD (1973) Malignant optic glioma of adulthood. Brain 96: 121–132

149. Huk W, Baer I (1980) A new targeting device for stereotaxic procedures within the CT scanner. Neuroradiology 19: 13–17

150. Hünig R, Walther E, Sauer R (1974) Die Strahlentherapie von ZNS-Tumoren bei Kindern und Jugendlichen. Strahlentherapie 147: 573–597

151. Ingraham DD, Bailey OT, Barker WF (1948) Medulloblastoma cerebelli: diagnosis, treatment and survivals, with a report of fifty-six cases. New Engl J Med 238: 171–174

152. Jellinger K (1972) "Frühe" Strahlenspätschäden des menschlichen Zentralnervensystems. Verh Dtsch Ges Path 56: 457–463

153. Jellinger K (1984) Häufigkeit und Charakteristik der zerebralen Karzinommetastasen. Akt Onkol 13: 49–79

154. Jellinger K, Volc D, Grisold W, Flament H, Vollmer R, Weiss R (1983) Kombinationsbehandlung maligner Gliome. Wien Klin Wochenschr 95: 407–416

155. Jenkin RDT (1982) Childhood ependymomas: radiation treatment results. In: Chang CH, Housepian EM (eds) Tumors of the CNS: modern radiotherapy in multidisciplinary management. Masson, New York, pp 384–432

156. Jenkin RDT (1969) Medulloblastoma in children: radiation therapy. Can Med Assoc J 100: 51–53

157. Jenkin RDT, Simpson WJK, Keen CW (1978) Pineal and suprasellar germinomas: results of radiation treatment. J Neurosurg 48: 99–107

158. Jennings AS, Liddle GW, Orth D (1977) Results of treating childhood Cushing's disease with pituitary irradiation. N Engl J Med 297: 957–962

159. Jereb B, Sundaresan N, Horten B, Reid A, Galicich JH (1981) Supratentorial recurrence in medulloblastoma. Cancer 47: 806–809
160. Kallmann RF (1974) The phenomenon of reoxygenation and its implications for fractionated radiotherapy. Radiology 105: 135–142
161. Kelly JP, Hannam TW, Giles GR (1979) The cytocidal action of metronidazole in combination with other neoplastic agents. Cancer Treat Rev [suppl] 6: 53–61
162. Kernohan JW, Sayre SP (1952) Tumors of the central nervous system. In: Atlas of tumor pathology, section X, fasc 35 and 37. Armed Forces Institute of Pathology, Washington, DC
163. Kernohan JW, Sayre GP (1956) Tumors of the pituitary gland and infundibulum, section 10, fasc 36. Armed Forces Institute of Pathology, Washington, DC, pp 7–57
164. Kim YH, Fayos JV (1977) Intracranial ependymomas. Radiology 124: 805–808
165. Kim TH, Chin HW, Pollan S, Hazel JH, Webster JH (1980) Radiotherapy of primary brain-stem tumors. Int J Radiat Oncol Biol Phys 6: 51–57
166. Kjellberg RN, Hanamura T, Davis KR, Lyons SL, Adams RD (1983) Bragg peak proton-beam therapy for arteriovenous malformations of the brain. N Engl J Med 309: 269–274
167. Kleinberg DL, Noel GL, Frantz AG (1977) Galactorrhea: a study of 235 cases, including 48 with pituitary tumors. N Engl J Med 28: 589–600
168. Kleinman GM, Schoene WC, Walshe TM, et al. (1978) Malignant transformation in benign cerebellar astrocytoma. J Neurosurg 49: 111–118
169. Kleinman GM, Hochberg FH, Richardson EP (1981) Systemic metastases from medulloblastoma: a report of two cases and review of literature. Cancer 48: 2296–2309
170. Kobayashi T, Kageyama N, Ohara K (1981) Internal irradiation for cystic craniopharyngioma. J Neurosurg 55: 896–903
171. Koos WT, Miller MH (1971) Intracranial tumors of infants and children. Mosby, St Louis
172. Kopelson G, Linggood RM, Kleinman GM (1982) Medulloblastoma in adults: improved survival with supervoltage radiation therapy. Cancer 49: 1334–1337
173. Kovacs K, Horvath E, Ezrin C (1971) Pituitary adenomas. In: Sommers DE (ed) Pathology annals, vol 2. Appleton-Century-Crofts, New York, pp 341–382
174. Kramer S (1969) Tumor extent as a determining factor in radiotherapy of glioblastoma. Acta Radiol 8: 111–117
175. Kramer S (1969) Radiation therapy in the management of brain tumors in children. Ann NY Acad Sci 159: 571–584
176. Kramer S (1973) Radiation therapy in the management of malignant gliomas. Seventh national cancer conference proceedings. Lippincott, Philadelphia, pp 823–826
177. Kramer S (1973) Indications for, and results of treatment of pituitary tumors by external radiation. In: Kohler PO, Ross GT (eds) Diagnosis and treatment of pituitary tumors. Excerpta Medica/American Elsevier, New York, pp 217–229
178. Kramer S, Lee KF (1974) Complications of radiation therapy: the central nervous system. Sem Oncol 9: 75–83
179. Krauseneck P (1984) Möglichkeiten und Grenzen der Chemotherapie maligner hirneigener Tumoren. G Fischer, S 209–216 (Verhandlungen der Deutschen Krebsgesellschaft, vol 5)
180. Krauseneck P, Mertens HG, Messerer G, Kleihues P, Bamberg M, Dittmann W, Gerhard L, Heuser K, Hobert U, Makoski HB, Poburski R, Ransmayr G, Richter E, Volc D (1986) German-Austrian study on malignant supratentorial gliomas. J Cancer Res Clin Oncol 111: 9 (abstract)
181 a. Kreuser ED, Schreml W, Potthoff PC, Keim HM, Neiß A, Schuster Ch (1984) Therapieergebnisse kombinierter und nichtkombinierter Modalitäten bei Hirnmetastasen solider Tumoren. Akt Onkol 13: 276–285

181. Kricheff JJ, Becker M, Schneck SA, Taveras JM (1964) Intracranial ependymomas. A study of survival in 65 cases treated by surgery and irradiation. Am J Roentgenol 91: 167–175
182. Kun LE (1983) Patterns of failure in tumors of the central nervous system. Cancer Treat Symp 2: 285–294
183. Kun LE, Mulhern RK, Crisco JJ (1983) Quality of life in children treated for brain tumors. Intellectual, emotional, and adacemic function. J Neurosurg 58: 1–6
184. Kun LE, Tang TT, Sty JR, et al. (1981) Primary cerebral germinoma and ventriculoperitoneal shunt metastasis. Cancer 48: 213–216
185. Kurup P, Reddy S, Henrickson FR (1980) Results of re-irradiation for cerebral metastases. Cancer 46: 2587–2589
186. Lampert PW, Davis RL (1964) Delayed effects of radiation on the human central nervous system. "Early" and "late" delayed reactions. Neurology 14: 912–917
187. Lang EF, Slater J (1964) Metastatic brain tumor. Results of surgical and nonsurgical treatment. Surg Clin N Am 44: 865–872
188. Laramore GF, Griffin TW, Gerdes AJ, Parker RG (1978) Fast neutron and mixed (neutron/photon) beam teletherapy for grades III and IV astrocytomas. Cancer 42: 96–103
189. Laws ER, Taylor WF, Clifton MB, Okazaki H (1984) Neurosurgical management of low-grade astrocytoma of the cerebral hemipheres. J Neurosurg 61: 665–673
190. Leibel SA, Sheline GE, Wara WM, Boldrey EB, Neilson SL (1975) The role of radiation therapy in the treatment of astrocytomas. Cancer 35: 1551–1557
191. Leibel SA, Wara WM, Sheline GE, Townsend JJ, Boldrey EB (1976) The treatment of meningiomas in childhood. Cancer 37: 2709–2712
192. Leksell L (1951) The stereotaxic method and radiosurgery of the brain. Acta Chir Scand 102: 316–319
193. Leksell L (1971) Stereotaxic and radiosurgery—an operative system. Charles C Thomas, Springfield, Ill
194. Leksell L, Backlund EO, Johansson L (1967) Treatment of craniopharyngiomas. Acta Chir Scand 133: 345–350
195. Levin VA, Freeman-Dove M, Landahl HD (1975) Permeability characteristics of brain adjacent to tumor in rats. Arch Neurol 32: 785–791
196. Levy LF, Elridge AR (1956) Astrocytomas of the brain and spinal cord. A review of 176 cases, 1940–1949. J Neurosurg 13: 413–443
197. Li, FP, Winston KR, Gimbrere K (1984) Follow-up of children with brain tumors. Cancer 54: 135–138
198. Lichter AS, Wara WM, Sheline GE, Townsend JJ, Wilson CB (1976) The treatment of craniopharyngiomas. Int J Radiat Oncol Biol Phys 2: 675–683
199. Lierse W (1985) Experimentelle Strahlenfolgen am Hirngewebe. In: Henck F, Scherer E (Hrsg) Strahlengefährdung und Strahlenschutz. Springer, Berlin Heidelberg New York Tokyo, pp 349–378 (Handbuch der medizinischen Radiologie, vol XX)
200. Lindgren M (1958) On tolerance of brain tissue and sensitivity of brain tumors to irradiation. Acta Radiol [suppl] 170: 1–73
201. Linfoot JA (1979) Heavy therapy: alpha particle therapy of pituitary tumors. In: Linfoot JA (ed) Recent advances in the diagnosis and treatment of pituitary tumors. Raven Press, New York, pp 245–267
202. Littman P, Jarrett P, Bilaniuk LT, Rorke LB, Zimmerman RA, Bruce DA, Carabell SC, Schut L (1980) Pediatric brain stem gliomas. Cancer 45: 2787–2792
203. Liu HM, Boggs J, Kidd J (1976) Ependymomas of childhood. Child's Brain 2: 92–110
204. Liwnicz B, Rubinstein L (1979) The pathways of extraneural spread in metastasizing gliomas: a report of 3 cases and critical review of literature. Hum Pathol 10: 453–467
205. Lloyd LA (1966) Gliomas of the optic nerve. Ophthalmologica 151: 260–271

206. Lücecke DK, Breustedt HJ, Brämswig J, Köbberling J, Saeger W (1982) Evaluation of surgically treated Nelson's syndrome. Acta Neurochir (Wien) 65: 3–13
207. Lutz B, Lüdecke DK (1983) Effect of proton beam radiation and conventional cobalt radiation as secondary treatment after surgical therapy of acromegaly. Proceedings of the 3rd European Workshop Pituitary Adenomas (abstract 20)
208. Mantravadi RVP, Phatak R, Bellur S, Liebner E, Haas R (1982) Brain stem gliomas: an autopsy study of 25 cases. Cancer 49: 1294–1296
209. Maor MH, Fields RS, Hogstrom KR, van Eys J (1985) Improving the therapeutic ratio of craniospinal irradiation in medulloblastoma. Int J Radiat Oncol Biol Phys 11: 687–697
210. Marks JE, Adler SJ (1982) A comparative study of ependymomas by site of origin. Int J Radiat Oncol Biol Phys 8: 37–43
211. Marks JE, Baglan RJ, Prassad SC, Blank WF (1981) Cerebral radionecrosis: incidence and risk in relation to dose, time, fractionation and volume. Int J Radiat Oncol Biol Phys 7: 243–252
212. Marsa GW, Gaffinet DR, Rubinstein J, Bagshaw MA (1975) Megavoltage irradiation in the treatment of gliomas of the brain and spinal cord. Cancer 36: 1681–1689
213. Marsa GW, Probert JC, Rubinstein CJ, Bagshaw MA (1973) Radiationtherapy in the treatment of childhood astrocytic gliomas. Cancer 32: 646–655
214. Marsden HB, Steward JK (1968) Tumors in children. Recent results in cancer research, vol 13. Springer, Berlin Heidelberg New York, pp 137–193
215. Martins AN, Johnston JS, Henry JM, Stoffel TJ, DiChiro G (1977) Delayed radiation necrosis of the brain. J Neurosurg 47: 336–345
216. Matson DD, Crigler JF (1969) Management of craniopharyngiomas in childhood. J Neurosurg 30: 377–390
217. McCullough DC, Epstein F (1985) Optic pathway tumors: a review with proposals for clinical staging. Cancer 56: 1789–1791
218. McFarland DR, Horwitz H, Saenger EL, Bahr GK (1969) Medulloblastoma—a review of prognosis and survival. Br J Radiol 43: 198–214
219. McKenzie AD, McIntosh HW (1965) Hyperpigmentation and pituitary tumor as sequelae of the surgical treatment of Cushing's syndrome. Am J Surg 110: 135–141
220. McKissock W, Payne KWE (1958) Primary tumors of the thalamus. Brain 81: 41–63
221. McNally NJ (1975) The effect of repeated small doses of radiation on recovery from sublethal damage by Chinese hamster cells irradiated in oxic or hypoxic conditions in the plateau phase of growth. Proceedings of the sixth LH Gray Conference 119
222. Mealey J, Hall PV (1977) Medulloblastoma in children: survival and treatment. J Neurosurg 46: 56–64
223. Miller NR, Iliff WJ, Green WR (1974) Evaluation and management of gliomas of the anterior visual pathways. Brain 97: 743–754
224. Mincer F, Meltzer J, Botstein C (1976) Pinealoma: a report of 12 irradiated cases. Cancer 37: 2713–2718
225. Molnar P, Blasberg RG, Horowitz M, Smith B, Fenstermacher J (1983) Regional blood-to-tissue transport in RT-9 brain tumors. J Neurosurg 58: 874–883
226. Montgomery AB, Griffin T, Parker RG, Gerdes AJ (1977) Optic nerve glioma: the role of radiation therapy. Cancer 40: 2079–2080
227. Moore TJ, Dluhy RG, Williams GH, Cain JP (1976) Nelson's syndrome: frequency, prognosis and effect of prior pituitary irradiation. Ann Int Med 85: 731–734
228. Mørk SJ, Lindegaard KF, Halvorsen TB, Lehmann EH, Solgaard T, Hatlevoll R, Harvel S, Ganz J (1985) Oligodendroglioma: incidence and biological behavior in a defined population. J Neurosurg 63: 881–889
229. Moss WT, Brand WN, Battifora H (1973) Radiation oncology, rationale, technique, results, 4th edn. Mosby, St Louis

230. MRC-Working Party (1983) A study of the effect of misonidazole in conjuction with radiotherapy for the treatment of grades 3 and 4 astrocytomas. Br J Radiol 56: 673–682
231. Müller W, Afra D, Schröder R (1977) Supratentorial recurrences of gliomas: Morphological studies in relation to time intervals with astrocytomas. Acta Neurochir (Wien) 37: 75–91
232. Mundinger F (1966) The treatment of brain tumors with radioisotopes. Prog Neurol Surg 1: 202–257
233. Mundinger F, Weigel K (1984) Long-term result of stereotactic interstitial curie-therapy. Acta Neurochir (Wien) [suppl] 33: 367–371
234. Neidhardt MK, Bamberg M, Riehm H (1986) Medulloblastoma, strategies for therapy. In: Riehm M (ed) Monographs in pediatrics, vol 18. Karger, Basel, pp 296–315
235. Neidhardt M, Greinacher I (1967) Über die Metastasierung von Medulloblastomen in Körperbereiche außerhalb des Zentralnervensystems. Ztschr Kinderheilk 101: 56–70
236. Neidhardt M, Habermalz HJ, Henze G, Langermann HJ (1982) Medulloblastomstudie der Gesellschaft für Pädiatrische Onkologie, ein Zwischenbericht. Klin Pädiat 194: 257–261
237. Nelson DH, Meankin JW, Thorn GW (1965) ACTH-producing pituitary tumors following adrenalectomy for Cushing's syndrome. Proc Roy Soc Med 52: 560–569
238. Norris DG, Bruce DA, Byrd RL, et al. (1981) Improved relapse-free survival in medulloblastoma. Neurosurgery 9: 661–664
239. Nüchel B, Andersen AP (1978) Medulloblastoma: treatment results. Acta Radiol Oncol Radiat Phys Biol 17: 305–311
240. Onoyama Y, Abe M, Takahashi M, Yabumoto E, Sakamoto T (1975) Radiation therapy of brain tumors in children. Radiology 115: 687–693
241. Onoyama Y, Ono K, Nakajima T, Hiraoka M, Abe M (1979) Radiation therapy of pineal tumors. Radiology 130: 757–760
242. Orth DN, Liddle GW (1971) Results of treatment in 108 patients with Cushing's syndrome. N Engl J Med 285: 243–247
243. Packer RJ, Sutton LN, Rorke LB, Zimmermann RA, Littmann P, Bruce DA, Shut L (1985) Oligodendroglioma of the posterior fossa in childhood. Cancer 56: 195–199
244. Pallis CA, Louis S, Morgan RL (1961) Radiation myelopathy. Brain 84: 460–479
245. Panitch HS, Berg BO (1970) Brain stem tumors of childhood and adolescence. Am J Dis Child 119: 465–472
246. Paoletti P, Knerich R, Butti G, Adinolfi D, Locatelli D, Robustelli della Cuna G, Cordero di Montezenola L, Schiffer D, Soffietti R, Nicolato A, Giunta D, Buonaristiani R, Scamoni C (1983) Italian cooperative study on malignant glial tumor therapy. In: Krauseneck P, Mertens HG (Hrsg) Therapie maligner Neoplasien des Gehirns. Perimed, Erlangen, S 46–49
247. Parker RG, Berry HC, Gerdes HJ, Soronen AJ, Shaw CM (1976) Fast neutron beam radiotherapy of glioblastoma multiforme. Am J Roentgenol 127: 331–335
248. Paterson E, Farr RF (1953) Cerebellar medulloblastoma: treatment by irradiation of the whole central nervous system. Acta Radiol (Stockh) 39: 323–336
249. Payne DG, Simpson WJ, Keen C, Platts ME (1982) Malignant astrocytoma. Hyperfractionated and standard radiotherapy with chemotherapy in a randomized prospective trial. Cancer 50: 2301–2306
250. Phillips TL, Cheline GE, Boldrey E (1964) Therapeutic considerations in tumors affecting the central nervous system: ependymomas. Radiology 83: 98–105
251. Pickren JW, Lopez G, Tsukada Y, Lane WW (1983) Brain metastases: an autopsy study. Cancer Treat Symp 2: 295–313
252. Pierre-Kahn A, Hirsch JF, Roux FX, Renier D, Sainte-Rose C (1983) Intracranial ependymomas in childhood: survival and functional results in 47 cases. Child's Brain 10: 145–156

253. Pistenma DA, Goffinet DR, Bagshaw MA, Hanbery JW, Eltringham JR (1975) Treatment of chromophobe adenomas with megavoltage irradiation. Cancer 35: 1574–1582

254. Pomarede R, Czernidow P, Finidori J, et al. (1982) Endocrine aspects and tumoral markers in intracranial germinoma: an attempt to delinate the diagnosis procedure in 14 patients. J Pediatr 101: 374–478

255. Posner JB (1977) Management of central nervous system metastases. Sem Oncol 4: 81–91

256. Price RA (1979) Histopathology of CNS leukemia and complications of therapy. Am J Pediat Hemat Oncol 1: 21–30

257. Price RA, Jamieson PA (1975) The central nervous system in childhood leukemia II. Subacute leukoencephalopathy. Cancer 35: 306–318

258. Raimondi AJ, Tomita T (1979) The disadvantages of prophylactic whole CNS postoperative radiation therapy for medulloblastoma. In: Paoletti P, Walker MD, Butti G, Knerich R (eds) Multidisciplinary aspects in brain tumor therapy. Elsevier/North-Holland Biomedical Press, Amsterdam, pp 209–218

259. Rao YTR, Medini E, Haselow RE, Jones Th, Levitt SH (1981) Pineal and ectopic pineal tumors: the role of radiation therapy. Cancer 48: 708–713

260. Rekate HL, Ruch T, Nulsen FE, Roessmann U, Spence J (1981) Needle biopsy of tumors in the region of the third ventricle. J Neurosurg 54: 338–341

261. Rich TA, Cassady JR, Strand RD, Winston KR (1985) Radiation therapy for pineal and suprasellar germ cell tumors. Cancer 55: 932–940

262. Richards GE, Wara WM, Grumbach MM, Kaplan SL, Sheline GE, Conte FA (1976) Delayed onset of hypopituitarism: sequelae of therapeutic irradiation of central nervous system, eye and middle ear tumors. J Pediatr 89: 553–559

263. Richmond IL, Wara WM, Wilson CB (1980) Role of radiation therapy in the management of craniopharyngiomas in children. J Neurosurg 6: 513–517

264. Ringertz N, Nordenstam H (1951) Cerebellar astrocytoma. J Neuropathol Exp Neurol 10: 343–367

265. Ringertz N, Reymond A (1949) Ependymomas and choroid plexus adenomas. J Neuropathol Exp Neurol 8: 355–380

266. Roberts M, German WJ (1966) A long-term study of patients with oligodendrogliomas: follow-up of 50 cases, including Dr. Harveys Cushing's series. J Neurosurg 24: 697–700

267. Robertson AG, Brewin TB (1980) Optic nerve glioma. Clin Radiol 31: 471–474

268. Rubin P, Kramer S (1965) Ectopic pinealoma: a radiocurable neuroendocrinologic entity. Radiology 85: 512–523

269. Rubinstein LJ (1972) Tumors of the central nervous system. In: Atlas of tumor pathology, 2nd series, fasc 6. Armed Forces Institute of Pathology, Washington, DC

270. Russell DS, Rubinstein LJ (1977) Pathology of tumors of the nervous system, 4th edn. Edward Arnold, London, pp 290–294

271. Rutten EHJM, Kazem I, Sloof JL, Walder AHD (1981) Post-operative radiation therapy in the management of brain astrocytoma: a retrospective study of 142 patients. Int J Radiat Oncol Biol Phys 7: 191–195

272. Samaan NA, Bakdash MM, Caderao JB, Cangir A, Jesse RH, Ballatyne AJ (1975) Hypopituitarism after external irradiation. Evidence for both hypothalamic and pituitary origin. Ann Intern Med 83: 771–777

273. Sack H, Calcanis A, Godehardt E, et al. (1982) Die postoperative Strahlenbehandlung von Astrozytomen Grad 3 und 4 mit dem Strahlensensibilisator Misonidazol. Strahlentherapie 158: 466–469

274. Salazar OM (1978) Primary brain tumors of the posterior fossa. In: Kagan AR, Gilbert HA (eds) Modern radiation oncology. Harper and Row, New York, pp 105–143

275. Salazar OM (1981) Primary malignant cerebellar astrocytomas in children: a signal for postoperative craniospinal irradiation. Int J Radiat Oncol Biol Phys 7: 1661–1665
276. Salazar OM (1983) A better understanding of CNS seeding and a brighter outlook for postoperatively irradiated patients with ependymomas. Int J Radiat Oncol Biol Phys 9: 1231–1234
277. Salazar OM, Castro-Vita H, Bakos RS, Feldstein ML, Keller B, Rubin P (1979) Radiation therapy for tumors of the pineal region. Int J Radiat Oncol Biol Phys 5: 491–499
278. Salazar OM, Rubin P (1976) The spread of glioblastoma multiforma as a determining factor in the radiation treated volume. Int J Radiat Oncol Biol Phys 1: 627–637
279. Salazar OM, Rubin P, Bassano D, Marcial VA (1975) Improved survival of patients with intracranial ependymomas by irradiation—dose selection and field extension. Cancer 35: 1563–1574
280. Salazar OM, Rubin P, Feldstein ML, Pizzutiello R (1979) High dose radiation therapy in the treatment of malignant gliomas: final report. Int J Radiat Oncol Biol Phys 3: 1733–1740
281. Salazar OM, Rubin P, McDonald JV, Feldstein ML (1976) High-dose radiation therapy in the treatment of glioblastoma multiforme: a preliminary report. Int J Radiat Oncol Biol Phys 1: 717–727
282. Salazar OM, Rubin P, McDonald JF, Feldstein ML (1976) Patterns of failure in intracranial astrocytomas after irradiation: analysis of dose and field factors. Roentgenology 126: 279–292
283. Salazar OM, van Houtte PJ, Bennett JM, Rubin P, Wheeler KT (1982) High-dose radiation therapy with low-dose (pulsed) BCNU in malignant gliomas: an Eastern Cooperative Oncology Group (ECOG) Report. Int J Radiat Oncol Biol Phys 8: 915–919
284. Salcman M, Samanas GM, Mena H, Monteiro P, Garcia J (1979) Whole-body hyperthermia: potential hazards in its application to glioblastoma. In: Paoletti P, Walker MD, Butti G, Knerich R (eds) Multidisciplinary aspects of brain tumor therapy. Elsevier/North-Holland Biomedical Press, Amsterdam New York Oxford, pp 197–208
285. Samaan NA, Leavens ME, Jesse JH, jr (1977) Serum prolactin in patients with "functionless" chromophobe adenomas before and after therapy. Acta Endocrinol 84: 449–460
286. Sauer R (1985) Klinik der Strahlenfolgen am Hirn- und Nervengewebe. In: Heuck F, Scherer E (Hrsg) Strahlengefährdung und Strahlenschutz. Springer, Berlin Heidelberg New York Tokyo (Handbuch der medizinischen Radiologie, vol XX, S 317–348)
287. Sauer R, Herbst M (1984) Hyperthermia for overcoming radioresistance—clinical experiences. Tumordiagnostik Therapie 5: 116–121
288. Sauer R, Hünig R (1975) Die Strahlentherapie von Hirnmetastasen. Strahlentherapie 150: 109–120
289. Sauer R, Pruy W (1986) Zur Radiotherapie von Hirnmetastasten — Untersuchungen zur Technik, Fraktionierung und Dosierung an Hand von 252 Fällen. Tumordiagnostik Therap 7: 45–51
290. Sauer R, Wenz S, Bär I: Therapie der Spongioblastome, Ergebnisse 1978–1983 (in Vorbereitung)
291. Scanlon PW, Taylor WF (1979) Radiotherapy of intracranial astrocytomas: analysis of 417 cases treated from 1960 through 1969. Neurosurgery 5: 301–308
292. Scholz W (1934) Experimentelle Untersuchungen über die Einwirkung von Röntgenstrahlen auf das reife Hirn. Z Neurol Psychiat 150: 765–785
293. Schryver A de, Greitz T, Forsby N (1976) Localized shaped field radiotherapy of malignant glioblastoma multiforme. Int J Radiat Oncol Biol Phys 1: 713–716

294. Schweisguth O (1979) Tumeurs solides de l'enfant. Flammarion Médecine-Sciences, Paris
295. Serri O, Rasio E, Beauregard H, Hardy J, Somma M (1983) Recurrence of hyperprolactinaemia after selective transphenoidal adenomectomy in women with prolactinomas. N Engl J Med 309: 280–283
296. Shalet SM, MacFarlane IA, Beardwell CG (1979) Radiation-induced hyperprolactinemia in a treated acromegalie. Clin Endocrin 11: 169–171
297. Shapiro WR (1982): Treatment of neuroectodermal brain tumors. Ann Neurol 12: 231–237
298. Sharma U, Tandon PN, Saxena KK, Singhal RM, Buruah JD (1974) Craniopharyngiomas treated by a combination of surgery and radiotherapy. Clin Radiol 25: 13–17
299. Sheline GE (1975) Radiation therapy of tumors of the central nervous system in childhood. Cancer 35: 957–964
300. Sheline GE (1977) Radiation therapy of brain tumors. Cancer 39: 873–881
301. Sheline GE (1981) Pituitary tumors: radiation therapy. In: Beardwell C, Robertson GL (eds) The pituitary. Butterworth, London, pp 106–139
302. Sheline GE, Boldrey E, Karlsberg P, Phillips TL (1964) Therapeutic considerations on tumors affecting the central nervous system: oligodendrogliomas. Radiology 82: 84–89
303. Sheline GE, Wara WM, Smith V (1980) Therapeutic irradiation and brain injury. Int J Radiat Oncol Biol Phys 6: 1215–1228
304. Shenkin HA (1965) The effect of roentgen-ray therapy on oligodendrogliomas of the brain. J Neurosurg 22: 57–59
305. Shin KH, Muller PJ, Geggie PHS (1983) Superfractionation radiation therapy in the treatment of malignant astrocytoma. Cancer 52: 2040–2043
306. Silverman CL, Simpson JR (1982) Cerebellar medulloblastoma: the importance of posterior fossa dose to survival and patterns of failure. Int J Radiat Oncol Biol Phys 8: 1869–1876
307. Simpson WJ, Platts ME (1976) Fractionation study in the treatment of glioblastoma multiforme. Int J Radiat Oncol Biol Phys 1: 639–644
308. Sinner W (1964) Strahlenspätschäden des Rückenmarks. Strahlentherapie 125: 219–238
309. Smalley SR, Schray MF, Laws E (1985) Impact of adjuvant radiation therapy following resection of solitary cerebral metastasis on survival and patterns of failure. Int J Radiat Oncol Biol Phys [suppl] 1: 158 (abstract)
310. Smith CE, Long DM, Jones TK, Levitt SH (1973) Medulloblastoma: an analysis of time-dose relationships and recurrence patterns. Cancer 32: 722–728
311. Smith NJ, El-Mahdi AM, Constable WC (1976) Results of irradiation of tumors in the region of the pineal body. Acta Radiol 15: 17–22
312. Solan MJ, Kramer S (1985) The role of radiation therapy in the management of intracranial meningiomas. Int J Radiat Oncol Biol Phys 11: 675–677
313. Soni SS, Marten GW, Pitner SE, Duenas DA, Powazek M (1975) Effects of central-nervous-system irradiation on neuropsychologic functioning of children with acute lymphocytic leukemia. N Engl J Med 293: 113–118
314. Stage WS, Stein JJ (1974) Treatment of malignant astrocytomas. Am J Roentgenol 120: 7–18
315. Stewart AM, Lennox EL, Sanders BM (1973) Group characteristics of children with cerebral and spinal cord tumors. Br J Cancer 28: 568–574
316. Strauß L, Sturm V, Georgi P, Schlegel W, Ostertag H, Clorius JH, van Kaick G (1982) Radioisotope therapy of cystic craniopharyngiomas. Int J Radiat Oncol Biol Phys 8: 1581–1585
317. Sturm V, Pastyr O, Schlegel W, Scharfenberg H, Zabel HJ, Netzeband G, Schabbert S, Berberich W (1983) Stereotactic computer tomography with a modified Riechert-

Mundinger device as the basis for integrated stereotactic neuroradiological investigations. Acta Neurochir (Wien) 68: 11–17

318. Sung DI, Harisiadis L, Chanf CH (1978) Midline pineal tumors and suprasellar germinomas: highly curable by irradiation. Radiology 128: 745–751

319. Sung, DI, Chang CH, Harisiadis L, Carmel PW (1981) Treatment results of craniopharyngiomas. Cancer 47: 847–852

320. Svien HJ, Mabon RF, Kernohan JW, Craig WM (1953) Ependymomas of the brain: pathologic aspects. Neurology 3: 1–15

321. Sweet DL, Hindler FJ, Hanlon K, Hekmatpanah J, Griem ML, Duda E, Mulligan B, Wollman RL (1979) Treatment of grade 3 and 4 astrocytomas with BCNU alone and in combination with VM 26 following surgery and radiation therapy. Cancer Treat Rep 63: 1707–1711

322. Symon L, Logne V, Jakubowski J (1982) The surgical treatment of craniopharyngioma. In: Brock M (ed) Modern neurosurgery. Springer, Berlin Heidelberg New York, pp 187–192

323. Szikla G, Schlienger M, Blond S, Daumas-Duport C, Missir O, Miyahara S, Musolino A, Schaub C (1984) Interstitial and combined interstitial and external irradiation of supratentorial gliomas. Results in 61 cases treated 1973–1981. Acta Neurochir (Wien) [suppl] 33: 355–362

324. Talairach J, Ruggiero G, Aboulker J, David M (1955) A new method of treatment of inoperable brain tumors by stereotaxic implantation of radioaktive gold—a preliminary report. Br J Radiology 28: 62–74

325. Tamulevicius P, Bamberg M, Scherer E, Steffer C (1981) Misonidazole as a radiosensitizer in the radiotherapy of glioblastoma and oesophageal cancer: Pharmacokinetic and clinical studies. Br J Radiol 54: 318–324

326. Tannock IF (1980) In vivo interaction of anti-cancer drugs with misonidazole or metronidazole: cyclophosphamide and BCNU. Br J Cancer 42: 871–880

327. Taveras JM, Mount LA, Wood EH (1956) The value of radiation therapy in the management of glioma of the optic nerves and chiasm. Radiology 66: 518–528

328. Tertsch D, Schon R, Ulrich FE, Alexander H, Horter V (1979) Pubertas praecox in neurofibromatosis of the optic chiasma. Acta Neurochir (Wien) [suppl] 28: 413–414

329. Thiel HJ, Huk WJ, Müller R, Sauer R (1983) Die computertomographiegeleitete stereotaktische interstitielle Therapie von Hirntumoren mittels temporärer oder permanenter Implantation von 125-Jod-seeds. Fortschr Röntgenstr 138: 348–355

330. Thiel HJ, Huk WJ, Müller R, Sauer R (1984) Inoperable Hirntumoren: Brachycurietherapie mit Jod-125-Seeds. Klinikarzt 13: 736–750

331. Thomsett MJ, Conte FA, Kaplan SL (1980) Endocrine and neurologic outcome in childhood craniopharyngioma: Review of effect of treatment in 42 patients. J Pediat 97: 728–735

332. Tönnis W, Walter W (1959) Das Glioblastoma multiforme. Bericht über 2611 Fälle. In: Loew F, Weber G (eds) Das Glioblastoma multiforme. Acta Neurochir (Wien) [suppl] 1: 40–62

333. Torkildsen A (1948) Should exstirpation be attempted in cases of neoplasm in or near third ventricle? Experiences with palliative method. J Neurosurg 5: 249–275

334. Tovi D, Schisano G, Liljeqvist B (1961) Primary tumors in the region of the thalamus. J Neurosurg 18: 730–740

335. Tribolet N de, Barrelet L (1977) Successful chemotherapy of pineoloma. Lancet ii: 1228–1229

336. Tovo MG, Minatel E, Veronesi A, Paoli A de, Franchin G, Roncadin M, Galligioni E, Tirelli U, Tumolo S, Grigolette E (1982) Radiotherapy of brain metastases: conventional versus concentrated treatment. Strahlentherapie 158: 20–22

337. Urtasun RC (1972) Cobalt 60 radiation treatment of pontine gliomas. Radiology 104: 385–387

338. Urtasun RC, Miller JDR, Frunchak V, Kozeol D (1977) Radiotherapy pilot trials with sensitizers of hypoxic cells: Metronidazole in supratentorial glioblastoma. Br J Radiol 50: 602–603

339. Vick NA, Khandekar JD, Bigner DD (1977) Chemotherapy of brain tumors. The "blood-brain barrier" is not a factor. Arch Neurol 34: 523–526

340. Walker MDE, Alexander E, jur, Hunt WE, Maccarty CS, Mahaley MS jr, Mealey J jr, Norrell HA, Owens G, Ransohoff J, Wilson CB, Gehan EA, Strike TA (1978) Evaluation of BCNU and/or radiotherapy in the treatment of anaplastic gliomas. J Neurosurg 49: 333–343

341. Walker MD, Green SB, Byar DP, Alexander E jr, Batzdorf U, Brooks WH, Hunt WE, Maccarty CS, Mahaley MS jr, Mealey J, Owens G, Ransohoff J, Robertson JT, Shapiro WR, Smith K R jr, Wilson CB, Strike TA (1980) Randomized comparisons of radiotherapy and nitrosoureas for the treatment of malignant glioma after surgery. N Engl J Med 303: 1323–1329

342. Walker MD, Strike TA (1979) A phase II evaluation of misonidazole in the treatment of malignant glioma. Proc Ass Cancer Res 20: 433

343. Walker MD, Strike TA, Sheline GE (1979) An analysis of dose-effect relationship in the radiotherapy of malignant gliomas. Int J Radiat Oncol Biol Phys 5: 1725–1731

344. Walther B, Gutjahr P (1982) Development after treatment of cerebellar medulloblastoma in childhood. In: Voth D, Gutjahr P, Langmaid C (eds) Tumors of the central nervous system. Springer, Berlin Heidelberg New York, pp 389–398

345. Wara WM, Jenkin DT, Evans A, Ertei I, Hittle R, Ortega J, Wilson CB, Hammond D (1979) Tumors of pineal and suprasellar region: childrens cancer study group treatment results 1960–1975. Cancer 43: 698–701

346. Wara WM, Sheline GE, Newman H, Townsend JJ, Boldrey EB (1975) Radiation therapy of meningiomas. Am J Roentgenol 123: 453–458

347. Weir B, Elvidge AR (1968) Oligodendrogliomas: an analysis of 63 cases. J Neurosurg 29: 500–505

348. West CR, Bruce DA, Duffner PK (1985) Ependymomas. Factors in clinical and diagnostic staging. Cancer 56 [suppl] 56: 1812–1816

349. West J, Maor M (1980) Intracranial metastases: behavioral patterns related to primary site and results of treatment by whole brain irradiation. Int J Radiat Oncol Biol Phys 6: 11–15

350. Westling P, Svensson H, Hele P (1972) Cervical plexus lesions following postoperative radiation therapy of mammary carcinoma. Acta Radiol Ther 11: 209–216

351. Whyte TR, Colby MY, Layton DD (1969) Radiation therapy of brain-stem tumors. Radiology 93: 413–421

352. Wilson CB (1977) Brain metastases: the basis for surgical selection. Int J Radiat Oncol Biol Phys 2: 169–172

353. Wilson CB, Dempsey LC (1978) Transsphenoidal microsurgical removal of 250 pituitary adenomas. J Neurosurg 48: 13–22

354. Yardeni D, Reichenthal E, Zucker G, Rubinstein A, Cohen M, Israeli CBJ, Shalit MN (1984) Neurosurgical managements of single brain metastasis. Surg Neurol 21: 377–384

355. Zeman W, Shidnia H (1976) Posttherapeutic radiation injuries of the nervous system. Reflections on their prevention. J Neurosurg 212: 107–115

356. Zimmerman HM, Netsky MG, Davidoff LM (1956) Atlas of tumors of the nervous system. Lea and Febiger, Philadelphia

357. Zülch KJ (1956) Biologie und Pathologie der Hirngeschwülste. In: Olivecrona H, Tönnis W (Hrsg) Handbuch der Neurochirurgie, vol III. Springer, Berlin-Göttingen-Heidelberg, S 1–702
358. Zülch KJ (1963) Morphologische Veränderungen an Geschwülsten nach Bestrahlung und Schädigungsmöglichkeiten am normalen Hirn. Strahlentherapie [suppl] 52: 47–62
359. Zülch KJ (1979) Histological typing tumors of the central nervous system. World Health Organization, Geneva

Author's address: Prof. Dr. R. Sauer, Direktor der Strahlentherapeutischen Klinik und Poliklinik, Universitätsstrasse 27, D-8520 Erlangen, Federal Republic of Germany.

6

Principles of Chemotherapy in Brain Neoplasia

Mary K. Gumerlock and *E. A. Neuwelt*

Department of Neurosurgery, The Oregon Health Sciences University, Portland, OR, U.S.A.

I. Introduction

For the neurooncologic clinician, brain tumors, be they primary or secondary, are a frustrating challenge. Successful therapy often is not achieved with surgery or radiation therapy. One is therefore faced with the choice of chemotherapy, itself currently a less than adequate answer. Also, for the neuroclinician, such a choice is at once intimidating. It is the purpose, then, of this chapter to put brain tumor chemotherapy into clinical perspective, beginning first with the basic principles of anticancer drug therapy, continuing through an organized schema of the currently available chemotherapeutic agents as applicable to neurooncology and applying these to the specific features of brain tumors. The focus is to work through various research angles to distill the clinically relevant perspectives of this vast subject.

II. Basic Principles

To understand the chemotherapeutic approach it is first necessary to have a working understanding of the principles of cancer growth and drug therapy. Many of these principles are not new, but become more fully appreciated as improved animal models are used in preclinical study.

A. Cell Cycle

A multicellular organism develops and grows through a series of regulated alterations in the life cycle of its cells. The basic cell cycle consists of four phases: gap (G_1), nucleic acid synthesis (S), gap (G_2), and mitosis (M). For any given cell or tissue the duration of S, G_2, and M is relatively constant while G_1 may show marked variability, being of short length in such tissue as bone marrow and gastrointestinal mucosa, moderate length in skin, and longer in liver or kidney. The designation G_0 is given to those cells not actively dividing (essentially permanent G_1 phase): nerve, heart, and muscle.

Cell Cycle

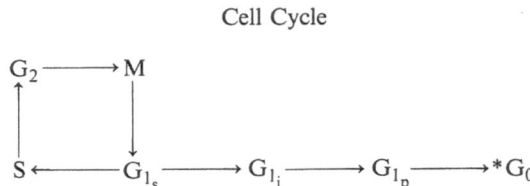

$*G_0$ Resting—nerve, heart, muscle.
G_{1_p} Prolonged—liver, kidney.
G_{1_i} Intermediate—skin.
G_{1_s} Short—bone marrow, gastrointestinal mucosa.

While the sequence $S \rightarrow G_2 \rightarrow M \rightarrow G_1$ is quite automatic, it remains unknown what triggers the critical $G_1 \rightarrow S$ transition, perhaps the central mystery of neoplasia. It is to these various cell cycle phases that nonsurgical treatment (both radiation and chemotherapy) is theoretically directed.

B. Tumor Cell Kinetics

Glial cell neoplastic growth has been studied both *in vitro* and *in vivo* measuring tritiated thymidine uptake as a marker of DNA synthesis. The tumor cell kinetics are characterized by several parameters including labeling index, cell cycle time, S-phase duration, growth fraction, theoretical doubling time, and cell loss[232]. These mathematically defined parameters require several assumptions including most importantly uniform rapid transport of the tritiated thymidine across the intact blood-brain barrier (BBB). This technique shows rare thymidine uptake in the glial nuclei of normal human brain[112a]. The kinetics of slow-growing brain tumors are more a function of a low growth fraction than of a long cell cycle[102, 103]. In more malignant gliomas the growth fraction is higher. With this technique, Hoshino differentiates glioblastoma multiforme from anaplastic astrocytoma with indices of 9 and 4%, respectively[102, 103]. Most recently, his study of medulloblastoma patients demonstrated a labeling index of 12%[104].

In general, a malignant glial tumor at diagnosis weighs approximately 100 g, containing 100 billion (10^{11}) cells[101, 232]. An optimistic 90% surgical removal leaves 10 g of tumor cells *in situ* or 10 billion (10^{10}) cells. If subsequent radiation therapy killed 99% of the remaining tumor burden, 100 million (10^8) cells would remain[232]. With approximately ⅓ of the tumor cell population proliferating and a cell cycle time of 2–3 days, one would then predict a doubling time of 7 days[101]. Fortunately while the estimates of tumor cell elimination by surgery and radiation are high, only 5–15% of such tumor is viable, thus effectively lengthening the clinically observed doubling time.

While doubling time and cell loss may have predictive value regarding the patient's prognosis, it is the growth fraction and cell cycle time which are theoretically important in developing a rational treatment plan. Given the above kinetics and the fact that effective chemotherapy should give a 2–3 log cell kill, tumor cell repopulation can be expected in 7–11 weeks[102]. Some would then note that after the initial chemotherapy cycle, a higher proportion of cells is viable and therefore tumor cell regrowth is faster after subsequent drug courses (3–4 weeks)[102, 103]. Normal cell repopulation then becomes a rate-limiting factor in determining chemotherapy cycle time. To be effective, chemotherapy must deliver *sufficiently high* concentrations of drug *long enough* for all the cells in the cycle to pass through the proliferative phase. Unfortunately, pushing either concentration or delivery time may increase drug toxicity.

While the above principles seem derived from a sound basis of experiments, and perhaps are followed in systemic cancer therapy, they may be based on a false assumption. To accurately assess brain (tumor or normal) cell kinetics, the marker substance must freely pass the BBB. If not, any results will be simply reflections of the differential permeability of that normally limited substance. Thymidine, a polar substance with a molecular weight of 242 daltons, does not freely penetrate the BBB. Furthermore, no specific transport of thymidine across that barrier (as for purine nucleosides) has been demonstrated, perhaps because the brain readily synthesizes pyrimidine nucleosides locally[26]. Spector and Eells[199] have demonstrated a transport system for thymidine across the blood-CSF barrier, the contribution of which seems minimal. Therefore not only is nucleic acid synthesis grossly underestimated, but also the differences as noted above between anaplastic astrocytoma, glioblastoma, and medulloblastoma are most likely only a measure of tumor-associated BBB alteration. To some extent this may actually explain why medulloblastoma is more responsive to chemotherapy than glioblastoma.

Another aspect of brain tumor growth is the fact that the tumor cell population is not a stable nor a homogenous population. Chromosomal studies of low and high grade astrocytomas show relative homogeneity of the former cell type compared to glioblastoma multiforme. High grade tumors show marked heterogeneity with numerous cell subpopulations. Initially, this heterogeneity was thought to be an "artifact" of cell culture studies, but in fact, *in vivo* sampling has yielded similar growth characteristics. Such a changing, heterogenous cell population promotes further growth and further ongoing drug resistance[193].

C. Anatomic Considerations

Unlike other more distensible areas of the body, the brain lies in a rigid skull, rather intolerant of volume increases. Thus tumor growth with its attendant mass effect will have increased pressure effects as well as tissue-destructive effects. The increased intracranial pressure may secondarily affect CSF circulation and rarely perhaps blood flow with additive deleterious effects. In addition, primary brain tumors are highly infiltrative. Thus the dividing tumor cells percolate through a relatively dormant environment of nondividing neurons and slowly proliferating, normal glial cells[54]. At least 5–10% of glioblastoma multiforme is multifocal[126].

This invasive behavior and lack of metastatic growth are hallmarks of primary CNS neoplasia. Attempts to correlate malignant invasive behavior with levels of 5'-nucleotidase, ornithine decarboxylase, and putrescine may yet prove clinically useful[120]. Inflammatory cells including mainly T cells are frequently seen within the primary tumor suggesting a local immune reaction, yet tumor invasion continues in the face of this reaction. On the other hand, Dick et al.[51] have described an interaction between lymphoid cells and cultured malignant glial cell lines which enhances protective cell coat production and may thus account for an apparant suppressor effect and malignant behavior.

If one is considering metastatic neoplasia, a further frequent problem is the multiplicity of lesions distributed primarily on the basis of tissue volume and proportional to cerebral blood flow. While metastatic tumors appear as frequently very well-circumscribed and easily-accessible lesions, there is a 30% local recurrence rate and generally the multiplicity and late detection preclude adequate surgical therapy[83a].

Perhaps the most unique anatomic aspect of brain tumors from the chemotherapeutic point of view is the BBB, a morphologic entity based on the brain capillary endothelial cell tight junctions[26, 178]. This structural barrier serves primarily a protective regulatory function constraining diffusion across capillaries in relation to lipid solubility and molecular weight. Brain tumor vascularity and the integrity of the BBB have long been debated. Suffice it to say that while each specific tumor nodule may have a variably permeable barrier, from the chemotherapeutic point of view, the state of the blood-brain and blood-tumor barriers must be factored into each drug delivery equation.

A number of tumor models have been developed to analyze blood-to-tissue transport of various drugs[94]. Regional capillary blood flow in tumor is decreased compared to normal brain especially in the central necrotic areas. However, a fairly consistent region of increased blood flow is seen at the junction of "tumor periphery" and "brain around tumor"[94]. This region also may show microscopic evidence of tumor infiltration. The blood-to-tissue transport constant (calculated as a measure of theoretical drug delivery across a barrier and dependent on blood flow, permeability, and capillary surface area) is variable, regionally within a single tumor, and from tumor to tumor in a single model. This constant cannot be correlated with histologic grade, tumor size or location, except for tumors in the meninges and choroid plexus[94]. Fenstermacher[65] cautions that "transfer constants are moderately difficult to measure, but their interpretation is frankly treacherous". Various membrane models to define the BBB have been developed with unclear clinical applicability at this point. No definite drug therapeutic advantage can be predicted, but it appears that barrier permeability is the rate-limiting factor.

Another aspect of brain tumor vascularity relates to tumor size and the large area of tumor necrosis. Whether tumor growth outstrips its blood supply or neoplastic vessels are occluded or tumor vessels shunt to changing regions[232], the end results are hypoxic regions and thus nonproliferating cells which are relatively immune to the effects of chemotherapeutic agents directed against cycling cells. In contrast to the tendency to increase their vascular volume, tumors also begin to compress their own capillaries, eventuating in tumor necrosis[77].

The idea postulated by Folkman[76] that tumor growth may be dependent on angiogenesis is perhaps distinctly evident in the marked capillary endothelial proliferation seen in glioblastoma multiforme. It appears that this tendency toward angiogenesis may well be related to tumor-derived stimulatory factors, angiogenesis factors[77]. Matsuno[138] has demonstrated such a tumor angiogenesis factor in cultured cells derived from 3 of 5 glioma lines and 3 of 4 meningioma lines, as well as in a lung carcinoma metastatic to brain. This angiogenic activity was stronger in the earlier cell passages, nondialyzable, and eliminated by ribonuclease or heating to 80 °C for 30 minutes[138]. Recent work suggests that not only does tumor-induced angiogenesis account for neovascularity but that macrophages infiltrating tumor may also induce such vascularity[77].

D. Prognostic Factors in Brain Tumors

The Brain Tumor Study Group (BTSG) and others have looked at various factors influencing prognosis, survival, and response to chemotherapy[41, 56]. The strongest recurrent influence on prognosis in brain tumor patients is *age*. Both Karnofsky performance scale[43] and tumor grade also have a positive prognostic effect, the former weighing more heavily.

Because of the difficulty in precise, consistent histopathologic characterization of tumors, prediction of biologic behavior has been difficult. Median survival in glioblastoma multiforme is eight months compared with 28 months in anaplastic astrocytoma[146]. Necrosis is a reliable indication of prognosis as perhaps are vascular endothelial proliferation and mitoses[81, 85, 146]. In analyzing clinical trials, care must be taken to differentiate patients with vascular endothelial proliferation and necrosis (glioblastoma) from those with anaplastic malignant high grade astrocytoma. A recent review of the BTSG trials also shows a statistically different survival between glioblastoma multiforme and anaplastic astrocytoma, subclassifying on the basis of necrosis[33]. Finally, it appears that patients with blood group A (either type A or type AB) have a decreased survival suggesting perhaps that those patients with anti-A antibodies may be able to mount a more effective immunologic defense against tumor cells[87]. To further support this idea, Epenetos *et al.*[62] describes a monoclonal antibody against epidermal growth factor receptor and blood group A antigen which bind *in vivo* to the tumor cells of a blood type 0 glioma patient.

In addition to the above prognostic factors, the BTSG found that duration of symptoms correlates directly with length of survival. Chang[41] reports that those patients with symptoms more than four months duration have a 39% 18-month survival while those with symptoms less than four months have an 11% 18-month median survival. While these factors influence survival, they do not have an effect on chemotherapeutic response. One factor, however, which does appear to influence response is the length of time from initial *diagnosis* to treatable *recurrence,* with tumor regression (increased survival) correlating with a prolonged time to that recurrence[56]. Neurooncologists are left then with the rather mundane conclusions that younger patients live longer than older patients and that tumor growth rate is probably not accelerated by chemotherapy.

E. Cancer Pharmacokinetics

In spite of the somewhat pessimistic conclusions above, brain tumor therapists are spurred by the gradual successes of systemic oncologists and are able to make use of their basic work. While many of the most prevalent forms of human cancer still resist effective chemotherapeutic intervention, some varieties have been influenced significantly by chemotherapy, including acute leukemia, Wilm's tumor, rhabdomyosarcoma and retinoblastoma in children, choriocarcinoma in women, Hodgkin's disease, diffuse histiocytic lymphoma, Burkitt's lymphoma, mycosis fungoides, and testicular carcinoma[1, 35]. In general, this chemotherapeutic success has not been realized though, when such "treatable" tumors have metastasized to the CNS.

Cancer chemotherapy is based on the fact that, since the chemotherapeutic agents act at the time of cell division, the fraction of cells killed is directly proportional to the number of cells dividing. This fraction of cells is also proportional to the length of the cell cycle (*i.e.*, a shorter cell cycle means a higher fraction of the total number of cells are in the dividing phase). Conversely, cells with long cycles tend to be rather resistant to both chemotherapy and radiation. Of note is the fact that *in vivo* cell cycles in any given tumor are not uniform. Historically, oncologists have used tumor doubling time as an estimate of cell cycle. This, however, does bear some caution as tumor size reflects not only tumor cell accumulation but also tumor cell loss and host inflammatory and immune responses[186]. Normal cells cycle in an automatic fashion and normal benign cell growth is kept under rigid control. One of the key differences between tumor and normal tissue is the stimulus of entry from G_1 phase into the S or synthesis phase. What triggers cells to move into this S-phase is unknown (oncogenes, perhaps). The biochemical events just after S-phase have been studied and it is in fact at this stage that most cancer chemotherapeutic agents work.

A basic tenet of any cancer chemotherapy is that the larger the tumor burden, the less effective the therapeutic maneuvers[50]. Such a principle is immediately obvious, but again, because of the nature of the organ involved (CNS) and the infiltrating growth pattern of these tumors, radical decompressive surgery and expert radiation therapy to an exquisitely sensitive tumor have only a minute effect on total tumor volume. However, in general within the constraints of CNS tumor location, maximal tumor resection should be undertaken to ultimately maximize the effect of chemotherapy[50]. However, the survival of glioblastoma patients undergoing limited versus radical tumor resection is similar suggesting, that at this time the nature of the disease (*infiltrative* brain tumor) itself takes precedence over current *focally* directed therapies.

In any treatment regime, cancer or not, the offending agents must be exposed to the drug in sufficient concentrations for a sufficient period of time, and regression response rates with effective drugs are extremely dose-dependent[185]. To be effective the drug must reach the sensitive cells in *lethal concentrations*. However, adequate serum concentrations do not insure adequate tissue concentrations, and this is further complicated in CNS malignancy by the BBB and the fact that CSF levels do not predict brain parenchymal levels[148]. The *length of time* tumor cells are exposed to adequate drug is as critical as concentration because many of the more effective chemotherapeutic agents are cell cycle specific, theoretically requiring cells to be in a particular phase to the operant. Cells, especially tumor cells, do not cycle synchronously and they spend the smallest fraction of time in their mitotic phase. Two consequences of inadequate drug delivery are suboptimal cell kill and possibly the induction of tumor resistance.

Because of the steep dose response curve, drugs must be given in the maximum tolerated amounts, just to the limits of toxicity[188]. While not a difficult course in treating systemic cancer where both disease and treatment can be devastating, such a concept is particularly dissatisfying in dealing with primary CNS malignancy in otherwise healthy patients. Conversely, it is difficult for patients feeling relatively well to accept a treatment course fraught with significant systemic toxicity. Furthermore, determining just those limits of toxicity with cytotoxic agents is difficult. Even in extremely inbred laboratory animals, lethal toxicity to cancer chemotherapeutic agents varies greatly, probably as a result of varying metabolic (activation, degradation, excretion) rates[185]. The combination of factors such as these makes dose determination just slightly better than arbitrary, yet an important aspect of chemotherapeutic success.

F. Chemotherapeutic Principles

Some of the concepts mentioned above can be summarized from the pharmacologic viewpoint.

1. Because a single cell can theoretically give rise to tumor sufficient to kill the host, it is necessary to destroy or inactivate every cell.

2. Emphasizing drugs is important, but the general status of the patient strongly influences chemotherapy (i.e., infection, previous radiation, nutritional and metabolic status, other complications).

3. Host defenses themselves can be tumoricidal.

4. Because the doubling time of tumors is constant during the logarithmic growth phase, host survival is inversely proportional to the number of malignant cells remaining at the termination of therapeutic measures.

5. Cell kill by antineoplastic agents is a first order kinetic phenomenon, i.e., a constant percentage rather than a constant number of cells is killed by any given therapeutic maneuver.

6. Most potent cytotoxic agents are cell cycle specific, acting at specific phases in the cell cycle, particularly when cells are undergoing mitosis. Thus tumors with a high growth fraction are most susceptible. These drugs act at DNA synthesis, transcription, or mitotic spindle formation.

7. This is a rapidly changing field requiring repeated reappraisals of the status of available agents.

G. Drug Classifications

To facilitate an understanding of the various available chemotherapeutic agents, the following section discusses various chemotherapeutic drug classifications. One approach is along the lines of classic pharmacology and considers chemical

Table 1. Chemotherapeutic agents

A. Alkylating agents
  1. nitrogen mustards
    a) cyclophosphamide
    b) mechlorethamine
    c) melphalan
    d) chlorambucil
  2. dacarbazine
  3. nitrosoureas
    a) carmustine (BCNU)
    b) lomustine (CCNU)
    c) semustine (Me-CCNU)
  4. streptozotocin
  5. thiotepa
 	
B. Antimetabolites
  1. folic acid analogs
    methotrexate (MTX)
  2. pyrimidine analogs
    a) fluorouracil (5-FU)
    b) cytarabine
  3. purine analogs
    a) mercaptopurine
    b) thioguanine
	C. Natural products
	  1. vinca alkaloids
	    a) vinblastine
	    b) vincristine
	  2. antibiotics
	    a) dactinomycin
	    b) doxorubicin
	    c) bleomycin
	    d) mithramycin
	    e) mitomycin
	  3. enzymes asparaginase
	
	D. Miscellaneous agents
	  1. cisplatin
	  2. hydroxyurea
	  3. procarbazine
	  4. etoposide
	  5. teniposide (VM-26)
	
	E. Hormones
	  1. tamoxifen
	  2. steroids

categories such as alkylating agents, antimetabolites, antibiotics and other natural products, enzymes, hormones, radioisotopes and miscellaneous drugs[35]. The following drug summaries are ordered along such a schema (Table 1).

Another method of classification is to consider the anticancer drugs based on the target to which the particular drug binds[186]. There are essentially four targets: nucleic acids, enzymes, microtubule spindle structure, and hormone receptors (Table 2). The first target, binding to nucleic acids, can occur through at least three mechanisms. Alkylation is a covalent linkage of drug to DNA; secondary DNA damage is cytotoxic. Chemotherapeutic drugs can also bind to nucleic acids via intercalation, drug insertion between two adjacent nucleotide bases. A third method of nucleic acid damage is direct modification of DNA structure with production of free aldehydes and single strand breakage, thus inhibiting DNA polymerase.

Enzymes are another target of chemotherapeutic agents. There are three enzymes susceptible to inhibition in the S-phase of the cell cycle: thymidylate synthetase, ribonucleic reductase, and DNA polymerase. These are specifically inhibited by 5-fluorouracil, hydroxyurea, and cytarabine. In addition, there are inhibitors of purine synthesis (mercaptopurine and thioguanine), pyrimidine synthesis (fluorouracil and cytarabine) and the folate reductase reaction (MTX). These agents are active against DNA synthesis and arrest the cell in the S-phase. Therefore, these agents are probably not active against cells which do not happen to enter the S-phase during the time when therapeutic levels of the drug are present.

Table 2. Chemotherapeutic agents

Drug	Cell Cycle	Binding Target	Plasma T½	CSF Penetration	Neurotoxicity
Cyclophosphamide	S	nucleic acid alkylation	3–10°	poor	×
Mechlorethamine	NS	nucleic acid alkylation	3°	poor	×
Melphalan	NS	nucleic acid alkylation	1.8°	poor	
Chlorambucil	NS	nucleic acid alkylation	1.5°	poor	
Dacarbazine	NS	nucleic acid alkylation	3–5°	poor	
Carmustine	NS	nucleic acid alkylation	70'	good	×
Lomustine	NS	nucleic acid alkylation	70'	good	
Streptozotocin	NS	inhibits DNA synthesis	15'	poor	
Thiotepa	NS	nucleic acid alkylation	short	fair	×
Methotrexate	S	enzyme inhib.: dihydrofolate reductase	2–4°	fair	×
Fluorouracil	S	enzyme inhib.: thymidylate synthetase	6–20'	good	×
Cytarabine	S	enzyme inhib.: DNA polymerase	7–20'	fair	×
Mercaptopurine	S	enzyme inhib.: purine synthesis	60'	poor	
Thioguanine	S	enzyme inhib.: purine synthesis	90'	poor	
Vinblastine	M	binds tubulin	2°	poor	
Vincristine	M	binds tubulin	2.5°	poor	×
Dactinomycin	NS	nucleic acid intercalator	36°	poor	
Doxorubicin	NS	nucleic acid intercalator	1.5–10°	poor	×
Bleomycin	G₁, G₂	DNA strand scission	2–4°	poor	
Mithramycin	NS	binds DNA, inhib. RNA synthesis	60'	fair	
Mitomycin	G₁, S	nucleic acid alkylation	30–45'	poor	
Asparaginase	G₁	depletes amino acid	5'	poor	×
Cisplatin	NS	nucleic acid intercalator	20–50'	poor	×
Hydroxyurea	S	enzyme inhib.: ribonucleotide reductase	2–4°	poor	
Procarbazine	S	nucleic acid alkylation	?	good	×
Etoposide	M, G₂	DNA strand scission	2–4°	poor	×
Tamoxifen	G₁	Hormone receptor binding	7–14°	?	

S = synthesis, WS = nonspecific, M = mitosis, G = gap.

A third target for chemotherapeutic agents involves the microtubule spindle structure. Vinblastine and vincristine act at this level. They interact with tubulin, the structural protein of microtubules, interrupting the cell cycle at the metaphase stage and arresting the cell in the M-phase.

The fourth target of chemocytotoxic agents is the hormone receptor. Active drugs first bind to specific cytoplasmic receptor proteins, and this hormone-receptor complex then translocates into the nucleus where it interacts with DNA. The exact cytotoxic mechanism of hormones is unknown.

Other methods of classification include categorizing the drugs as to metabolic site of action—purine or pyrimidine synthesis, DNA synthesis, RNA synthesis, protein synthesis, structure (microtubules) or function (enzyme)—or as to phase of cell cycle interference (S-G_2-M-G_1). A final classification is based on particular tumor sensitivity (which drugs are specifically active against a given tumor type). With this classification, some would list no drugs in the brain tumor category[35]. On a somewhat more optimistic note, others consider chemotherapy for brain tumors as having moderate efficacy using such drugs as MTX, nitrosourea, vincristine, mechlorethamine, procarbazine, and prednisone[1].

III. Specific Therapeutic Agents

Because of the frustrating situation of brain tumor chemotherapy, most of the available drugs have been tried in patients with CNS neoplasm. Such a catalog of agents and barrage of information can be overwhelming for the clinician. The following categorization of drugs attempts a logical and useful reference (Tables 1 and 2, Figs. 1–5). Each of the agents is commercially available (approved, not experimental) and each has been used in brain tumor therapy.

A. Alkylating Agents

1. Nitrogen Mustards

a) Cyclophosphamide

Cyclophosphamide (Fig. 1), a nitrogen mustard, is usually considered an alkylating agent. The drug is metabolized to active products by hydroxylation (4-hydroxy-cyclophosphamide) and aldehyde formation (aldophosphamide), presumably via the hepatic microsomal enzyme cytochrome P450 system. These are further metabolized in the tumor cells. The cytotoxic action of this drug is presumed to result from DNA alkylation, however the exact mechanism of action is unknown. Because the drug is metabolized in the liver, its half life may be shortened by such drugs as phenobarbital which induce the metabolizing enzymes. Hemorrhagic cystitis is commonly seen in association with cyclophosphamide therapy. Toxicity relates to destruction of rapidly growing tissues and therefore affects the bone marrow, gastrointestinal system, and skin. Other side effects include carcinogenesis and occasionally cardiac failure; the syndrome of inappropriate antidiuretic hormone has been seen in patients receiving higher doses. Response is seen in malignant lymphomas, multiple myeloma, leukemia, mycosis fungoides, neuro-blastoma, ovarian carcinoma, retinoblastoma and carcinoma of the breast. The drug also has immunosuppressive effects and is used in nonneoplastic conditions of altered immune reactivity. More recently it has been shown to enhance humoral immunity in patients with advanced metastatic disease[15].

In the treatment of brain tumors, cyclophosphamide has been most useful in combination therapy in protocols for treatment of both primary and metastatic CNS neoplasia[148, 153, 165–167, 204, 207]. Because the drug is activated in the liver, it is not useful for direct intra-arterial administration. Recurrent pediatric medulloblas-toma, glioma, and germ cell tumors have responded to high dose cyclophosphamide[4], and it has been used in combination with doxorubicin, MTX, CCNU, and cisplatin for treating the rare peripheral metastatic glioma[173].

b) Mechlorethamine

Another nitrogen mustard analog, mechlorethamine (Fig. 1), is also a biological alkylating agent which inhibits rapidly proliferating cells. Toxicity from this drug consists of the expected systemic and marrow suppressive effects. Shortly after intravenous injection this drug undergoes chemical transformation, combines with its reactive products, and is undetectable in its native form in the serum. It is used in the treatment of Hodgkin's disease, lymphosarcoma, myelocytic or lymphocytic leukemia, polycythemia vera, mycosis fungoides and bronchogenic carcinoma.

Mechlorethamine is the agent first used in brain tumor chemotherapy. As an intracarotid infusion, it was given in combination with intravenous sodium thiosulfate rescue to decrease hematologic complications. There were a significant number of intracranial complications with this early regimen[10, 174]. A randomized trial in pediatric recurrent brain tumors with and without mustard in combination with vincristine, procarbazine, and prednisone showed more effect but more toxicity using mechlorethamine[36]. Systemic administration is associated with significant neurotoxicity: acute encephalopathy, cerebellar syndrome, and peri-pheral neuropathy[235]. Histologic changes include diffuse neuronal degeneration, gliosis and perivascular fibrosis especially in the subcortical white matter[209].

c) Melphalan

Melphalan (Fig. 1) was developed to specifically utilize the principle that tumor cells rapidly metabolizing L-phenylalanine and tyramine should show enhanced uptake of such a drug. It is actively transported by two amino acid carrier systems, but whether there is preferential uptake in malignant cells is unknown. The drug acts by intracellular alkylation and DNA crosslinking and does not cross the BBB well[93]. As with the other alkylating agents, side effects include myelosuppression, nausea, vomiting, gonadal destruction, and carcinogenesis. Ariel reported hemipa-resis following intracarotid injection in three patients[10]. Wilson et al.[205] have used the drug in limited intraarterial trials. Its primary use is in the treatment of multiple myeloma, malignant melanoma, and epithelial ovarian carcinoma, and perhaps CNS metastatic disease.

d) Chlorambucil

Chlorambucil (Fig. 1) is an orally administered congener of melphalan, that is extensively bound to plasma and tissue proteins with poor CSF penetrations. In addition to the usual hematologic and gastrointestinal side effects, interstitial pneumonia, a peripheral neuropathy and secondary malignancies are described. Generalized seizures have been reported in children[231] and dose-related focal seizures are described in adults[145]. The drug is used in treatment of hematopoietic malignancies. Only limited effectiveness has been demonstrated against glioblastoma multiforme.

2. Dacarbazine

Dacarbazine (Fig. 1) is metabolized by the hepatic microsomal system. Though considered primarily an alkylating agent, it is a purine analog and may also act by inhibition of DNA synthesis. A third possible mechanism of action is interaction with sulfhydryl groups. Although the drug may gain some access to the CSF, little has been reported in the way of CNS toxicity. The drug is indicated in the treatment of metastatic malignant melanoma and Hodgkin's disease. Decarbazine has been evaluated in patients with gliomas, neuroblastoma and recurrent medulloblastoma; response rate as a single agent has been disappointing[59]. The drug continues under trial in comparison with BCNU and procarbazine, and may be more effective with less toxicity than the other drugs.

3. Nitrosoureas

The third category of alkylating agents is the nitrosourea group, used quite extensively in the treatment of primary brain tumors. These are lipid soluble agents which alkylate and cross-link DNA. Delayed cumulative bone marrow suppression is a significant toxic effect. The two most common nitrosoureas, carmustine (BCNU) and lomustine (CCNU), are in wide use in the treatment of brain tumors.

BCNU (Fig. 1) appears to cross the BBB readily and has been used in the treatment of glioblastoma, brain stem glioma, medulloblastoma, astrocytoma, ependymoma and metastatic brain tumors[59]. It is also used in the treatment of multiple myeloma, Hodgkin's disease and other lymphomas. Side effects are hematopoietic and gastrointestinal with a transient increase in liver enzymes. Pulmonary fibrosis has been described.

CCNU (Fig. 1) as a single agent appears to be less effective than BCNU although it has the advantage of oral administration. It crosses the BBB readily, acts as an alkylating agent, and may also inhibit key enzymatic processes.

Intracarotid administration of BCNU has been associated with marked neurotoxicity and retinal toxicity. While these were initially felt to be related to the ethanol vehicle, further studies revealed that similar neurotoxic effects remained with a nonalcohol-based drug[90, 121, 182]. This issue is not resolved. These effects may in fact be more related to nonuniform drug delivery as a result of laminar flow and secondary drug streaming than to drug or diluent alone[20].

In evaluating nitrosourea therapy in glioblastoma patients, the BTSG determined a 37.5 week survival for patients undergoing surgery and irradiation

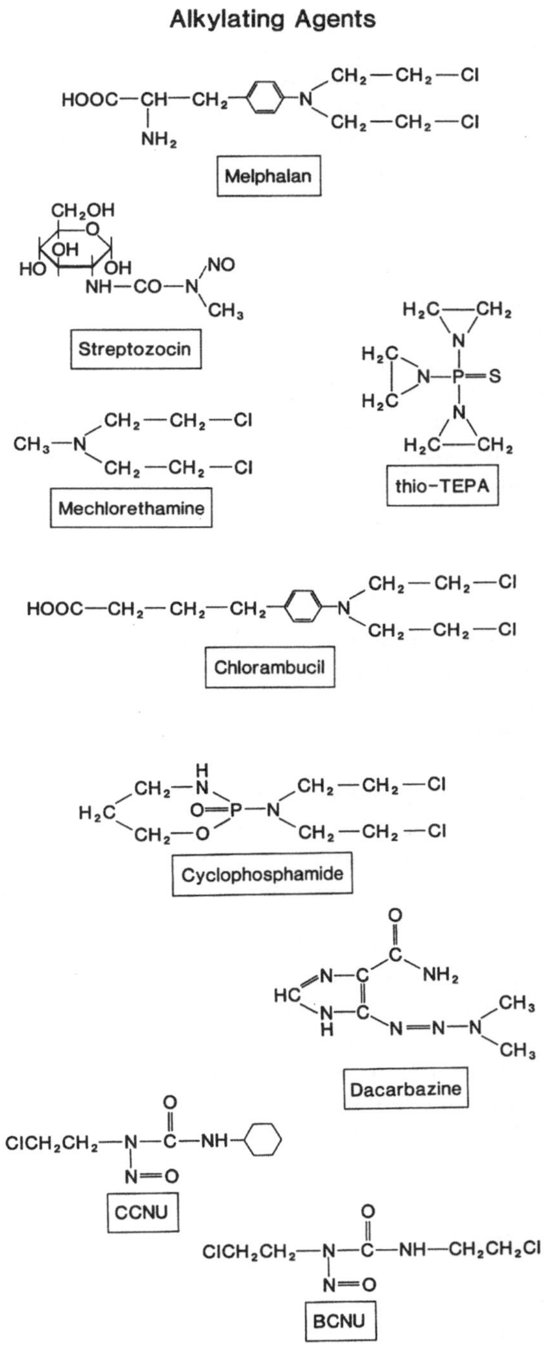
Alkylating Agents
Melphalan
Streptozocin
thio-TEPA
Mechlorethamine
Chlorambucil
Cyclophosphamide
Dacarbazine
CCNU
BCNU

Fig. 1

compared to a 40.5 week survival following surgery, radiation, and BCNU. This difference was determined statistically insignificant[222].

Because of their ability to penetrate the BBB nitrosoureas are a major part of most brain tumor therapy protocols. Intraarterial BCNU has been used as a single agent or in combination with cisplatin and epidophyllotoxin (VP-16)[206, 228]. There is a suggestion that early (6–8 hours after surgery) nitrosourea administration may have a therapeutic advantage[34].

4. Streptozotocin

Streptozotocin (Fig. 1), a naturally occurring nitrosourea antibiotic, inhibits DNA synthesis and affects all stages of the mammalian cell cycle. The drug also has insulin-like properties and has been used in the treatment of metastatic pancreatic islet cell carcinoma, as well as melanoma, carcinoid, and lymphoma. No specific neurotoxicity has been described. This drug has shown significant antineoplastic activity against murine ependymoblastoma[221] and is currently in clinical trial by the BTSG where a randomized four-armed study with streptozotocin, BCNU, and radiation shows no difference in these treatment regimens[88]. It has also been used in the treatment of brain metastases.

5. Thiotepa

Thiotepa (Fig. 1) has a radiomimetic action thought to be secondary to release of radicals which disrupt the DNA bonds (as does irradiation). One of the principal bonds disrupted is the N-7 position of guanine. Cell replication is altered. Thiotepa may also be described as mutagenic in that it causes chromosomal aberrations which increase with the age of the patient; it is also carcinogenic. Alkylating agents such as this (cell cycle independent) may have an advantage against more slowly proliferating tumors. Toxicity is again primarily bone marrow suppression. The drug is usually given intravenously, but some have preferred to inject the drug directly into the tumor mass. Early use of this drug intraarterially has been described for both primary and metastatic brain tumors in both carotid and vertebral circulations[46, 135]. Intrathecal thiotepa has shown some effect (with minimal toxicity) in patients with CNS leukemia[226] and in children with recurrent disseminated medulloblastoma[124]. Either with or without other intrathecal agents (MTX, cytarabine) it has produced short-term stabilization of disease. Edwards et al.[58] found no response in its use as a single agent against malignant gliomas. Some use of this drug in conjunction with BBB disruption has been described in dogs and in patients studied with magnetic resonance imaging[71].

B. Antimetabolites

1. Folic Acid Analogs

Methotrexate (MTX)

MTX (Fig. 2) interrupts cell reproduction by competitive inhibition of dihydro-folate reductase. Reduced folates are necessary cofactors in purine and pyrimidine biosynthesis. MTX binds to the dihydrofolate reductase (DHFR) enzyme, thus ultimately depleting the tetrahydrofolate pools intracellularly. Ultimately dihydrofolate then accumulates. This accumulated substrate can then compete with MTX for binding to the DHFR enzyme. Thus, high levels of free intracellular MTX are necessary for ongoing interference with the inhibited enzyme. Intracellular MTX is subject to the addition of glutamyl residues, thus resulting in "polyglutamated" antifolates which penetrate cellular membranes poorly. Polyglutamates enhance MTX toxicity by "trapping" the drug intracellularly and also by inhibiting thymidylate synthetase[35, 83].

MTX is a highly ionized molecule which diffuses readily throughout the total body water. Adequate CSF levels are difficult to achieve. The drug is transported intracellularly via a carrier-mediated transport system, and acts in the S-phase of the cell cycle. For this drug to be most effective, the cell population should be in the logarithmic rather than plateau phase of growth. MTX is used in treatment of choriocarcinoma, leukemias, breast cancer, lymphoma, various pediatric tumors and has been used rather extensively in brain tumor (primary and metastatic) therapy. Toxicities include bone marrow suppression, oral mucositis, interstitial pneumonitis, renal failure and multiple CNS toxicities: encephalopathy, myelopathy, arachnoiditis.

The early trials of MTX in brain tumor patients utilized intraarterial infusions; the drug was also given topically at surgery and instilled via Ommaya reservoir[60]. High dose systemic MTX treatment of glioma patients has also been described with questionable response[52].

2. Pyrimidine Analogs

a) Fluorouracil (5-FU)

The pyrimidine analogs form another group of antimetabolite chemotherapeutic agents. 5-FU (Fig. 2) is a synthetic pyrimidine antimetabolite. The drug appears to flow through the phosphorylation pathways and binds covalently with thymidylate synthetase. Though the exact mechanism of action is unknown, it is felt that the drug interferes with RNA processing and function, and is more lethal to logarithmically growing cells.

An interesting phenomenon associated with fluorouracil has been described. Pretreating with MTX and other purine synthesis inhibitors enhances 5-FU activity (*i.e.*, a sequence-dependent synergism develops), perhaps by increasing cellular pools of phosphoribosyl pyrophosphate[66]. The therapeutic index is also improved with allopurinol and thymidine. The drug is used primarily in treating carcinomas of the gastrointestinal tract, choriocarcinoma, and breast cancer. Severe gastrointestinal toxicity is noted as is bone marrow suppression.

Neurologic toxicity, including a cerebellar syndrome and myelopathy, has been reported after intrathecal administration[225]. The cerebellar syndrome (ataxia, unsteady gait, slurred speech and nystagmus) is felt to be related more to peak plasma levels of drug rather than cumulative dosing, and is reversible with discontinuation of the drug. Confusion, seizures and lethargy have also been reported. It is interesting that a report of intraventricular fluorouracil producing high levels of CSF drug showed no adverse neurologic effect[45]. The neurotoxicity is

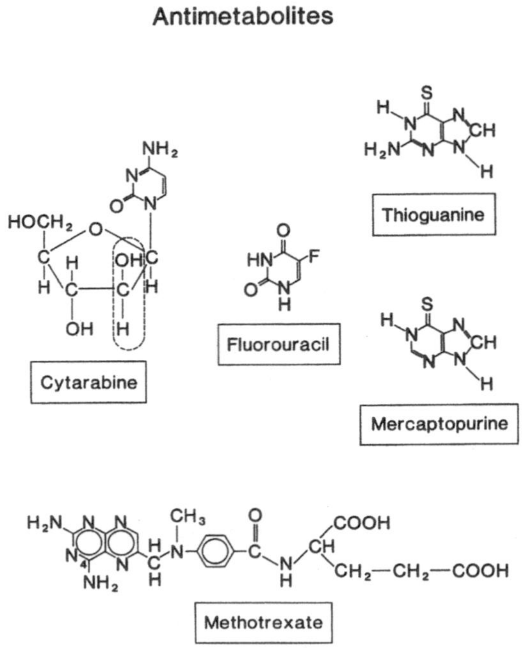

Antimetabolites

Fig. 2

related to Krebs cycle interference by systemically-produced fluoroacetate and increased plasma citrate levels[117]. Purkinje cell and mitochondrial abnormalities are described[235].

A randomized study of the drug in glioblastoma patients following surgery and irradiation was without benefit[221]. The drug has also been instilled directly into the tumor bed without prolongation of survival. There is some suggestion that in combination with BCNU it may have some effect against astrocytomas.

b) Cytarabine

Cytarabine (Fig. 2), an arabinose containing nucleoside, has its mechanism of action in base pair substitution leading to abnormal stacking of the bases, hence nucleic acid dysfunction. It may also be an inhibitor of DNA polymerase, as well as the RNA-dependent DNA polymerase (*i.e., reverse transcriptase*). Resistance to this S-phase specific drug can develop by induction of the enzyme cytidine deaminase. Even though the drug penetrates the BBB somewhat, direct intrathecal injection has been used in treating meningeal neoplasms. However, because of significant toxicity, this regimen has been replaced by equally effective systemic dosing[8]. Cytarabine also has immunosuppressive effects. In addition to its action at the S-phase there is some suggestion that it blocks progression of cells from the G_1 phase entering into the S-phase. The drug has been used in lymphoma and the intrathecal treatment of meningeal leukemia, and is frequently used in combination chemotherapy. Toxicities include bone marrow suppression, gastrointestinal and hepatic dysfunction. A specific toxicity syndrome has been described with the onset of fever, myalgia, bone pain, chest pain, maculopapular rash, conjunctivitis and malaise 6–12 hours following medication[210]. Neurotoxicity has included cerebral and cerebellar dysfunction with personality changes and somnolence at higher drug doses. The cerebellar toxic effects appear cumulative[14, 107a], and autopsy pathology shows extensive Purkinje cell damage[55].

3. Purine Analogs

The purine analog antimetabolites include 6-mercaptopurine and 6-thioguanine (Fig. 2). These drugs represent the subsitution of a thiol group for a hydroxyl group in the purine ring. Intracellularly, the drugs are converted to active nucleotide by the enzyme hypoxanthineguanine phosphoribosyl transferase. Base pair substitution in DNA then occurs. Mercaptopurine toxicity may be excessive if given in the presence of allopurinol because the drug is metabolized via the xanthine oxidase pathway. It is primarily used in leukemia, and has not been effective in lymphomas or other solid tumors. It is not particularly effective in prophylaxis of CNS leukemia, even though it can theoretically penetrate the BBB[140]. Patients receiving mercoptopurine display decreased cellular hypersensitivities and impaired induction of immunity to infectious agents. As with many other antineoplastic agents, mutagenesis and carcinogenesis are potential and human chromosomal abberrations have been seen. Thioguanine is administered orally and is also used in the combination treatment of leukemia. Toxicity includes bone marrow suppression and gastrointestinal toxicity.

C. Natural Products

1. Vinca Alkaloids

The naturally occurring vinca alkaloids, vincristine and vinblastine (Fig. 3), are derivatives of the periwinkle plant, a species of myrtle. They are considered spindle poisons and act by binding to tubulin, a structural intracellular protein, entering the cells via an energy-dependent carrier-mediated transport system. While the drugs act similarly, vinblastine is limited by its bone marrow toxicity and vincristine by its neurotoxicity. The drugs are cell cycle specific and block mitosis with metaphase arrest.

Vinblastine is used primarily in combination with bleomycin and cisplatinum for germ cell tumors (intracranial and peripheral). It has also been used in the treatment of lymphoma, neuroblastoma, eosinophilic granuloma, choriocarcinoma, and breast cancer. Toxicity is primarily bone marrow suppression and may be dose-limiting. Neurologic effects include temporary mental depression, paresthesias, loss of deep tendon reflexes, occasionally headaches, convulsions, and psychosis. Dysfunction of the autonomic nervous system has also been reported.

The well-known neurotoxicity of vincristine may be based on its more lipophilic nature and thus its ability to penetrate neural tissue, both central and peripheral. The drug binds to microtubules and interferes with axoplasmic transport. A dose-related peripheral neuropathy is well described. Loss of reflexes are quite characteristic and may not return following discontinuation of the drug. Motor strength resolves, albeit slowly, and paresthesias will usually disappear. Various cranial neuropathies have been described with vincristine. These are usually bilaterally symmetric and they involve the facial, oculomotor or recurrent laryngeal nerves[114]. Autonomic neuropathy is also not uncommon with vincristine including colicky abdominal pain and constipation. Vincristine only rarely affects the bladder. Orthostatic hypotension is an uncommon, but reported complication[39]. Symptoms of encephalopathy include seizures, and a cerebellar picture of ataxia and athetosis (cerebellar/basal ganglia). Vincristine may induce hyponatremia (syndrome of inappropriate antidiuretic hormone). The toxicity may be aggravated in patients who are elderly, in patients receiving previous radiation therapy, and in patients with pre-existing neurologic disease. Accidental intrathecal administration of vincristine has led to severe and sometimes fatal myeloencephalopathies[198, 230]. Electrophysiologically, the vincristine peripheral neuropathy is felt to be an axonal degeneration. These observations have been confirmed pathologically and the axonal nature of this neuropathy includes loss of microtubules and proliferation of abnormal aggregates of neurofilaments. Nerve cell changes have been described in the medulla[31].

2. Antibiotics

a) Dactinomycin

Dactinomycin (Fig. 3) binds to DNA and blocks RNA polymerase and RNA-dependent DNA polymerase; it also may bind to DNA by intercalating between base pairs on the double helix. The drug does not cross the BBB and has a serum half life of approximately 36 hours, probably secondary to slow release from binding sites.

Much evidence exists that the phenomenon of "radiation recall" exists following dactinomycin administration—a severe inflammatory reaction developing in sites previously irradiated[186]. Such reactions may be severe and life threatening, but the effect may be used to advantage in tumors partially responsive to radiation with a combined lower dose of dactinomycin and lower dose of radiation. This drug has also been used in isolation perfusion techniques to minimize systemic drug exposure, while increasing the dose over usual systemic concentrations. This drug is used in the treatment of Wilm's tumor, rhabdo-myosarcoma and germ cell tumors. Other bony and soft tissue tumors have been treated with dactinomycin via the regional perfusion method. The usual toxic side effects of anticancer therapy are noted.

b) Doxorubicin

Doxorubicin (adriamycin) is an anthracycline ring structure (Fig. 3). This, like the preceding drug, acts by specific intercalation of the planar ring structure into the double helix, thus inhibiting nucleic acid synthesis. It is used in soft tissue tumors including Wilm's tumor, neuroblastoma, sarcomas and breast carcinomas. Cardiac toxicity is prominent, with two types of myopathy[186]. The first is an acute form with abnormal EKG changes especially ST-T wave alterations and arrhythmias. There is an acute reversible reduction of ejection fraction 24 hours after a single dose of this drug. A second, chronic, cumulative dose-related toxicity manifests with congestive heart failure. Cardiac biopsies are positive for myocardial toxicity. This is a dose-dependent phenomenon and is aggravated in patients who have had prior cardiac radiation or have received cyclophosphamide[186]. Like many other cytotoxic agents doxorubicin may induce hyperuricemia secondary to rapid lysis of neoplastic cells.

Because of its poor lipid solubility and high molecular weight, doxorubicin has limited penetration of the BBB and thus little clinically neurotoxicity. Cytofluorescent techniques show that the drug localizes in the nuclei of neurons and glia and regions lacking a BBB—area postrema, pineal, median eminence, neurohypophysis, choroid plexus[18]. In the peripheral nervous system the drug localizes in the superior cervical ganglia and dorsal root ganglia[19]. High doses in animal models have shown neuronal necrosis. A fatal necrotizing angiopathy with doxorubicin and some of its derivatives has been seen in monkeys after intrathecal or intraventricular administration. Patients receiving an analog in Spain suffered massive brain edema and coma after intracarotid administration[29]. Administration in conjuction with BBB disruption resulted in severe neurotoxicity in dogs[151]. A phase II study with adriamycin as a single agent in relapsed malignant gliomas failed to show any response[142]. The drug is used in combination therapy for both systemic and metastatic disease and has been used in the rare instance of extracranial glial metastasis[173]. An anti-tumor synergy between doxorubicin and verapamil has been described[187].

c) Bleomycin

Bleomycin (Fig. 3) is a copper-chelating glycopeptide, a mixture of small molecular weight peptides. The drug acts primarily by causing chain fragmentation of the DNA molecules. It causes this scission by intercalating between guanine-cytosine base paits. While cells in all phases of the cell cycle are susceptible to the cytotoxic effects of bleomycin, they are maximally susceptible when exposed during the G_1 phase. In addition, bleomycin has a cell synchronization effect at the G_2 phase (post-DNA synthesis). The drug has minimal myelosuppressive toxicity but does have unusual pulmonary toxicities. An acute idiosyncratic pulmonary toxicity, most likely a hypersensitivity immune reaction, is seen even with low dose treatment[12]. The chronic pulmonary toxicity with bleomycin manifests as decreased pulmonary function tests, fine rales, cough and diffuse bibasilar infiltrates that can progress to a fatal pulmonary fibrosis. Ready availability of oxygen fosters the development of superoxide radicals in the pulmonary parenchyma thus leading to toxicity, either a subacute or chronic interstitial pneumonitis. Other antineoplastic agents may potentiate the drug toxicity, which is a cumulative-dose-related side-effect with safe upper limits ranging from 150–360 units depending on patient age. Bleomycin has been used systemically in combination chemotherapy with a few responses in malignant gliomas and medulloblastomas. Results of brain tumor treatment with bleomycin are still inconclusive. Patients with primary intracranial germ cell tumors respond to the combination bleomycin-vinblastine-cisplatin chemotherapy but pulmonary toxicity can limit success[160].

Natural Products

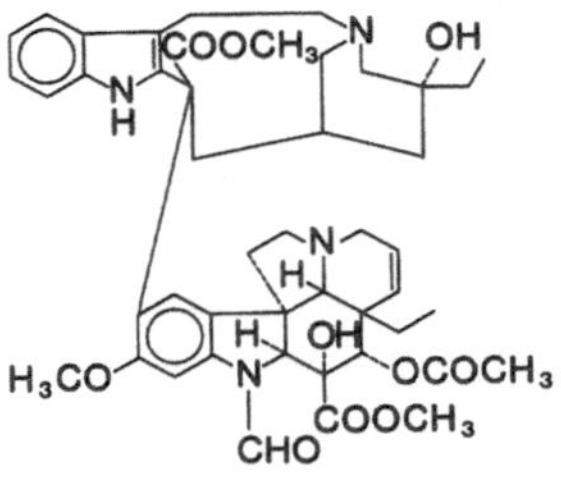

Vincristine

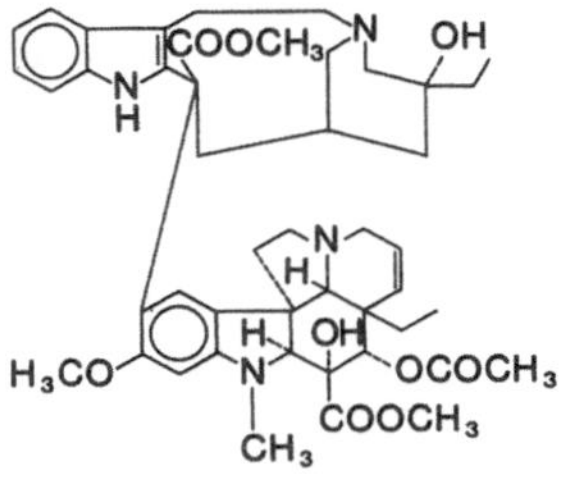

Vinblastine

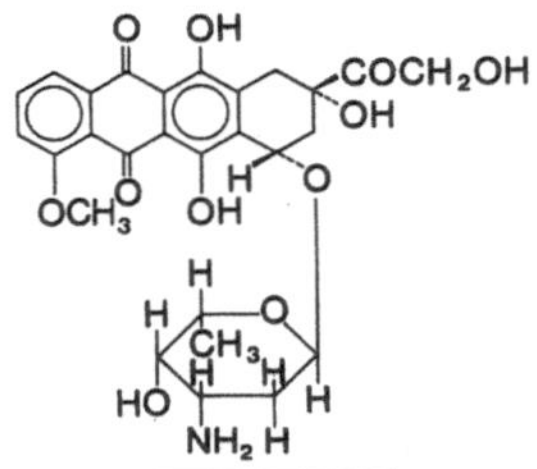

Doxorubicin

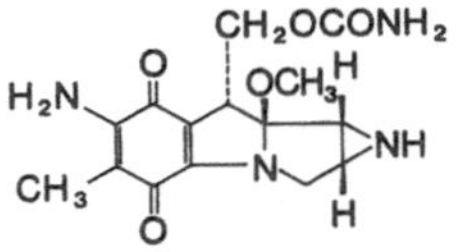

Mitomycin

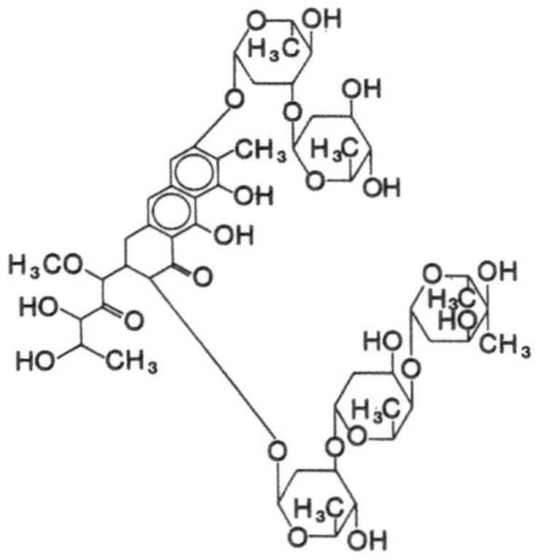

Mithramycin

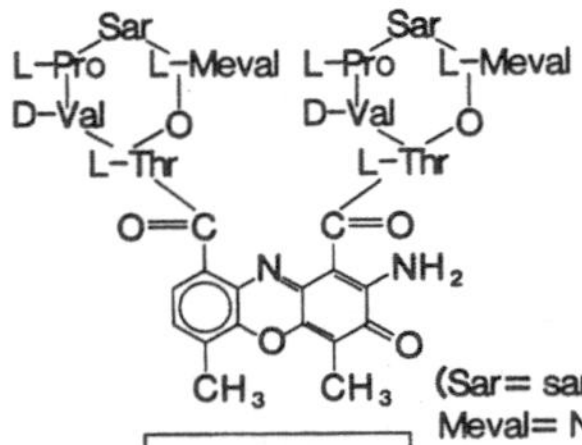

(Sar = sarcosine,
Meval = N–methylvaline)

Dactinomycin

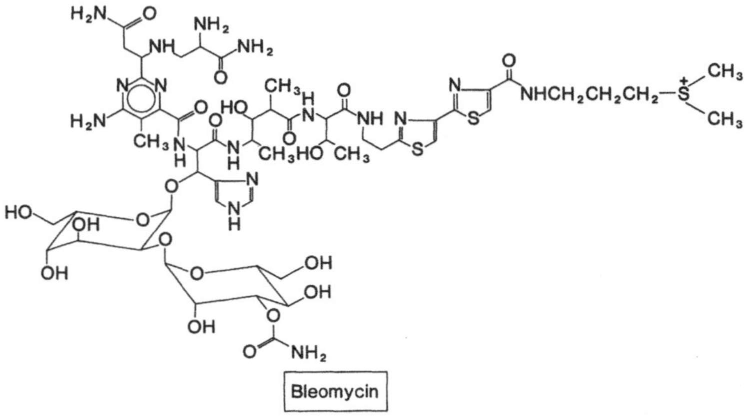

Fig. 3

Morantz et al.[144] describe a Phase I trial of bleomycin in recurrent malignant brain tumors. The drug is given via Ommaya reservoir directly into the tumor bed without apparent toxicity. This, in combination with cranial radiation, did prolong survival. Takahashi et al.[211] report the use of intracyst bleomycin for craniopharyngioma treatment with definite improvement.

Systemic toxicity is less with such intratumoral therapy. Animal toxicity from intraventricular bleomycin results in elevated CSF protein levels, and a necrotizing vasculitis precludes such use in clinical trials[125, 154, 155].

d) Mithramycin

Mithramycin (Fig. 3), another antibiotic, has an effect on osteoclasts and decreases calcium production; it, therefore, is used in treating malignant hypercalcemia. The presumed mechanism of action is binding to DNA and inhibition of RNA synthesis. Toxicity includes a dose-related syndrome of abnormal platelet function and decreased coagulation factors that may manifest initially as epistaxis. In treating Paget's disease, mithramycin reduces alkaline phosphatase activity. It is also used in the treatment of germ cell tumors, especially the embryonal cell type.

Evaluation of mithramycin in early clinical trials suggested activity against intracranial neoplasia, however, further study failed to show an effect against glioblastoma multiforme[221]. Intracarotid administration resulted in hemiplegia[139]. Gastrointestinal hemorrhage is a significant complication of the use of this drug intravenously, and intracranial hemorrhage into tumor has been reported[59]. Although mithramycin has been measured in the CSF, its molecular weight (> 1,000 daltons), poor lipid solubility, and high plasma protein affinity all contribute to its exclusion across the blood-brain barrier (BBB).

e) Mitomycin

Mitomycin-C (Fig. 3) is activated in vivo to alkylate and cross-link DNA. Renal failure and microangiopathic hemolytic anemia have been documented. Pulmonary fibrosis (similar to bleomycin toxicity) and potentiation of doxorubicin-induced cardiac failure have also been noted, as has cumulative myelosuppression. This drug acts during the late G_1 phase and in the early S-phase. The drug is activated in areas of low redox potential and may thus be useful in intratumoral/intracyst treatment, where oxygen tension and/or pH may be decreased[107]. The drug is selectively toxic to hypoxic tumor cells even at relatively low doses, while at higher doses, superoxide radical formation will damage the more oxygenated tumor cells[53]. The drug has been used in treating the brain metastases of large cell lung and oat cell carcinoma[113].

3. Enzymes

Asparaginase

Asparaginase is an enzyme catalyzing the hydrolysis of L-asparagine, the nonessential amino acid synthesized from L-aspartate in normal tissues. Because the enzyme catalyzing asparagine synthesis is present in only very low concentrations in certain malignant tissues, these tumor cells depend on uptake of L-asparagine itself.

L-asparaginase therefore exerts its tumoricidal effect by depleting the circulating pools of L-asparagine, one of the amino acids necessary for protein synthesis. The drug exerts a rapid enzymatic effect. It appears that CSF L-asparagine levels are depleted despite the fact that L-asparaginase remains primarily in the intravascular space with poor CNS penetration[186]. The drug has an interesting array of clinical toxicities including hypersensitivity in 5–20% of patients. The effects of interference with protein synthesis include hypoalbuminemia, coagulation factor deficiency, and hypothyroidism. Confusion, stupor and acute pancreatitis have also been reported. L-asparaginase has immunosuppressive activity, inhibiting antibody synthesis. It also appears to interfere with delayed hypersensitivity and lymphocyte transformation. The drug is used in combination with cytarabine for its synergistic effect in the treatment of CNS leukemia[8].

D. Miscellaneous Agents

1. Cisplatin

Cisplatin (Fig. 4) is an inorganic, heavy metal complex with broad spectrum antitumor activity[129]. The drug attacks negatively charged (nucleophilic) sites on the DNA molecules especially the N-7 position of guanine, thus producing intra- and interstrand cross-links. The drug is cell-cycle nonspecific and actually acts similarly to the alkylating agents. The drug is used in the treatment of germ cell tumors, bladder carcinomas and more recently brain tumors. Prominent nephrotoxicity, with decreased renal blood flow and glomerular filtration rate, is associated with coagulative necrosis of the distal tubular epithelium. Preinfusion hydration is necessary to prevent renal failure. Magnesium wasting and asymptomatic hypomagnesemia are common findings but may manifest with seizures or tetany[30,-74]. In addition to its cytotoxic effects, cisplatin is a radiosensitizer and has been used synergistically with cranial radiation[202].

Cisplatin is well-known for its ototoxic side effects which may be dose-limiting. The mechanism is poorly understood, and perhaps based on the loss of hair cells in the organ of Corti. A peripheral neuropathy, primarily sensory, with paresthesias and dysesthesias, and disturbances of vibratory sensation and proprioception has been described. Motor neuropathy is usually not significant. In contrast to the ototoxicity, which does not improve with discontinuation of the drug, most of the signs and symptoms of the peripheral neuropathy are transient. There are variable reports on the cumulative doses which produce electrophysiologic or clinical symptoms. A number of electrophysiological reports have described absent sensory nerve amplitudes and delayed latencies[114]. Polyphasic and prolonged compound nerve action potentials have also been described. Pathologically, the most frequent effect is a segmental demyelination[219]. Cisplatin belongs to the heavy metal series and peripheral neuropathy has been described in heavy metal poisoning. Two reports of retrobulbar neuritis in patients with cisplatin and one patient with papilledema both resemble similar toxicities with other heavy metals.

Recent trials with intracarotid infusions of cisplatin in brain tumor patients has resulted in augmented neurotoxicity including focal or generalized encephalopathy and retinal blindness. A single patient with cortical blindness and seizures was found to have CSF cisplatin levels equal to blood levels for 18 days postinfusion[16]. This is interesting given the fact that cisplatin does not cross the BBB well. Lowering the dose decreased both toxicity and effectiveness. Neuwelt *et al.*[154] have demonstrated that intraarterial administration in dogs caused severe neurotoxicity and the drug itself appeared to open the BBB. Intravenous use of this drug in combination chemotherapy for recurrent brain tumor continues with some success in pediatric brain tumors[191], and it is under trial in combination with radiation in adult glioma patients[48].

Attempts to decrease toxicity have led to the use of thiosulfate to inactivate cisplatin as a rescue technique. Rescue has been used in association with intraperitoneal cisplatin in the treatment of ovarian carcinoma and malignant ascites but the protective effect is limited to the nephrotoxicity[105, 136].

2. Hydroxyurea (HU)

HU (Fig. 4) is an analog of urea which acts primarily by inhibition of the enzyme ribonucleotide reductase, thus decreasing the availability of nucleic acids necessary for DNA synthesis. HU has been used in combination with radiation therapy as a radiation sensitizer in the treatment of malignant brain tumors. The drug itself does not appear to be neurotoxic. Two early clinical trials in malignant glioma patients demonstrated a significant amount of tumor necrosis[59]. Further trials with HU in combination with radiation therapy followed by other chemotherapy combination drug regimens are in process[7, 23].

3. Procarbazine

Procarbazine (Fig. 4) is a monoamine oxidase (MAO) inhibitor. It is used in the treatment of lymphomas and brain tumors. The drug itself is not cytotoxic but is activated to potentially toxic derivatives. These are thought to be primarily alkylating intermediates and free radicals causing DNA damage. The exact mechanism of action of procarbazine is unknown but there is some suggestion that there is suppression of mitosis as a result of prolonged interphase. Because of the MAO inhibitor potential of this drug, patients ingesting foods high in tyramine are at risk for acute hypertensive crises. The drug also has a disulfiram-like effect in patients ingesting alcohol. It may potentiate the effect of sedative hypnotic drugs secondary to competitive metabolism at the hepatic microsomal enzyme cytochrome P450 site. To minimize this synergism one is cautioned in the use of such agents as barbiturates, antihistamines, narcotics, hypertensive agents or phenothiazines. There is rapid equilibration between plasma and CSF after oral administration.

CNS toxicity, more apparent with intravenous than oral administration manifests with paresthesias, myalgias, neuropathies and confusional states. Although procarbazine is somewhat related to isoniazid, the peripheral neuropathies have not been reversed with the administration of pyridoxine[225]. Orthostatic hypotension is reported in patients receiving procarbazine[114]. Central effects, including disorders of consciousness, have been seen in approximately 30% of the patients and peripheral neuropathies in approximately 17% of the patients[225]. A sensitivity to catecholamines and ataxia have also been described. Procarbazine used as a single agent has been shown to be effective against primary malignant brain tumors[119]. The drug is frequently used in combination brain tumor chemotherapy. Combinations with vincristine, CCNU and prednisone[218] or with vincristine and prednisone (+ /— mechlorethamine)[36] have shown some responses. The drug is also used with MTX and cyclophosphamide in clinical BBB disruption protocols[153, 165–167]. Intravascular hemolysis and the appearance of Heinz-Ehrlich inclusion bodies in red cells have been described in patients taking procarbazine[186].

4. Etoposide

Etoposide (Fig. 4) is a derivative of podophyllotoxin, a drug which inhibits tubulin polymerization. However, the etoposide derivative appears to function by interaction with DNA and production of DNA strand breaks, acting at the G_2 portion of the cell cycle. Two different dose-dependent responses have been seen: at high concentrations, lysis of cells entering mitosis is observed; at low concentrations, the cells are inhibited from entering the prophase[186]. This drug does not interfere with microtubular assembly. Since nucleic acid strand breaks can be repaired by most cells, the drug cytotoxicity is enhanced by inhibition of DNA repair with such agents as caffeine or chloroquine. The drug is felt to be more effective if administered frequently rather than as a single dose[170].

Drug distribution is of interest because of the suggestion that etoposide is active against brain tumors. There is variable distribution of the drug and its metabolites in the CSF[177]. Pharmacokinetic studies after administering a dose of 100 mg/nm^2 IV. show that etoposide penetrates the CSF poorly, but mean drug levels of 1.0 and 1.8 μg/g are seen in brain tumor (primary and metastatic) tissue[203]. Because etoposide induces chromosomal abnormalities it must be considered a carcinogen. Temporary hypotension following rapid intravenous injection of this drug has been noted in a number of patients. The only frequent toxicity is myelosuppression.

Miscellaneous Agents

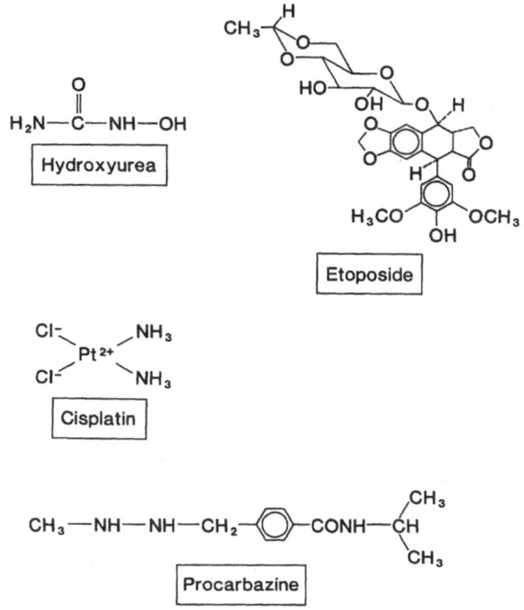

$$H_2N-\overset{O}{\underset{||}{C}}-NH-OH$$

Hydroxyurea

Etoposide

$$\underset{Cl^-}{\overset{Cl^-}{\diagdown}}Pt^{2+}\underset{NH_3}{\overset{NH_3}{\diagup}}$$

Cisplatin

$$CH_3-NH-NH-CH_2-\bigcirc-CONH-\overset{CH_3}{\underset{CH_3}{\overset{|}{C}H}}$$

Procarbazine

Fig. 4

In combination with vincristine there is a synergistic neurotoxicity, a severe neuropathy with muscle atrophy and paralytic ileus which develops in approximately one-third of the patients[186]. The drug has substantial activity in small cell carcinoma of the lung, testicular cancer, lymphoma, and leukemia. A few responses have been seen in uterine cancer, Wilm's tumor, rhabdomyosarcoma, prostate, and thyroid cancer. A phase II trial in recurrent malignant brain tumors has shown some response[214]. Spigelman *et al.*[200, 201] describe intracarotid etoposide modifying the BBB yet intraarterial administration in brain tumor therapy is under clinical investigation[67].

E. Hormones

1. Tamoxifen

This drug is an antiestrogen and its use is based on the principle that certain breast cancer cells (primarily those with estrogen receptors) depend on the presence of estrogen for their growth. The drug blocks the uptake of estrogen by binding to estrogen receptors, which complex is then transported into the cell to bind with nuclear chromatin. The drug may also bind to cytoplasmic receptors or compete with estradiol for binding to cytoplasmic endoplasmic reticulum. It blocks cells in the early G_1 phase. The drug is given orally and appears more effective in menopausal women. It is used in the treatment of disseminated breast carcinoma.

Adverse reactions include hot flashes, nausea, and vomiting. An increase in response rate is reported when the drug is combined with an inhibitor steroid production such as aminoglutethimide[180]. Insufficient data are available to correlate response rate with receptor status. There have also been some trials of tamoxifen combined with chemotherapeutic agents such as the cyclophosphamide-MTX-fluorouracil protocol suggesting an increased therapeutic benefit[180].

As with all of the drugs discussed in this chapter, the question comes as to whether this drug is effective in intracranial disease: does the drug cross the BBB effectively? An interesting case report documents regression of cerebral metastases with tamoxifen treatment following previous treatment with 2,400 rads cranial radiation[38].

When discussing estrogen receptors, the neurooncologist immediately wonders whether such an antiestrogen might have clinical benefit in the management of meningiomas given the various reports of hormone receptors in these tumors. An *in vitro* study of cultured meningioma cells showed that cells were stimulated in the face of estradiol or tamoxifen alone; the combination of these drugs showed an inhibition of the estradiol-stimulated growth[110]. The clinical significance of hormone receptors in meningiomas remain controversial.

2. Steroids

Perhaps the drug to have had the most significant effect in the management of brain tumor patients has been the corticosteroid. While its effect is primarily an anti-edema action rather than oncolytic effect, dramatic improvement in the patient's neurologic state has ensued over hours to days after beginning treatment. As with all the other chemotherapeutic agents, toxicity appears. Steroids alter mood and may lower the threshold for seizures[235]. Iatrogenic Cushing's syndrome and its attendant morbidity is not uncommon. Steroid myopathy is superimposed on primary neurologic deficit. Gastrointestinal bleeding and impairment of host defenses may complicate therapy, as may glucose intolerance requiring insulin. A variety of corticosteroids including prednisone, methylprednisolone, hydrocortisone, and dexamethasone have all been used to benefit these patients. Dexamethasone has less mineralocorticoid (salt-retaining) side effects and more anti-inflammatory effects and is therefore most widely used. Measurements of brain sodium and water content as well as ultrastructural studies of brain and tumor biopsies in patients treated with and without steroids suggest that the steroidal effect is a result of the reduction of cerebral edema[131]. Lieberman[127] describes the use of "high dose corticosteroids" in treating brain tumor patients unresponsive to "conventional" steroid doses. They define a conventional methylprednisolone dose as 80–120 mg/day (16–24 mg/day dexamethasone) and describe the use of high dose 200–2,000 mg/day methylprednisolone (40–400 mg/day dexamethasone) over a 21 day course. They noticed increasing effect with increasing methylprednisolone up to 1,000 mg/day but no difference between 1,000 mg and 2,000 mg/day.

With regard to the oncolytic effect of steroids, human glioblastoma cells grown in culture have been inhibited with high dose methylprednisolone or dexamethasone[221]. The drug is used for its lympholytic effect in the treatment of primary CNS lymphoma[153, 165]. Epidural metastatic disease may respond to the oncolytic effect of steroids[176]. The BTSG clinically addressed the question of oncolytic effect of steroids in a four-armed randomized study comparing methylprednisolone ($400\,mg/m^2/day$ for seven days with three weeks off) with BCNU, procarbazine, and BCNU plus methylprednisolone[87]. This study suggested that steroids in this regimen resulted in significantly decreased survival, particularly when used as a single agent. They also detracted from the single agent BCNU effect.

The mechanism of "vasogenic edema" associated with brain tumors is unknown but may be the result of increased intracapillary pressure[40]. Likewise the effective action of steroids is not understood. Dexamethasone closes the BBB when measured in the C_6 glioma model by quantitative autoradiography. Some authors, however, suggest that the action of dexamethasone is to reduce the extracellular space and decrease bulk flow of plasma-derived tumor fluid without a direct change in capillary permeability[21, 223]. Using a rabbit model, Weissman and Grossman[227] showed that dexamethasone decreases the amount of Evan's blue extravasation in tumor-bearing cerebral hemispheres, suggesting perhaps a relation between BBB disruption and tumor edema. Neuwelt and Frenkel[152] shown that steroids interfere with the enhanced drug delivery seen after BBB disruption. Suffice it to say, steroids are an effective mainstay in CNS tumor treatment.

IV. Practical Pharmacologic Considerations

A. Combination Chemotherapy

Initial combination drug therapy began with the empiric use of a single agent with subsequent addition of agents from different classes [*i.e.,* cyclophosphamide (alkylating agent), MTX (antifolate), and 5-FU (antipyrimidine)]. More recently, a growing understanding of anticancer drug pharmacology has spurred study of combinations based on theoretical (or observed) drug interactions[229]. With the various drug combinations, one is ultimately attempting to find synergism just as with antimicrobial combinations, wherein the net effect of several drugs is more than the sum of their effects. As it turns out, drug synergy in the patient is not predicted by the results of tissue culture studies, as clinical synergy most likely represents the added interplay of drug effect and host immunity. Finally, it must be noted that the same combination of drugs may at times be antagonistic and at other times synergistic based on changes in drug dose ratios, drug sequencing or scheduling[106, 229].

One effect of drug combination can be *biochemical modulation* such that giving one drug enhances the action of a second drug. Many of the drugs are metabolized into active forms *in vivo* and, as biochemical pathways are quite intertwined, one drug may affect several pathways indirectly. Such an example is the fact that cytarabine uptake and effectiveness can be attenuated by MTX, fluorouracil and thymidine. However, if exogenous purines are given with MTX and cytarabine, the combination becomes synergistically cytotoxic[109]. MTX can also enhance the conversion of 5-FU to its respectibe nucleotide and this combination of MTX and a pyrimidine analog can actually overcome the resistance of tumor cells to a single agent. Conversely, vincristine and etoposide can enhance the activating metabolism of MTX[223].

Most of the cytotoxic agents act by inhibition of biochemical pathways. Compound drug synergy multiplies this inhibition in a sequential, concurrent, complementary, or concerted manner. Examples of each are well-described by White et al.[229]. Hydroxyurea acts *sequentially* with fluorouracil to thus inhibit the pyrimidine base substrate and its enzyme thymidylate synthetase[143]. An example of *concurrent* inhibition, interrupting two alternate pathways in the synthesis of a metabolite, is theoretically possible by combining hydroxurea and cytarabine. *Complementary* inhibition involves the combination of an alkylating agent to damage DNA and an antimetabolite to block further DNA synthesis or repair; examples of such include combining MTX with doxorubicin and either cytarabine, cisplatin or etoposide. By inhibiting DNA repair, accumulated genetic mutations can result in "error amplification"[83] and thus increased cytotoxicity. *Concerted* inhibition involves drug interference at several sites along the biochemical pathway simultaneously. Combining thymidine with fluorouracil, MTX, and cytarabine allows the biochemical modulation of thymidine to interfere with the cytotoxicity of the other drugs. By interfering with drug degradation and thus prolonging the plasma half-life of these agents, thymidine added to the treatment regimen increases toxicity[116].

The synergistic effect of drug combinations may be schedule-dependent such that timing and sequencing drug delivery may account for variable responses in clinical trials[106]. Cell cycle specific (S-phase) drugs such as cytarabine, MTX and hydroxurea are particularly effective during the tumor's rapid recovery phase of DNA synthesis following inhibition by a previous drug[229]. Synchronization of the tumor cell population has been demonstrated with cytarabine and vincristine[212]. There are animal data suggesting enhanced survival if MTX precedes 5-FU by 1–6 hours. Several mechanisms for this synergy are postulated[66]. There is also a schedule-dependency between L-asparaginase and MTX such that pretreating with L-asparaginase just prior to MTX diminishes/inhibits the MTX effect, but if this latter drug is delayed until there has been a postasparaginase recovery of DNA synthesis, the MTX effect is enhanced[37, 137]. One might postulate such effects with other drug combinations.

Most of the anticancer agents are operant inside the cell. Lipophilic drugs such as etoposide, dactinomycin, vincristine, doxorubicin, and vinblastine can interact with the cell membrane and thus alter permeability of other cytotoxic agents[236]. Verapamil can increase vincristine uptake[215], and vincristine given 24–48 hours after MTX displays synergism by inhibiting this latter's efflux without affecting influx[86]. Probenecid also inhibits cellular MTX efflux[196]. Another synergistic effect is noted between vinblastine and bleomycin. The effect of bleomycin is significantly enhanced if vinblastine is administered 6–8 hours prior to the administration of bleomycin. This schedule permits more cells to be arrested during metaphase, the cell cycle stage at which bleomycin acts[229].

Competitive plasma protein binding may occur between cytotoxic drugs and with other medications. Particularly important for the neurooncologist is the fact that liver microsomal enzymes are induced by phenobarbital, a drug widely used in brain tumor patients. Cyclophosphamide is more rapidly activated following administration of barbiturates.

In brain tumor chemotherapy, relatively few drug combinations have been tried. An interesting experience to again emphasize dosing and scheduling is the experience of the BTSG where the BCNU—procarbazine study initially failed. Laboratory work suggested larger doses of BCNU, and adding procarbazine 4–8 days later resulted in increased effect and reduced toxicity. Given the significant number of chemotherapeutic agents, the potential for combinations is numerous, and when one considers dosage ranges and drug sequencing, the number of trials becomes awesome.

Edwards et al.[59] have reviewed the various published protocols between 1969 and 1980 and note that much of the literature is anecdotal. Others more recently have developed new methods of discussing response, remission, and survival noting their subjectivity and thus poor inter-trial comparability. Edwards et al.[59] also call for evaluation of new combinations, new dosages, and new drug scheduling. They recommend the use of low molecular weight, highly lipid soluble cell-cycle nonspecific agents in combination to maximize effectiveness. Others argue for cell-cycle specific drugs effective in different phases.

Thus many sources suggest that, because of differential tumor cell sensitivity in a heterogenous cell population, combination chemotherapy will ultimately be required for effective brain tumor control. An exciting example of such an approach is the combination eight drug regimen which includes vincristine, CCNU, procarbazine, HU, cisplatin, cytarabine, cyclophosphamide (or dacarbazine) and methylprednisolone. This new regimen includes lipid and water soluble drugs, cell-cycle specific and nonspecific drugs in sequences to enhance combined cytotoxicity[7, 23, 183]. By giving all drugs in a 24-hour period, multiple myelosuppressive effects may not be additive. An additional advantage is that the drug course precedes radiation therapy. As with all chemotherapy trials, it remains too early to accurately evaluate results and come to significant conclusions.

B. Drug Resistance

Normal cells have not yet been shown to develop resistance to anticancer agents, while tumor cell resistance takes a number of forms[186]. Resistance to alkylating agents develops via at least two methods: either loss of the capacity to transport drug across the cell membranes or by synthesis of larger quantities of sulfhydryl-containing proteins which avidly bind alkylating agents. Resistance to those drugs which modify DNA structure (bleomycin) develops as an increased ability to repair such modified DNA.

There are three methods of resistance that can develop to the enzyme inhibitors. These include increased amounts of the target enzyme, increased degradation of the inhibitory drug, or alternative biochemical pathways. Resistance can also develop on the basis of enhanced drug extrusion (anthracyclines, vinca alkaloids, dactinomycin) or gene amplification. MTX resistance can be threefold: 1. impaired or defective transport of MTX into cells, 2. altered forms of the enzyme dihydrofolate reductase with decreased affinity for the inhibitor MTX, and 3. increased intracellular dihydrofolate reductase.

Resistance can develop as tumor cells require less of a specific metabolic product (asparaginase). Cytarabine resistance develops as increased drug inactivation. Tumor cells can be resistant to 5-FU on the basis of insufficient drug activation.

At the more basic level, drug resistance is beginning to correlate with chromosomal abnormalities. Stimulation of DNA synthesis, a characteristic of BCNU-resistant cells, correlates with a hyperploidy of chromosome 22[193]. The phenomenon of "pleomorphic drug resistance" describes the ability of cancer cells to be cross-resistant to a number of agents either spontaneously or after exposure to a single drug (doxorubicin, vinca alkaloids, dactinomycin)[49]. While such pleomorphic resistance thwarts clinical treatment, it happens that development of resistance may be associated with increased sensitivity to cyclophosphamide and steroids and may correlate with extra-chromosomal DNA and/or alteration of membrane proteins[49].

Of further interest is the observation from cell culture lines that doxorubicin and vincristine resistance can be reversed with calcium channel blockers such as verapamil[215]. Although the mechanism is unknown, a clinical trial with verapamil and doxorubicin is underway.

C. Neurotoxicity

A number of chemotherapeutic agents used in the treatment of both primary and secondary CNS malignancies have occasional and sometimes frequent neurotoxic side effects. Because the patient's primary disease itself may well manifest progression and regression based on neurologic changes, it is important for any clinician to be aware of the potential neurotoxic side effects which may well aggravate the patient's underlying neurologic condition. Such a situation might mimic progressive neurologic tumor-induced deterioration and it is important, therefore, to differentiate these. Furthermore, metastatic disease, in addition to its local neurologic effects, may manifest any one of a number of "paraneoplastic syndromes" including: encephalomyelitis, cerebellar cortical degeneration, peripheral neuropathy, myopathies, myastenia, myotonia, polymyositis, cerebrovascular disorders, and paraproteinemia[97]. The neurologic syndromes caused by the various antineoplastic agents, either alone, or in combination, cover the gamut of neurologic disease from diffuse encephalopathy to specific neuropathies (Table 3). There may be acute or chronic presentations; some effects are dose-related, others appear more idiosyncratic. Some respond to drug discontinuation or reduction. For the most part, the mechanism of these neurotoxicities is unknown. Given that neural cells are primarily in G_0, the neurotoxic effects are unlikely to be the result of direct antineoplastic action (nucleic acid alkylation or enzyme inhibition), but may be more the result of membrane and transport interference (anticancer drugs also bind to hormone receptors and the microtubule structure). This point actually assumes even more importance considering that optimal membrane integrity and cellular transport are probably the dominant activities of neural cells.

The drugs notorious for neurotoxicity include MTX, cisplatin, vincristine, 5-FU, asparaginase, procarbazine, doxorubicin, cytarabine, etoposide, and intracarotid BCNU. Other drugs less commonly have associated neurotoxic effects. A

Table 3. Neurotoxic syndromes

---

1. Neuropathies
   Chlorambucil
   Cisplatin
   Cytarabine
   Etoposide
   Fluorouracil
   Mechlorethamine
   Procarbazine
   Vinca alkaloids

2. Myopathies
   Steroids
   Vincristine

3. Arachnoiditis/myelopathy/encephalomyelopathy
   Cytarabine
   Methotrexate
   Thiotepa

4. Acute encephalopathies
   Asparaginase
   Carmustine
   Chlorambucil
   Cisplatin
   Cyclophosphamide
   Cytarabine
   Fluorouracil
   Mechlorethamine
   Methotrexate
   Procarbazine
   Vincristine

5. Chronic encephalopathies
   Cytarabine
   Methotrexate

6. Acute cerebellar syndrome
   Carmustine
   Fluorouracil
   Mechlorethamine
   Procarbazine
   Vincristine

7. Syndrome of inappropriate antidiuretic hormone
   Cyclophosphamide
   Vincristine

---

comprehensive review of this subject by Kaplan and Wiernik delineates the reports and theories for each of the drugs[114].

1. Peripheral Neuropathy

Drug-induced peripheral neuropathies represent a confusing disease category (Table 4). Cranial nerves or distal nerves may be affected as may the autonomic nervous system. Peripheral neuropathy has been classified descriptively (sensory, sensorimotor) or pathophysiologically (axonal degeneration, demyelination, uncertain). These various classifications make no attempt at etiologic explanation.

The peripheral neuropathy seen with *cisplatin* is a bilaterally symmetric, predominantly sensory neuropathy associated with paresthesias and dysesthesias involving both the upper and lower extremities. Vibratory and position sense are the most affected[114]. Deep tendon reflexes are decreased but present, and the neuropathy is generally reversible. The marked proprioceptive abnormality makes one wonder about neurotoxicity at the cord level. However, nerve conduction studies suggest a sensorimotor peripheral neuropathy with unobtainable sensory nerve action potentials, polyphasic and widened nerve action potentials and prolongation of the nerve fiber relative refractory period. Just as there is clinical reversal of symptoms, the nerve conduction changes are reported to be reversible as well. Such findings suggest demyelination as the mechanism of the peripheral neurotoxicity[213]. Pathologic correlation has been variable with one report showing scattered destruction of myelin sheaths and intact axons suggestive of a segmental demyelination process[219] while another report showed mixed myelin sheath and axonal lesions[114]. As cisplatin is considered a member of the heavy metal group one might suggest that the same mechanism in heavy metal peripheral neuropathy may be operant in cisplatin neuropathy[114].

The characteristic peripheral neuropathy of *vincristine* is manifest early and consistently with loss of deep tendon reflexes in the lower extremities. Drug continuation may result in more symptomatic neurotoxicity including muscle pain, weakness, gait disturbances and sensory impairment. In some sense the weakness appears out of proportion to the sensory deficit. A single dose of vincristine may result in reflex abnormalities which resolve in one to three months. Neither thiamine nor B_{12} therapy has been found to be of benefit in treating the vincristine neuropathy[114]. Vincristine toxicity results in axonal degeneration. Electrophysiologic studies show minimal impairment of nerve conduction velocities in the face of a severe neuropathy; histology confirms axonal loss. Ultrastructurally there is a loss of microtubules and proliferation of neurofilaments.

Procarbazine, mechlorethamine, etoposide and cytarabine have all been associated with peripheral neuropathies as well. The mechanism of these neuropathies is unknown. It is interesting that the mechlorethamine neurotoxicity may be improved with pyridoxine therapy while the procarbazine peripheral neuropathy, which tends to come on after several weeks of oral therapy, appears to be unaffected by pyridoxine even though procarbazine itself is somewhat chemically related to isoniazid, the toxicity of which can be treated with pyridoxine. Both these drugs have been shown to lower pyridoxal phosphate *in vivo*[225]. Etoposide has been associated with a rare peripheral neuritis.

Cranial neuropathies have been reported with fluorouracil, cisplatin, and vincristine. Those associated with cisplatin include ototoxicity, a vestibular neuronitis and retrobulbar neuritis. Cranial neuropathies with vincristine include a recurrent laryngeal nerve paresis affecting the vocal cords, oculomotor nerve dysfunction, facial palsy and optic neuropathy. All the cranial nerve findings tend to be bilateral and reversible on discontinuation of therapy[114].

An autonomic neuropathy may be an early manifestation of vincristine toxicity with constipation and abdominal pain. Bladder atony and orthostatic hypotension have been described. Autonomic effects are also seen with procarbazine, and orthostatic hypotension has been described in some 8% of patients receiving this drug alone[114].

Table 4. Antineoplastic drug-induced neuropathies

A. Cranial
     cisplatin
     fluorouracil
     vincristine
	2. Descriptive presentation
	     a) Sensory
	         cisplatin
	         procarbazine
	         vincristine

B. Peripheral
     1. Pathophysiologic etiology
         a) Axonal degeneration
             vincristine
         b) Demyelination
             cisplatin
         c) Uncertain
             chlorambucil
             cytarabine
             etoposide
             procarbazine
	b) Sensorimotor
	         vincristine
	
	C. Autonomic
	     etoposide
	     procarbazine
	     vincristine

2. Myopathy

Steroid myopathy is seen in approximately 7% of those patients receiving steroids, and occurs more frequently as patients requiring dexamethasone live longer. The onset is usually insidious, and within several months of beginning therapy patients present with atrophy and symmetric proximal weakness. While this myopathy may slowly respond to drug discontinuation, such is often not feasible in brain tumor patients. Vincristine has been associated with a toxic myopathy, clinically apparent with weakness, atrophy, and muscle pain, and histologically described with necrosis, myofibrillary disruption, and autophagocytosis[111, 235].

3. Arachnoiditis/Myelopathy

An acute meningeal irritation/arachnoiditis has been described with intrathecal drug administration, particularly MTX. This syndrome begins 3–4 hours following infusion and may last up to three days. It includes all of the signs and symptoms of meningitis including fever, stiff neck, headache, nausea, vomiting, lethargy, and CSF pleocytosis, and occurs in up to 60% of patients, both those treated prophylactically and those with meningeal disease[114]. This has been described for MTX, cytarabine, and thiotepa in combination and separately.

A paraplegic syndrome, either permanent or temporary, has also been described with each of the three drugs. This may be the result of demyelination or perhaps direct toxicity. It is seen with several drug preparations, with and without preservatives, with and without dilution using water, saline, or Elliott's B solution[82]. It is seen in patients treated prophylactically and in those with central nervous system disease. Pathologically, areas of necrosis and gliosis are described at the base of the brain, along the spinal cord, and at the root entry zones[114]. Elevated levels of myelin basic protein have been reported suggesting an early and direct effect on the myelin sheath following MTX, cytarabine, and hydrocortisone[42]. Neither the arachnoiditis nor the myelopathy are specifically related to radiation treatment or intracranial radiation. Accidental intrathecal vincristine results in an ascending neurotoxicity with eventual death[198, 230].

4. Acute Encephalopathy

An acute encephalopathy has been the key neurotoxic syndrome associated with asparaginase use. Lethargy, confusion, seizures and hallucinations, usually transient have been described[230]. An acute encephalopathic syndrome progressing even to coma has also been described with MTX. Cytarabine either alone in high dose or in combination with MTX has been implicated in a reversible dose-limiting acute encephalopathy[11a]. Procarbazine as a monoamine oxidase inhibitor can manifest with CNS depression and altered level of consciousness. An encephalopathic syndrome has also been described with cyclophosphamide[114]. Intracarotid mechlorethamine has produced seizures, coma, and death[225]. 5-FU used in conjunction with allopurinol is associated with an encephalopathy manifesting seizures, hemiparesis, and brain stem dysfunction[114]. Coma, parkinsonism, and visual disturbances have also been noted[111]. Seizures and papilledema acutely with systemic cisplatin have been reported, and intracarotid drug has also resulted in permanent neurologic deficits[16]. While confusion, delirium, and coma have been described with vincristine, additional chemotherapy or metabolic misbalance may have been responsible[114].

Intracarotid infusion of BCNU has been associated with a number of neurotoxic events including an acute diffuse hemispheric encephalopathy[78, 90, 114]. Pathologically, a necrotizing arteriolitis has been noted with intracarotid nitrosourea infusion[114]. This neurotoxicity, initially thought to be secondary to the alcohol diluent, is now considered possibly the result of nonuniform drug delivery secondary to drug streaming as a result of laminar flow[20, 90, 121, 182]. This is seen especially with superselective catheterization for intracarotid infusion distal to the ophthalmic artery. High dose BCNU systemically without cranial radiation can produce a dramatic encephalomyelopathy[32].

5. Chronic Encephalopathy

Beginning in the early 1970's a chronic encephalopathic syndrome associated with MTX administration, primarily intrathecal or intraventricular, has been described. The syndrome initially involves a clinical picture of confusion, somnolence, irritability, ataxia, dementia, tremor and seizures. Over time, this can progress to include spasticity, quadriparesis, visual disturbances, other focal findings, coma, and death. It has been described as transient, progressive, or permanent[114]. Discrete multifocal areas of coagulative necrosis are seen in the white matter. There is associated gliosis but lack of inflammatory reaction. Axonal damage is also noted[111, 114]. This has since been recognized as a disseminated, necrotizing leukoencephalopathy. The pure syndrome itself usually lacks vascular changes and this is to be differentiated from an associated postradiation vascular damage also described. Elevated levels of myelin basic protein and β_2 microglobulin have been described[114]. This syndrome is seen with cranial radiation alone, intrathecal MTX alone, and intravenous MTX alone as well. Any combination of these three treatment modalities does increase the percent of patients developing this syndrome. The most toxic combination is intravenous MTX combined with intracranial radiation and intrathecal MTX, with 45% of leukemic patients thus treated developing the syndrome[22]. In addition, it appears that the sequence of administration (*i.e.*, the radiation therapy prior to MTX) has a major contribution to developing this syndrome. There have been no documented reports of delayed leukoencephalopathy in patients who received MTX therapy prior to radiation and not resumed[22]. The CT abnormality consists of low density regions paraventricularly, ventricular and subarachnoid dilatation. There may or may not be calcification in the central white matter. Delayed encephalopathy has also been described with intrathecal thiotepa, cytarabine, and high dose systemic BCNU[111].

The mechanisms responsible for the cytarabine or MTX neurotoxicity are unknown. Demyelination is a major factor in both the myelopathic syndrome and as a contributing aspect to the leukoencephalopathy. Abnormalities of CSF dynamics may contribute to persistently elevated CSF drug levels and hence a propensity for neurotoxicity. The ability of vincristine to augment the CSF levels of MTX has also been described but the mechanism is not understood[86]. The interaction of cranial radiation and MTX may have as its basis endothelial damage and disruption of the BBB after radiation therapy. This seems unlikely in the face of growing experience with BBB disruption and subsequent MTX infusion without any apparent evidence of leukoencephalopathy[148, 152, 153, 165–167]. Another potential mechanism of toxicity relates to the dihydrofolate reductase identified in human brain tumors. It is quite possible that with inhibition of this enzyme, a subsequent cellular accumulation of dihydrofolate might be toxic to the brain[2, 114]. In addition, MTX-induced inhibition of tetrahydrobiopterin, a cofactor in biogenic amine and serotonin synthesis may contribute to a MTX-induced neurotoxic syndrome on the basis of decreased availability of these neurotransmitters[114].

Monitoring drug-induced leukoencephalopathy has been difficult. Certain CT scan changes may be seen as may elevations of myelin basic protein and/or β_2 microglobulin. However, none of these are consistent and all may be normal in patients with clinical leukoencephalopathy. More recently MRI has demonstrated cerebral demyelination periventricularly in patients with combination radiation/chemotherapy[80].

6. Acute Cerebellar Syndrome

An acute cerebellar syndrome has been described with 5-FU and procarbazine as well as BCNU and vincristine. An ataxic syndrome with agitation may result from vincristine administration. This neurotoxicity, though, appears to be synergistic with the combined addition of 5-FU and cyclophosphamide.

The characteristic cerebellar syndrome with 5-FU consists of slurred speech, nystagmus and dizziness as well as dysmetria, truncal and extremity ataxia and gait difficulty. This syndrome is not related to cumulative dose but rather to the plasma level of the drug[225]. This is usually reversible. Pathologically the cerebellar lesions include chromatolysis of neurons in the olive and dentate nucleus. There is also a diffuse neuronal cell loss in the granular layer[114]. An important clinical point is that cerebellar toxicity must not be confused with either direct tumor effects or, in fact, the remote effects of cancer which commonly affect the cerebellum. Ataxia is described with the use of procarbazine. Loss of equilibrium and ataxia have also been reported with intravenous BCNU therapy. Intention tremor, ataxia and vertigo may be seen with mechlorethamine[114]. Recently a patient receiving high dose cytarabine developed a fatal cerebellar syndrome and was found to have extensive Purkinje cell loss at autopsy[55]. There is clinical evidence that the cytarabine effect on the cerebellum is cumulative[14].

7. Syndrome of Inappropriate Antidiuretic Hormone

The syndrome of inappropriate antidiuretic hormone (SIADH) has been described with the use of vincristine and cyclophosphamide. Cyclophosphamide causes a transient decrease in free-water clearance and urine volume with subsequent decreased serum sodium concentration. It has been argued whether the mechanism is ADH release from the hypothalamic/pituitary axis or whether it is ectopic ADH or an ADH-like kidney effect[114]. This effect is observed 4–12 hours after cyclophosphamide administration and may last up to 20 hours. The administration of vincristine has also resulted in hyponatremia resulting from inappropriate ADH secretion. Seizures with the hyponatremia after vincristine administration have been reported[114].

V. Histopathologic Effects of Brain Tumor Chemotherapy

As chemotherapy (either with or without, preceding or following radiation therapy) becomes more acceptable in brain tumor treatment, it will become increasingly important to understand drug effects on both tumor and normal brain. This will be important in choosing the most effective agents and will be necessary in evaluating CNS toxicity. Because chemotherapy has usually followed radiation, it has been difficult to define histopathologic changes that are solely the result of chemotherapy. However, recent reviews by Jellinger[111, 112] of the pathologic changes seen in tumors as well as the neuropathology associated with CNS toxicity syndromes defines the changes as distinctly as possible. The changes seen in glioblastomas treated with CCNU or polychemotherapy (cyclophosphamide, vincristine, mechlorethamine, prednisone) included significant increase in giant cells, monstrous cells, nuclear inclusions, and nuclear hyperchromasia[112]. While necrosis and vascular changes were increased, these did not reach statistical significance; cellularity, pleomorphism and mitoses were decreased. Tumor-associated cystic cavities have been seen following therapy, and may themselves produce significant mass effect.

Toxic changes in the nontumor CNS have been described clinically; histopathologically they take several forms. Disseminated necrotizing leukoencephalopathy following intravenous vincristine and intrathecal MTX shows coagulation necrosis focally but extending to confluence without inflammatory response[112]. Demyelination and axonal swelling and damage, astrocytosis, and white matter status spongiosis are also seen along with Rosenthal fibers in the cortex and brain stem[31]. Fibrinoid vascular necrosis is also described, but in most reports this has been observed only with combined radiation and chemotherapy[112].

However, Burger et al.[32] also described a similar encephalomyelopathy following systemic high dose BCNU without cranial irradiation. Their patients had the above pathologic changes prominent in pons, corpus callosum and spinal cord white matter. In addition they demonstrated fibrinoid necrosis following the limbic system (temporal lobes, insula, amygdala, and hypothalamus).

Subpial necrosis of brain and spinal cord gray matter, either diffuse or sharply demarcated, without evidence of vascular changes or inflammation, has been seen in nonirradiated patients treated with intrathecal MTX, thiotepa, or cytarabine[112]. Intrathecal drugs can result acutely in subpial edema[31], and perhaps the lepto-meningeal fibrosis seen frequently in leukemic patients is the similar result of a chronic insult. Cerebral atrophy is seen following intrathecal MTX and correlates with illness duration. The myelopathy described with intrathecal drugs shows anterior horn necrosis as well as white matter demyelination. Mineralizing microangiopathy and the dystrophic calcification seen with MTX are not described with chemotherapy in the absence of radiation[114].

Neuroaxonal dystrophy in the long tracts and medulla is seen at autopsy in patients receiving systemic vincristine; nerve cell bodies in the medulla also show central neuronal chromatolysis[31]. These changes may be the retrograde result of a vincristine peripheral neuropathy. Other histopathologic changes seen in association with chemotherapy, including central pontine myelinolysis and the changes of Wernicke's encephalopathy, may well be the result of metabolic and/or nutritional insult rather than chemotherapeutic agents.

VI. Modes of Drug Administration

As with many aspects of neurooncology, therapeutic approaches have been designed along the lines of general oncology. Chemotherapy for systemic disease emphasizes control of metastases, a key part of most malignancies. Thus adequate tissue exposure against such metastases is required throughout the body. Hence an emphasis on high dose intravenous drug administration. In contrast, primary brain malignancy spreads within the CNS only 5% of the time and extracranial metastases are very rare, $\sim 0.1\%$ incidence[126]. Thus chemotherapy against brain neoplasia need not necessarily focus on systemic delivery except with regard to drug exposure and toxicity.

In an attempt to circumvent the problem of the BBB, higher doses of anticancer drugs are given with attendant increased toxicity. This has generated a number of unique attempts to maximize the concentration × time ($C \times T$) parameter while minimizing systemic drug toxicity. Current studies also define the role of bolus dosing and continuous infusion. Such novel approaches are particularly justified in primary brain tumor therapy because this disease rarely leaves the CNS.

A. Intraarterial Administration

The rationale of intraarterial chemotherapy infusion involves augmentation of an increased "peak concentration over infusion time". This route of administration offers an advantage over the conventional intravenous route only during the initial first passage; thereafter the intraarterial concentrations are similar to intravenous levels. If rates of biotransformation, metabolism, and excretion during the first pass are high, a larger amount of drug can be delivered to the brain for a similar degree of systemic toxicity. This route of drug administration was pioneered using mechlorethamine in the 1950's with disappointing results [10]. In attempts to decrease toxicity, researchers developed an elaborate method of vessel isolation-perfusion using carotid arteries and jugular veins. Toxicity of the procedure itself with thromboembolic and bleeding complications as well as increased CNS and ocular toxicity dampened enthusiasm for this route of drug administration. However, more recently renewed efforts at this approach have led to evaluation of a number of agents: MTX, vincristine, vinblastine, mechlorethamine, melphalan, BCNU, cisplatin, etoposide, and tenoposide. Also reminiscent of the past experience is the new discussion of improving therapeutic ratio by intraarterial drug infusion and removal of drug by dialysis, another sound theory yet to be clinically proven [47, 172].

With intraarterial infusions there are several factors that influence drug uptake, toxicity and effectiveness. The tissue partition coefficient measures the capacity of a given tissue to uptake drug. Drug-tissue interaction is affected by protein binding, membrane transport, and extracellular diffusion [205]. A decrease in cerebral blood flow will enhance the effective arterial concentration in that slow blood flow allows for higher tissue drug extraction. This extraction fraction measures the rate of blood-brain exchange [64, 205]. Perhaps the most important parameter, though, for promoting the possible advantage of intraarterial administration over intravenous administration is the rate of systemic drug breakdown or clearance; delivery of a more rapidly metabolized or excreted drug will be enhanced by intraarterial administration [64]. Certain drugs have the property of rapid intravascular degradation; with intraarterial drug delivery this property is an advantage in that it limits systemic exposure to the drug and therefore has decreased systemic toxicity.

However, in intraarterial injections it is not systemic toxicity but rather local toxicity which limits use. Balloon catheterization with superselective arterial drug delivery has the advantage of increased selective drug delivery but has the attendant risk of thromboembolic complications and cerebral ischemia [205]. Slow continuous infusions may have a therapeutic advantage over rapid bolus in that the latter affords higher drug concentration and hence increased toxicity compared to the former. The concentration × time (C × T) parameter is not affected by infusion rate [205].

The use of intraarterial mechlorethamine by Mahaley and Woodhall resulted in a significant number of patients who died from drug-induced cerebral edema [205]. Other agents tried then via this technique were melphalan, cyclophosphamide and thiotepa. Intra-arterial MTX both with and without BBB disruption has been used. A single patient with a meningiosarcoma was treated with intraarterial fluorouracil [205]. Intracarotid vincristine has resulted in ipsilateral conjunctival toxicity as well as ophthalmoplegia, and, in patients with prior cranial radiation, severe local CNS toxicity. Wilson *et al.*[232] has used both intracarotid and vertebral artery infusions of vinblastine with some tumor response.

Intracarotid cisplatin has been studied extensively by Stewart *et al.*[202, 206]. Neurologic toxicity as well as retinal toxicity with blindness has been reported. Besides cisplatin another major chemotherapeutic agent under study with intra-carotid infusion is BCNU, which can produce neurologic dysfunction and an associated vasculitis[206]. Greenberg *et al.*[90] describes retinal vasculitis in nine of 36 patients treated with intraarterial BCNU; unexpected white matter necrosis was seen in seven patients. Others note a higher incidence of symptomatic leukoencephalopathy[78]. The associated retinal toxicity was reported less often with supraophthalmic infusion and the use of another drug vehicle. It appears however that these two modifications of the BCNU chemotherapy program have not improved the therapeutic ratio. More recent work with flow models suggests that some of the toxicity with intraarterial chemotherapy may result from drug streaming and nonuniform drug delivery[20].

Intracarotid mithramycin has been given as has doxorubicin[139]. Etoposide intra-arterially is currently under clinical trial. The drug appears well-tolerated; toxicity in 12 patients included transient lethargy in one and a grand mal seizure in another[67].

Intraarterial therapy with a combination of BCNU, cisplatin, and tenoposide has shown some effect as has each of the agents alone[68, 69, 206]. Again problems with diluent toxicity are seen with BCNU and cisplatin. Transient marked cardio-respiratory depression was seen with vertebral artery infusions of BCNU and tenoposide[206].

Stewart *et al.*[208] have also used intracarotid mitomycin in treating patients with primary and metastatic brain tumors. While neurotoxicity and ocular side effects were significant at doses of $18 \, mg/m^2$, further study is underway at a lower dose. More recent drug protocols for intracarotid delivery include a combination of mithramycin and vincristine. Other studies combine BCNU with vincristine followed by oral procarbazine and a combination of BCNU with either cisplatin or etoposide. These combinations have been associated with transient decreased neurologic function.

Further emphasizing the importance of drug delivery, Stewart *et al.*[208] have observed, as has Neuwelt *et al.*[161] with other drugs, that tumor bridging two circulations, one infused and one not, showed regression on the treated side and progression in the untreated hemisphere. Intraarterial chemotherapeutic protocols have reported initial tumor response but subsequent tumor progression, suggesting the emergence of drug resistance. Alternatively, one might argue that BBB permeability is high initially with attendant good drug delivery intraarterially. However, as the tumor responds, BBB permeability is likely to decrease with subsequent impaired drug penetration. Thus, what appears as drug resistance, may in fact simply be inadequate drug delivery.

Intraarterial chemotherapy with the currently available drugs has the potential for significant local toxicity although it may limit systemic toxicity. It is therefore important to determine which drugs can be used without significant local toxicity but with a diminution in systemic toxicity. Several methods for further direct arterial catheterization are under investigational trial.

B. Intrathecal Administration

This method of chemotherapeutic administration has developed as an attempt to deliver larger or polar drugs past the BBB. However, there are several limitations. Initial clinical and experimental work has involved lumbar subarachnoid injection. Such a method may not allow uniform drug distribution and intraventricular flow is frequently limited. Furthermore, the tumor itself may interfere with CSF flow or be relatively isolated from the CSF, precluding adequate drug delivery (Fig. 5). Finally, the tumor may be of sufficient mass that herniation risk prohibits lumbar puncture. To circumvent the problems of lumbar injection, cisternal and/or intraventricular installation have been used. The latter, via an Ommaya reservoir, also lends itself to more prolonged infusion. Assured CSF administration and more even drug distribution are also advantages of the intraventricular route, not to mention apparent increased drug efficacy[175]. Intrathecal agents most commonly used include MTX, cytarabine and thiotepa.

CSF pharmacokinetics are sufficiently different that each drug should be evaluated independently. For instance, while MTX has a serum half life of 45 minutes, its CSF half life is approximately 4½ hours[92, 175]. Drug penetration intraparenchymally is limited, being maximum for MTX to a depth of 3.2 mm at one hour[92, 175]. Because the depth of drug penetration is somewhat influenced by perfusion time, Wilson conducted a 36-hour perfusion study which, though abandoned temporarily, may have some applicability to treatment of meningeal carcinomatosis[232]. Drug distribution in the CSF is influenced by a number of factors including bulk CSF flow, diffusion through the extracellular spaces of the brain and spinal cord, transport across the choroid plexus, removal by CSF absorption, and diffusion from the extracellular space into the capillaries of the CNS[175].

In evaluating drugs for CSF installation a number of factors should be considered. First, from experience with MTX it appears that toxicity is proportional to drug dose. An ideal drug should be slowly cleared from the CSF with rapid extracellular distribution and slow uptake by the capillaries. Nonpolar lipid-soluble agents such as the nitrosoureas readily diffuse across brain capillaries thus having a very short CSF half-life and limited use via this route. In intrathecal therapy, CSF protein content which can be both advantageous and disadvantageous. Elevated CSF protein may be associated with significant drug binding and thus decreased amounts of free CSF drug. Conversely, elevated levels of CSF protein may interfere with normal CSF absorption affording more prolonged CSF drug levels.

To implement the important concentration × time effect, Poplack et al.[175] have studied a method to allow minimal but prolonged tumoricidal levels of MTX in the CSF. Via an Ommaya reservoir, instead of the single intraventricular injection, a series of injections every 12 hours over a 72-hour period maintains a therapeutic level for the 72-hour period as opposed to approximately 32 hours with the single injection. This intermittent technique may also be associated with less neurotoxicity. Another attempt to maintain CSF drug levels would be to decrease CSF clearance. Drug clearance is via CSF reabsorption, diffuse bulk CSF flow, transport across cell membranes, and absorption into capillaries. Probenecid, an inhibitor of the active transport of MTX, has been used clinically to prolong CSF MTX levels presumably by inhibiting the drug's active transport across the choroid plexus[175]. One might also postulate the use of acetazolamide to decrease CSF production and thus reduce the bulk flow and turnover of CSF and intrathecal drugs[175].

The ventriculo-lumbar CSF perfusion method of drug therapy has been investigated by both Poplack and Wilson[179]. The theoretical advantage of this method is that the CSF will be exposed to prolonged high levels of drug with supposedly less systemic absorption and thus less systemic toxicity. The latter aspect of systemic/CSF concentration ratios has not been well-investigated to date.

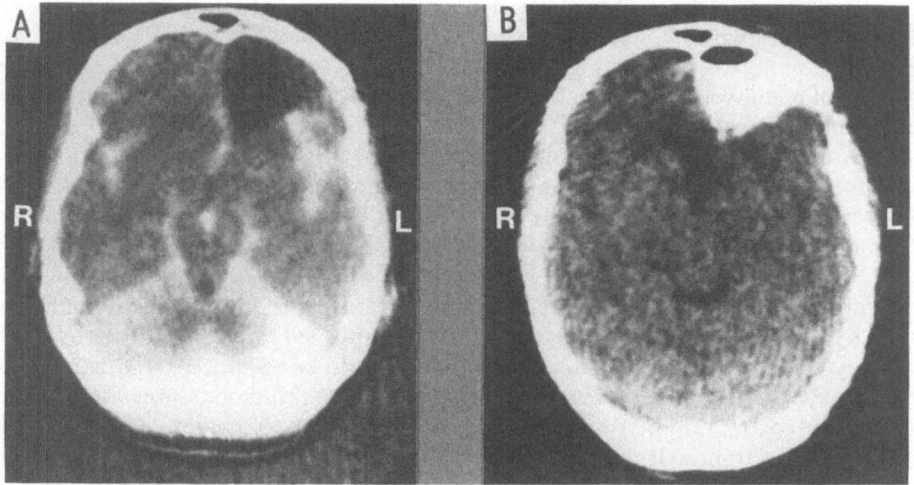

Fig. 5. Patient with left frontal glioma. *A* CT scan one hour after intrathecal administration of metrizamide. The entire intracranial subarachnoid space is filled with metrizamide except the tumor cavity in the left frontal region. The contrast agent is not able to diffuse beyond the pial margins of that tumor cavity. *B* CT scan after the percutaneous intracranial infusion of metrizamide into the tumor cavity. The contrast agent is not able to escape from the tumor cavity into either the subarachnoid space or the ventricular system. Reprinted with permission[147]

While intrathecal therapy and maintenance of CSF drug levels has a certain intellectual appeal, it is well to remember that CSF levels have no correlation with parenchymal and tumor drug levels. This route then has limited use, except perhaps in the case of pure carcinomatous meningitis.

C. Intratumoral Administration

Another method for bypassing the BBB is direct installation of chemotherapeutic agents into the tumor bed and/or into associated tumor cysts (Fig. 5). Use of the Ommaya reservoir or an adapted tumor cyst device allows for direct installation of several chemotherapeutic agents. If a cyst is part of this tumor complex, access to tumor fluid and ongoing biochemical analysis is available. Kinetic drug studies can also be performed. The more recent development of the Ommaya tumor cyst device allows the tumor bed cavity to persist. This catheter device remains patent until tumor regrowth essentially engulfs it. Tumor cyst device contents may be aspirated for culture, cytology, and other studies.

Thusfar, the agents administered via this route include MTX, 5-FU and BCNU[175]. There are certain technical limitations to such a chemotherapeutic approach. Water-soluble drugs are likely to diffuse slowly throughout the extracellular space. More lipid soluble agents are likely to diffuse back across the barrier into the systemic circulation. Either of these limitations will therefore require a large drug dose to overcome the diffusion problem. Avellanosa et al.[11] describes the installation of bleomycin and mitomycin into high-grade gliomas and tumor cavities without significant success but shows histopathologic evidence of liquefaction necrosis and nonuniform drug distribution. Morantz et al.[144] describe the use of bleomycin in conjunction with systemic BCNU to be more effective than either modality alone.

More recently Takahashi et al.[211] reported the postoperative intratumor injection of bleomycin in patients with craniopharyngioma. He found the drug to be particularly more effective in cystic rather than in solid or mixed tumors. Craniopharyngiomas as an epithelial tumor are known to take up bleomycin very well. Intracystic installation of bleomycin is also associated with tumor cell degeneration and decreased secretion of cystic fluid. Systemic exposure and thus toxicity is less with intratumoral bleomycin as compared to intravenous drug[205]. It remains to be seen whether such an approach would be applicable to other tumor types associated with cysts or with other agents such as thiotepa known to have an effect on extracranial tumor-associated malignant effusions. The use of intracyst/intratumor drugs presupposes a focal disease process and is therefore somewhat limited in most primary brain tumors, especially as diffusion to surrounding brain is quite limited.

D. Liposome Drug Delivery

Another method of achieving an adequate drug concentration over a sufficient period of time has been the use of liposomes as drug carriers. This technology first requires the incorporation of antimitotic drugs into the liposomes. Liposomes are phospholipid vesicles formed by the dispersion of bilayer lipid lamellae. These micelles can be inverted such that the polar region is inside and the nonpolar phospholipid tails are outside thus allowing increased lipid solubility and membrane penetration. These liposomes can be formed of varying sizes. Recent work incorporates such drugs as bleomycin and vincristine into liposomes of 0.1–15 micron diameter[73]. Such drug-containing liposomes can then act as a depot for slow drug release. The use of this drug delivery method in rats has demonstrated prolonged levels of bleomycin intracerebrally with liposome-entrapped bleomycin compared to free bleomycin. Additionally, low urine and serum drug levels in the liposome-treated rats are noted[72]. MTX entrapped in cholesterol liposomes has been studied in primates resulting in a higher average brain concentration than injection of free MTX[205]. While this particular method of CNS chemotherapy has not reached the clinical stage, and may be limited by the amount of drug packageable, it represents a unique approach to both penetrating the BBB and maintaining prolonged tissue concentrations.

VII. Blood-Brain Barrier Disruption (BBBD)

Multiple methods of enhancing the amount of drug delivered to CNS tumors have been developed with variable toxicity and varying effect. Also as mentioned above, one of the unique aspects of tumors within the CNS is the presence of the BBB, an anatomic and physical barrier to substances within the bloodstream. A unique though quite rational approach to the problem of chemotherapeutic drug delivery therefore has been drug administration concurrent with transient reversible BBBD.

In the 1940's Broman and Olsson[27, 28] demonstrated reversible opening of the BBB with iodinated contrast agents (these are hyperosmolar). This observation largely lay dormant until Rapoport began his elaborate studies on rats, rabbits, and monkeys detailing the physico-chemical parameters of the BBB and its role in the passage of substances from the blood to the CNS extracellular space[178]. He has described the methods of using hyperosmolar mannitol, urea, or arabinose to reversibly open the BBB, temporarily opening the tight junctions, thus precipitating transient unregulated entry of circulating substances into the CNS. Neuwelt *et al.* subsequently applied these observations and techniques to the clinically relevant problem of chemotherapeutic drug delivery in animals and then to patients with primary and metastatic CNS tumors[148–159, 161, 162, 165–167].

How do the basic principles outlined above apply to this choice of therapeutic modality? First of all, the concept of a BBB in tumors has been debated and studied from various angles. Suffice it to say that the state of the BBB in tumors differs anatomically and physicochemically *to a varying degree* from tumor nodule to tumor nodule, from tumor type to tumor type, and within any given single focus of tumor. The state of the BBB in tumors, though, becomes a moot point because substances diffuse from areas of high concentration to areas of lower concentration to the point of equilibrium. Therefore, even if a tumor has complete absence of a BBB, because the barrier remains intact in the surrounding brain parenchyma (thus inhibiting drug delivery in the CNS tissue), any immediate increased concentration of drug to the tumor rapidly diffuses out to equilibrate with the remaining CNS (the "sink effect"). Thus any concentration advantage is lost too quickly to be effective. The technique of BBBD provides an increased and more uniform drug delivery, decreases the tendency toward rapid diffusion, and therefore, allows tumor exposure to a higher concentration of drug for a longer period of time (concentration × time). As this exposes the normal CNS to much higher concentrations of anticancer agents, one must be alert to increased toxicity secondary to this increased drug exposure. One balances the potential morbidity of the BBBD and possible drug toxicity against therapeutic gain.

The technique of reversible osmotic BBBD is detailed by Neuwelt *et al.*[150, 152, 157, 159] in both animals and patients, and involves opening of the BBB in the distribution of one circulation (a carotid or vertebral artery). The exact distribution of disruption is therefore dependent on the flow as determined by these vessels and the circle of Willis. One selects then left carotid, right carotid, or vertebral arterial distribution pertinent to tumor location. For those tumors in the border zone areas, 2 disruptions may be performed sequentially over 2 days. Attempt at three sequential disruptions has not been described, but all three circulations have been modified, two at a time sequentially over two days and repeated at monthly intervals.

To obtain reversible disruption of the BBB, a hyperosmolar saturated solution of 25% mannitol is injected at sufficient rate and volume to essentially replace blood flow. Studies have shown that such an infusion must continue for approximately 30 seconds, at which time the threshold event of disruption occurs[178]. Because the degree and extent of BBBD can be variable, one must document the disruption. Rapaport[178] describes the use of Evans blue as a marker in animal studies. Neuwelt et al.[156] evaluated the use of iodinated contrast agent and radioisotope for BBBD documentation. In clinical studies, while CT scanning with contrast is anatomically more sensitive, radionuclide brain scanning is a reproducible and semiquantitative technique with possibly less toxicity.

Table 5. Osmotic blood-brain barrier disruption protocol

---

 1. Preoperative medication—Valium 10 mg PO
 2. Intubation/general anesthesia
 3. Diuresis with Lasix 10 mg IV
 4. Catheterization of selected artery (carotid or vertebral)
 5. Cytoxan 15–30 mg/kg IV (10 minutes prior to BBBD)
 6. Hyperventilation with 100% O_2 (3–5 minutes)
 7. Atropine, valium and pentothal
 8. Mannitol infusion (over 30 seconds)
 9. ^{99m}Tc-glucoheptonate 25 μCi (5 minutes after BBBD)
10. Methotrexate 1–5 gm IA (over 10–15 minutes)
11. Procarbazine 100 mg PO qd × 14 days
12. Leucovorin 20 mg PO q6° × 5 days (begun at 36 hours)

The procedure is performed under general endotracheal anesthesia (Table 5). Patients undergo retrograde catheterization via the femoral artery (Seldinger technique) and the selected artery is cannulated. The procedure carries the attendant risks of thromboembolic ischemia or infarction, symptomatic in less than 0.6% of procedures. BBBD allows for nonselective entry (for a period of approximately 30 minutes) of substances previously excluded from the CNS and tumor. Monitoring of the patient's peri-procedure medications is therefore mandatory.

Is chemotherapeutic agent delivery enhanced with BBBD? Initial studies in the rat and dog document BBBD with Evans blue and/or CT scanning. Following barrier modification, intracarotid infusion of MTX results in markedly increased levels of intraparenchymal drug as measured by tissue assay[149, 150]. Further studies including CSF assay confirm the fact that CSF drug levels have little correlation with brain tissue levels. While studies in the rat are limited to the carotid circulation, dog experiments have permitted application of the technique clinically to the posterior fossa. This modality results in enhanced MTX delivery of 10–50-fold over nondisruption intravenous drug delivery.

These studies document increased drug delivery to normal brain. To compare antitumor agent delivery to intracerebral and systemic tumor, a nude rat—human lung tumor model has been used to show enhanced MTX delivery to intracerebral tumor and brain around tumor with osmotic BBBD[164]. Further work in the avian sarcoma virus rat glioma model demonstrates increase drug delivery (with barrier modification) to tumor and the whole ipsilateral hemisphere[152, 158]. The same model is also used to evaluate the effect of steroids on BBBD, a significant factor as most patients are treated with steroids. Steroid administration greatly reduces the increased drug delivery obtained with BBBD. This might well be predicted as steroids have a tendency to stabilize membranes and are known to decrease CT contrast enhancement of tumors. Final parameters to consider in maximizing drug delivery are route of administration (intraarterial over intravenous) and the fact that moderate hypocarbia (mean pCO_2 28 mm Hg) maximizes drug delivery with BBBD in rats[152, 159].

Having established the parameters of BBBD and subsequent MTX delivery, Neuwelt has evaluated other chemotherapeutic agents. In the absence of BBBD, doxorubicin levels in the rat and dog cerebrum are undetectable, however following BBBD, increased drug is assayed but significant neurotoxicity, including necrosis and hemorrhagic infarcts even at subtherapeutic drug levels, precludes the clinical use of this drug[151]. Intracarotid infusion of cisplatin without osmotic BBBD resulted in Evans blue staining suggestive that the drug itself modifies the barrier[154]. Spigelman et al.[200, 201] report similar results with etoposide.

Bleomycin and fluorouracil also display significant neurotoxicity in the dog when administered intracarotid in association with BBBD[154, 155]. While the bleomycin brain concentrations remain quite variable, osmotic BBBD results in a tenfold increase in 5-FU brain concentration over that in controls. Cyclophosphamide infusion (given IV prior to BBBD to permit hepatic activation) results in no neurotoxicity; the parenchymal levels of radioactivity with and without BBBD are similar, but it is unclear how much activated drug is present. Again, using the avian sarcoma virus rat glioma model, Neuwelt has shown that cyclophosphamide penetrates normal brain and to a greater extent, brain tumor; 5-FU also penetrates normal brain and tumor, but to a lesser degree[158]. Bleomycin and MTX levels in tumor and surrounding brain are quite variable.

Clinical experience with BBBD and chemotherapy extends over 92 patients and 614 procedures. Included are patients with malignant glial tumors, primary CNS lymphoma, metastatic disease. An important observation early in our clinical series emphasizes the effect of adequate drug delivery and suggests that chemotherapy in conjunction with BBBD may approach such "adequate" delivery. Five patients (glioblastoma multiforme, primary CNS lymphoma, metastatic breast carcinoma) demonstrated clinical and radiographic evidence of tumor regression in the face of single circulation BBBD and drug delivery. However, these patients each developed new progressive tumor in brain regions supplied by vessels other than the disrupted cerebral circulation (Fig. 6)[161]. Such an experience has led us to obtain

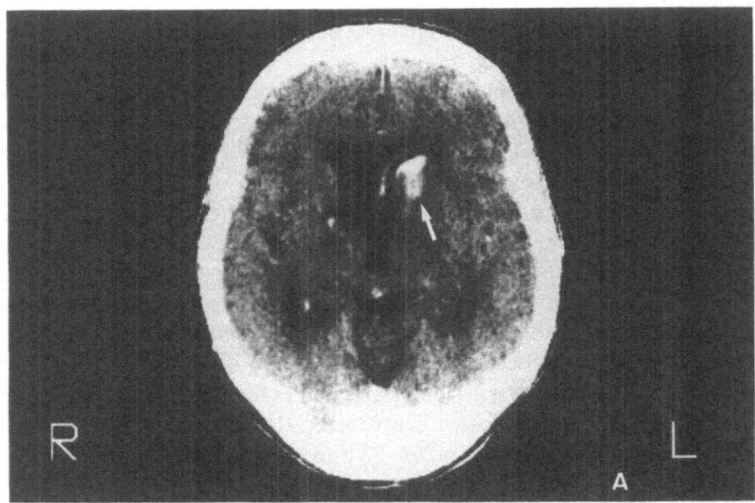

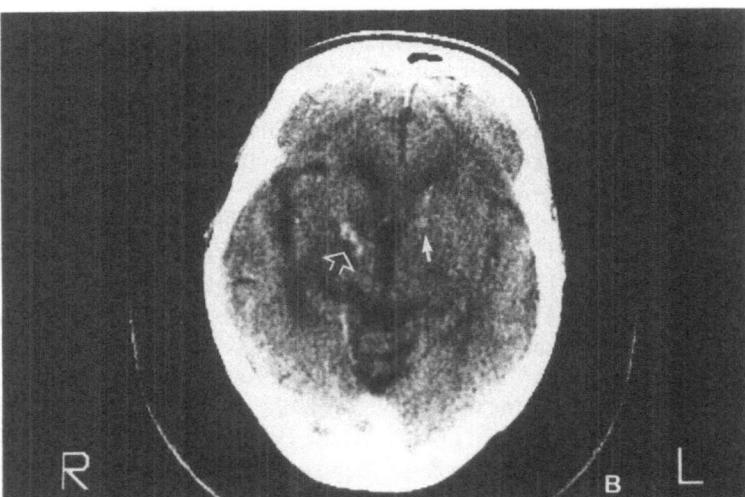

Fig. 6. Patient with primary CNS lymphoma. *A* transverse CT (enhanced) at the level of the lateral ventricles six months after operation and radiation for the treatment of a right basal ganglion lesion. The lesion (arrow) in the left cerebral hemisphere compressing the left lateral ventricle developed after radiation. *B* CT (enhanced) one month after the first course of chemotherapy with barrier modification. There is marked reduction in the left cerebral hemispheric lesion (white arrow), but a recurrent lesion in the right cerebral hemisphere adjacent to the lateral and third ventricles is seen (open arrow). Reprinted with permission[161]

sequential disruptions of all three circulations in those disease processes likely to have diffuse CNS malignancy. Neurotoxicity is minimal with this chemotherapeutic regimen.

VIII. Drug Rescue Techniques

Using the principles of drug delivery one attempts to enhance clinical effect by maximizing the dosage of a cytotoxic drug and the duration of exposure to that drug. Dose limitation is frequently extraneural toxicity. In an effort to provide more effective treatment, the current practice of "high-dose" chemotherapy has been developed. The rationale for such treatment is to improve drug delivery to relatively protected body areas (i.e., the CNS and CSF) or to improve drug delivery to poorly perfused tumors. Such high-dose chemotherapy may also circumvent or prevent tumor cell resistance. To counteract the attendant increased host toxicity from such high-dose chemotherapy, various rescue techniques have been developed. One method available is to alter the drug schedule. Another method is administration of an antidote, either concomitant with or sequential to the administration of the chemotherapeutic agent.

The prototype drug rescue regimen is the use of leucovorin (formyltetrahydrofolate) with MTX to reduce MTX toxicity. The mechanisms of rescue with this regimen include competitive interaction for a common membrane transport carrier, replacement of reduced folate, and hence enhanced competition because of increased dihydrofolate pools. Another method of MTX rescue is the administration of thymidine and purine. Uridine rescue has been used in combination with 5-FU, as have leucovorin and folinic acid[137]. One method of combatting cytarabine toxicity is to alter its dosage schedule. One might consider the practice of hydrating patients prior to cyclophosphamide administration to prevent renal toxicity as another method of "rescue".

Cisplatin administration requires that patients be prehydrated; the drug is given with concomitant mannitol-induced diuresis as prophylaxis against nephrotoxicity. Another "rescue" involves the administration of systemic thiosulfate in conjunction with intraperitoneal cisplatin in the treatment of ovarian carcinoma and malignant ascites[105, 136]. The thiosulfate protects against nephrotoxicity, and at a higher dose, reduces thrombocytopenia. The mechanism of such protection is unknown. Recall also the early experience with intracarotid mechlorethamine used with intravenous thiosulfate for bone marrow protection[174].

Since bone marrow toxicity represents a dose-limiting factor in the use of BCNU for primary brain tumor treatment, neurooncologists in the last 5 years have investigated the use of autologous bone marrow transplant (ABMT) rescue in conjunction with chemotherapy[70, 100]. Several small series report the use of BCNU with ABMT. High dose etoposide has also been given in conjunction with bone marrow rescue[115]. While there may be some increased survival, toxicity associated with the procedure is not insignificant. Furthermore, while limiting bone marrow toxicity, such a selective method of rescue allows for increased pulmonary and hepatic toxicity[70].

Another attempt to "rescue" systemic toxicity involves essentially an "isolated perfusion" approach. Pioneered by the initial investigators in brain tumor chemotherapy, this method, tried recently with BCNU and an extraction hemoperfusion columm, results in decreased systemic drug levels and less hematopoietic toxicity in three rhesus monkeys[172].

Perhaps a novel approach to drug rescue is the use of antibody against the particular chemotherapeutic agent to bind and hopefully inactivate said drug. Such a method of chemotherapy rescue is particularly applicable to brain tumor therapy where systemic toxicity is limiting, and systemically administered antibody can bind peripheral drug with limited access to CNS drug. Preliminary results in our laboratory using a rat model and MTX as well as antiMTX antisera suggests serum drug binding of at least 90%. Such an approach may well be useful with other agents in neurooncology.

IX. Radiation Sensitizers

In an effort to improve brain tumor treatment, attempts have been made to potentiate the cytotoxic effects of radiation on tumor without increasing damage to normal brain. One approach has been an effort to synchronize the cell cycle of tumor cells prior to radiation using such combinations as ACNU, epipodophyllo-toxin, and vincristine. Described by Takakura[212], the rationale of this "synchronized chemo-radiotherapy" is to potentiate the radiation effect.

Bromouridine, a thymidine analog, is incorporated into DNA and may thus increase radiosensitivity. Tumor cell uptake of bromouridine is enhanced by giving MTX or 5-FU to block the normal thymidine pathway. The bromouridine is given intracarotid because this drug is rapidly dehalogenated by the liver and intracarotid infusion increases local concentration approximately 11- to 16-fold[184]. Its use in patients with malignant glioma has not added benefit[60]. The Japanese studies describe intrathecal bromouridine administration via Ommaya reservoir in patients with metastatic brain tumors or carcinomatous meningitis, in conjunction with radiation and systemic antimetabolite (MTX or 5-FU) chemotherapy[212].

Metronidazole acts to radiosensitize hypoxic cells. Several clinical trials with this agent did not significantly influence the median survival with radiation alone. Peripheral neuropathy is a potential side effect of metronidazole and misonidazole, respectively[60, 139a].

A similar agent, misonidazole, is currently under investigation in patients with high grade glioma. Studied in patients with systemic tumors, the drug had a 12% peripheral neuropathy incidence and a 9% incidence of central neurotoxicity; however, this neurotoxicity rate was less in patients receiving dexamethasone or phenytoin[224].

The most promising agent is hydroxyurea, a chemotherapeutic agent in its own right. This drug figures prominently in a number of current brain tumor protocols including the "8 in 1" protocol, in combination with BCNU, and in combination with procarbazine, CCNU, and vincristine. Used as a single agent with radiation, this drug produced significant tumor necrosis and prolonged survival[108]. Cisplatin, also part of the "8 in 1" protocol, has been described to act synergistically with cranial radiation as a "radiosensitizer"[48, 99, 202].

X. Monoclonal Antibodies

Monoclonal antibodies (MAbs) directed against human tumor-associated antigens are under investigation as diagnostic and therapeutic vehicles. Extensive research continues in defining their use as target-seeking carriers of radiation (for imaging and therapy) or chemotherapeutic agents in systemic tumors. Molecular weight and antigen-antibody kinetics influence the use of such agents chemotherapeutically. While intact antibody retains greater antigen affinity, better and more rapid tumor localization is achieved with F(ab')$_2$ fragments[220]. Because the MAbs are primarily of mouse origin, there is concern that patients treated with these foreign proteins will be susceptible to a serum sickness syndrome. Limited clinical studies suggest that human antimurine antibodies develop rather rapidly in a significant number of patients, but the clinical relevance of this has not been fully determined[190]. To date, toxicity from such antimouse antibodies has been negligible. While *in vitro* progress continues, difficulties with *in vivo* selectivity have hampered clinically significant advances. Intratumoral cell heterogeneity accounts for part of this discrepancy. Other factors affecting tumor localization include vascular permeability (MAb delivery), surface antigen modulation by the tumor (binding sites) and antibody affinity.

As might be predicted, the blood-brain barrier presents an additional factor to consider in MAb delivery to intracranial tumors. While Fab fragments have a molecular weight of approximately 50,000 these MAbs may range up to molecular weight 10^6 (*i.e.,* IgM). Brain tumor permeability limits agents of higher molecular weight. Neuwelt reports three patients in whom brain tumor visualization with ^{99m}Tc-albumin (molecular weight 69,000) was less than brain scan tumor visualization with the more conventional ^{99m}Tc-glucoheptonate (molecular weight 226)[169]. Neuwelt et al.[163] has also described the delivery of MAb to dog brain and CSF both with and without osmotic BBB modification. Such studies as well as pharmacokinetic studies of MAb delivery to rat brain[168] are important preliminary experiments prior to clinical treatment with MAb-associated compounds.

In an attempt to enhance the therapeutic ratio in brain tumor treatment, MAbs are under investigation as specific drug carriers for melphalan, MTX, chlorambucil, and the anthracyclines[25]. In these studies, attempts are being made to maintain high drug tumor levels and reduce systemic toxicity. Early work with MTX has been limited by solubility difficulty and poor cell membrane crossing[25]. An antibody-chlorambucil conjugate has been developed but *in vivo* mouse tumors were not inhibited[25]. Somewhat better results have been achieved conjugating anthracyclines to anti-alphafetoprotein with delayed *in vivo* tumor growth in rats[25]. Improvements are yet needed in immunolocalization and drug conjugation to maitain *active* chemotherapeutic agent at a specific site.

XI. Special Cases in CNS Tumor Therapy

A. Primary CNS Lymphoma

The clear efficacy of chemotherapy in the management of systemic lymphoma, particularly the large cell type, has resulted in a variety of trials of cytoreductive agents in the management of primary CNS lymphoma. Steroids are the most commonly utilized drug; they can produce a decrease in mass effect by altering cerebral edema and may have a lympholytic effect. Steroid responses are transient yet the change as measured by CT scan may be dramatic. However, steroids may mask the extent of tumor by stabilizing the BBB and thus reducing contrast enhancement.

Although partial responses have been obtained in most series, no drug nor combination of drugs administered systemically has resulted in complete remission with significant prolongation of life. In most series the use of conventional chemotherapeutic agents including the nitrosoureas, procarbazine, cytarabine, cyclophosphamide, bleomycin, vincristine, and doxorubicin shows only modest efficacy [17, 63, 98, 122, 132, 207]. The most consistent results have been achieved with high dose MTX: 45% achieved a complete response and 36% a partial response though only 3 had responses sustained for greater than one year [2, 197]. Loeffler et al [128] noted a 44 month median survival in those patients treated with chemotherapy and radiotherapy compared to 14 months in those without drug therapy.

The BBB is a key factor affecting drug delivery to malignant lymphoma as well as other tumors in the CNS. Evidence for this is seen in a report where two patients developed CNS involvement while in complete remission from systemic lymphoma on multiagent chemotherapy (cyclophosphamide, doxorubicin, vincristine, and prednisone) [96]. Similarly, the observation that there can be extensive tumor burden at autopsy despite little or no enhancement on CT scan further emphasizes the importance of the BBB. Another point suggesting the problem of drug delivery is the fact that high-dose rather than conventional dose MTX administration is needed for any definitive response.

Efficacy of drug therapy administered following BBB modification is emphasized by tumor regression in the areas of brain supplied by the artery through which the drugs are given. In our own series two primary CNS lymphoma patients had CT documentation of tumor progression in untreated brain regions concurrent with tumor regression in areas of BBB. This observation coupled with the fact that CNS lymphoma is frequently multifocal, and extensive disease may not be evident on CT scan, has led us to now routinely treat CNS lymphoma patients with sequential BBBD and chemotherapy in all circulations. Durable responses have been seen only in those patients treated with several courses of therapy after documentation of complete response by CT scan.

It does appear possible to achieve complete remission, by clinical and CT criteria, in a high proportion of patients with primary CNS lymphoma, even without the use of radiation therapy. Our one year survival of 75% can be compared to the average 57% one year survival in series of patients undergoing radiation [165]. The administration of chemotherapy rather than radiation therapy may be less neurotoxic, and radiation can be administered subsequent to chemotherapy in patients who fail to respond and may possibly be less toxic when administered in this fashion [5].

B. Primitive Neuroectodermal Tumors

Primitive neuroectodermal tumors (PNETs) may arise intracranially or at more peripheral nervous system sites. As a group they have a tendency to disseminate along the CSF pathways. They may exhibit varying degrees of differentiation. The undifferentiated PNET of the cerebellum, medulloblastoma, is the most common pediatric malignant brain tumor. Other PNETs include medulloepithelioma, neuroblastoma, polar spongioblastoma, pineoblastoma, ependymoblastoma, retinoblastoma, and esthesioneuroepithelioma[13].

The therapeutic approach to such tumors includes early surgery to make a diagnosis, treat symptoms of mass effect, decrease tumor bulk, and provide time for further therapy. Whether surgery alters cell kinetics by stimulating quiescent cells to become more malignant is unknown at this time. Further therapy for these tumors includes radiation, usually craniospinal. In general, PNETs are radiosensitive, and in contradistinction to gliomas, may also be quite chemosensitive. Most drug protocols are designed for medulloblastoma, and have shown responses in recurrent tumors but not as adjuvant therapy[4, 7, 44]. Because of the tendency for these tumors to disseminate and metastasize, attempts are made to stage patients prior to adjuvant therapy. Patients with disseminated disease and patients under four years of age have a poor prognosis[7].

More promising protocols for treatment of such tumors include most recently the "8 in 1" regimen, an exciting multidrug approach with some early success in very unfavorable patients[7, 23]. Other important protocols are the procarbazine-BCNU-vincristine[124] and the cyclophosphamide-hydroxyurea combinations[5]. Intrathecal MTX, cytarabine, and thiotepa are used either individually or in combination[60]. Because of the significant marrow suppression which attends pediatric craniospinal irradiation these intrathecal agents have also been used with systemic chemotherapy. A mechlorethamine-vincristine-prednisone-procarbazine combination is under investigation for medulloblastoma as well[7]. Additionally cisplatin and etoposide or the Einhorn regimen of vinblastine, bleomycin and cisplatin are anticipated to be useful. Combination chemotherapy (MTX, cyclophosphamide, and procarbazine) with BBBD is under trial.

As the toxicity of radiation therapy becomes more apparent and frequently recognized, the use of preradiation chemotherapy seems more reasonable. Gradually, the chemotherapeutic regimens are being tried concomitant with or prior to radiation and as responses are seen in both the low risk patients and in those with a hopeless prognosis, a bolder first-line chemotherapeutic approach can be expected.

C. Germ Cell Tumors

Successful chemotherapeutic treatment of intracranial germ cell tumors has been limited until, extrapolating from the experience of Einhorn with testicular tumors[61], Neuwelt and Frenkel[160] used combination chemotherapy with vinblastine, cisplatin and bleomycin to improved response. This "Einhorn regimen" has been used with success in patients with CNS germinoma (pineal or suprasellar) primary or metastatic[160, 195]. When these tumors secrete markers (β-human chorionic gonadotropin or α-fetoprotein), CSF levels may be followed to monitor chemotherapeutic response and recurrence. When there is a concern about bleomycin-induced pulmonary toxicity, the combination cisplatin and etoposide may provide similar treatment potential[160]. This latter regimen has also been used in refractory or relapsing germ cell tumors[24].

Logothetis *et al*[130] report the use of doxorubicin, cisplatin, and bleomycin in the treatment of germ cell brain metastasis; patients with a single metastasis did significantly better than those with multiple metastases or diffuse leptomeningeal carcinomatosis. Allen *et al*[6] have treated recurrent or relapsing CNS germ cell tumors with a combination of vinblastine, bleomycin, cyclophosphamide, dactinomycin and cisplatin. The Japanese Intracranial Germ Cell Tumor Study Group, using cisplatin, vinblastine, and bleomycin both with and without radiation find significant response to adjuvant drug therapy without radiation in the nonrecurrent cases (Matsutani, presented at the 8th International Congress of Neurosurgery). Recurrent cases have a better response to combination radiation/chemotherapy.

Speculation as to the chemotherapeutic response in germ cell tumors raises the possibility of exquisite tumor sensitivity to drug despite the reduced CNS drug exposure secondary to the BBB. Conversely, these tumors are densely enhancing and may lack an intact BBB especially as the suprasellar germinoma derives its vascular supply from the anterior pituitary which lacks such a barrier. Likewise, pineal region germinomas demonstrate a similar phenomenon. Intraparenchymal germ cell metastases most likely are subject to BBB dynamics, yet they also demonstrate a clinical response similar to primary CNS germ cell tumors.

D. Brain Metastases

In reviewing the literature, one realizes that chemotherapy for metastatic brain tumors presents an inconclusive picture. As brain metastases are usually part of a disseminated disease, systemic chemotherapy is of paramount importance. Yet at a time when systemic chemotherapeutic advances are being made, rare success is noted in intracranial metastatic disease. Furthermore, in CNS metastases, systemic chemotherapy may control peripheral disease in the face of thriving CNS malignancy. The BBB again remains a significant hurdle in brain tumor chemotherapy, primarily influencing the pharmacokinetic behavior of these drugs. Thus, differences between drug delivery to subcutaneous and brain tumors are again the result of lipid solubility, protein binding, ionization fraction, and molecular weight. Despite a relative BBB lack in metastatic tumors, drug delivery differs between intracerebral and subcutaneous tumor[164].

As with primary tumor the BBB poses a problem to be circumvented in treatment of metastatic disease. One method of circumvention, less feasible in multiple brain metastases than in a single tumor, is the introduction of drug directly into the tumor itself. Another method, that of direct intrathecal administration, is discussed above. The technique of reversible alteration of the BBB in more than one arterial distribution lends itself to treatment of multiple metastases[166]. A fourth method to circumvent the barrier is chemical modification of existing drugs and synthesis of new agents that particularly penetrate the BBB[92]. However, agents which are too lipophilic are technically difficult to administer. One chemical modification method is to mask the polar groups of agents already in use and then enzymatically retransform the drug within the brain. This "prodrug" could then be coupled to an inert carrier for more specific CNS uptake. Such a concept has been in use for dopamine and testosterone, and experiments applying such a technique to anticancer agents are underway[92]. As with systemic tumors, combination therapy will likely have therapeutic advantage. A final concept borrowed from systemic oncology but applicable in CNS tumor treatment, both primary and metastatic, is the idea of "consolidation chemotherapy", continued treatment of patients for a specific time following evidence of remission[92]. Such efforts in patients with leukemias have resulted in significantly longer remission times.

The use of high dose chemotherapy for brain metastases has been debated, particularly in the absence of systemic disease. Previously treated with radiation alone, these tumors have responded to such drugs as mitomycin, doxorubicin, etoposide, cisplatin, and the Einhorn regimen of bleomycin, cisplantin and vincristine in addition to the more usual nitrosoureas and procarbazine. Rosner et al[181] report on 66 patients with metastatic breast disease treated with chemotherapy alone; 34 of 66 (52%) patients showed active response to various combinations of cyclophosphamide, 5-FU, MTX, vincristine, and doxorubicin though median survival in these responders was only 13 months. Brain metastases from lung carcinoma have also been treated with a variety of systemic agents. Small cell tumors are particularly radio- and chemo-sensitive and have been treated with doxorubicin, cisplatin, etoposide, CCNU, cyclophosphamide, vincristine, and MTX[217]. Kantarjian reports on four patients with metastatic lung carcinoma treated with chemotherapy alone (combinations of cisplatin, etoposide, cyclophosphamide, doxorubicin, and vincristine) and good response[113]. Combining the principles of treatment for brain tumors as outlined above with the drugs particularly suited for the metastatic tumor and adapted to maximize CNS delivery diffusely should improve results.

XII. Experimental Drugs

The emphasis in this review chapter has been on the current clinically available drugs relevant to the treatment of brain neoplasia. These 27 drugs represent those agents widely available, the current distillation of some 40,000 compounds per year, screened for possible chemotherapeutic use. This review would not be complete however without mentioning several of the potentially promising experimental agents (Table 6).

Table 6. Pertinent experimental drugs

Dianhydrogalactitol
Diaziquone
Fludarabine
Neocarzinostatin
Nitrosoureas
ACNU
PCNU
Prednimustine
Spiromustine
Teniposide
Triazinate
Vindesine

Teniposide (VM-26), an epipodophyllotoxin-like etoposide, causes DNA strand breakage (Fig. 7). Drug trials show activity against intracranial disease even when used as a single agent and in patients with recurrent disease following nitrosourea therapy[59]. Garbino[84] reports a statistically significant increased median survival in patients with pure glioblastoma multiforme associated with minimal reversible hematologic, hepatic, and neurologic toxicity. Intracarotid use of the drug both as a single agent and in combination with intraarterial BCNU and cisplatin has been described[206]. Tenoposide may have activity against the primitive neuroectodermal tumors as well.

A synthetic lipid soluble quinone, 2,5-diaziridinyl-3,6-biscarboethoxyamino-1,4-benzoquinone (diaziquone, AZQ), was found to be active in experimental intracerebral tumors and has since been used in clinical trials as a single agent against malignant glioma (Fig. 7). A modest response was seen and more recently, the drug has been evaluated for intraarterial use and in combination with a nitrosourea[89, 91, 189]. Haid, however, notes that while diaziquone in recurrent disease had a moderate response, those patients previously treated with nitrosoureas did not respond[95]. Furthermore, with diaziquone therapy, initial tumor enlargement may precede response. Intraventricular administration for treatment of meningeal leukemia showed no evidence of neurotoxicity[237].

Dianhydrogalactitol, one of the hexitol epoxides, is active against animal ependymoblastoma, neuroblastoma and other primitive neuroectodermal tumors[123]. An early clinical trial against high grade astrocytoma showed no significant difference in survival duration compared with radiation alone[59], while more recent trials showed a median survival of 67 weeks when combined with radiation therapy[192]. This drug, like diaziquone crosses the BBB readily.

An antitumor antibiotic, neocarzinostatin, has a strong cytotoxicity against cultured glioblastoma but does not cross the BBB. Theoretically, Maeda et al.[133] feel such a combination would limit CNS toxicity. However, given the chemotherapeutic principles as discussed above as well as the poor correlation between cell culture and clinical response, one might be skeptical about the eventual success of this drug[193].

Nitrosoureas possess both alkylating and carbamylating activity. It is the former that correlates with anti-tumor effect but as alkylating activity increases, lipid solubility decreases. The carbamylation reaction results in covalent bond formation between isocyanate (a decomposition product of nitrosoureas) and proton-losing reactants. This reaction is felt to explain some of the drug toxicity. Based on these observations, efforts at rational drug analog development and selection have yielded two agents, 3-[(4-amino-2-methyl-5-pyrimidinyl)methyl]-1-(2-chloroethyl)-1-nitrosourea (ACNU) and 1-(2-chloroethyl)-3-(2,6-dioxo-3-piperidyl)-1-nitrosurea (PCNU) (Fig. 7). However, at this point there is little to recommend these over the conventional nitrosoureas. ACNU is both water and lipid-soluble and has been used extensively in Japan for treatment of malignant brain tumors. A small study comparing intravenous and intraarterial drug administration showed postoperative survival to be slightly higher in the intra-arterial group[234]. The drug is widely distributed with retention in tumor tissue but relatively low levels are seen in brain and CSF. Japanese cooperative studies showed

Experimental Agents

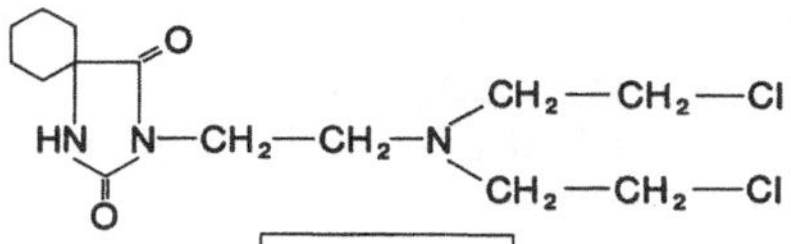

Spiromustine

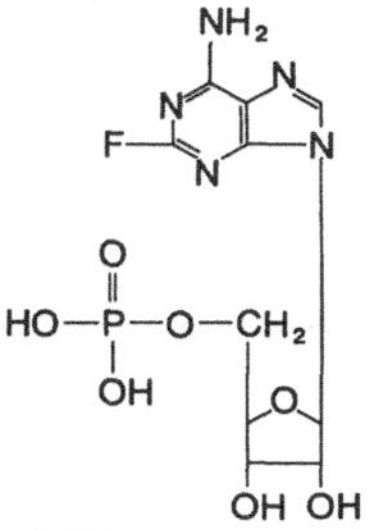

Fludarabine

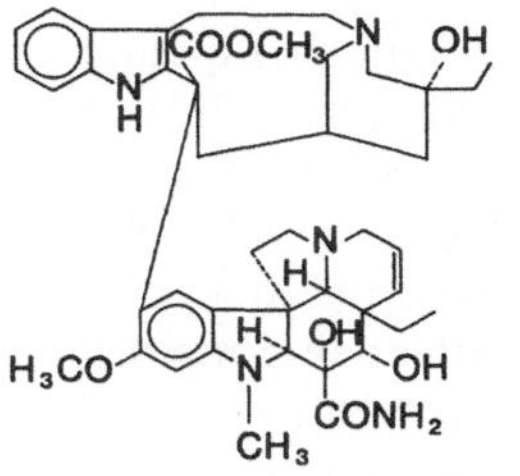

Vindesine

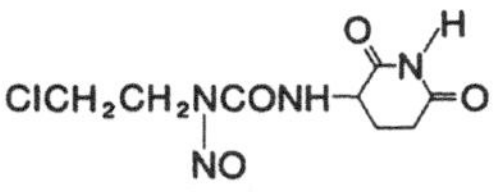

PCNU

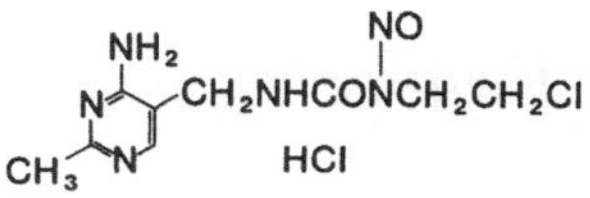

ACNU

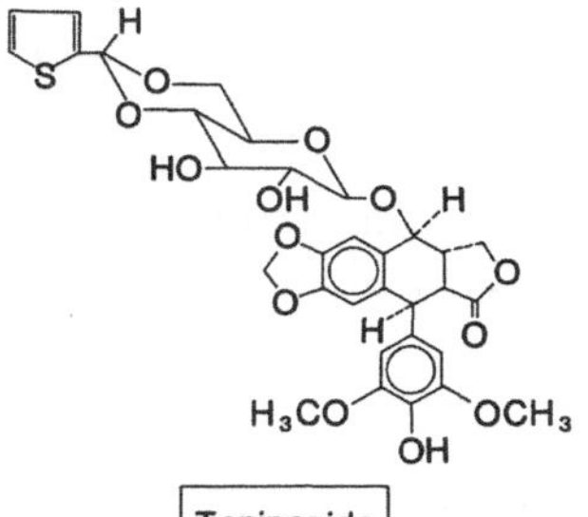

Teniposide

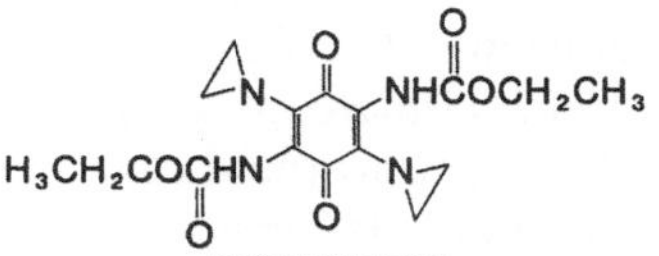

Diaziquone

Fig. 7

a 34–48% response rate in brain tumors[171]. Hematologic toxicity, which may be cumulative, is the dose-limiting factor.

Intrathecal ACNU may be useful in carcinomatous meningitis but may be associated with diffuse gliosis along the cortical surface[216]. PCNU has an octanol/water partition coefficient of 0.4 which theoretically is optimal for CNS delivery. Small clinical pilot studies have shown a response in half the patients[79]. The drug is relatively more toxic than BCNU.

Other experimental agents under trial in primary brain tumor protocols include triazinate (Baker's antifol), a potent dihydrofolate reductase inhibitor[57], and vindesine (Fig. 7), a lipid soluble vinca alkaloid reported to cause less neurotoxicity than vincristine even in previously treated patients[3].

Prednimustine and spiromustine represent chemical combinations synthesized to potentially enhance the therapeutic ratio of the individual drugs given separately. Prednimustine is a chlorambucil ester of prednisolone, lipid-soluble with increased intracellular uptake, used in the adjuvant treatment of glioblastoma; there is little effect in prolonging survival[9]. Spiromustine (Fig. 7) combines properties of alkylating agents and diphenylhydantoin for a low molecular weight, lipid soluble antitumor agent with major neurologic toxicity—ataxia, vertigo, lethargy, paresthesias. Substantial cytotoxic activity against intracerebral-implanted tumors in mice has been demonstrated[75, 194]. Early clinical trials are underway.

Fludarabine (Fig. 7) is a fluorinated and phosphorylated derivative of vidarabine, exerting its metabolic effect at DNA synthesis. Early phase clinical studies are ongoing and include patients with primary brain tumors[118].

XIII. Drug Protocols

Before discussing some of the currently prominent multiagent chemotherapy protocols, the current work of Maheley[134] in synthesizing the status of brain tumor chemotherapy bares emphasis. He defines effective trials as those with at least 20 patients having at least a 30% response, surviving for at least 35 weeks. Using this definition, BCNU, PCNU, tenoposide, procarbazine, streptozotocin, and vincristine are "effective" in treating recurrent gliomas while such drugs as CCNU, cisplatin, mithramycin, thiotepa, hydroxurea, doxorubicin, MTX, dacarbazine, and triazinate have yet to fulfill the criteria.

Mahaley[134] then goes on to note that the use of multiple agents has yet to be proven more effective than single drug therapy. Using his same criteria, some of the "effective" drug combinations include BCNU-5-FU, CCNU-tenoposide, CCNU-tenoposide-doxorubicin, CCNU-procarbazine-vincristine, CCNU-vincristine-MTX, CCNU-5-FU-HU-mercaptopurine, and cisplatin-cytarabine. Of note is the fact that all except the last protocol contain a nitrosourea. A number of protocols exist for new glioma patients including chemotherapy, with or without radiation therapy, with or without radiation sensitizers.

Jellinger[112] advocates polychemotherapy and compares a number of trials. Most recent results study radiation alone, polychemotherapy alone, or their combination[218]. Drugs include CCNU, procarbazine, vincristine, MTX and methylprednisone. Patients treated with chemotherapy alone had a mean survival of 13.2 months and those treated with the combination survived a mean of 19.1 months[218]. Adverse side effects included the expected hematologic and gastrointestinal toxicity as well as polyneuropathy, intratumoral hemorrhage, radionecrosis, infection (abscess/encephalitis) and hydrocephalus. Not infrequently the patients developed cerebral cysts associated with tumor and tissue necrosis. These responded transiently to surgical decompression, but if they ruptured into the ventricles, patients deteriorated rapidly with fatal generalized tumor seeding[111, 218].

Similar drug combinations for recurrent pediatric brain tumors include the use of vincristine, procarbazine, and prednisone with or without mechlorethamine[36]. Nine of 54 patients receiving mechlorethamine responded while six of 52 without nitrogen mustard responded. The former regimen was more toxic and the difference in response not statistically significant.

Bleyer et al[23], working primarily with pediatric patients has developed a multi-agent chemotherapy protocol giving eight drugs in one day ("8 and 1" regimen). The drug dosages are reduced to limit toxicity. In patients with PNETs, two courses of chemotherapy are given prior to radiation therapy with the intent to further delay radiation therapy if such a regimen shows results[7, 23]. The drugs include methylprednisolone, vincristine, CCNU, HU, cisplatin, cytarabine, procarbazine, and cyclophosphamide (medulloblastoma, other PNETs) or dacarbazine (gliomas). This particular regimen was chosen to affect the heterogenous subpopulations of malignant cells and their varying chemosensitivities and resistances. By giving multiple myelosuppressive agents in less than 24 hours one may avoid additive toxicity. Lipid- and water-soluble agents, cell cycle-specific, -nonspecific, and -independent drugs are included. Sequences and combinations to enhance cytotoxicity are used: vincristine before cyclophosphamide, cytarabine after cisplatin, and HU with cytarabine and alkylating agents. While long-term follow-up is not yet available, response rates of 57–67% are seen[7, 23]; these are unfortunately transient. Rozenthal et al[183] reports the use of this protocol in nine adult patients with high-grade astrocytoma (uses dacarbazine not cyclophosphamide) with a 92% response by radiographic criteria.

Recurrent medulloblastoma and other pediatric brain tumors have been treated with a combination of procarbazine, CCNU, and vincristine[44]. While the drug has shown response in this and other series, myelosuppression is a limiting factor particularly in those patients with previous craniospinal radiation. Delaying the procarbazine and reducing its dose relative to the nitrosourea may reduce myelosuppression while maintaining the antineoplastic effect[44].

In 1974 Einhorn[61] instituted a regimen of cisplatin, vinblastine, and bleomycin in the treatment of testicular cancer, with an extremely high remission rate. Reasoning from the fact that intracranial germinomas (pineal and suprasellar) as well as other pineal region germ cell tumors are derived for the same stem cell as testicular seminoma, Neuwelt instituted treatment of such CNS tumors with the same regimen[160]. Though these drugs ordinarily have limited penetrance across the BBB, germinomas frequently are lacking such a barrier and prove to be quite chemosensitive.

Finally, the unique approach of multiagent chemotherapy in association with BBBD deserves mention. This ongoing protocol has analyzed data on 38 patients with glioblastoma multiforme[167], 12 patients with primary CNS lymphoma[165], and patients with intracranial metastatic disease[166]. For patients with glioblastoma, median survival is 19 months and 33% are alive at two years. The patients with CNS lymphoma have a 73% one-year survival and a 33% two-year survival. Seven patients with metastatic brain tumors, including malignant melanoma, breast, lung and testicular carcinoma have been treated in this protocol.

XIV. Conclusion

With some 30 years experience in general antineoplastic chemotherapy and some 20 years experience with brain neoplasia, where does the neuroclinician stand? We have accumulated a substantial amount of data on malignant cell cycles and tumor cell kinetics with tight experimental constructs, however little is extrapolative to *in vivo* malignancy, and for CNS tumors even the methodology may be lacking with a failure to account for the BBB and the CSF circulation. General anatomic parameters regarding the infiltrative primary brain tumor and the multifocal metastatic disease have been defined, but it is only recently that we have recognized our failure to consider these in treatment protocols. Perhaps the most drastic example of this are the separate observations of Neuwelt and Stewart of tumor regression in a focally treated CNS circulation with simultaneously observed tumor progression in an adjacent untreated region[161, 206].

We have accepted the importance of age and performance status in predicting eventual outcome in glioma patients, but until recently have frequently combined patients with anaplastic astrocytoma and glioblastoma multiforme, two entities histologically distinguishable with statistically distinct natural histories, perhaps crediting therapeutic success for what is simply natural outcome. Little is known about the host's role in treating such neoplasia, let alone the detrimental effect of those *immunosuppressive* agents we call *antineoplastic*. Drug pharmacokinetic clinical observations are currently based on plasma and perhaps CSF concentrations with little known about brain tumor and surrounding parenchymal drug levels.

Elaborate drug classifications have been developed based on biochemical definition, metabolic site of action, or tumor susceptibility. Major emphasis is placed on delivering adequate amounts of drug for sufficient lengths of time, but we fail to realize that we have only assumptions at this point regarding these parameters in patients, and furthermore have no means to account for interpatient metabolic variability, a large enough problem in syngeneic animal studies (let alone patients!) to thwart almost all pharmacokinetic conclusions. Given the fact of tumor cell population heterogeneity and the propensity to develop drug resistance, we begin to realize the necessity of "multi-agent" therapy. This at once compounds the metabolic equation, requiring consideration of drug synergism and antagonism; but again our conclusions are frequently based on assumptions rather than clinically-derived data.

In addition, we have yet to clearly define the histologic effects of treatment in the face of progressive disease. Is the demyelination or necrosis adjacent to tumor the result of our drugs, previous or concurrent radiation, or the disease itself?

Defining toxicity and risk-benefit ratios requires an almost impossible sorting of probably overlapping effects, both clinically and histopathologically.

The specific chemotherapeutic agents are directed against rapidly dividing cells—tumor cells and also normal cells of the bone marrow and gastrointestinal system; hence their effect and their toxicity. But what about the fact that 12 of 27 (48%) of the agents here discussed for brain tumor treatment are associated with some form of neurotoxicity, the mechanisms of which are elusive? Perhaps the potential for drug rescue (currently available for but a few agents) could be expanded.

Can we draw any generalizations from what is currently known about the available drugs and treatment regimens? It seems that intrathecal MTX in association with radiation therapy results in a high incidence of leukoencephalopathy yet MTX with BBB disruption is not associated with such. Intracarotid infusion of BCNU has significant toxicity not seen with MTX; drug streaming is the implicated mechanism, perhaps accentuated by poor drug solubility. Cisplatin and hydroxyurea are both cytotoxic in their own right and enhance radiation effects. Direct intra-tumor drug installation may be beneficial in treating tumor-associated cysts with bleomycin; perhaps thiotepa, cisplatin, cytarabine, and mechlorethamine would be useful in this manner too. The exact role of steroids, and specifically which steroids remains to be defined.

Without sufficient success to direct our approach, we are currently forced to almost randomly pursue a variety of antineoplastic agents, combinations, and routes of administration, usually based on untestable assumptions. When we discuss drug delivery to tumor, we often do not consider beyond its immediate fate, given surrounding normal brain, the BBB, and CSF circulation. Current clinical studies cannot be compared or in fact even evaluated due to a lack of concordance on simple definitions of treatment protocol, response, valid study groups, or data analysis.

Emphasizing the role of the BBB in defining adequate drug delivery has resulted in a clinically feasible new approach to brain tumor chemotherapy. Current results with BBBD and subsequent multi-agent drug administration establishes this treatment regimen as an alternative to other drug protocols. The observation that intracarotid cisplatin and etoposide may themselves disrupt the BBB suggests the potential use of etoposide (cisplatin may be too neurotoxic) as an alternative to mannitol in BBB modification prior to further drug delivery.

As safe, adequate, and rational chemotherapy develops, the role of radiation treatment (prominent only by default) is called up for risk-benefit analysis. Advances in molecular biology have established monoclonal antibodies in brain neoplasia diagnosis and treatment. The role of oncogenes in CNS tumorogenesis suggests the more prominent use of such agents as cytarabine and dactinomycin (inhibitors of reverse transcriptase) in progressive chemotherapy.

But where does this leave the neuroclinician? One has the responsibility to avail patients of progressive therapy, "experimental" though it be, for this is the often unspoken desire of those with such a futile disease. To justify such a course one must be assured of ongoing improvement in the risk-benefit ratio, of a therapy scientifically based in facts, medically sound and fiscally responsible.

Acknowledgments

Special thanks to Ms. Suellen Hill for her editorial comments and to Ms. Patricia Butler for her secretarial assistance.

References

1. Abramowicz H (1985) Cancer chemotherapy. Med Lett Drugs Ther 27: 13–20
2. Abelson HT, Kufe DW, Skarin AT, *et al.* (1981) Treatment of central nervous system tumors with methotrexate. Cancer Treat Rep 65: 137–140
3. Alavi JB, Weiler CB, Bruno LA (1984) Phase II evaluation of vindesine in the treatment of malignant glioma. Cancer Treat Rep 68: 807–808
4. Allen JC, Helson L (1981) High-dose cyclophosphamide chemotherapy for recurrent CNS tumors in children. J Neurosurg 55: 749–756
5. Allen JC, Helson L, Jereb B (1983) Preradiation chemotherapy for newly diagnosed childhood brain tumors: a modified phase II trial. Cancer 52: 2001–2006
6. Allen JC, Bosl G, Walker R (1984) Chemotherapy trials in recurrent CNS germ cell tumors. Proc Am Soc Clin Oncol 3: 325
7. Allen JC (1985) Childhood brain tumors. Current status of clinical trials in newly diagnosed and recurrent disease. Pediatr Clin North Am 32: 633–651
8. Amadori S, Papa G, Avisati G, *et al.* (1984) Sequential combination of systemic high-dose ara-C and asparaginase for the treatment of central nervous system leukemia and lymphoma. J Clin Oncol 2: 98–101
9. Andersen J, Christensen L, Kongsholm H (1984) Phase II trial of prednimustine in glioblastoma multiforme. Cancer Treat Rep 68: 795–797
10. Ariel IM (1961) Intra-arterial chemotherapy for metastatic cancer to the brain. Am J Surg 102: 647–650
11. Avellanosa A, West C, Barua N, Patel A (1984) Intracavitary combination chemotherapy of recurrent malignant glioma via Ommaya shunt—A pilot study. Proc Am Soc Clin Oncol 2: 234
11 a. Barnett MJ, Ganesan TS, Waxman JH, *et al.* (1985) Central nervous system toxicity of high-dose cytosine arabinoside. Sem Oncol 12 [suppl] 3: 227–232
12. Bauer KA, Skarin AT, Balikian JP, *et al.* (1983) Pulmonary complications associated with combination chemotherapy programs containing bleomycin. Am J Med 74: 557–563
13. Becker LE, Hinton D (1983) Primitive neuroectodermal tumors of the central nervous system. Human Pathol 14: 538–550
14. Benger A, Browman GP, Walker IR, Preisler HD, Goldberg J (1985) Clinical evidence of a cumulative effect of high-dose cytarabine on the cerebellum in patients with acute leukemia: a leukemia intergroup report. Cancer Treat Rep 69: 240–241
15. Berd D, Maguire HC, Mastrangelo MJ (1984) Potentiation of human cell-mediated and humoral immunity by low-dose cyclophosphamide. Cancer Res 44: 5439–5443
16. Berman IJ, Mann MP (1980) Seizures and transient cortical blindness associated with cisplatinum (II) diamminedichloride (PDD) therapy in a thirty year old man. Cancer 45: 764–766
17. Berry MP, Simpson WJ (1981) Radiation therapy in the management of primary malignant lymphoma of the brain. Int J Radiat Oncol Biol Phys 7: 55–59
18. Bigotte L, Arvidson B, Olsson Y (1982) Cytofluorescence localization of adriamycin in the nervous system. I. Distribution of the drug in the central nervous system of normal adult mice after intravenous injection. Acta Neuropathol (Berl) 57: 121–129

19. Bigotte L, Arvidson B, Olsson Y (1982) Cytofluorescence localization of adriamycin in the nervous system. II. Distribution of the drug in the somatic and autonomic peripheral nervous systems of normal adult mice after intravenous injection. Acta Neuropathol (Berl) 57: 130–136

20. Blacklock JB, Wright DC, Dedrick TL, et al. (1985) Drug streaming during intraarterial chemotherapy. Sixth international conference on brain tumor research and therapy, Asheville (abstract)

21. Blasberg RG, Nakagawa H, Patlak CS, Groothuis DR (1985) Dexamethasone reduces tumor and brain extracellular space: Effects on edema propagation. J Neuro-Oncol 2: 227

22. Bleyer WA, Griffin TW (1980) White matter necrosis, mineralizing microangiopathy, and intellectual abilities in survivors of childhood leukemia. In: Gilbert HA, Kagan AR (eds) Radiation damage to the nervous system. A delayed therapeutic hazard. Raven Press, New York, pp 155–174

23. Bleyer WA, Milstein J, Balis F, et al. (1983) "8 drugs in 1 day" chemotherapy for brain tumors: a new approach and rationale for preradiation chemotherapy. Med Pediatr Oncol 11: 213

24. Bosl GJ, Yagoda A, Golbey RB, Whitmore W, et al. (1985) Role of etoposide-based chemotherapy in the treatment of patients with refractory or relapsing germ cell tumors. Am J Med 78: 423–428

25. Bourdon MA, Coleman RE, Bigner DD (1984) The potential of monoclonal antibodies as carriers of radiation and drugs for immunodetection and therapy of brain tumors. Prog Exp Tumor Res 28: 79–101

26. Bradbury M (1979) The concept of a blood-brain barrier. J Wiley, New York

27. Broman T, Olsson O (1948) The tolerance of cerebral blood-vessels to a contrast medium of the diodrast group. Acta Radiol 30: 326–342

28. Broman T, Olsson O (1949) Experimental study of contrast media for cerebral angiography with reference to possible injurious effects on the cerebral blood vessels. Acta Radiol 31: 321–334

29. Brugarolas A, Garcia de Sola R, Bravo G, et al. (1980) Intra-arterial quelamycin in the treatment of glioblastoma. Proc Am Assoc Cancer Res 21: 346

30. Buckley JE, Clark VL, Meyer TJ, Pearlman NW (1984) Hypomagnesemia after cisplatin combination chemotherapy. Arch Intern Med 144: 2347–2348

31. Budka H (1982) Pathology of encephalopathies induced by treatment or prophylaxis of neoplastic lesions of the nervous system. In: Hildebrand J, Gangji D (eds) Treatment of neoplastic lesions of the nervous system. Pergamon Press, New York, pp 45–50

32. Burger PC, Kamenar E, Schold SC, et al. (1981) Encephalomyelopathy following high-dose BCNU therapy. Cancer 48: 1318–1327

33. Burger PC, Vogel FS, Green SB, Strike TA (1985) Glioblastoma multiforme and anaplastic astrocytoma: Pathologic criteria and prognostic implications. Cancer 56: 1106–1111

34. Butti G, Knerich R, Tanghetti B, et al. (1984) Perioperative carmustine chemotherapy for malignant brain tumors. Cancer Treat Rep 68: 1505–1506

35. Calabresi P, Parks RE (1985) Chemotherapy of neoplastic diseases. In: Gilman AG, Goodman LS, Gilman A (eds) The pharmacological basis of therapeutics. Macmillan, New York, pp 1240–1306

36. Cangir A, Ragab AH, Steuber P, et al. (1984) Combination chemotherapy with vincristine (NSC-67574), procarbazine (NSC-77213), prednisone (NSC-10023) with or without nitrogen mustard (NSC-762) (MOPP vs OPP) in children with recurrent brain tumors. Med Ped Oncol 12: 1–3

37. Capizzi RL, Nichols R, Mullins J (1972) Long-term survival of leukemic mice by therapeutic synergism between asparaginase and methotrexate. Fed Proc 31: 553

38. Carey RW, Davis JM, Zervas NT (1981) Tamoxifen-induced regression of cerebral metastases in breast carcinoma. Cancer Treat Rep 65: 793–795
39. Carmichael SM, Eagleton L, Ayers CR, et al. (1970) Orthostatic hypotension during vincristine therapy. Arch Intern Med 126: 290–293
40. Casanova MF (1984) Vasogenic edema with intraparenchymatous expanding mass lesions: A theory on its pathophysiology and mode of action of hyperventilation and corticosteroids. Med Hypotheses 13: 439–450
41. Chang CH, Horton J, Schoenfeld D, et al. (1983) Comparison of postoperative radiotherapy and combined postoperative radiotherapy and chemotherapy in the multidisciplinary management of malignant gliomas. Cancer 52: 2297–1007
42. Clark AW, Cohen SR, Nissenblatt MJ, Wilson SK (1982) Paraplegia following intrathecal chemotherapy: neuropathologic findings and elevation of myelin basic protein. Cancer 50: 42–47
43. Coscarelli C, Heinrich RL, Ganz PA (1984) Karnofsky performance status revisited: Reliability, validity and guidelines. J Clin Oncol 2: 187–193
44. Crafts DC, Levin VA, Edwards MS, Pischer TL, Wilson CB (1978) Chemotherapy of recurrent medulloblastoma with combined procarbazine, CCNU, and vincristine. J Neurosurg 49: 589–592
45. Dakhil S, Ensminger W, Strother V, et al. (1981) Pharmacokinetics of intraventricular 5-fluoro-2-deoxiuridine (FUDR) in patients with meningeal neoplasia. Proc Am Assoc Cancer Res 22: 178
46. Davis PL, Shumway MH (1961) Thio-tepa in treatment of metastatic cerebral malignancy. JAMA 175: 714–175
47. Dedrick RL, Oldfield EH, Collins JM (1984) Arterial drug infusion with extra-corporeal removal. I. Theoretic basis with particular reference to the brain. Cancer Treat Rep 68: 373–380
48. Delaney WE, Antoniades J (1985) Combination radiation/cisplatinum for adult malignant gliomas. Proc Am Soc Clin Oncol 4: 522
49. De Vita VT (1985) Principles of chemotherapy. In: DeVita ST, Hellman S, Rosenberg SA (eds) Cancer: principles and practice of oncology. JB Lippincott, Philadelphia, pp 257–285
50. De Vita VT (1983) The relationship between tumor mass and resistance to chemotherapy. Cancer 1: 1209–1220
51. Dick SJ, Macchi B, Papazoglou S, et al. (1983) Lymphoid cell glioma cell interaction enhances cell coat production by human gliomas: Novel suppressor mechanism. Science 220: 739–742
52. Djerassi I, Kim JS, Reggev A (1985) Response of astrocytoma to high-dose methotrexate with citrovorum factor rescue. Cancer 55: 2741–2747
53. Doll DC, Weiss RB, Issell BF (1985) Mitomycin: Ten years after approval for marketing. J Clin Oncol 3: 276–286
54. Duffy PE (1983) Astrocytes: normal, reactive, and neoplastic. Raven Press, New York
55. Dworkin LA, Goldman RD, Zivin LS, Fuchs PC (1985) Cerebellar toxicity following high-dose cytosine arabinoside. J Clin Oncol 3: 613–616
56. Eagen RT, Scott MS (1983) Evaluation of prognostic factors in chemotherapy of recurrent brain tumors. J Clin Oncol 1: 38–44
57. Eagen RT, Dinapoli RP, Hermann RC, Groover RV, Layton DD (1984) Carmustine and Baker's antifol combination chemotherapy for primary brain tumors progressive after irradiation and chemotherapy. Cancer Treat Rep 68: 431
58. Edwards MS, Levin VA, Seager ML, Pischer TL, Wilson CB (1979) Phase II evaluation of thioTEPA for treatment of central nervous system tumors. Cancer Treat Rep 63: 1419–1421

59. Edwards MS, Levin VA, Wilson CB (1980) Brain tumor chemotherapy: An evaluation of agents in current use for phase II and III trials. Cancer Treat Rep 64: 1179–1205

60. Edwards MS, Levin VA, Seager ML, Wilson CB (1981) Intrathecal chemotherapy for leptomeningeal dissemination of medulloblastoma. Child's Brain 8: 444–451

61. Einhorn LH (1980) Chemotherapy of metastatic seminoma. In: Einhorn H (ed) Testicular tumors: management and treatment. Masson, New York, pp 151–167

62. Epenetos AA, Courtenay-Luck N, Pickering D, et al. (1985) Antibody guided irradiation of brain glioma by arterial infusion of radioactive monoclonal antibody against epidermal growth factor receptor and blood group A antigen. Br Med J 290: 1463–1466

63. Ervin T, Canellos GP (1980) Successful treatment of recurrent primary central nervous system lymphoma with high-dose methotrexate. Cancer 45: 1556–1557

64. Fenstermacher J, Gazendam J (1981) Intra-arterial infusions of drugs and hyperosmotic solutions as ways of enhancing CNS chemotherapy. Cancer Treat Rep 65: 27–37

65. Fenstermacher JD (1985) Current models of blood-brain transfer. Trends in Neurosciences 8: 449–453

66. Fernandes DJ, Bertino JR (1980) 5-fluorouracil-methotrexate synergy: Enhancement of 5-fluorodeoxyuridylate binding to thymidylate synthase by dihydropteroyl polyglutamates. Proc Natl Acad Sci 77: 5664–5667

67. Feun LG, Wallace S, Lee F, et al. (1983) Phase I trial of intracarotid VP-16-213 (Etoposide) in patients with intracerebral tumors. Proc Am Soc Clin Oncol 2: 238

68. Feun LG, Wallace S, Yung WKA, et al. (1984) Phase I-II trial of intracarotid (IC) BCNU and cisplatin in patients with intracerebral tumors (ICT). Proc Am Soc Clin Oncol 3: 999

69. Feun LG, Lee YY, Yung WKA (1985) Phase II trial of intracarotid (IC) BCNU and cisplatin (DDP) in malignant brain tumors. Proc Am Soc Clin Oncol 4: 585

70. Fingert HJ, Hochberg FH (1984) Megadose chemotherapy with bone marrow rescue. Prog Exp Tumor Res 28: 67–78

71. Finlay JL, Knipple J, Turski P, et al. (1985) Pharmacokinetic studies of thio-tepa in dogs following delivery by various routes. Sixth international conference on brain tumor research and therapy, Asheville (abstract)

72. Firth G, Oliver AS, McKeran RO (1984) Studies on the intracerebral injection of bleomycin free and entrapped within liposomes in the rat. J Neurol Neurosurg Psychiat 47: 585–589

73. Firth G, Oliver AS, McKeran RO (1984) Studies on the use of antimitotic drugs entrapped within liposomes and of their action on a human glioma cell line. J Neurol Sci 63: 153–165

74. Flombaum CD (1984) Hypomagnesemia associated with cisplatin combination chemotherapy. Arch Intern Med 144: 2336–2337

75. Flora KP, Cradock JC, Kelley JA (1982) The hydrolysis of spirohydantoin mustard. J Pharm Sci 71: 1206–1211

76. Folkman J (1984) What is the role of endothelial cells in angiogenesis? Lab Invest 51: 601–604

77. Folkman J (1985) Tumor angiogenesis. Adv Cancer Res 43: 175–203

78. Foo S-H, Ransohoff J, Berenstein A, Choy I-S (1985) Intra-arterial BCNU chemotherapy for malignant gliomas. J Neurosurg 62: 458–459

79. Friedman MA (1981) Phase I and II studies of PCNU. In: Prestayko AW, et al. (eds) Nitrosoureas: current status and new development. Academic Press, New York, pp 379–386

80. Frytak S, Earnest F, O'Neill BP, Lee RE (1985) Nuclear magnetic resonance scanning (NMRS) for neurotoxicity (NT) in long term survivors of carcinoma (CA). Proc Am Soc Clin Oncol 4: 515

81. Fulling KH, Garcia DM (1985) Anaplastic astrocytoma of the adult cerebrum. Cancer 55: 928–931

82. Gagliano RG, Costanzi JJ (1976) Paraplegia following intrathecal methotrexate. Cancer 37: 1663–1668

83. Galivan J, Nimec Z (1984) Effects of folic acid on hepatoma cells containing methotrexate polyglutamates. Cancer Res 43: 551–555

83 a. Gamache FW, Galicich JH, Posner JB (1980) Treatment of brain metastasis by surgical extirpation. In: Weiss L, Gilbert HA, Posner JB (eds) Brain metastasis. G. K. Hall, Massachusetts, pp 390–414

84. Garbino CE, Gordon-Firing S (1984) Adjuvant chemotherapy with VM 26 in glioblastoma multiforme. Proc Am Soc Clin Oncol 3: C997

85. Giangaspero F, Burger PC (1983) Correlations between cytologic composition and biologic behavior in the glioblastoma multiforme. Cancer 52: 2320–2333

86. Goldman ID, Fyfe M (1974) The mechanism of action of methotrexate: II. Augmentation by vincristine of inhibition of deoxyribonucleic acid synthesis by methotrexate in Ehrlich ascites tumor cells. Mol Pharmacol 10: 275–282

87. Green SB, Byar DP, Walker MD, et al. (1983) Comparisons of carmustine, procarbazine, and high-dose methylprednisolone as additions to surgery and radiotherapy for the treatment of malignant glioma. Cancer Treat Rep 67: 121–132

88. Green SB, Byar DP, Strike TA, et al. (1984) Randomized comparisons of BCNU, streptozotocin, radio-sensitizer, and fractionation of radiotherapy in the postoperative treatment of malignant glioma (Study 7702), Proc Am Soc Clin Oncol 3: C 1018

89. Green SB, Byar DB, Strike TA, et al. (1985) Randomized phase II comparison of PCNU and AZQ for the treatment of primary brain tumors (Study 8120). Proc Am Soc Clin Oncol 4: C 558

90. Greenberg HS, Ensminger W, Chandler WF, et al. (1984) Intra-arterial BCNU chemotherapy for treatment of malignant gliomas of the central nervous system. J Neurosurg 61: 423–429

91. Greenberg HS, Ensminger W, Layton P, Gebarski S, Meyer MB (1984) A phase 1–2 evaluation of intra-arterial diaziquone (AZQ) for malignant tumors of the central nervous system. Proc Am Soc Clin Oncol 3: C 1003

92. Greig NH (1984) Chemotherapy of brain metastases: Current status. Cancer Treat Rev 11: 157–186

93. Greig NH, Sweeney DJ, Rapaport SI (1985) Inability of dimethyl sulfoxide to increase brain uptake of water-soluble compounds: Implications to chemotherapy for brain tumors. Cancer Treat Rep 69: 305–312

94. Groothuis DR, Molnar P, Blasberg RG (1984) Regional blood flow and blood-to-tissue transport in five brain tumor models. Prog Exp Tumor Res 27: 132–153

95. Haid M, Khandekar JD, Christ M, et al. (1985) Aziridinylbenzoquinone in recurrent, progressive glioma of the central nervous system. Cancer 56: 1311–1315

96. Hawkey CJ, Toghill PJ (1984) The need for prophylactic treatment to the central nervous system in patients with aggressive non-Hodgkin's lymphoma. Postgrad Med J 59: 283–297

97. Henson RA, Urich H (1982) Cancer and the nervous system: the neurological manifestations of systemic malignant disease. Blackwell, London

98. Herbst KD, Corder MP, Justice GR (1976) Successful therapy with methotrexate of a multicentric mixed lymphoma of the central nervous system. Cancer 38: 1476–1478

99. Herchbergs A, Sahar A, Tadmor R, Brenner HJ (1985) Primary cerebral neoplasia—Rapid performance status improvement (upgrading) following hypofractionated radiation combined with cisplatinum. Proc Am Soc Clin Oncol 4: C 516

100. Hochberg FH, Parker LM, Takvorian T, Canellos GP, Zervas NT (1981) High-dose BCNU with autologous bone marrow rescue for recurrent glioblastoma multiforme. J Neurosurg 54: 455–460

101. Hoshino T, Wilson CB, Rosenblum, ML, Baker M (1975) Chemotherapeutic implications of growth fraction and cell cycle time in glioblastoma. J Neurosurg 43: 127–135

102. Hoshino T (1979) The cell kinetics of gliomas: its prognostic value and therapeutic implications. In: Paoletti P, Walker MD, Butti G, Knerich R (eds) Multidisciplinary aspects of brain tumor therapy. Elsevier/North-Holland, New York, pp 105–112

103. Hoshino T, Wilson CB (1979) Cell kinetic analyses of human malignant brain tumors (gliomas). Cancer 44: 956–962

104. Hoshino T, Kobayashi S, Townsend JJ, Wilson CB (1985) A cell kinetic study on medulloblastomas. Cancer 55: 1711–1713

105. Howell SB, Pfeifle CE, Wung WE, Olshen RA (1983) Intraperitoneal cis-diamminedichloroplatinum with systemic thiosulfate protection. Cancer Res 43: 1426–1431

106. Hrushesky WJM (1984) Chemotherapy timing: an important variable in toxicity and response. In: Perry MC, Yarboro JW (eds) Toxicity of chemotherapy. Grune and Stratton, New York, pp 449–477

107. Hu E, Howell SB (1984) Pharmacokinetics of intraarterial mitomycin C in humans. Cancer Res 43: 4474–4477

107 a. Hwang TL, Yung WKA, Estey EH, Fields WS (1985) Central nervous toxicity with leigh-dose Ara-C. Neurology 35: 1475–1479

108. Irwin L, George F, Pitts F (1975) Hydroxyurea and radiation therapy in primary intracranial malignant glial tumors. Proc Am Assoc Cancer Res 16: 243

109. Jackson RC, Harkrader RJ (1981) Synergistic and antagonistic interactions of methotrexate and 1-β-D-arabinofluranosyl-cytosine in hepatoma cells. Biochem Pharmacol 30: 223–229

110. Jay JR, MacLaughlin DT, Riley KR, Martuza RL (1985) Modulation of meningioma cell growth by sex steroid hormones in vitro. J Neurosurg 62: 757–762

111. Jellinger K (1983) Pathologic effects of chemotherapy. In: Walker MD (ed) Oncology of the nervous system. M Nijhoff, Boston, pp 285–340

112. Jellinger K (1985) Changes induced in anaplastic gliomas and brain tissue as a result of treatment. In: Voth D, Krauseneck P (eds) Chemotherapy of gliomas. De Gruyter, Berlin, pp 153–176

112 a. Johnson HA, Haymaker WE, Rubini JR, et al. (1960) A radioautographic study of a human and glioblastoma multiforme after the in vivo uptake of tritiated thymidine. Cancer 13: 636–642

113. Kantarjian H, Farah PAM, Spitzer G, Murphy WK, Valdivieso M (1984) Systemic combination chemotherapy as primary treatment of brain metastasis from lung cancer. Southern Med J 77: 426–430

114. Kaplan RS, Wiernick PH (1984) Neurotoxicity of antitumor agents. In: Perry MC, Yarbro JW (eds) Toxicity of chemotherapy. Grune and Stratton, New York, pp 365–431

115. Kessinger A (1984) High dose chemotherapy with autologous bone marrow rescue for high grade gliomas of the brain: a potential for improvement in therapeutic results. Neurosurgery 15: 747–750

116. Kirkwood JM, Ensminger W, Rosowsky A, et al. (1980) Comparison of pharmacokinetics of 5-fluorouracil and 5-fluorouracil with concurrent thymidine infusions in a phase I trial. Cancer Res 40: 107–113

117. Koenig H (1970) Biochemical basis for fluorouracil neurotoxicity: The role of Krebs cycle by inhibition by fluoroacetate. Arch Neurol 23: 155–160

342 Mary K. Gumerlock and E. A. Neuwelt:

118. Kuhn J, von Hoff DD, *et al* (1983) Phase I trial of 2-fluoro-ara-AMP (NSC 312887). Fourth NCI-EORTC symposium on new drugs in cancer therapy, Brussels

119. Kumar ARV, Renaudin J, Wilson CB, *et al.* (1974) Procarbazine hydrochloride in the treatment of brain tumors. J Neurosurg 40: 365–371

120. Laerum OD, Bjerkvig R, Steinsvag SK, de Ridder L (1984) Invasiveness of primary brain tumors. Cancer Metastasis Rev 3: 223–236

121. Layton PB, Greenberg HS, Stetson PL, Ensminger WD, Gyves JW (1984) BCNU solubility and toxicity in the treatment of malignant astrocytomas. J Neurosurg 60: 1134–1137

122. Letendre L, Banks PM, Reese DF, *et al.* (1982) Primary lymphoma of the central nervous system. Cancer 49: 939–943

123. Levin VA, Wheeler KT (1982) Chemotherapeutic approaches to brain tumors: Experimental observations with dianhydrogalactitol and dibromodulcitol. Cancer Chemother Pharmacol 8: 125–131

124. Levin VA, Vestnys PS, Edwards MS, *et al.* (1983) Improvement in survival produced by sequential therapies in the treatment of recurrent medulloblastoma. Cancer 51: 1364–1370

125. Levin VA, Byrd D, Sikic BI, *et al.* (1985) Central nervous system toxicity and cerebrospinal fluid pharmacokinetics of intraventricularly administered bleomycin in beagles. Cancer Res 45: 3810–3815

126. Levin V, Choucair A, Davis RL, *et al.* (1985) Development of CNS "metastases" in patients with glioblastoma multiforme and other anaplastic gliomas while undergoing therapy. Sixth international conference on brain tumor research and therapy, Asheville (abstract)

127. Lieberman A, le Brun Y, Glass P, *et al. (1977)* Use of high dose corticosteroids in patients with inoperable brain tumours. J Neurol Neurosurg Psychiat 40: 678–682

128. Loeffler JS, Ervin TJ, Mauch P, *et al.* (1985) Primary lymphomas of the central nervous system: Patterns of failure and factors that influence survival. J. Clin Oncol 3: 490–494

129. Loehrer PJ, Einhorn LH (1984) Cisplatin. Ann Intern Med 100: 704–713

130. Logothetis CJ, Samuels ML, Trindade A (1982) The management of brain metastases in germ cell tumors. Cancer 49: 12–18

131. Long DM, Hartmann FJ, French LA (1969) The response of human cerebral edema to glucosteroid administration—An electron microscopic study. Neurology 31: 521–528

132. Mackintosh FR, Colby TV, Podolsky WJ, *et al.* (1982) Central nervous system involvement in non-Hodgkin's lymphoma: an analysis of 105 cases. Cancer 49: 586–595

133. Maeda H, Sano Y, Takeshita J, *et al.* (1981) A pharmacokinetic simulation model for chemotherapy of brain tumor with an antitumor protein antibiotic, neocarzinostatin: theoretical considerations behind a two-compartment model for continuous infusion via an internal carotid artery. Cancer Chemother Pharmacol 5: 243–249

134. Mahaley MS (1985) Summary of clinical trials of chemotherapy and conventional radiation therapy in the treatment of patients with primary malignant brain tumors. Sixth international conference on brain tumor research and therapy, Asheville (abstract)

135. Mark VH, Kjellberg RN, Ojemann RG, Slolway AH (1960) Treatment of malignant brain tumors with alkylating agents. Neurology 10: 772–776

136. Markman M, Cleary S, Howell SB (1985) Nephrotoxicity of high-dose intracavitary cisplatin with intravenous thiosulfate protection. Eur J Cancer Clin Oncol 21: 1015–1018

137. Martin DS, Stolfi RL, Sawyer RC, Spiegelman S, Young CW (1983) Improved therapeutic index with sequential N-phosphonacetyl-L-aspartate plus high-dose

methotrexate plus high-dose 5-fluorouracil and appropriate rescue. Cancer Res 43: 4653–4661

138. Matsuno H (1981) Tumor angiogenesis factor (TAF) in cultured cells derived from central nervous system tumors in humans. Neurol Med Chir 21: 765–773

139. Mealey J, Chen TT, Pedlow E (1970) Brain tumor chemotherapy with mithramycin and vincristine. Cancer 26: 260–367

139 a. Melgaard B, Hansen HS, Kamieniecka Z, Paulson OB, Pedersen AG, Tang X, Trojaborg W (1981) Misonidazole neuropathy: A clinical electrophysiological and histological study. Ann Neurol 12: 10–17

140. Mellett LB (1977) Physicochemical considerations and pharmacokinetic behavior in delivery of drugs to the central nervous system. Cancer Treat Rep 61: 527–531

141. Mendenhall NP, Thar TL, Agee OF, et al. (1983) Primary lymphoma of the central nervous system. Cancer 52: 1993–2000

142. Mooney C, Thomas DGT, Souhami RL (1983) Adriamycin in the treatment of relapsed primary malignant brain tumors. Eur J Cancer Clin Oncol 19: 1037–1038

143. Moran RG, Danenberg PV, Heidelberger C (1982) Therapeutic response of leukemic mice treated with fluorinated pyrimidines and inhibitors of deoxyuridylate synthesis. Biochem Pharmacol 31: 2929–2935

144. Morantz RA, Kimler BF, Vats TS, Henderson SD (1983) Bleomycin and brain tumors. J Neuro-Oncol 1: 249–255

145. Naysmith A, Robson RH (1979) Focal fits during chlorambucil therapy. Postgrad Med J 55: 806

146. Nelson JS, Tsukada Y, Schoenfeld D, et al. (1983) Necrosis as a prognostic criterion in malignant supratentorial, astrocytic gliomas. Cancer 52: 550–554

147. Neuwelt EA, Diehl JT, Hill SA, Marvilla KR (1979) Use of metrizamide computerized tomographic cisternography in the evaluation of patients with malignant glioma for immunotherapy. Neurosurgery 5: 576–582

148. Neuwelt EA, Frenkel EP, Diehl J, et al. (1980) Reversible osmotic blood-brain barrier disruption in humans: Implications for the chemotherapy of malignant brain tumors. Neurosurgery 7: 44–52

149. Neuwelt EA, Frenkel EP, Rapaport S, Barnett P (1980) Effect of osmotic blood-brain barrier disruption on methotrexate pharmacokinetics in the dog. Neurosurgery 7: 36–43

150. Neuwelt EA, Glasberg M, Diehl J, Frenkel EP, Barnett P (1981) Osmotic blood-brain barrier disruption in the posterior fossa of the dog. J Neurosurg 55: 742–748

151. Neuwelt EA, Pagel M, Barnett P, Glasberg M, Frenkel EP (1981) Pharmacology and toxicity of intracarotid adriamycin administration following osmotic blood-brain barrier modification. Cancer Res 41: 4466–4470

152. Neuwelt EA, Frenkel EP (1982) Osmotic blood-brain barrier disruption as a means of increasing chemotherapeutic agent delivery to the central nervous system: animal and clinical studies. In: Hildegrand J, Gangji D (eds) Treatment of neoplastic lesions of the nervous system. Pergamon Press, New York, pp 129–133

153. Neuwelt EA, Balaban E, Diehl J, Hill S, Frenkel E (1983) Successful treatment of primary central nervous system lymphomas with chemotherapy after osmotic blood-brain barrier opening. Neurosurgery 12: 662–671

154. Neuwelt EA, Barnett PA, Glasberg M, Frenkel EP (1983) Pharmacology and neurotoxicity of cis-diamminedichloroplatinum, bleomycin, 5-fluorouracil, and cyclophosphamide administration following osmotic blood-bran barrier modification. Cancer Res 43: 5278–5285

155. Neuwelt EA, Glasberg M, Frenkel E, Barnett P (1983) Neurotoxicity of chemotherapeutic agents after blood-brain barrier modification: Neuropathological studies. Ann Neurol 14: 316–324

156. Neuwelt EA, Specht HD, Howieson J, *et al.* (1983) Osmotic blood-brain barrier modification: Clinical documentation by enhanced CT scanning and/or radionuclide brain scanning. AJNR 4: 907–913

157. Neuwelt EA (1984) Therapeutic potential for blood-brain barrier modification in malignant brain tumors. Prog Exp Tumor Res 28: 51–66

158. Neuwelt EA, Barnett PA, Frenkel EP (1984) Chemotherapeutic agent permeability to normal brain and delivery to avian sarcoma virus-induced brain tumors in the rodent: Observations on problems of drug delivery. Neurosurgery 14: 154–160

159. Neuwelt EA, Barnett PA, McCormick CI, Frankel EP (1984) Osmotic blood-brain barrier modification: Parameters effecting drug delivery. In: Caciagli F, Giacobini E, Paoletti R (eds) Developmental neuroscience: physiological, pharmacological and clinical aspects. Elsevier, New York, pp 173–179

160. Neuwelt EA, Frenkel EP (1984) Germinomas and other pineal tumors: chemotherapeutic responses. In: Neuwelt EA (ed) Diagnosis and treatment of pineal region tumors. Williams and Wilkins, Baltimore, pp 332–343

161. Neuwelt EA, Hill SA, Frenkel EP (1984) Osmotic blood-brain barrier modification and combination chemotherapy: concurrent tumor regression in areas of barrier opening and progression in brain regions distant to barrier opening. Neurosurgery 15: 362–366

162. Neuwelt EA, Rapaport SI (1984) Modification of the blood-brain barrier in the chemotherapy of malignant brain tumors. Fed Proc 43: 214–219

163. Neuwelt EA, Barnett PA, McCormick CI, Frenkel EP, Minna JD (1985) Osmotic blood-brain barrier modification: Monoclonal antibody, albumin, and methotrexate delivery to cerebrospinal fluid and brain. Neurosurgery 17: 419–423

164. Neuwelt EA, Frenkel EP, d'Agostino AN, *et al.* (1985) Growth of human lung tumor in the brain of the nude rat as a model to evaluate antitumor agent delivery across the blood-brain barrier. Cancer Res 45: 2827–2833

165. Neuwelt EA, Frenkel EP, Gumerlock MK, *et al.* (1986) Developments in the diagnosis and treatment of primary CNS lymphoma: A prospective series. Cancer 58: 1609–1620

166. Neuwelt EA, Hill SA (1986) Chemotherapy administered in conjunction with osmotic blood-brain barrier modification in patients with brain metastases. J Neurooncol (in press)

167. Neuwelt EA, Howieson J, Frenkel EP, Specht D, Weigel R, *et al.* (1986) Therapeutic efficacy of multiagent chemotherapy with drug delivery enhancement by blood-barrier modification in glioblastoma. Neurosurgery 19: 573–582

168. Neuwelt EA, Minna J, Frenkel E, Barnett PA, McCormick CI (1986) Osmotic blood-brain barrier opening to IgM monoclonal antibody in the rat. Am J Physiol 250: R 875–R 883

169. Neuwelt EA, Specht HD, Hill SA (1986) Permeability of human brain tumor to ^{99m}Tc-glucoheptonate and ^{99m}Tc-albumin: Implications for monoclonal antibody therapy. J Neurosurg 65: 194–198

170. O'Dwyer PJ, Leyland-Jones B, Alonso MT, Marsoni S, Wittes RE (1985) Etoposide (VP-16-213): Current status of an active anticancer drug. New Engl J Med 312: 692–700

171. Ogawa M (1981) Current status of nitrosoureas under development in Japan. In: Prestayko AW, *et al.* (eds) Nitrosoureas: current status and new developments. Academic Press, New York, pp 399–410

172. Oldfield EH, Dedrick RL, Chatterji DC, *et al.* (1985) Arterial drug infusion with extracorporeal removal. II. Internal carotid carmustine in the rhesus monkey. Cancer Treat Rep 69: 293–303

173. Oster MW (1979) Combination chemotherapy for extracranial metastases of a primary malignant cerebral neoplasms. Cancer Treat Rep 63: 1417–1418

174. Owens G (1969) Intraarterial chemotherapy of primary brain tumors. Ann NY Academy Sci 159: 603–607

175. Poplack DG, Bleyer WA, Horowitz ME (1980) Pharmacology of antineoplastic agents in cerebrospinal fluid. In: Wood JH (ed) Neurobiology of cerebrospinal fluid I. Plenum Press, New York, pp 561–578

176. Posner JB, Howieson J, Cvitkovic E (1977) "Disappearing" spinal cord compression: Oncolytic effect of glucocorticoids (and other chemotherapeutic agents) on epidural metastases. Ann Neurol 2: 409–413

177. Postmus PE, Holthius JJM, Haaxma-Reiche G, et al. (1984) Penetration of VP 16-213 into cerebrospinal fluid after high-dose intravenous administration. J Clin Oncol 2: 215–220

178. Rapoport SI (1976) Blood-brain barrier in physiology and medicine. Raven Press, New York

179. Riccardi R, Bleyer WA, Poplack DG (1983) Enhancement of delivery of antineoplastic drugs into cerebrospinal fluid. In: Wood JH (ed) Neurobiology of cerebrospinal fluid II. Plenum Press, New York, pp 453–466

180. Rose C, Mouridsen HT (1984) Treatment of advanced breast cancer with tamoxifen. Recent Results Cancer Res 91: 230–242

181. Rosner D, Nemoto T, Pickren J, Lane W (1983) Management of brain metastases from breast cancer by combination chemotherapy. J Neuro-Oncol 1: 131–137

182. Ross RL, Kapp JP, Hochberg F, et al. (1983) Solvent systems for intracarotid 1,3-Bis-(2-chloroethyl)-1-nitrosourea (BCNU) infusion. Neurosurgery 12: 512–514

183. Rozenthal J, Trump D, Finlay J, et al. (1985) Pilot study of eight-drugs-in-one-day chemotherapy for high-grade astrocytomas. Sixth international conference on brain tumor research and therapy, Asheville (abstract)

184. Russo A, Gianni L, Kinsella TJ, et al. (1984) Pharmacological evaluation of intravenous delivery of 5-bromodeoxyuridine to patients with brain tumors. Cancer Res 44: 1702–1705

185. Schabel FM, Griswold DP, Corbett TH, Laster WR (1984) Increasing the therapeutic response rates to anticancer drugs by applying the basic principles of pharmacology. Cancer 54: 1160–1167

186. Schilsky RL, Yarbro JW (1984) Pharmacology of antineoplastic drugs. In: Perry MC, Yarbro JW (eds) Toxicity of chemotherapy. Grune and Stratton, New York, pp 21–59

187. Schnur G, Choy M, Stirling M, et al. (1984) Hemodynamic consequences of combined adriamycin-verapamil administration. Proc Am Soc Clin Oncol 3: C95

188. Schold SC, Carincross JG, Bullard DE (1984) Chemotherapy of primary brain tumors. In: Wilkins RH, Rengachary S (eds) Neurosurgery. McGraw-Hill, New York, pp 1143–1153

189. Schold SC, Friedman HS, Bjornsson TD, Falletta JM (1984) Treatment of patients with recurrent primary brain tumors with AZQ. Neurology 34: 615–619

190. Schroff RW, Foon KA, Beatty SM, Oldham RK, Morgan AC (1985) Human anti-murine immunoglobulin responses in patients receiving monoclonal antibody therapy. Cancer Res 45: 879–885

191. Sexauer C, Kahn A, Burger P, et al. (1984) Cisplatinum in recurrent pediatric brain tumors: A phase II study. Proc Am Soc Clin Oncol 3: 329

192. Shapiro WR, Byrne TN (1983) Chemotherapy of brain tumors—Basic concepts. In: Walker MD (ed) Oncology of the nervous system. M Nijhoff, Boston, pp 65–100

193. Shapiro WR (1985) Cell biology of primary brain tumors. Paper presented at the meeting of the American Academy of Neurology, Dallas

194. Shoemaker DD, O'Dwyer PJ, Marsoni S, et al. (1983) Spiromustine: a new agent entering clinical trials. Invest New Drugs 1: 303–308

195. Siegal T, Pfeffer MR, Catane R, *et al.* (1983) Successful chemotherapy of recurrent intracranial germinoma with spinal metastases. Neurology 33: 631–636

196. Sirotnak FM, Moccio DM, Hancock CH, *et al.* (1981) Improved methotrexate therapy of murine tumors obtained by probenecid-mediated pharmacological modulation of the level of membrane transport. Cancer Res 41: 3944–3949

197. Skarin AT, Zukerman KS, Pitman SW, *et al.* (1977) High-dose methotrexate with folinic acid in the treatment of advanced non-Hodgkin lymphoma including CNS involvement. Blood 50: 1039–1947

198. Slyter H, Liwnicz B, Herrick MK, *et al.* (1980) Fatal myeloencephalopathy caused by intrathecal vincristine. Neurology 30: 867–871

199. Spector R, Eells J (1984) Deoxynucleoside and vitamin transport into the central nervous system. Fed Proc 43: 196–200

200. Spigelman MK, Zappulla RA, Goldberg JD, *et al.* (1984) Effect of intracarotid etoposide on opening the blood-brain barrier. Cancer Drug Delivery 1: 207–211

201. Spigelman MK, Zappulla RA, Johnson J, *et al.* (1984) Etoposide-induced blood-brain barrier disruption. J Neurosurg 61: 674–678

202. Stewart DJ, Leavens M, Maor M, *et al.* (1982) Human central nervous system distribution of cis-diamminedichloroplatinum and use as a radiosensitizer in malignant brain tumors. Cancer Res 42: 2474–2479

203. Stewart DJ, Hugenholtz RH, Dennery J (1984) VP-16 (VP) and VM-26 (VM) penetration into human brain tumors (BT). Proc Am Assoc Cancer Res 24: 527

204. Stewart DJ, Russel N, Atack EA, Quarrington A, Stolbach L (1983) Cyclophosphamide, doxorubicin, vincristine, and dexamethasone in primary lymphoma of the brain: A case report. Cancer Treat Rep 67: 287–291

205. Stewart DJ (1984) Novel modes of chemotherapy administration. Prog Exp Tumor Res 28: 32–50

206. Stewart DJ, Grahovak Z, Benoit B, *et al.* (1984) Intracarotid chemotherapy with a combination of 1,3-bis(2-chlorethyl)-1-nitrosourea (BCNU), cis-diaminedichloroplatinum (Cisplatin), and 4'-O-demethyl-1-O-(4,6-O-2-thenylidene-β-D-glucopyranosyl) epipodophyllotoxin (VM-26) in the treatment of primary and metastatic brain tumors. Neurosurgery 15: 828–833

207. Stewart DJ, Russell N, Atack EA, Quarrington A, Stolback L (1984) Cyclophosphamide, doxorubicin, vincristine, and dexamethasone in the treatment of bulky CNS lymphoma. J Neuro-Oncol 2: 289

208. Stewart DJ, Grahovaz Z, Maroun J, *et al.* (1985) Intraarterial (IA) chemotherapy (CT) for brain tumors (BT). Proc Am Soc Clin Oncol 4: C 513

209. Sullivan KM, Storb R, Shulman HM, *et al.* (1982) Immediate and delayed neurotoxicity after mechlorethamine preparation for bone marrow transplantation. Ann Int Med 98: 182–189

210. Syndran AC (1981) The cytosine arabinoside (Ara-C) syndrome. Med Ped Oncol 9: 257–264

211. Takahashi H, Nakazawa S, Shimura T (1985) Evaluation of postoperative intratumoral injection of bleomycin for craniopharyngioma in children. J Neurosurg 62: 120–127

212. Takakura K, Sano K, Hojo S, Hirano A (1982) Metastatic tumors of the central nervous system. Igaku-Shoin, Tokyo New York

213. Thompson SW, Davis LE, Kornfeld M, Hilgers RD, Standefer JC (1984) Cisplatin neuropathy: Clinical, electrophysiologic, morphologic and toxicologic studies. Cancer 54: 1269–1275

214. Tirelli U, d'Incalci M, Canetta R, *et al.* (1984) Etoposide (VP-16-213) in malignant brain tumors: A phase II study. J Clin Oncol 2: 432–437

215. Tsuruo T, Iida H, Tsukagoshi S, *et al.* (1981) Overcoming of vincristine resistance in P 388 leukemia *in vivo* and *in vitro* through enhanced cytotoxicity of vincristine and vinblastine by verapamil. Cancer Res 41: 1967–1972

216. Ushio Y (1985) Intrathecal ACNU against leptomeningeal dissemination of tumor: experimental study. Sixth international conference on brain tumor research and therapy, Asheville (abstract)

217. Vermorken JB, Stam J, Karim AB, *et al.* (1983) Treatment of small cell lung cancer (SCLC) utilizing two alternating combination chemotherapy regimens. Proc Am Soc Clin Oncol 2: 785

218. Volc D, Jellinger K, Grisold W, *et al.* (1985) Combined radiation and polychemotherapy (COMP) in the postoperative treatment of high-grade supratentorial gliomas. In: Voth D, Krauseneck P (eds) Chemotherapy of gliomas. De Gruyter, Berlin, pp 341–352

219. Von Hoff DD, Reichert CM, Cuneo R, *et al.* (1979) Demyelinization of peripheral nerves associated with cis-diamminedichloroplatinum (II) (DDP) therapy. Proc Am Assoc Cancer Res 20: 367

220. Wahl RL, Parker CW, Philpott GW (1983) Improved radioimaging and tumor localization with monoclonal F(ab'). J Nuc Med 24: 316–325

221. Walker MD, Weiss HD (1975) Chemotherapy in the treatment of malignant brain tumors. Adv Neurol 13: 149–191

222. Walker MD, Green SB, Byar DP, *et al.* (1980) Randomized comparisons of radiotherapy and nitrosoureas for the treatment of malignant glioma after surgery. New Engl J Med 303: 1323–1329

223. Warnke P, Groothuis D, Kuruvilla A, *et al.* (1985) The effect of corticosteroids on drug delivery parameters in experimental brain tumors. Sixth international conference on brain tumor research and therapy, Asheville (abstract)

224. Wasserman TH, Stetz J, Phillips TL (1981) Radiation therapy oncology group clinical trials with misonidazole. Cancer 47: 2382–2390

225. Weiss HD, Walker MD, Wiernik PH (1974) Neurotoxicity of commonly used antineoplastic agents (parts I and II). New Engl J Med 291: 75–81

226. Weiss HD, Wiernick PH, Walker MD (1974) Intrathecal N, N', N''-Triethylenethiophosphoramide [Thio-TEPA (NSC 6396)] in the treatment of malignant meningeal disease phase I–II study. Proc Am Assoc Cancer Res 15: 257

227. Weissman D, Grossman S (1985) Temporal development of peritumoral brain edema in rabbit VX 2 brain tumors. Sixth international conference on brain tumor research and therapy, Asheville (abstract)

228. West CR, Avellanosa AM, Barua NR, Patel A, Hong CI (1983) Intra-arterial 1,3-Bis(2-chlorethyl)-1-nitrosourea (BCNU) and systemic chemotherapy for malignant gliomas: A follow-up study. Neurosurgery 13: 420–426

229. White JC, Fernandes DJ, Capizzi RL (1984) Pharmacologic approaches to combination chemotherapy. In: Perry MC, Yarbro JW (eds) Toxicity of chemotherapy. Grune and Stratton, New York, pp 61–99

230. Williams ME, Walker AN, Bracikowski JP, *et al.* (1983) Ascending myeloencephalopathy due to intrathecal vincristine sulfate: a fatal chemotherapeutic error. Cancer 51: 2041–2047

231. Williams SA, *et al* (1978) Seizures: significant side effect of chlorambucil therapy in children. J Peds 93: 516–518

232. Wilson CB, Levin V, Hoshino T (1982) Chemotherapy of brain tumors. In: Youmans JR (ed) Neurological surgery. W B Saunders, Philadelphia, pp 3065–3095

233. Yalowich JC, Fry DW, Goldman ID (1982) Teniposide (VM-26)—and etoposide (VP-16-2132)-induced augmentation of methotrexate transport and polyglutamylation in Ehrlich ascites tumor cells *in vitro*. Cancer Res 42: 3648–3653

234. Yamashita J, Handa H, Tokuriki Y, *et al.* (1984) Intra-arterial ACNU therapy for malignant brain tumors. J Neurosurg 59: 424–430
235. Young DF, Posner JB (1980) Nervous system toxicity of the chemotherapeutic agents. In: Vinken PJ, Bruyn GW (eds) Handbook of clinical neurology. North-Holland, New York, pp 91–129
236. Zager RF, Frisby SA, Oliverio VT (1973) The effects of antibiotics and cancer chemotherapeutic agents on the cellular transport and antitumor activity of methotrexate in L 1210 murine leukemia. Cancer Res 33: 1670–1676
237. Zimm S, Collins JM, Curt GA, O'Neill D, Poplack DG (1984) Cerebrospinal fluid pharmacokinetic of intraventricular and intravenous aziridinylbenozquinone. Cancer Res 44: 1698–1701

Authors' address: Prof. Dr. Mary K. Gumerlock, The Oregon Health Sciences University, Department of Neurosurgery L 472, 3181 SW Sam Jackson Park Road, Portland, OR 97201, U.S.A.

7

Results of Chemotherapy of Malignant Brain Tumors in Adults

P. Krauseneck and *H. G. Mertens*

Department of Neurology, University of Würzburg, Federal Republic of Germany

1. Diagnostics

The aim of this article is to review the results of modern chemotherapy and multiple agent trials in the treatment of malignant brain tumors in adults. As introduction a brief outline of diagnostic methods is given, and some remarks on time schedule and pecularities of follow-up examinations and treatment evaluation are made to allow a more critical appraisal of the clinical results.

1.1. Clinical Findings

Table 1 shows the most common symptoms [123, 186] which usually quickly prompt to CT scanning and the tumor diagnosis is made. Only if, in the beginning, symptoms are restricted to personality changes or emotional disorders is the diagnosis difficult and may be missed for longer time. This particularly occurs with slowly growing frontal tumors (meningiomas!). Therefore, patients showing continuing psychic

Table 1. The frequency of symptoms at diagnosis of cerebral gliomas

Symptoms	McKeran and Thomas 1980 (%)	Walker *et al.* 1980 (%)
Headache	71	55
Epilepsy	54	36
Mental change	52	35
Hemiparesis	43	46
Dysphasia	27	24
Impaired consciousness	25	?

changes, especially chronic depression, should be subjected to CT scanning even if the EEG findings are unremarkable. It is especially important to pinpoint exactly the begin of the disease since the duration of symptoms is of prognostic importance and contributes to the decision of therapy[26, 66].

1.2. Laboratory Findings

In primary brain tumors, laboratory findings are usually not diagnostic at all. In primary cerebral lymphomas one or several classes of immunoglobulins may be suppressed, resulting in low serum levels. Rarely is an increase in serum immunoglobulin found pointing to a possible systemic spreading of the lymphoma.

In secondary malignancies to the brain the well-known changes in the blood chemistry as in cancer of other sites occur. In case of positive tumor markers in the serum (CEA, human choriongonadotropin [HCG], etc.) these can also be used for monitoring of the brain involvement.

1.3. Cerebrospinal Fluid

Primitive neuroectodermal tumors (PNETs), particularly medulloblastomas, often produce polyamines (putrescine, spermidine, spermine) in sufficient quantities to provide a reliable monitoring by the CSF levels[9, 35, 121, 144]. Since an increase in putrescine in the CSF often precedes tumor recurrence, earlier treatment becomes possible. More important is the screening of the CSF for dissemination of tumor cells, because a positive finding always indicates progressive and widespread disease with the need for intrathecal cytostatic treatment and—where available—systemic cytostatic therapy. A positive finding does not require proof of malignant cells but in patients with known malignancy the combination of (multiple) neurologic symptoms and elevated protein in the CSF is sufficient to make the diagnosis of leptomeningeal cancer if an infection, solid tumors and metabolic disturbances can be excluded[146]. The progress in the treatment of systemic cancer has achieved longer survival and hence more frequent involvement of the nervous system. Therefore, to rule out carcinomatous meningosis, CSF examination should be done routinely in patients with acute leucemias, malignant non-Hodgkin's lymphomas and metastasizing disease of breast and lung or melanoma, or if neurological signs or symptoms are present in a patient with known malignant disease. CT scan and MRI can often only give hints to meningeal or ventricle wall involvement even when malignant cells in the CSF have been demonstrated[7]. Since patients with malignant brain tumors also live longer with aggressive therapy and may experience several relapses, leptomeningeal carcinomatosis or seeding of glioma cells can occur more often. In recent autopsy series up to 75% leptomeningeal metastases were found in malignant gliomas[20, 53, 134, 135, 142]. Particularly in cases where the tumor is located in the vicinity of the CSF pathways, examination of the CSF should be performed. Cell markers such as GFAP, S-100, cytokeratin or panels of monoclonal antibodies help defining the origin of the tumor cells[102]. CSF examination is important in patients where a primary cerebral lymphoma is suspected. This diagnosis may be missed for months by CT scan, MRI or even biopsy while malignant cells in the CSF—often only found after repeated CSF sampling—confirm the diagnosis [17, 90, 91, 125].

1.4. EEG

Classical findings are focal slow waves in the theta and/or delta range corresponding to the tumor site often accompanied by paroxysmal changes. Spreading to adjacent areas or to the contralateral side is common, not always dependent on brain edema. The EEG is no more relevant for making the diagnosis of a brain tumor but remains useful as a screening test in patients with unspecific signs or symptoms. In the follow-up the EEG is helpful to identifiy neurologic side effects of the treatment *e.g.* metabolic encephalopathies or in differentiating tumor recurrence from postoperative changes in patients with equivocal CT findings and is necessary in assessing the risk of seizures after successful tumor therapy.

1.5. Radioisotopic Brain Scan

The conventional technetium scans are replaced more or less completely by the CT scan. However, new tracers like iodine-125-amphetamine are possibly more sensitive than the CT scan for certain tumor types such as primary cerebral lymphomas. Radioactive labeled monoclonal antibodies may be a new tool to identify tumor areas in the brain in the future [10, 21, 102, 117, 169].

1.6. Positron-Emission Tomography (PET)

PET scanning is not available now for individual routine diagnostics, but has provided new basic insights with brain tumors [18, 41, 122, 149]. For instance it was shown that there are no hypoxic areas in gliomas but that oxygen consumption is low although sufficient oxygen is supplied. So, the hypothetic rationale for some radiosensitizing substances like metro- and misonidazole could not be confirmed. Only with PET the differentiation of radiation necrosis and tumor regrowth may be possible by measuring the low glucose metabolism in necrotic areas [41, 143]. In the future it might be possible to determine the metabolic parameters and the status of the BBB of an individual patient's tumor and to adapt to these the delivery of cytostatic agents.

1.7. Angiography

In contrast to some benign tumors, *e.g.* angioblastoma or meningioma, in malignant brain tumors the angiography adds little to the CT scan in defining the tumor type. In glioblastoma the typical early filling of veins or lacunar contrast depots may be present or not. Metastatic tumors may present the same features and even the phase of luxury perfusion after ischemic stroke may mimic these "typical" angiographic findings. Digital subtraction angiography (DSA) provides better imaging but no higher diagnostic accuracy. In special cases selective or highly-selective catheter techniques contribute to better diagnostic validity. Preoperative embolization of highly vascularized tumors, especially meningiomas because of their blood supply via the external carotid artery, is possible with the new catheters.

1.8. Computer-assisted Tomography (CT)

The revolutionary impact of this new X-ray technique on the diagnostics of brain tumors need not be described in detail. Most of the malignant brain tumors show a hypodense area in the native scan with surrounding edema, often extending finger-like into the white matter and sparing the cortex and basal ganglia. After contrast enhancement usually irregular ring structures become visible demarcating the tumor from surrounding brain and often comprising a necrotic pseudocystic inner area (Fig. 1). Homogenous contrast enhancement is usually seen in smaller lesions, in lymphomas (Fig. 2), in some gliomas of the corpus callosum, in some kinds of metastases and in a variety of benign tumors such as meningiomas. Primary hyperdense tumors (without contrast enhancement) are usually meningiomas, hypernephroid carcinomas, gemistocytic low grade gliomas or lymphomas. Isodense tumors can only be seen after enhancement. Therefore contrast-enhanced CT scan is mandatory if a brain tumor is suspected.

In intrinsic brain tumors, as a rule, the grade of malignancy corresponds to the extent of contrast enhancement and of surrounding edema, but as much as 20–30% of low grace gliomas show contrast enhancement[99a].

All these typical findings are no reliable criteria for an individual tumor. Even combinations of typical findings in CT scan, angiography and EEG may be

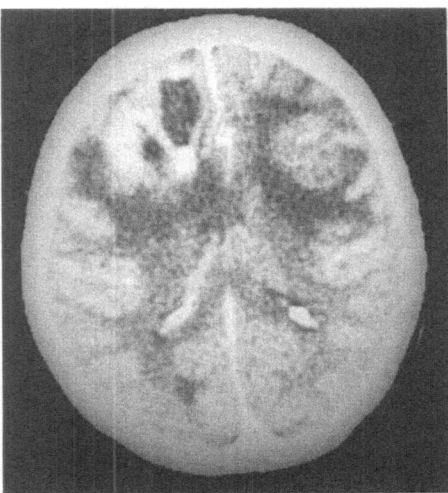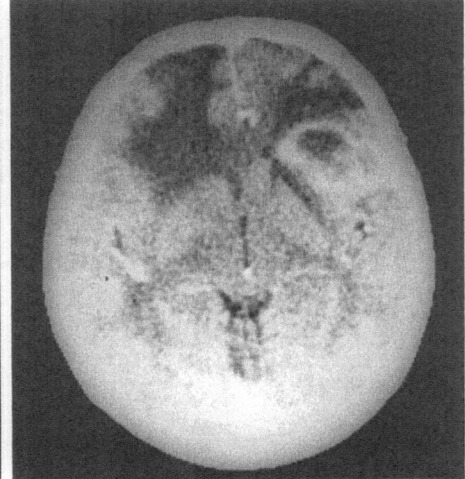

Fig. 1. Multifocal glioblastoma multiforme with pseudocystic necrotic inner area and finger-like edema into the white matter (biopsy proven). This picture is undistinguishable from brain metastases

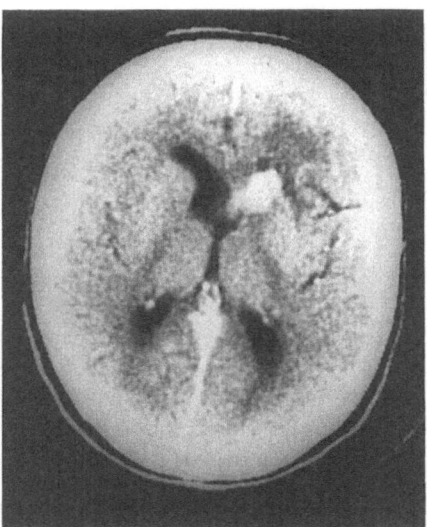

Fig. 2. Typical picture of a primary CNS lymphoma after contrast enhancement. In the native scan only a small hypodense area was seen. Note the intrinsic diffuse growth with little or no mass effect

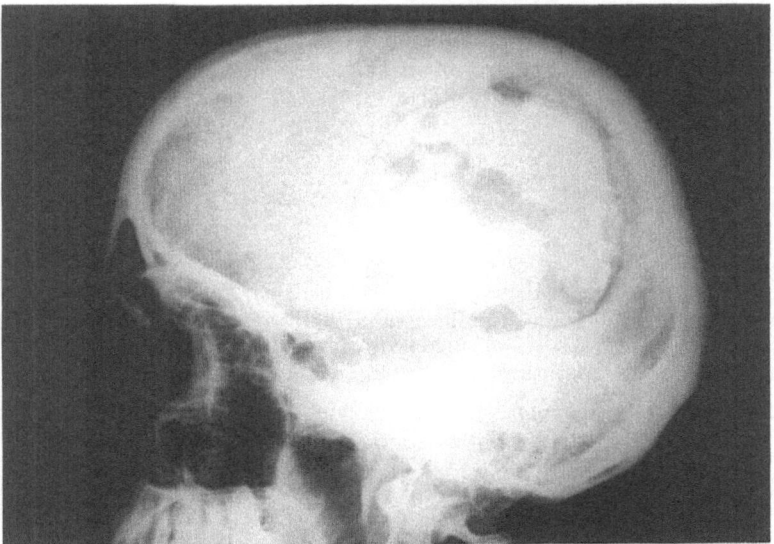

Fig. 3. Osteomyelitis of the bone flap causing a small hypodense area with questionable contrast enhancement in the CT scan and a slight hemiparesis. No recurrence of the anaplastic oligodendroglioma until two years later

misleading. Pitfalls are, *e.g.* some weeks old hematomas, abscesses, inflammatory lesions of multiple sclerosis or hemorrhagic infarcts. A variety of factors influence the contrast enhancement of a tumor, *e.g.* quantity and method of application of the contrast medium, amount of steroids administered, osmotherapy, disturbances of the BBB by trauma, local (*e.g.* of the bone flap (Fig. 3)] or systemic infection,

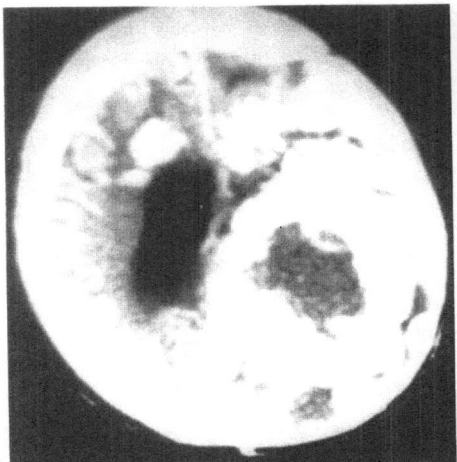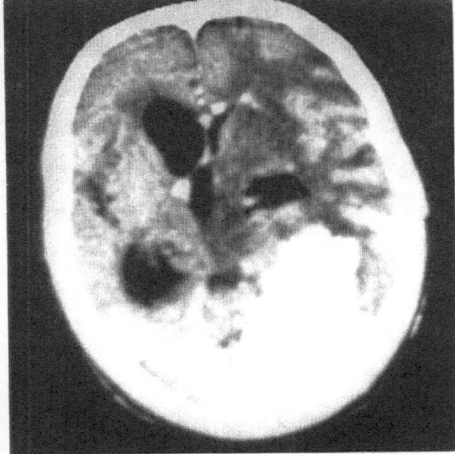

Fig. 4. Huge, monstrous relapse of a malignant ependymoma after several operations and combined radio-/chemotherapy. Note the distinct periventricular calcifications. The patient survived this final relapse for one year

epileptic seizures, etc.[98]. This must be kept well in mind when CT scans are evaluated.

Calcifications can be seen in all tumor types if efficient therapy achieved a longer lasting regression of the tumor (*cf.* Fig. 4).

1.9. Nuclear Magnetic Resonance Imaging (MRI)

In comparison with the CT scan the known advantages of the MRI take effect particularly on tumors near the basis of the skull and in the initial stage of low grade gliomas. The density of these gliomas can hardly be distinguished from the normal brain tissue, so that CT findings may be ambiguous or negative when in the MRI the lesion is already plain (Fig. 5). The sensitivity of MRI for brain tumors is considerably higher and extends from more than 90% sensitivity of the CT scan to nearly 100%, but specificity is not as good and the nature of a known lesion often has to be clarified by other methods.

1.10. Biopsy

As mentioned above, even very "characteristic" findings of the imaging techniques may be misleading and therefore no harmful therapy—like irradiation or cytostatic treatment—should be done without histologic proof either in the CSF or the tissue sampling. Now biopsies in every brain area are possible due to improvement of the diagnostic and stereotactic tools. Open biopsies should be considered only in superficial lesions. The stereotactic biopsies should sample along the biopsy axis several small tissue pieces of the brain adjacent to the tumor, at the edges and in the

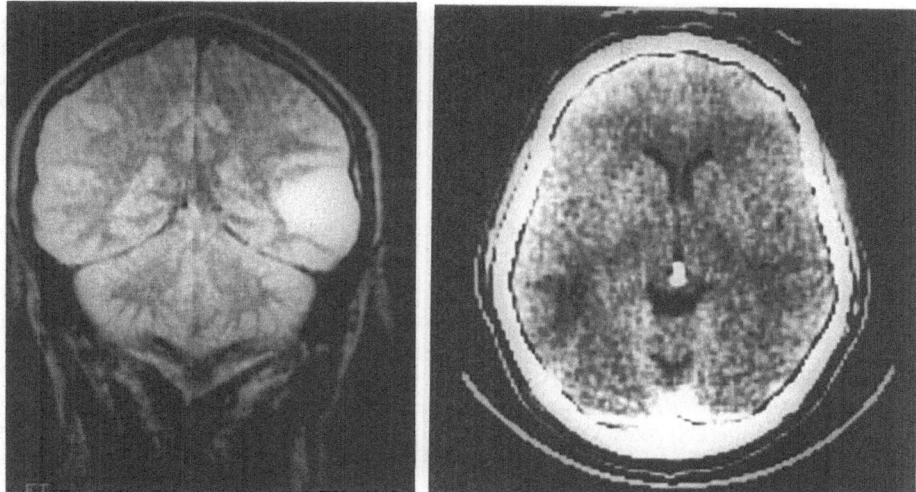

Fig. 5. An astrocytoma grade 2 is well demarcated in the MRI scan whereas in the CT scan only a small irregular hypodense area is seen

core of the tumor. This procedure provides correct neuropathologic diagnosis in about 90% of the cases, even to the grade of malignancy (*e.g.*[19]). The rate of complications is low ($< 5\%$) and the rate of mortality is well below 1%. Instead of an increasingly extending work-up for a possible primary tumor, early stereotactic biopsy is easier for the patient and may save valuable time.

1.11. Follow-Up Examinations

In the evaluation of treatment efficacy CT scan and MRI are not as accurate as in making the diagnosis. Postoperatively, hemorrhages and contrast enhancement of zones of reparation at the margins of the operative site make the evaluation difficult, especially as this unspecific contrast enhancement may last for several months. Contrast enhancement depends strongly on the concomitant dose of steroids and may be suppressed almost completely by very high doses. Inflammation of adjacent tissues can provoke contrast enhancement of the tumor area, *e.g.* osteomyelitis of the bone flap. Edematous reactions after grand mal seizures or trauma can resemble tumor progression[98].

The crucial question, if after radiotherapy or longer periods of successful chemotherapy, there is viable tumor remaining can often not be answered by a single CT scan and even not by MRI, as scar tissue, necrotic or cystic areas and reactive gliosis may be undistinguishable from tumor mass[156]. With MRI demyelinization after radiation or as sequelae of chronic elevated intracranial pressure show similar spin echos as infiltrating tumor. The same problems arise in defining radiation necrosis, even with biopsies. Tumor necrosis and viable tumor

Table 2. Recommended time table for routine follow-up examinations in brain tumors

---

WHO grade 1:
  Clinical examination and CT scan with contrast enhancement 1, 6, and 12 months postoperatively.
  Further evaluation only if new symptoms occur.

WHO grade 2:
  Clinical examination and CT scan with contrast enhancement 1 month postoperatively, then every 3 months for 1 year, then at least once a year.

WHO grades 3 and 4:
  CT scan with contrast enhancement within 72 hours after surgery to define tumor rest (later on zones of reparation will also enhance), 1 month postoperatively and then every 3 months for 2 years, then every 6 months. Clinical examination every 6 weeks. CSF cytology postoperatively or at diagnosis and every 6 months, if tumor is situated adjacent to the CSF pathways.

---

areas may well occur simultaneously after aggressive therapy[22, 87]. Repeating the CT scan after some weeks or months often settles the question but the tumor may grow in the meantime or undue therapy will have been started. So, in spite of great progress in making the diagnosis of a brain tumor, exact evaluation of the effects of treatment on the tumor often remains difficult and unsatisfactory. Therefore, regular CT examinations are necessary. Table 2 gives recommendations for a time schedule dependent on the tumor type.

EEG is helpful and economic but does not replace CT or MRI scanning in tumor assessment.

CSF examination every 6 months is recommended in patients with remaining tumor masses after the initial therapy to rule out secondary leptomeningeal involvement.

For at least one year clinical examination of the patient should be done every six weeks, since sophisticated evaluation of the clinical course of the patients is necessary. Patients under prolonged steroid medication or/and cytostatic treatment tend to develop latent chronic and uncommon infections especially of the lungs, which worsen the patient's shape and simulate tumor progression. Other causes of deterioration not related to the tumor can be endocrinological problems such as insufficiency of the thyroid or adrenal glands. Toxic reactions, *e.g.* intolerance of phenytoin, paraneoplastic syndromes or vitamin deficiencies may also be misleading, *e.g.* Wernicke encephalopathy[98].

1.12. Neurotoxicity

An essential aim of the fine-mesh follow-up examinations consists in early recognition of serious side-effects and preventing permanent damage. In BCNU, to a much higher percentage than previously supposed, exists the danger of interstitial pneumonia with permanent limitation of lung function or of a lethal lung fibrosis. BCNU treatment should, therefore, be executed only with regular check-ups of the lung function, *i.e.* before every new application. A certain prognosis of the risk of lung fibrosis is possible using the formula given by Aronin *et al.*[6], in which the patient's age, total dosis, application intervals and previous pulmonary disorders are of importance. These authors recommend that the total dose not exceed 1,500 mg/m² BCNU. Our own experience has shown that it is necessary to discontinue BCNU therapy when, during the lung function examinations, the diffusion capacity for CO (as the most sensitive parameter) sinks lower than 50% or, when the total lung capacity falls off to below 50% of the original value[160].

Frequent cases of polyneuropathy from cisplatinum and especially vincristine must also be pointed out. This requires discontinuance of the medication if motor paresis sets in. Sensitive dysesthesia can usually be brought about by applying carbamazepine to make it more bearable for the patient. After long-term chemotherapy a permanent light to moderate bone marrow depression is inevitable and must be chanced. However, concerning hemotological toxicity the treatment strategies vary a great deal, so that, for example, in US studies cytostatics are reduced at a leucocyte nadir under 2,500/µl, whereas in the Austro-German study a reduction in dosis was not made till a nadir of below 1,500 µl. The influence of such more or less aggressive modes of chemotherapy on the efficacy and rate of side-effects is still unclear.

Neurotoxic side-effects presenting as encephalopathy have also been described in BCNU and procarbazine[88, 93]. However, they were not reported in randomized studies of conventional, intravenous or oral application[4, 33, 48—52, 68, 69, 77, 107, 108, 176, 184–186]. A possible explanation is that the separation of tumor-caused symptoms is very difficult.

Considerable neurotoxic lesions with development of dementia have been observed following intra-arterial BCNU administration in the current study of the American BTSG. This forced a reduction of the BCNU dosis from the second cycle onwards from 200 mg/m² to 100 mg/m². The risk of dementia developing during the normal intravenous or oral chemotherapy according to the data presented is low, whereas high-dose irradiation with 60 Gy whole brain or high doses of BCNU, methotrexate or cytosine-arabinoside treatment could involve the risk of demential development[8, 43, 75, 93]. In high-dose chemotherapy acute reactions (stroke-like syndrome) or the development of a leukoencephalopathy occur within a few months. Radiation damage after a total dosis of up to 60 Gy does not occur until the second year of treatment, so that only a small number of patients with malignant gliomas and metastases lives long enough to suffer this complication[87, 88, US-BTSG].

Recurrence should be defined as a clear-cut enlargement of the tumor in the CT scan (at least 20–25% increase of tumor volume) *and* an unequivocal worsening of the clinical status, because changes in one parameter only are unreliable.

1.13. Neuropathological Classification

One of the most crucial points for the indication of chemotherapy is an exact neuropathological diagnosis. Several classifications and grading systems are used and a "glioblastoma" of the Kernohan system does not necessarily correspond to a "glioblastoma" of the Ringertz (1950) or Zülch (1952) or WHO (1979) classification (see Jellinger, this volume). Conflicting results of clinical trials in some cases can be explained by different neuropathological criteria or insufficient grading. Thus gliomas grade II (WHO), *i.e.* oligodendrogliomas, fibrillary, protoplasmatic and gemistocytic astrocytomas, after operation have a *median* life expectancy of 5 or more years[99a], whereas patients with gliomas grade III, *i.e.* anaplastic astrocytomas/oligodendrogliomas, even with aggressive multimodal therapy live in the median less than 2 years and the grade IV gliomas, *i.e.* glioblastoma multiforme less than 10 months[24, 25]. The grading system cited here is that of the WHO[191], which should be considered the binding compromise of the different systems. Even within this system differences of interpretation exist as to the transition of grade II to III or III to IV. Therefore, a valid study must have a central pathological review committee deciding on the eligibility and classification of the cases.

A neuropathologic reference evaluation should be searched for also in cases of malignant brain tumors with equivocal histologic features before starting chemotherapy. Not only the malignancy, *i.e.* the grading, of a brain tumor determines the choice of therapy but even more important is the exact tumor type for developing an appropriate treatment strategy. Not all grade IV tumors necessarily require chemotherapy and the choice of cytostatic agents in some respect depends on the neuroectodermal or mesodermal origin of the tumor because in mesodermal tumors no efficacious BBB will be present and agents not penetrating the BBB will be appropriate, and *vice versa*.

For the WHO grading for the most important tumor types see Jellinger (this volume).

2. Results and Indications of Chemotherapy

2.1. Preliminary Remarks

There are only two brain tumor types which until now have been studied so systematically that quantitative assessment of the efficacy of chemotherapy is possible: malignant gliomas in adults and medulloblastomas in children. Other rare tumors were treated with chemotherapy but not in randomized, well controlled trials limited to a few years. The big multi-center studies on malignant gliomas cited below demonstrated a very heavy impact of prognostic factors, *e.g.* age, on the treatment outcome. These factors influence the results of treatment groups in terms of survival more than the application of cytostatic agents or even radiotherapy. Studies of small numbers of patients or those done retrospectively are unable to control the prognostic factors and therefore are with respect to the survival times of little relevance for the evaluation of chemotherapy. However, with respect to response rates even small studies may be important if the diagnosis of the special tumor type and grade and recurrence is well established, a clear and reasonable definition of "response" is meticulously followed and the treatment setting was completely standardized.

Many studies do not fulfill these criteria and the published papers often do not give enough details to allow a critical appraisal of the study design. The evaluation of such early clinical trials should therefore imply an appraisal of the reliability of the data and should not be a mere listing of results, although personal bias may influence such an evaluation.

For this reason the reader will find below only a selection of phase II and III studies, mainly those from the cooperative groups of the US and Europe.

2.2. Malignant Gliomas

2.2.1. Phase III Trials

For his own appraisal of the following results of big studies the reader should be aware of the fact that 250 patients in each treatment arm are necessary to get a 80% probability to prove a statistically significant ($p < = 0.05$) difference of 20% in survival times, *e.g.* for malignant gliomas a prolongation to 14.4 months of the best known median survival time of 12 months.

That means, that even some of the randomized cooperative trials may have missed great differences in survival times and therefore in many studies it was only demonstrated that chemotherapy does not have a dramatic effect, but an assessment of the real effect was hardly possible.

It should be remembered that proving the efficacy of radiation therapy took very many years, even though it more than doubled the median survival for malignant glioma patients. Not until the second cooperative randomizing study by the US BTSG could the final proof be brought that radiation helps[184, 185]. This study made it possible for the first time for chemotherapy to be qualitatively and quantitatively appraised. The results achieved then with BCNU as cytostatic substance are, in principle, still valid today (see Table 3). The importance of chemotherapy in malignant gliomas can best be seen in Fig. 6. This combined

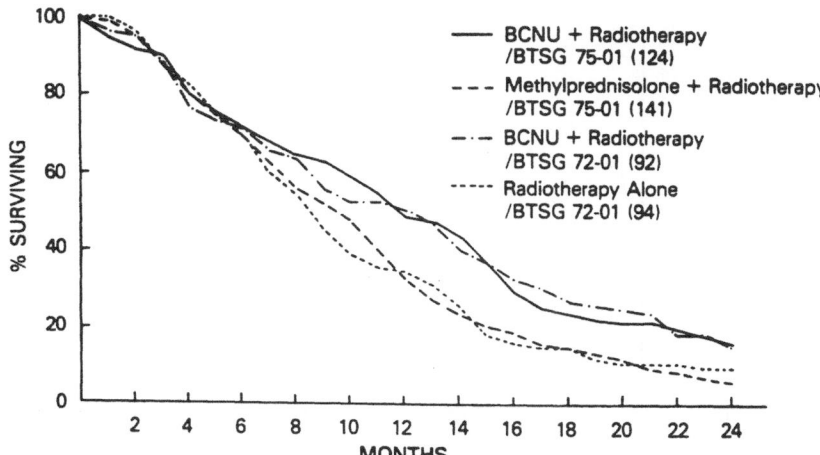

Fig. 6. The effect of adiuvant chemotherapy with the most effective substance BCNU in malignant gliomas in adults is demonstrated in this picture, combining the results of two consecutive studies of the US BTSG. Since the methylprednisolone treatment was not effective, a comparison of radiotherapy alone with additional BCNU treatment is possible[68]

Table 3. Results of randomized phase-III studies of malignant supratentorial gliomas—median survival times

Authors	References	Number of patients	MST (weeks)	18 months (%)+	Comments
Walker et al. 1978	185	222			
Support		31	14	0	RT, RT + BCNU
BCNU		51	19	4	significantly better than supportive care
RT		68	36	4	
RT + BCNU		72	35	19	
Walker et al. 1980	186	358			
Methyl-CCNU		81	24	10	meCCNU alone
RT		94	36	15	significantly less effective
RT + meCCNU		91	42	23	
RT + BCNU		92	51	27	
Green et al. 1983	68	527			
RT + corticoid*		141	40	15	RT + BCNU, RT + procarbazine
RT + procarbazine		128	47	29	significantly better than RT + corticoid*
RT + BCNU		124	50	24	
RT + BCNU + corticoid*		134	41	23	
Green et al. 1984	69	557			
RT + BCNU		(152)	44	16	no significant difference among
RT 2 × daily + BCNU		(154)	45	25	treatment arms
RT + BCNU + misonidazole		(151)	40	16	
RT + BCNU + streptozotocin		(146)	43	25	
US-BTSG 1986 (unpublished)[1]		571			
RT + BCNU/procarbazine		196	~50	?	
RT + BCNU + HU/procarbazine + VM 26		190	~50	?	
RT + BCNU		185	~50	?	

All before-mentioned US BTSG studies: RT = 60 Gy whole brain

	Ref	n			
EORTC brain tumor group 1976	[47]	81			positive patient selection: no corticosteroids allowed, high Karnofsky scores required ($\geq 70\%$)
RT + CCNU adjuvant		45	43	?	
RT + CCNU after relapse		36	62	?	
EORTC brain tumor group 1981	[50]	116			
RT + CCNU ± VM 26 after relapse		55	61	30	
RT + CCNU + VM 26 adjuvant		61	58	30	
EORTC brain tumor group 1983	[51]	163			RT = 40 Gy whole brain + 20 Gy tumor boost
RT		81	51	28	
RT + misonidazole		82	50	28	
EORTC brain tumor group 1986 (unpublished preliminary results)[2]		213			
RT		105	~52		
CCNU + VM 26 + RT after 3 months		108	~52		
Scandinavian glioblastoma study group 1985	[4]	244			RT only 40 or 50 Gy small subgroups
RT (40 Gy, high fractions) ± CCNU		57	43	~20	
+ misonidazole ± CCNU		62			
RT (50 Gy, 5 ×/wk) ± CCNU		61			
+ misonidazole ± CCNU		64			
German-Austrian brain tumor group (Krauseneck et al. 1986) (unpubl. preliminary results)	[99a]	250			RT = 40 Gy whole brain + 20 Gy tumor boost age limit ≤ 70; more aggressive chemotherapy
RT + BCNU		113	~62	~44	
RT + BCNU + VM 26		116	~62	~44	

Table 3 (continued)

Authors	References	Number of patients	MST (weeks)	18 months (%)[+]	Comments
Italian cooperative group (Paoletti et al. 1983)	141	126			
RT + BCNU		66	54	24	
RT + CCNU		60	50	23	RT = 60 Gy whole brain
Japanese brain tumor chemotherapy study group (Takakura et al. 1986)	176	77			
RT anaplastic astrocytoma (AA)		18	148	65	younger patients; only patients with demonstrable tumor in the postoperative CT scan; no steroids; variable RT (50–60 Gy); significant advantage for ACNU only for response rate, not for survival.
RT glioblastoma (Gbl)		19	60	13	
RT + ACNU AA		14	200	75	
RT + ACNU Gbl		26	52	20	
Radiation therapy oncology group/ Eastern cooperative oncology group (Chang et al. 1983)	33	554			
RT (60 Gy whole brain)		148	43	19	in the age group 40–60 years chemotherapy significantly better; no other significant differences
RT + 10 Gy tumor boost		105	36	22	
RT + BCNU		165	43	29	
RT + MeCCNU + DTIC		136	42	24	

[+] % surviving 18 months; * high-dose methyl prednisolone; [1] cited from Mahaley 1986; [2] cited from Chatel 1986; (...) randomized pts., not all evaluable.

SURVIVAL PERIOD - AFTER OPERATION

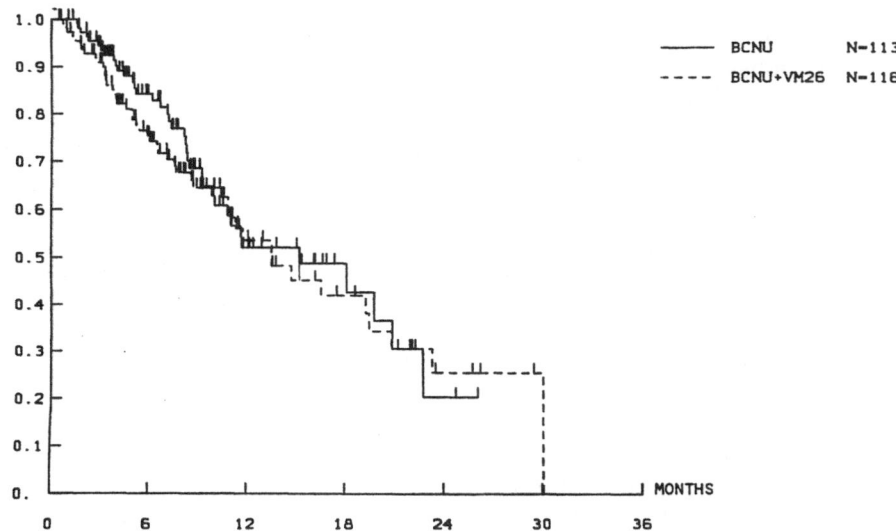

Fig. 7. Preliminary results of the German-Austrian multicenter trial of malignant gliomas. No difference is seen between BCNU monotherapy and the combination of BCNU and VM 26. All patients were operated on and were irradiated with 40 Gy to the whole brain plus 20 Gy to the tumor site. The slightly better results than in the US studies may be explained by more aggressive chemotherapy, age limit (< = 70 years) and/or Karnofsky limit (> = 50%)

representation[68] of two consecutive studies by the US BTSG illustrates the effect of BCNU chemotherapy applied in addition to surgery and radiation:
— The additional chemotherapy clearly improves the results.
— The therapeutic gain is relatively slight and does not benefit all patients.
Put simply, one can say that approx. 30% of the patients have an unfavorable prognosis, die quickly within 6 months and do not profit from the chemotherapy; in 40 to 50% of the cases the chemotherapy prolongs the survival period by one to several months and, for 20 to 30% there is a chance of long-term survival.
Table 3 shows how achievements in randomized studies have so far not been improved upon by polychemotherapy or the combination with a radiosensitizer.
Next to BCNU only methyl CCNU, streptozotocine and procarbazine have proved similarly effective[33, 68, 69, 105, 108]. ACNU also possibly fits into this category, where the Japanese study altogether clearly differs from the rest[176, 182]. The additional dosage of VM-26 every 6 weeks brought no improvement of the results[50]. While EORT's better results in 1976 and 1981 could be explained by positive patient selection, the starting conditions in the German-Austrian study are comparable with those of the American study (see Fig. 7). The slight proportion of patients over 70 years old or a Karnofsky value under 50 in the American studies, which were eliminated in the German-Austrian study because of their bad prognosis, may be responsible for some of the variation. Other differences lie only

in the aggressive carrying through of chemotherapy (lower nadirs of the blood parameter allowed, chemotherapy cycles are scheduled every 6 instead of 8 weeks) and the less extensive radiotherapy.

The results of the CCNU treatment are contradictory. Earlier positive studies with partly longer survival times than in BCNU (*e.g.*[47, 152]) stand in opposition to the lack of proof of efficacy in the randomized studies of the EORTC and the Scandinavian BTSG[48, 50, 77]. A randomized Italian study showed that CCNU is inferior to BCNU[141]. A possible cause for this is the less sure application of CCNU because of its exclusively oral administration. Moreover, the varied criteria for admittance in the studies must be taken into consideration. The requirements concerning general health are not uniform and the lowest Karnofsky limit varies between 40–50 and 70% (*e.g.* EORTC). The EORTC studies also have the particularity that only patients not receiving cortisone therapy are admitted.

Also, the result of the first study done by EORTC in 1976, that the use of CCNU was only significantly better after relapse but not as adjuvant therapy, was not confirmed in the follow-up study in 1978 with the combination of CCNU and VM-26.

The most recent study of the US-BTSG applies a sandwich therapy, *i.e.* primarily alternating effective substances to avoid development of resistance, which unfortunately has so far not brought any improvement of the results[118].

The important question, whether corticosteroids also have a cytostatic or life-prolonging effect, was answered in the negative by the US BTSG[68]. At least, in the high, once-weekly doses the adjuvant application of corticosteroids was, if anything, sooner harmful, as also could be seen in the many complications through infections.

Studies which measure not the survival time but the time to tumor progression (free interval) (see Table 4) are not so reliable in their statements, as the goal criteria are not absolutely clearly measurable. Moreover, in the studies of the San Francisco group[104-114] it must be taken into consideration that, in the in itself sensible separate evaluation of glioblastomas and anaplastic astrocytomas, important variations in nomenclature play a part. These authors differentiate between mildly, moderately, and highly anaplastic astrocytomas, so that here a series of astrocytomas may be seen as malignant which elsewhere are defined as low grade and will not be treated cytostatically. As a result of a broader glioblastoma definition the American randomized studies show a higher portion of glioblastomas (85–90%) than the European (70–80%). Results in the German-Austrian study show that the prognosis of an intermediary group grade 3–4 does not differ from that of a pure glioblastoma group, which fact supports the American conception.

The EORTC studies on free interval[47, 48, 50] show a slight, but not significant, advantage for the CCNU and the CCNU plus VM-26 groups respectively over its radiation therapy. Misonidazole proves ineffective here also[51]. The results reported by Levin *et al.*[107, 108, 112, 114] are less consistent, but agree essentially with the EORTC results concerning glioblastomas and show no advantage in the applied polychemotherapy schemata. The efficacy of hydroxyurea as radiosensitizer could not be proved[107] and, in exact analysis of the data, the advantage of the modified combination procarbazine, CCNU and vincristine over BCNU/hydroxyurea only in the anaplastic astrocytomas is not convincing[114]. No good studies on vincristine

Table 4. Results of randomized phase-III studies of malignant supratentorial gliomas —free interval/time to tumor progression

Authors	Reference	Number	FI* (weeks) (median)
EORTC brain tumor group 1978	48	81	
RT		36	31.0
RT + CCNU		45	34.5
EORTC brain group 1981	50	116	
RT		55	30.7
RT + CCNU + VM 26		61	39.0
EORTC brain tumor group 1983	51	163	
RT		81	30.0
RT + misonidazole		82	30.0
EORTC brain tumor group 1986 (unpublished preliminary results)[1]		213	
RT		105	28.0
CCNU + VM 26 + RT after 3 months		108	32.0
Western cancer study group (Levin *et al.* 1979)	107	99	
RT + HU + BCNU glioblastoma		35	41.0
RT + HU + BCNU anaplastic astrocytoma		18	50.0
RT + BCNU glioblastoma		26	31.0
RT + BCNU anaplastic astrocytoma		20	72.0
Northern California oncology group (Levin *et al.* 1985)	113	148	
RT + HU + BCNU glioblastoma		40	32.0
RT + HU + BCNU anaplastic astrocytoma		36	77.0
RT + HU + PCV glioblastoma		36	31.0
RT + HU + PVC anaplastic astrocytoma		36	123.0
Northern California oncology group (Levin *et al.* 1985) (not published in detail)	114		
RT + FU + CCNU + HU + misonidazole + procarbazine + vincristine + BCNU/FU in glioblastoma		?	42.0

* FI = free interval in weeks, HU = hydroxyurea; PCV = procarbazine, CCNU, vincristine; FU = 5-fluorouracil, [1] = cited from Chatel 1986.

have been done which prove its efficacy in gliomas[60], so that in view of the lack of liquor patency, its application in gliomas is hardly justified—especially because of the known neurotoxicity of this substance.

The results of a further sandwich therapy with 7 substances[113] as reported so far do not, unfortunately, stand out much against the earlier reports.

The good results of the retrospective and nonrandomized study by Jellinger *et al.*[86] with the COMP protocol, above all concerning the 2- and 3-year survival

Table 5. Special retrospective studies of malignant gliomas

Authors	References	Number of patients	MST (weeks)	18 months (%)	
Jellinger 1986	90				
Support		280	20	5	
RT 40–60 Gy		67	53	16	
CCNU, VCR, procarbazine, MTX (= COMP)		69	57	19	38–70% had second surgery
RT (60 Gy) + COMP		43	60	40	
		101			
Krauseneck et al. 1985, patients without tumor resection	97	88			
RT (40 + 20 Gy)		15	25	0	
RT (40 + 20 Gy) + BCNU		23	31	9	
RT (40 + 20 Gy) + BCNU + bleomycine		50	20	12	—severe pulmonary toxicity

MST = median survival time in weeks; VCR = vincristine, MTX = methotrexate.

Table 6 a. The relative importance of selected prognostic factors in studies of the US BTSG

Gehan and Walker 1977 [66]		regression coefficient [+]
Radiotherapy		—1.001
Age		+ 0.3649
Seizures × cranial nerve disturbances		—0.4416
BCNU		—0.4040
Encapsulated tumor		—0.6923
Parietal location		+ 0.3636
Walker *et al.* 1978 [185]		MST (weeks)
Karnofsky rating	> 90%	33.0
	50–80%	25.0
	< 50	13.0
Walker *et al.* 1980 (9 factors) [186]		death rate*
Age	< 45	0.42
Age	45–54	0.76
Age	55–64	1.20
Age	> 65	1.41
Duration of symptoms (months)	< 4	0.98
	4–6	0.96
	> 6	0.49
Histopathologic category		
glioblastoma		0.96
other malignant glioma		0.44
Karnofsky rating	10–40%	1.52
	50–60%	1.04
	70–80%	· 0.70
	90–100%	0.55
Green *et al.* 1983 [69] (16 factors)		death rate*
Resection type	biopsy	0.96
	subtotal	0.73
	total	0.66
	total + lobectomy	0.39
History of arteriosclerosis	yes	1.39
	no	0.68
Consciousness level	abnormal	1.28
	normal	0.64

[+] Negative regression coefficient is favorable. * Death rate = number of deaths per 10 patient months.

times not included in Table 5, likewise allow no conclusion as to the superiority of polychemotherapy. The results presented correspond to those of the German-Austrian or the Japanese study with a BCNU or ACNU monotherapy. As methotrexate in the dosage applied and vincristine do not cross the blood-brain barrier, efficacy of this treatment must be ascribed more to CCNU and procarbazine. An essential point in this study is also that it emphasizes the

Table 6b. Statistically significant prognostic factors in the studies of the US BTSG

	Walker et al. 1976	Walker et al. 1978	Walker et al. 1980	Green et al. 1983
Age	+	+	+*	+*
Karnofsky rating		+	+*	+*
Tumor grading			+*	+*
Tumor location		+		+
Extent of surgical removal		+		+
Consciousness level				+*
Duration of symptoms	+	−	+*	+*
Cranial nerve abnormality		+		+
Seizures		+	+	+
Personality change			+*	−
Motor disorder			+	+
Sensory disorder				+
Speech disorder				+
Blood type				+*
History of arteriosclerosis				+
History of cancer				+
White-cell count pre treatment				+*
Platelet-count pre treatment				+*
Headache			+	
Necrotic tumor			+	

* These factors were independent and necessary to predict survival in the Weibuell model.

importance of a second or even third operation for these patients with unfavorable prognosis.

In a retrospective, nonrandomized study[97] (Table 5), as was to be expected, there were shorter survival times for inoperable patients, but in both chemotherapy groups there was, happily, a not inconsiderable number of longer survivals. A sorrowful experience in polychemotherapy with BCNU and bleomycine at the beginning of the study in 1977/78 was the unknown synergism of these two substances in the causing of an interstitial pneumonia with possibly lethal pulmonary fibrosis.

2.2.2. Prognostic Factors

The enormous importance of prognostic factors becomes obvious in Table 6a, which also allows the inclusion of radiotherapy and BCNU treatment as prognostic factors when analyzing the early study 69-01 of the US BTSG. Irradiation is indeed clearly shown to be the most important prognostic parameter, but age, tumor site and type of neurological symptoms are just as important as the BCNU treatment. Also the later studies show the express dependency of the survival rate on the factors age, Karnofsky, value, grade of malignancy, duration of symptoms, consciousness level or even a history of arteriosclerosis. The extent of surgery is

SURVIVAL PERIOD - AGE

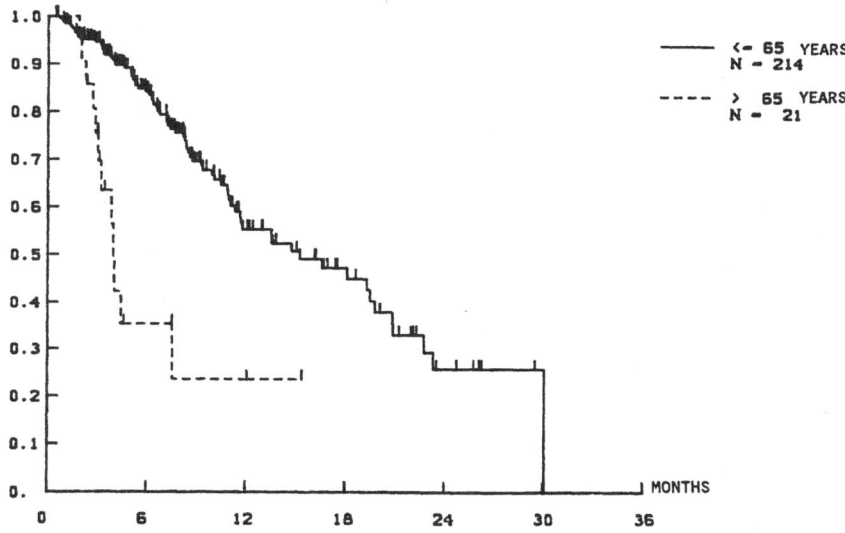

Fig. 8. Even in the age group 65–70 years old approx. 20% have a chance of longer survival while the overall prognosis in this age group is clearly worse than in younger patients

important, but in no way more important than the afore-mentioned factors and it is not presented in all studies as an important factor (Table 6 b).

This variability of the factors from study to study, shown in Table 6 b, decreases their usefulness. Fairly good prognosis of the life expectancy for a group of patients[68, 186] can indeed be made, but for the concrete therapy decision in individual patients these factors have only a limited usefulness. Moreover, also in the groups with very unfavorable prognosis there are some few patients who survive longer and clearly profit from the therapy. Thus, the dilemma remains for the time being that, for example, in the age group of 65–70 years, many patients must be treated without therapeutic gain in order not to omit the chance of longer survival for approximately 20% of the cases (Fig. 8). Further knowledge of the prognostic factors and the individual risks of side-effects in the glioma patients will, in the future, make a better patient selection or, at least an early well-founded discontinuation of therapy possible.

2.2.3. Phase II Studies in Malignant Gliomas

In this type of study, the survival time is an unsuitable parameter of the success of therapy. The purpose of these studies is to examine in proportionately few patients, down to a number of 15, the tumor remission rates to new substances. Only when in phase-II studies the tested substance proves to be comparably or better effective than the already known substances, is there any sense in measuring in a randomized phase-III study under strictly controlled conditions also the survival time as most important therapy parameter.

Table 7. Phase-II studies for recurrent gliomas—single agent therapy

	Dose	Number	% Glioblastoma	% Resp.*	Author
BCNU	$80\,mg/m^2 \times 3$	25	75	44	Wilson et al. 1970
		30	100	53	Fewer et al. 1972
		12	0	58	Fewer et al. 1972
CCNU	$120\text{–}130\,mg/m^2 \times 1$	19	100	26	Fewer et al. 1972
		19	90	21	Rosenblum et al. 73
		28	?	28	EORTC 1978
		16	60	19	EORTC 1981
MeCCNU	$220\,mg/m^2 \times 1$	15	?	13	Young et al. 1973
		28	?	50	Levine et al. 1974
		29	?	28	Tranum et al. 1975
Procarbazine	$150\text{–}200\,mg/m^2\ 30$	36	72	22	Kumar et al. 1974
	$150\text{–}200\,mg/m^2\ 30$	27	?	52	Wilson et al. 1976
	$150\text{–}200\,mg/m^2\ 30$ (after CCNU)	17	?	0	EORTC 1981
DTIC	$900\,mg/m^2 \times 5$	20	15	25	Levin et al. 1975
	$175\,mg/m^2 \times 5\text{–}10$	8	50	63	Taylor et al. 1975
AZQ	$17.5\,mg/m^2 \times 2$	20	?	30	Aroney et al. 1982
	$20\,mg/m^2 \times 2$	15	73	53	Curt et al. 1982
	$6\text{–}8\,mg/m^2 \times 5$	25	76	52	Feun et al. 1984
	$8\text{–}15\,mg/m^2 \times 3\text{–}5$	27	41	26	Schold et al. 1984
	$15\text{–}20\,mg/m^2/w \times 4$	17	?	24	Decker et al. 1985
	$8\,mg/m^2 \times 5$	34	50	47	EORTC 1985
	$30\,mg/m^2 \times 1$	28	29	39	Haid et al. 1985
	$5.5\,mg/m^2 \times 5$	23	?	39	Maral et al. 1985
Cis-Platinum	$35\,mg/m^2 \times 3$	31	30	13	Stewart et al. 1983
	$60\text{–}120\,mg/m^2\,i.a.$	22	82	45	Feun et al. 1984

Substance	Dose	n	%	%	Reference
Methotrexate	5–2,200 mg/kg + C.F.**	11	27	73	Djerassi et al. 1985
	27–522 mg/kg + C.F.**	6	83	17	Shapiro, W. R. 1977
VM 26	130 mg/m^2/w × 4	20	50	70	Gerosa et al. 1981
	100–130 mg/m^2/w × 6–8	23	?	38	Sklansky et al. 1974
	100–130 mg/m^2/w (after BCNU)	20	?	35	Kessinger et al. 1979
VP 16	50–100 mg/m^2 × 5	18	?	50	Tirelli et al. 1984
	900 mg/m^2 × 3	4	100	75	Wolff et al. 1983
DDMP	75 mg/m^2/w × 5 + C.F.**	29	55	38	EORTC 1980
Cytosin-arabinoside	150 mg/m^2 × 4	7	57	72	Krauseneck et al. 1984
Interferon-beta	1–6 Mio U/d × ? (—56) i.v	54	?	22	Sano et al. 1982
	3 Mio U/d × ? (—64) i.tu	5	100	0	Otsuka et al. 1984
	0.3–6 Mio U/d × ? i.tu, i.th	20	100	40	Nagai and Arai 1984
	10 Mio U/d iv + 1 Mio itu × 10–30	12	100	8	Duff et al. 1986
Interferon-alpha-HU-Leu	0.05–3 Mio U/d i.m	8		25	Hirakawa et al. 1983
	3–9 Mio U/d × 30 i.m	12	100	8	Boethius et al. 1983
	1 Mio U/d × 10–60 i.tu/i.th	17	59	12	Nakagawa et al. 1984
	1.6–9 Mio U/2 d × 20 i.tu	3	0	33	Obbens et al. 1985
Interferon-alpha-HU-Ly	3–6 Mio U/d × ? i.m	3	100	33	Nagai and Arai 1984
	10–30 Mio U/m^2/d × 30 i.v, i.m	17	53	41	Mahaley et al. 1985
Interferon-alpha-recomb. A	3–54 Mio U/d × 3 i.m	9	100	22	Nagai and Arai 1984
	3–50 Mio U/d × 30 i.m	39	36	10	Takakura et al. 1985
Interferon-gamma	0.01–0.025 Mio U/d × 28 i.tu	6	?	17	Nagai and Arai 1985
	0.075–0.125 Mio U/3 d × 10 i.tu	3	0	33	Smith et al. 1984
Interferon-gamma-recomb.	0.25–2.0 Mio U/d × 28 it.u	6	?	17	Nagai and Arai 1985

* Response = "objective" response + stable disease. ** C.F. = citrovorum factor rescue.

The requirements which are to be demanded of a phase II study are completely different from those of a phase-III study.

These requirements are:

1. Monotherapy (when there is insufficient information on the efficacy of a substance) or polychemotherapy (combination only of substances known for their efficacy), in no case a combination with other forms of therapy;

2. defined, uniform tumor histology, where a certain heterogeneity within a tumor type is allowed, *e.g.* glioma grade III and IV, primary treatment or relapse treatment. A mixture of different tumor types, *e.g.* the inclusion of ependymoma or metastases is not usable;

3. clear, objectifiable response criteria;

4. sufficient duration of treatment so that the effect of the applied therapy can at all be measured. In an examination of a cytostatic drug a stipulation is recommended, that at least two complete chemotherapy cycles must be survived. In this type of study it is not purposeful to evaluate a patient as a therapy failure who, for example, dies one week after application of chemotherapy;

5. well-standardized and exactly registered accompanying therapy. In brain tumors especially the good symptomatic effect of the accompanying cortisone therapy must be strictly controlled;

6. systematic coverage of the side-effects.

Only relatively few studies fill these basic prerequisites. Often in a study design a mixture of phase-II and phase-III occurs, which makes a clear statement on the response rate and on the survival time impossible.

In Table 7 only such studies are included which quote a rather well-defined response rate, whereas studies which only measured survival time were not taken into consideration. The selection of studies also took place under the aspect that the comparison of well-tried substances with those still being tested should be made possible. The results in intraarterial cytostatica application are dealt with elsewhere (see Gumerlock and Neuwelt, this volume). The current US BTSG study will eventually render a reliable estimation of its value.

Older studies (1976 and earlier) did not have regular CT checks at their disposal and therefore had to use the radioisotopic brain scan for course checks. Their statements have somewhat less strong evidence. The definition of "response" are very varied. Therefore, all patients showing no progression, *i.e.* "complete" or "partial" response, "stable disease", "no change" are combined as "response" in Table 7 to enable a possibly better comparison. The quoted response rates therefore lie partly above those cited by the authors and represent an optimistic evaluation. As glioblastomas (WHO grade IV) respond less well than "other malignant gliomas" (WHO grade III) the proportion of glioblastomas was as far as possible, quoted. As, however, many of the mentioned studies only incompletely fulfil the above list of criteria the result is still a diversiform picture for most substances. A realistic evaluation of the efficacy of the meanwhile "classic" substances, nitrosoureas and procarbazine, lies without doubt in the region of 25–50% of objective remissions. The table shows that newer substances are by no means more effective.

DTIC has, so far, was tested as a single substance only in a phase II study[178]; in combination[33] no additive effect was recognized. The liquor patency is slight (14% of blood level).

The new lipophil quinone derivative AZQ (azaridinylbenzoquinone) probably represents an acquisition, while the previous cytostatics from the group of antibiotics—so highly effective in general oncology—remained ineffective in intrinsic brain tumors, what is to ascribe to lack of penetration of the BBB.

Cisplatinum does not penetrate the intact BBB and we shall have to wait and see whether the originally moderately optimistic reports are confirmed. It is, at present, being tested in a phase III study by the EORTC essentially as radiosensitizer[34].

The cell cycle specific substances methotrexate, VM-26, VP 16, DDMP and cytosine-arabinoside can only in high dosage penetrate the BBB. However, cytosine-arabinoside achieves also in low dosage through a longer infusion time of at least 2 hours a CSF level of 40% of blood level, and DDMP also essentially better penetrates into the CSF than the mother substance methotrexate. Partial defects of BBB could be the explanation for remissions observed with other substances in lower doses (see Table 7), although in the randomized phase III studies so far no additive effect for VM-26 in addition to BCNU, CCNU or procarbazine could be shown (see above). High dose Ara-C or methotrexate application in grams doses is very toxic and not favorable for a cytostatic combination therapy.

Interferons have not come up to expectations in brain tumors either. The response rates are slight and the toxicity is relatively high (Table 7). Single obvious remissions, however, point to a certain therapeutic potential. This is of importance because a completely different therapeutic principle exists in cytostatics. Use of interferons in a combination therapy is conceivable.

Response rates in combination therapy seem altogether more favorable (Table 8). As far as the listed combinations could be tested in randomized checks in phase-III studies (Tables 3 and 4) the results were almost all disappointing and not superior to a BCNU monotherapy. It is, indeed, doubtful whether vincristine, adriamycine[73, 81, 108, 147] and the bolus injection of cytosine-arabinoside[172] are at all of use.

In summary, at this time it has to be said that promising new substances—also those outside the already mentioned series—are, unfortunately, not available. Previous studies with polychemotherapy have brought no progress. The possibilities of a meaningful combination of cytostatics have, so far, been limited, as the highly effective substances of general oncology (adriamycine and the other antibiotics, cyclophosphamide and derivatives, cisplatinum) do not penetrate the BBB. The development of new penetrating substances (AZQ, various platinum derivatives) promises, however, an improvement of therapeutic possibilities in the future. The previous combinations of substances with very similar therapeutic mechanism (BCNU/CCNU with procarbazine) or lack of liquor patency (vincristine, methotrexate, adriamycine, cisplatinum, 5-FU, VM-26) and only short-term application of cell cycle specific drugs (long-term application reaches more cells in the sensitive phase of the cycle) were not optimal, so that a higher efficacy of improved combination schemata with the available substances is quite probable. The inclusion of more recent pharmacokinetic knowledge and a better understanding of the BBB will be helpful here.

Table 8. Phase-II studies for recurrent gliomas—multiple agent therapy

	Number	% Glioblastoma	% Resp.*	Authors	References
CCNU + VCR + methotrexate	22	60	36	Hildebrand et al. 1975	81
CCNU + VCR + procarbazine	38	29	53	Gutin et al. 1975	73
CCNU + VCR + procarbazine (modif.)	46	26	61	Levin et al. 1980	108
CCNU + VM 26 + ADM	43	?	72	Pouillart et al. 1976	147
AZQ + procarbazine	96	40	42	Duke/UNC 1986 unpub.[1]	
AZQ + BCNU	67	47	40	Duke/UNC 1986 unpub.[1]	
Cisplatinum + cytosine-arabinoside	25	81	64	Stewart et al. 1984	172
BCNU + FU	29	19	76	Levin et al. 1979	107

* Response = "objective" response + stable disease. [1] Cited from Mahaley 1986.

Table 9. Results of chemotherapy in primary cerebral malignant lymphoma in comparison to radiotherapy

Authors	Reference	Number grade	% high >40 Gy	% RT (m)	(MST) with chemoth.	Number of pts. response	MST+(m)/
Bogdahn et al. 1986	17	10	60	50	11	4	13
Doreen et al. 1986		8	50	75	10	—	—
Helle et al. 1984	78	17	71*	88	16	5	22
Jellinger and Slowik 1986	91	34	53		17		
Letendre et al. 1982	103	17	94*	65	24	4	no resp.[1]
Loeffler et al. 1985	115	10	90*	90	14.5[2]	5	23
MacIntosh et al. 1982	116	5	100*	100	16/10[3]	—	—
Neuwelt et al. 1983	132	3	?	67	12[4]	3	3 resp.
Stewart et al. 1983	171	1	?	—	—	1	1 resp.

* Rappaport classification: unfavorable prognosis. [1] Two patients with stable disease but no clear response of relapse after radiotherapy. [2] All 4 survivors had intrathecal chemotherapy. [3] Two differing data given. [4] ia and iv chemotherapy + blood-brain-barrier disruption. MST (m) = median survival time in months (all patients); MST+ (m) = median survival time in months (only patients with chemotherapy).

2.3. Malignant Ependymomas (WHO Grades III and IV)

These tumors have a better prognosis in adult patients than in children and show, corresponding to their origin, an express tendency to metastasize into the liquor. A postoperative intrathecal prophylactic cytostatic dose outside of the period of radiotherapy is therefore generally to be recommended. In children, an adjuvant chemotherapy corresponding to the medulloblastoma schemata as tested in current studies, in adults corresponding to a glioblastoma schema, is recommended[3, 35, 111]. Because of the low number of cases special studies for this type of tumor are hardly possible, so that we have to revert to well-documented single cases. In adults the prognosis is obviously more favorable than in malignant gliomas.

2.4. Primary Cerebral Malignant Lymphomas

Although primary cerebral lymphomas have in recent years been clearly more often diagnosed (CT scan!) and probably as a result of favoring factors (organ transplants, long-term immunosuppression, AIDS) will also really increase, the classification is still frequently insufficient and, above all, diversiform. It is, however, agreed that the prognosis in primary cerebral site is always unfavorable, so that WHO prefers the malignancy grades IV or III. (For details see Jellinger this volume). The vast majority of the primary CNS lymphomas are non-Hodgkin's lymphomas of B-cell origin.

Jellinger and Slowik[91] showed in their 34 patients that the immunocytomas defined in the Kiel classification as low grade come off considerably better with 30 months median survival time than the high-grade immunoblastomas or lymphoblastomas with a median survival of 6–7 months. Secondary CNS involvement of systematic non-Hodgkin lymphomas has a considerably worse prognosis with about 2 months median survival time. Untreated primary CNS lymphomas lead within a few weeks to death[1, 17, 65, 78, 91, 101, 103, 115, 116, 158].

Corticosteroids have a very good symptomatic effect and can render the tumor invisible in CT in a short time, which can be considered as a diagnostic pointer[183]. This phenomenon must not lead to a delay in radiotherapy if histology is certain. The prophylactic dose of antiepileptic drugs is recommended as acute irreversible deteriorations were seen with status epilepticus. Systematic studies on chemotherapy of these tumors are not available as they respond at first very well to radiotherapy and are rare. Systemic chemotherapy protocols used till now are very varied and therefore not included in Table 9. Moderately high dosed methotrexate has a good effect[79, 85]. The results of additional chemotherapy compared with only radiotherapy, compiled in Table 9, turn out somewhat more favorable. Although comparison tests are lacking, written reports[17, 103, 115] and our own experience indicate that before and after radiation intrathecal chemoprophylaxis with Ara-C or methotrexate should be applied. In up to 2/3 of the cases the cytological evidence of lymphoma cells in the liquor is successful[17, 91], not seldom even after normalization of the CT findings. Therefore, in diagnostic lumbar punctures we administer 40 mg/m^2 Ara-C prophylactically. The high rate of a liquor cell dissemination can be explained by the fact that the perivascular spaces are to be regarded as origin of the tumor.

Experimental studies on the BBB in lymphomas have not been carried out. The lack of neovascularization, the occasional lack of contrast enhancement and the good cortisone effect indicate an extremely intact BBB, so that CSF penetrating substances are recommended for the chemotherapy. In the USA a randomized study with high-dose methotrexate and in Germany/Austria one with radiation and Ara-C are in preparation.

2.5. Medulloblastomas in Adults

Medulloblastomas in adults are seldom found. In most cases they are young adults around 20 years old. The tumors are almost always of the desmoplastic subtype and have a better prognosis than in children[2, 14, 16, 35, 154].

Since an adjuvant chemotherapy could not achieve a clear effect even in the rapidly progressing tumors in children[3], it cannot be recommended for adults. Medulloblastomas, as tumors directly adjacent to the CSF spaces, have a strong tendency to disseminate malignant cells so that in children the neuraxis is also to be radiated. The value of this action, which causes a considerable reduction in bone marrow reserves, has not been proved in adults. It can, possibly, be replaced by an intrathecal chemoprophylaxis with Ara-C or methotrexate. Regular CSF cytological tests postoperatively and prophylactic intrathecal cytostatic therapy outside the radiation period is to be recommended, likewise in the lymphomas.

Well-tried substances for systemic chemotherapy are the nitrosoureas, procarbazine, dibromodulcitol[3, 61, 110, 111]. Melphalan is possibly a specially suitable alkylanting agent[62].

Levin et al.[110] calculated a prolongation of the median survival time by 29 months after appearance of the recurrence by applying aggressive polychemotherapy.

2.6. Pinealoblastomas

These tumors are rare in adults except for Japan[175]. Together with the medulloblastomas they are classified as primitive neuroectodermal tumors (PNET).

This would correspond to a relatively high sensitivity to radio- and probably also chemotherapy. As there is limited chemotherapeutic experience with pinealoblastomas[159] only the application of a medulloblastoma schema and the intrathecal postoperative prophylaxis with continuing monitoring of the liquor cytology can be recommended. It might be preferable to apply systemic chemotherapy only in relapse.

2.7. Germ Cell Tumors

These tumors outside the CNS show a high sensitivity to radio- and chemotherapy[92, 131, 159, 175], especially if they produce human choriongonadotropin. A special sensitivity of these tumors to methotrexate is known. Rustin et al. 1986[155] attribute their very good results with a combination of cisplatinum, vincristine, bleomycine, methotrexate alternating with dactinomycin, cyclophosphamide and etoposide also to the application of a high intravenous methotrexate dose in combination with intrathecal methotrexate: 8 out of 10 patients with brain metastases and 1 out of 2 patients with primary intracranial germ cell tumors survived with no evidence of disease. These tumors also tend to disseminate liquor cells and even to metastasize over a possible shunt system[177], so that here also CSF monitoring and intrathecal prophylaxis is necessary (see also Gumerlock and Neuwelt, this volume).

2.8. Brain Metastases

Chemotherapy for brain metastases was considered for a long time to be ineffective as the appearance of brain metastases was observed during a current but otherwise successful chemotherapy (e.g.[145]), therapeutic attempts on patients mostly in rapid systemic progression showed no success and because regression of the metastases could not previously be proved in CT. The few systematic studies with a sole chemotherapy can be summarized in one table (Table 10).

With an aim to prolonging the survival time it can be seen that the efficacy of chemotherapy altogether corresponds roughly to that of radiotherapy or that of surgery alone (see also[173]). The remission rates of radiotherapy of 60% are, on the contrary, only reached in the chemosensitive breast carcinomas. The prolongation of the survival time can also be explained by the fact that about 50% of the patients do not die of brain metastases but of a progression of the primary tumor.

Chemotherapy is evidently effective, while the more recent cisplatinum schemata can produce complete remissions even in lung carcinomas (own observations). Chemotherapy fails where also for the treatment of the primary no good cytostatics are available, such as for melanomas and renal carcinomas. A polychemotherapy aimed at the primary is clearly more effective than a CSF penetrating monotherapy (see Table 11).

At the onset of neovascularization, when the brain metastases reach a certain size (approx. 1 cm diameter), the BBB is destroyed and no longer forms an obstacle for chemotherapy[11]. For the formation of brain metastases the BBB is, however, of importance as, behind its protection, micrometastases can develop which at first cannot be reached by the systemic chemotherapy because of the existing barrier[145].

The antiestrogen tamoxifen penetrates the CSF and single cases of a regression of a brain metastasis with breast carcinomas using solely hormone therapy have been described[30, 36].

The combination of chemotherapy with radiotherapy (see Table 11) considerably raises the remission rates, the survival times are, however, not clear, which is understandable because of the systemic progression which cannot easily be influenced. Patients, who can be operated on for a solitary brain metastasis, and who can be treated postoperatively with cytostatics and/or radiotherapy, have the best prognosis whereby these patients' prognosis also depends greatly on the primary tumor[27–29, 31, 32, 37, 64, 69, 96, 120, 124, 133, 147, 150, 153, 165, 173].

Table 10. Results of chemotherapy of brain metastases

Author	References	Protocol	Tumor	N	Resp.	MST
Hildebrand et al. 1975	81	CCNU/VCR/MTX	lung carcinoma	20	1	1.5
			breast carcinoma	11	5	6
			melanoma	5	0	1.5
Pouillart et al. 1976	147	CCNU/ADM/VM26	lung carcinoma	13	3	2.5
			breast carcinoma	8	6	8.0
			others	9	3	3.5
Markesbery et al. 1978	120	ADM/DEX, MIT/DEX	mixed	21	?	4.0
Krauseneck et al. 1980	96	CPM/MTX/PRED	lung carcinoma	9	4	3.0
			breast carcinoma	11	7	5.0
			others	11	4	3.0
Shapiro 1980	165	BCNU/CCNU	lung carcinoma	12	3	3.0
			breast carcinoma	3	0	3.0
			melanoma	12	3	6.0
Conte et al. 1982	37	CCNU/ADM/VM26	lung carcinoma	14	5	5.5*
			breast carcinoma	8	5	5
			others	10	3	3.5
Mende et al. 1983	124	5-FU/ADM/CPM + tamoxifen	breast carcinoma	11	10	15.0
Rosner et al. 1983	153	CPM/5-FU/PRED/MTX/ VCR, CPM/ADM/PRED	breast carcinoma	66	34	7
Madajewicz et al. 1981		BCNU ia + others iv	lung carcinoma	25	12	4
			melanoma	10	0	<4
Krauseneck et al. 1986	99	adapted to primary	miscell.	22		7
Unpublished		not adapted to primary	miscell.	17		3

N = number of patients; Resp. = number of responders ("objective" remission); MST = median survival time in months. ADM = adriamycine; CPM = cyclophosphamide; Dex = dexamethasone; Mit = mitolactol; PRED = prednisone; VCR = vincristine. * Refers to all patients not only to the evaluable ones.

Table 11. Results of combined radio- and chemotherapy of brain metastases

Author	Protocol	Tumor	Number	Resp. (%)	MST
Robustelli della Cuna et al. 1979	5,500 c Gy + BCNU/CCNU	lung carcinoma	44	10 (23)	4.5
		breast carcinoma	27	14 (52)	7.5
		others	31	16 (52)	6.0
Chan et al. 1980	4,000 c Gy ADM + CCNU + (CPM)	lung carcinoma	22	22 (100!)	8.0
Casimir et al. 1981	4,000 c Gy + ADM + Ftorafur + Dibromodulcitol	breast carcinoma	61	32 (52)	11.0

Resp. = "objective" response; MST = median survival time in months.

2.9. Leptomeningeal Cancer, Neoplastic Meningosis

Here, it is probably useful to distinguish between 3 types:

1. The terminal type with very unfavorable prognosis, which occurs within the framework of a rapidly developing systemic illness with general metastasization;

2. the metastatic type with doubtful prognosis, which appears after a stable course of illness as complication or primary manifestation of a progredient tumor with neurological symptoms;

3. the transient type with, under certain conditions, favorable prognosis, which is discovered in spite of lacking, or slight, neurological symptoms within the framework of routine diagnostics, for example postoperatively or during treatment of tumors close to the CSF pathways.

For the transient form the emphasis of therapy lies in prophylaxis for which the administration of the usual dosage of 12–15 mg/m^2 methotrexate or 30 mg/m^2 Ara-C every 2–3 weeks 3–6 times intrathecally (!) is sufficient. In acute leukemia and lymphoblastic non-Hodgkin lymphomas this prophylaxis must be carried out, in *metastasizing* melanomas, breast and lung carcinomas it must be considered. Moreover, prophylaxis as mentioned above, is to be recommended in malignant gliomas situated close to the CSF pathways, in malignant ependymomas, in PNET and in intracranial germ cell tumors. In solid brain metastases a meningosis often also occurs so that a short-term intrathecal prophylaxis (2–3 injections) is of use.

For the metastatic form the intensive intrathecal therapy with 2–3 injections per week of methotrexate, Ara-C or alternating must be complemented with a systemic cytostatic therapy in order to achieve a permanent success[43]. In this form of metastasization also more than 50% of the patients die of the systemic effects of their disease. Not infrequently the meningosis has a main site of involvement with focal neurological deficits. Here an additional radiation of this region (30–40 Gy in

Table 12. Survival in meningosis neoplastica

Author	[Reference]	Primary	Number	Resp. (%)	MST (m)
Wasserstrom *et al.* 1982	[187]	breast	46	28 (61)	7.2
		lung	23	9 (39)	4.0
		melanoma	11	2 (18)	3.6
		others	10	3 (30)	6.3
Theodore and Gendelman 1981	[179]	breast	21	9 (43)	3.0
		lung	5	2 (40)	3.0
		melanoma	5	1 (20)	3.0
		others	2	2 (100)	7.5
Yap *et al.* 1982	[189]	breast	40	27 (68)	5.8
Grisold *et al.* 1984	[71]	breast	5	4 (80)	6.1
Eyre and Sause 1985	[56]	breast	15	6 (40)	6.0
		lung	2	0	0.8
		melanoma	3	0	1.7

Resp. = "objective" responder; MST = Median survival time in months.

2–4 weeks) can help. This should also always be carried out when in the CT scan involvement of the subarachnoid spaces becomes visible[7]. A prolongation of the survival time (2–4 weeks without treatment) to several months with single longtime survivors is possible (Table 12) where the primary tumor is likewise of considerable prognostic importance[28, 43, 46, 56, 63, 71, 76, 146, 151, 168, 179, 187, 189].

In the terminal form insofar as neurological deficits exist few, highly dosed intrathecal injections are recommended to achieve a rapid and often dramatic palliation.

The side-effects of intrathecal cytostatica doses can be serious in single cases[12, 55]. In spite of doubling the afore-mentioned dosage, however, we have not observed any permanent damage to our patients (Table 13). In our opinion it is essential to use pure electrolyte solutions without bacteriostatic or other additives and to dilute them with a buffer solution (Elliot B) to 10 to 20 ml. With a correct needle position the injection is given very slowly, in ventricular dosing always using a perfusor, and must be interrupted immediately at any sign of side-effects. The addition of corticosteroids (Table 13) reduces the side-effects significantly. Other authors have

Table 13. Side effects of intrathecal cytostatic treatment [97, 99]. No permanent complications were observed. More than 80% of the side effects were restricted to signs of meningeal irritation

	MTX	MTX + Triam.	Triam.	Ara-C	Ara-C + Triam.
First injection					
Number of pat.	17	35	151	46	20
Age (years)	18–75	15–71	14–71	18–72	22–74
Age (median)	44	47	39	39	59.5
Site of injection:					
Lumbar	10	29	150	40	19
SOP	2	6	1	5	1
Ventricular	5	—	—	1	—
Dose (mg)	5–50	5–50/ 40–120	40–120	40–120	40–120/ 40–80
Dose (median)	18	25/40	80	100	60/40
All side-effects	41%	9%	9%	35%	0%
Multiple injections					
N patients	17	35	151	46	20
N injections	47	154	494	128	94
Side effects per patients	47%	29%	15%	57%	30%
Side effects per injections	19%	10%	6%	31%	7%

MTX = methotrexate, Triam. = triamcinolone crystaline suspension, Ara-C = cytosine-arabinoside.

administered doses of up to 3 mg/kg body weight without toxicity[43, 54, 161], but the very high doses were injected only once a week[161].

Of methotrexate it is known that the elimination out of the liquor is subjected to strong fluctuations if the meninges are affected[12, 76]. In severe affection with disordered CSF circulation under certain circumstances toxic levels remain locally for a long time which can then cause neurotoxic damage.

Therefore, in intensive intrathecal treatment a determination of the CSF level of methotrexate should be carried out. This is also necessary in the "concentration × time" method suggested by Bleyer and Poplack[13], where, after ventricular injection of 10 mg methotrexate, 1 mg is then injected every 12 hours to maintain a therapeutic CSF level for 72 hours. But even with this technique considerable fluctuations of the CSF levels occur.

The application of a ventricle catheter with Ommaya[137] or Rickham reservoir is advantageous when there is a chance of stabilization and the need for a longer intrathecal treatment exists as higher cytostatic levels in the ventricle and a better distribution is achieved. The rate of complications is, however, higher than in lumbal therapy.

3. Summary and Conclusions

The diagnostics of brain tumors in recent years has decisively improved as to neuroimaging techniques or a more specified and uniform neuropathologic evaluation. Only on this basis was an exact appraisal of the chemotherapy of malignant brain tumors and elaboration of better treatment strategies possible.

The diagnostic problems being essential solved, the follow-up evaluation may yet be difficult, since costly equipment like PET is available only in a few places and both the CT scan and the MRI are not reliable in classifying abnormal findings generated by the treatment or by remaining tumor mass. The influence of concomitant therapies like steroids or osmotic agents is also not always clearly comprehensible and therefore equivocal evaluations of clinical course or CT and MRI images occur. But, all in all, we are now well able to define the effects of chemotherapy, even if these are often of small magnitude or short-lived.

Thus, a more important drawback of today's clinical brain tumor research becomes apparent: consensus on study design and the best way to report the results is insufficient or, respectively, existing rules are insufficiently followed. Since, as demonstrated above, the efficiency of chemotherapy is low with the common malignant brain tumors and dramatic effects are only seen in singular cases, studies with small numbers of patients or ill-defined response criteria must produce contradictory results, because the influence of the prognostic factors is so strong (see Fig. 9). So, maximum utilization of the clear-cut existing therapeutic potential of chemotherapy was not yet possible. However, in recent years a tendency to accept uniform international standards and to analyze more thoroughly the applied treatment schedules and study results becomes obvious and will lead to better and clearer results of chemotherapy using the already available drugs.

As to the rare malignant brain tumors, a personal bias in the recommendation of chemotherapy is inevitable due to lack of sufficient data. For the malignant gliomas and the brain metastases however, clear treatment outlines can be given:

SURVIVAL PERIOD - DIFFERENT CENTRES

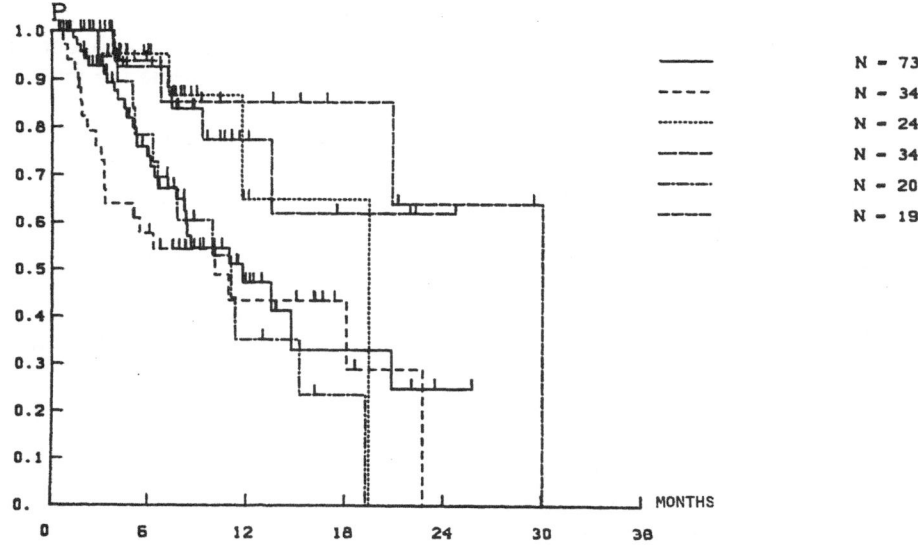

Fig. 9. Survival times in various centers in the German-Austrian randomized multicenter trial of malignant gliomas. Note the remarkable different survival curves in spite of highly standardized, identical treatment. The numbers of patients in each center correspond to those usually treated in single center or pilot studies

In malignant gliomas (WHO grades III and IV, *i.e.* anaplastic astrocytoma, anaplastic oligodendroglioma, anaplastic oligoastrocytoma, glioblastoma multiforme) *adjuvant* chemotherapy with a nitrosourea (BCNU, streptozotocine, possibly PCNU) or procarbazine should be given since it achieves a prolongation of the median survival time for 4–12 weeks to 50–60 weeks and a 3–4-fold increase of the percentage of patients living more than 18 months to about. 30(–40)%. This is true, however, only for patients not older than 70 years (possibly 65 years) with a Karnofsky performance status of at least 50% (*i.e.* they are able to care for themselves but need considerable assistance) and without serious concomitant diseases. Only one not otherwise confirmed study with relatively few cases[47] indicates a possible advantage in delaying chemotherapy until relapse. This issue has not been studied sufficiently, since the closely related problem of clearly defining a tumor rest postoperatively is not settled and hence it is difficult to decide if a therapy is really "adjuvant" or treats remaining tumor.

With brain metastases chemotherapy has meanwhile proved to achieve objective remissions and to prolong median survival time. This is valid for solid brain metastases and, with the special delivery techniques, for meningosis neoplastica also. Therefore, in all primary tumors for which an efficacious chemotherapy regimen is available, additional cytostatic treatment of brain metastases is clearly to be recommended if the patient is in a condition to allow aggressive therapy.

With all other malignant brain tumors the efficacy of *adjuvant* chemotherapy is not proven due to lack of data of systematic studies. However, for all these tumor types remissions of recurrences are reported to be achieved by chemotherapy. Therefore, chemotherapy must be considered an important component of treatment for these tumors, too, and may even be used as first-line therapy for certain chemosensitive tumors like medulloblastomas[110].

On the other hand, for very radiosensitive tumors like germinomas the best strategy might be to withhold chemotherapy until relapse. These issues cannot be settled until these rare tumors are collected and treated systematically in larger centers to allow treatment evaluation within a few years.

As a rule, intrinsic malignant brain tumors and lymphomas should be treated by drugs penetrating the BBB fairly well, whereas metastatic tumors or malignant tumors of mesenchymal origin like sarcomas or the rare malignant meningiomas are not expected to have a BBB and can be treated with the drugs well-tried for these tumors in general oncology.

The intrathecal cytostatic therapy or prophylaxis has proved to be a *conditio sine qua non* for long-term survival in acute leucemias in children. Regular CSF examinations in other malignancies, also in primary brain tumors, demonstrate a much higher incidence of leptomeningeal involvement than previously supposed. This is partly due to the increasing survival times and successfully treated relapses resulting from the aggressive multimodal modern treatment approaches in cancer patients. Since the intrathecal cytostatic therapy used properly has hardly severe side-effects it should be applied more extensively especially as prophylactic treatment, as mentioned above with the special tumor types. This may offer longer survival for those patients primarily successfully treated or having been stabilized after relapse.

Acknowledgement

The authors thank Mrs. B. Herrmann and Mrs. M. Vesely for excellent secretarial assistance.

References

1. Aabo K, Walbom-Jorgensen S (1986) Central nervous system complications by malignant lymphomas: Radiation schedule and treatment results. J Radiat Oncol Biol Phys 12: 197–202
2. Afra D, Lázár L, Slowik F (1979) Combined treatment of medulloblastomas in adults. In: Paoletti P, Walker MD, Butti G, Knerich R (eds) Multidisciplinary aspects of brain tumor therapy. Elsevier/North-Holland, pp 177–188
3. Allen JC, Bloom J, Ertel I, Evans A, Hammond D, Jones H, Levin V, Jenkin D, Sposto R, Wara W (1986) Brain tumors in children: Current cooperative and institutional chemotherapy trials in newly diagnosed and recurrent disease. Semin Oncol 13: 110–122
4. Andersen AP (1981) Scandinavian glioblastoma study group: Combined modality therapy of operated astrocytomas grade III and IV. Confirmation of the value of postoperative irradiation and lack of potentiation of bleomycin on survival time. Cancer 47: 649

5. Aroney RS, Kaplan RS, Salcman M, Montgomery E, Wiernik PH (1982) A phase II trial of AZQ (NSC 182986) in patients with recurrent primary or metastatic brain tumors. Abstract, ASCO Meeting

6. Aronin PA, Mahaley MS jr, Rudnick SA, Dudka L, Donohue JF, Selker RG, Moore P (1980) Prediction of BCNU pulmonary toxicity in patients with malignant gliomas. N Engl J Med 303: 183–188

7. Ascherl GF jr, Hilal SK, Brisman R (1981) Computed tomography of disseminated meningeal and ependymal malignant neoplasms. Neurology 31: 567–574

8. Barnett MJ, Ganesan TS, Waxman JH, Richards MA, Smith BF, Rohatiner AZS, Dhaliwal HS, Slevin ML, Lister TA (1985) Neurotoxicity of high-dose cytosine arabinoside. Prog Exp Tumor Res 29: 177–182

9. Bateman DE, McDermott J, Hughes DR, Edwardson JA (1986) The selective release of polypeptides from human glioma cell cultures and their possible modification by dexamethasone. Abstract, International meeting on brain oncology, Rennes, p 11

10. Behnke J, Mach JP, Buchegger F, Carrel S, Delaloye B, de Tribolet N (1986) In vivo localization of radiolabelled monoclonal antibody in human gliomas. Abstract, International meeting on brain oncology, Rennes, p 22

11. Blasberg R, Patlak C (1979) Metastatic brain tumors: local blood flow and capillary permeability. Neurology 29: 547

12. Bleyer WA, Drake JC, Chabner BA (1973) Neurotoxicity and elevated cerebrospinal-fluid methotrexate concentration in meningeal leukemia. N Engl J Med 289: 770–773

13. Bleyer WA, Poplack DG, Simon RM (1978) "Concentration × Time" methotrexate via a subcutaneous reservoir: A less toxic regimen for intraventricular chemotherapy of central nervous system neoplasms. Blood 51: 835–842

14. Bloom HJG (1982) Medulloblastoma in children: Increasing survival rates and further prospects. Int J Radiat Oncol Biol Phys 8: 2023–2027

15. Boethius J, Blomgren H, Collins VP, Greitz T, Strander H (1983) The effect of systemic human interferon-alpha administration to patients with glioblastoma multiforme. Acta Neurochir (Wien) 68: 239–251

16. Boettcher HD, Wagner W, Haverkamp U, Schadel A (1983) Zum Auftreten und zur Prognose des Medulloblastoms im Erwachsenenalter. Strahlentherapie 159: 143–146

17. Bogdahn U, Bogdahn S, Mertens HG, Dommasch D, Wodarz R, Wünsch PH, Kühl P, Richter E (1986) Primary non-Hodgkin's lymphomas of the CNS. Acta Neurol Scand 73: 602–614

18. Brooks DJ, Beaney RP, Thomas DGT (1986) The role of positron emission tomography in the study of cerebral tumors. Semin Oncol 13: 83–93

19. Brucher JM (1983) Stereotaxic biopsies of the brain. In: Krauseneck P, Mertens HG (Hrsg) Therapie maligner Neoplasien des Gehirns. Perimed, Erlangen, S 26–28

20. Bryan P (1974) CSF seeding of intra-cranial tumours: A study of 96 cases. Clin Radiol 25: 355–360

21. Budka H, Majdic, Knapp W (1985) Cross-reactivity between human hemopoietic cells and brain tumors as defined by monoclonal antibodies. J Neuro-Oncol 3: 173–179

22. Burger PC, Dubois PJ, Schold SC jr, Smith KR jr, Odom GL, Crafts DC, Giangaspero F (1983) Computerized tomographic and pathologic studies of the untreated, quiescent, and recurrent glioblastoma multiforme. J Neurosurg 58: 159–169

23. Burger PC (1983) Pathologic anatomy and CT correlations in the glioblastoma multiforme. Appl Neurophysiol 46: 180–187

24. Burger PC, Vogel FS, Green SB, Strike TA (1985) Glioblastoma multiforme and anaplastic astrocytoma. Cancer 56: 1106–1111

25. Burger PC (1986) Malignant astrocytic neoplasms: Classification, pathologic anatomy, and response to treatment. Semin Oncol 13: 16–26

26. Byar DP, Green SB, Strike TA (1983) Prognostic factors for malignant glioma. In: Walker MD (ed) Oncology of the nervous system. M Nijhoff, Boston, pp 379–396
27. Cairncross JG, Chernik NL, Kimm JH, Posner JB (1979) Sterilization of cerebral metastases by radiation therapy. Neurology 29: 1195–1202
28. Cairncross JG, Posner JB (1983) The management of brain metastases. In: Walker MD (ed) Oncology of the nervous system. M Nijhoff, Boston, pp 341–378
29. Cascino TL, Byrne TN, Deck MDF, Posner JB (1983) Intraarterial BCNU in the treatment of metastatic brain tumors. J Neuro-Oncol 1: 211–218
30. Carey RW, Davis JM, Zervas NT (1981) Tamoxifen-induced regression of cerebral metastases in breast carcinoma. Cancer Treat Rep 65: 793–795
31. Casimir M, Yap HY, di Stefano A, Hortobagyi GN, Blumenschein GR (1981) The influence of combined modality treatment on the survival of breast cancer patients with brain metastases. ASCO Abstracts, C-427
32. Chan PYM, Byfield JE, Campbell T, Sladoff L, Rao AR (1980) Combined chemotherapy and irradiation in the treatment of brain metastases from lung cancer. In: Weiss E, Gilbert HA, Posner JB (eds) Brain metastasis. Hall, Boston
33. Chang CH, Horton J, Schoenfeld D, Salazer O, Perez-Tamayo R, Kramer S, Weinstein A, Nelson JS, Tsukada Y (1983) Comparison of postoperative radiotherapy and combined postoperative radiotherapy and chemotherapy in the multidisciplinary management of malignant gliomas. Cancer 52: 997–1007
34. Chatel M (1986) EORTC chemotherapeutic trials in malignant brain gliomas. Abstract 14th Int Cancer Congr, Budapest, p 294
35. Cohen ME, Duffner PK (1984) Brain tumors in children. Raven Press, New York
36. Colomer R, Fuentes R, Boada M, Rubio D (1986) Regression of brain metastases from breast cancer with tamoxifen. Abstr 14th Int Cancer Congr, Budapest, p 470
37. Conte PF, Guerrasio A, Bumma C, Giaccome C, Musella R, Lombard GF, Distefano FF, Calciati A (1982) VM 26, adriamycine and CCNU combination chemotherapy in metastatic brain tumours. In: Hildebrand D, Gangji D (eds) Treatment of neoplastic lesions of the nervous system. Pergamon Press, Oxford New York, pp 161–164
38. Curt GA, Schilsky R, Kelly J, Kufta C, Smith B, Thomas C, Young RC (1982) Phase II study of aziridinylbenzoquinone (AZQ) in high grade gliomas. Abstract, ASCO meeting
39. Darling JL, Bradley NJ, Pilkington GJ, Lantos PL, Thomas DGT (1984) Differential effects of human leukocyte (IFN-gamma) and fibroblast (IFN-beta) derived interferons on human glioma cell cultures in vitro. Neuropathol Appl Neurobiol 10: 309
40. Decker DA, Sarraf MA, Kresge C, Austin D, Wilner HI (1985) Phase II study of aziridinylbenzoquinone (AZQ: NSC-182986) in the treatment of malignant gliomas recurrent after radiation. J Neuro-Oncol 3: 19–21
41. Di Chiro G (1985) Brain imaging of glucose utilization in cerebral tumors. In: Sokoloff L (ed) Brain imaging and brain function. Raven Press, New York, pp 185–197
42. Djerassi I, Kim JS, Reggev A (1985) Response of astrocytoma to high-dose methotrexate with citrovorum factor rescue. Cancer 55: 2741–2747
43. Dommasch D, Przuntek H, Grüninger W, Mertens HG (1976) Intrathecal cytostatic chemotherapy of meningitis carcinomatosa. Eur Neurol 14: 178
44. Donoso JA, Samson F (1984) Mechanisms of neurotoxicity of anticancer drugs. In: Blum K, Manzo L (eds) Neurotoxicology. Marcel Dekker, New York Basel
45. Duff TA, Borden E, Bay J, Phepmeier J, Sielaff K (1986) Phase II trial of interferon-β for treatment of recurrent glioblastoma multiforme. J Neurosurg 64: 408–413
46. Ehya H, Hajdu SI, Melamed MR (1981) Cytopathology of non lymphoreticular neoplasms metastatic to the central nervous system. Acta Cytol 25/6: 599–610

47. E.O.R.T.C. Brain Tumor Group (1976) Effect of CCNU on survival rate of objective remission and duration of free interval in patients with malignant brain glioma—first evaluation. Eur J Cancer 12: 41–45

48. E.O.R.T.C. Brain Tumor Group (1978) Effect of CCNU on survival rate of objective remission and duration of free interval in patients with malignant brain glioma—final evaluation. Eur J Cancer 14: 851–856

49. E.O.R.T.C. Brain Tumor Group (1980) Effect of DDMP (2, 4-diamino-5-3', 4'-dichlorophenyl-6-methylpyrimidine) on brain tumors. A phase II study. Europ J Cancer 16: 1639–1640

50. E.O.R.T.C. Brain Tumor Group (1981) Evaluation of CCNU, VM-26 plus CCNU, and procarbazine in supratentorial brain gliomas. J Neurosurg 55: 27–31

51. E.O.R.T.C. Brain Tumor Group (1983) Aberle HG, Brotchi J, Lemaire M, Calliauw L, Chatel M, de Barsy T, Longueville J, de Tribolet N, Bernasconi S, Garfield J, Punt J, Gonzales D, Greiner R, Haefliger LM, Haferkamp G, Hery M, Hildebrand J, Regnier R, Resche F, Bourdin S, Dalesio O, Solbu G: Misonidazole in radiotherapy of supratentorial malignant brain gliomas in adult patients: A randomized double-blind study. Eur J Cancer Clin Oncol 19/1: 39–42

52. E.O.R.T.C. (1985) Effect of AZQ (1,4-cyclohexadiene-1,4-diacarbamic acid-2,5-bis(1-aziridinyl)-3,6-dioxodiethylester) in recurring supratentorial malignant brain gliomas—a phase II study. Eur J Cancer Clin Oncol 21/1: 143–146

53. Erlich SS, Davis RL (1978) Spinal subarachnoid metastasis from primary intracranial glioblastoma multiforme. Cancer 42: 2854–2864

54. Ettinger LJ, Freeman AI, Creaven PJ (1978) Intrathecal methotrexate overdose without neurotoxicity. Cancer 41: 1270–1273

55. Ettinger LJ (1982) Pharmacokinetics and biochemical effects of a fatal intrathecal methotrexate overdose. Cancer 50: 440–450

56. Eyre HJ, Sause WT (1985) Treatment of meningeal carcinomatosis with irradiation plus intrathecal methotrexate: A Southern Oncology Group study, ASCO Proc 4: 149

57. Feun LG, Stewart DJ, Maor M, Leavens ME, Savaraj N, Burgess MA, Yung WKA, Benjamin RS (1983) A pilot study of cisdiamminedichloroplatinum and radiation therapy in patients with high grade astrocytomas. J Neuro-Oncol 1: 109–113

58. Feun LG, Yung WKA, Leavens ME, Burgess MA, Obbens EA, Bedikian AY, Savaraj N, Stewart DJ, Benjamin RS, Fields WS, Bodey GP (1984) A phase II trial of 2,4,-diaziridinyl 3,6-bis(carboethoxy amino)1,4-benzoquinone (AZQ, NSC 182986) in recurrent primary brain tumors. J Neuro-Oncol 2: 13–17

59. Feun LG, Wallace S, Stewart DJ, Chuang VP, Yung WKA, Leavens ME, Burgess MA, Savaraj N, Benjamin RS, Young SE, Tang RA, Handel S, Mavligit G, Fields WS (1984) Intracarotid infusion of cis-diamminedichloroplatinum in the treatment of recurrent malignant brain tumors. Cancer 54: 794–799

60. Fewer D, Wilson CB, Boldrey EB, Enot KJ, Powell MR (1972) The chemotherapy of brain tumors. Clinical experience with carmustine (BCNU) and vincristine. JAMA 222/5: 549–552

61. Friedman HS, Schold SC jr (1985) Rational approaches to the chemotherapy of medulloblastoma. Neurol Clin 3: 843–853

62. Friedman HS, Colvin OM, Ludeman SM, Schold SC jr, Boyd VL, Mulhbaier LH, Bigner DD (1986) Experimental chemotherapy of human medulloblastoma with classical alkylators (in press)

63. Fulton DS, Levin VA, Gutin PH, Edwards MSB, Seager ML, Stewart J, Wilson B (1982) Intrathecal cytosine arabinoside for the treatment of meningeal metastases from malignant brain tumors and systemic tumors. Cancer Chemother Pharmacol 8: 285–291

64. Galicich JH, Sundaresan N, Thaler HT (1980) Surgical treatment of single brain metastasis. Evaluation of results by computerized tomography scanning. J Neurosurg 53: 63–67
65. Gastaut JA, Grisoli F, Vincentelli F, Peragut JC, Maraninchi D, Andrac L, Carcassonne Y (1982) Intracranial malignant lymphoma. In: Hildebrand D, Gangji D (eds) Treatment of neoplastic lesions of the nervous system. Pergamon Press, Oxford New York, pp 149–155
66. Gehan EA, Walker MD (1977) Prognostic factors for patients with brain tumors. Natl Cancer Inst Monogr 46: 189–195
67. Gerosa MA, di Stefano E, Olivi A (1981) VM-26 monochemotherapy trial in the treatment of recurrent supratentorial gliomas: Preliminary report. Surg Neurol 15/2: 128–134
68. Green SB, Byar DP, Walker MD, Pistenmaa DA, Alexander E jr, Batzdorf U, Brooks WH, Hunt WE, Mealey J jr, Odom GL, Paoletti P, Ransohoff J II, Robertson JT, Selker RG, Shapiro WR, Smith KR jr, Wilson CB, Strike T (1983) Comparisons of carmustine, procarbazine, and high-dose methylprednisolone as additions to surgery and radiotherapy for the treatment of malignant glioma. Cancer Treat Rep 67/2: 123–132
69. Green SB, Byar DP, Strike TA, Alexander E jr, Brooks WH, Burger PC, Hunt WE, Mealey J jr, Odom GL, Paoletti P, Pistenmaa DA, Ransohoff J II, Robertson JT, Selker RG, Shapiro WR, Smith KR jr (1984) Randomized comparisons of BCNU, streptozotocin, radiosensitizer, and fractionation of radiotherapy in the postoperative treatment of malignant glioma (study 7702). ASCO Proc 3: 260
70. Green SB, Byar DB, Strike TA, Burger PC, Mahaley MS, Mealey J jr, Pistenmaa DA, Ransohoff J II, Robertson JT, Selker RG, Shapiro WR, VanGilder JC (1985) Randomized phase II comparison of PCNU and AZQ for the treatment of primary brain tumors (study 8120). ASCO Proc 4: 143
71. Grisold W, Weiss R, Jellinger K (1984) Klinik und zytologische Diagnostik der meningealen Neoplasien. In: Heyden HW von, Krauseneck P (Hrsg) Hirnmetastasen. Zuckschwerdt, München Bern Wien (Aktuelle Onkol 13, S 85–103)
72. Groothuis DR, Molnar P, Blasberg RG (1984) Regional blood flow and blood-to-tissue transport in five brain tumor models. Implications for chemotherapy. In: Brain tumor biology. Karger, Basel, pp 32–153 (Prog Exp Tumor Res, vol 24)
73. Gutin PH, Wilson CB, Kumar ARV, Boldrey EB, Levin V, Powell M, Enot KJ (1975) Phase II study of procarbazine, CCNU, and vincristine combination chemotherapy in the treatment of malignant brain tumors. Cancer 35: 1398–1404
74. Haid M, Khandekar JD, Christ M (1985) Aziridinylbenzoquinone in recurrent, progressive glioma of the central nervous system. Cancer 56: 1311–1315
75. Hande KR, Stein RD, McDonough DA, Greco FA, Wolff SN (1982) Effects of high-dose cytarabine. Clin Pharmacol and Therapeutics 31/5: 669–674
76. Hanson B, Malarme M, Abele R, Regnier R, Hildebrand J (1982) Treatment results in neoplastic meningitis. In: Hildebrand J, Gangji D (eds) Treatment of neoplastic lesions of the nervous system. Pergamon Press, Oxford New York, pp 59–61
77. Hatlevoll R, Lindegaard KF, Hagen S, Kristiansen K, et al. (1985) Combined modality treatment of operated astrocytomas grade 3 and 4. Cancer 56: 41–47
78. Helle TL, Britt RH, Colby TV (1984) Primary lymphoma of the central nervous system. J Neurosurg 60: 94–103
79. Herbst KD, Corder MP, Justice GR (1976) Successful therapy with methotrexate of a multicentric mixed lymphoma of the central nervous system. Cancer 38: 1476–1478
80. Heyden HW von, Krauseneck P (Hrsg) (1984) Hirnmetastasen. Zuckschwerdt, München Bern Wien (Aktuelle Onkologie 13)

81. Hildebrand J, Brihaye JM, Wagenknecht L, Michel J, Kenis Y (1975) Combination chemotherapy with CCNU, vincristine and methotrexate in primary and metastatic brain tumors. Eur J Cancer 11: 585–587

82. Hildebrand J, Brihaye J, Wagenknecht JM, Kenis Y (1975) Combination therapy with CCNU, vincristine and methotrexate in primary and metastatic brain tumors. Eur J Cancer 11: 585–587

82 a. Hildebrand J, Gangji D (eds) (1982) Treatment of neoplastic lesions of the nervous system. Pergamon Press, Oxford New York

83. Hildebrand J (1985) Current status of chemotherapy of brain tumours. Prog Exp Tumor Res 29: 152–166

84. Hirakawa K, Ueda S, Nakagawa Y, Suzuki K, Fukuma S, Kita M, Imanishi J, Kishida T (1983) Effect of human leukocyte interferon on malignant brain tumors. Cancer 51/11: 1976–1981

85. Hochberg FH, Miller G, Schooley RT, et al. (1983) CNS lymphoma related to Epstein-Barr virus. N Engl J Med 309: 745–749

86. Jellinger K, Volc D, Grisold W, Flament H, Vollmer R, Weiss R (1983) Kombinationsbehandlung maligner Gliome. Wien klin Wschr 95/12: 407–416

87. Jellinger K (1983) Histologische Klassifikation und therapiebedingte Veränderungen. In: Krauseneck P, Mertens HG (Hrsg) Therapie maligner Neoplasien des Gehirns. Perimed, Erlangen, S 15–25

88. Jellinger K (1983) Pathologic effects of chemotherapy. In: Walker MD (ed) Oncology of the nervous system. M Nijhoff, Boston, pp 285–340

89. Jellinger K (1984) Häufigkeit und Charakteristik der zerebralen Karzinommetastasen. In: Heyden HW von, Krauseneck P (Hrsg) Hirnmetastasen. Zuckschwerdt, München Bern Wien (Aktuelle Onkologie 13, S 49–79)

90. Jellinger K (1986) Present limits of conventional treatment for malignant brain tumors. In: Hatanaka H (ed) Boron-neutron capture therapy for tumors. Nishimura, Tokyo, pp 309–349

91. Jellinger K, Slowik F (1986) Primary non-Hodgkin lymphomas of the central nervous system. J Neuro-Oncol (in press)

92. Jenkin RDT, Simpson WJK, Keen CW (1978) Pineal and suprasellar germinomas. J Neurosurg 48: 99–107

93. Kaplan RS, Wiernik PH (1984) Neurotoxicity of antitumor agents. In: Perry MC (ed) Toxicity of chemotherapy. Grune & Stratton, London, pp 365–433

94. Kessinger A, Lemon HM, Foley JF (1979) VM-26 as a second drug in the treatment of brain gliomas. Cancer Treat Rep 63: 511–512

95. Krauseneck P, Mertens HG (Hrsg) (1983) Therapie maligner Neoplasien des Gehirns. Perimed, Erlangen

96. Krauseneck, P (1984) Chemotherapie von Hirnmetastasen. In: Heyden HW von, Krauseneck P (Hrsg) Hirnmetastasen. Zuckschwerdt, München Bern Wien. (Aktuelle Onkologie 13, S 167–179)

97. Krauseneck P, Mertens HG, Richter E, Schmidt M, Halves E, Bogdahn U, Kappos L, Seybold D (1985) Combined chemotherapy of inoperable and operable malignant gliomas. In: Voth D, Krauseneck P (eds) Chemotherapy of gliomas. De Gruyter, Berlin New York, pp 353–359

98. Krauseneck P, Seybold D, Mertens HG (1985) Pseudo-recurrence in malignant brain tumors. In: Voth D, Krauseneck P (eds) Chemotherapy of gliomas. De Gruyter, Berlin New York, pp 283–290

99. Krauseneck P, Dommasch D, Dienst P, Bogdahn U, Kappos L, Seybold D, Mertens HG (1985) Intrathekale Verträglichkeit von Cytosin-Arabinosid. Verh Dt Ges Neur 3: 500–504

390   P. Krauseneck and H. G. Mertens:

99 a. Krauseneck P, Richter E, Dittmann W, Müller HA, Ködel B, Bogdahn U (1986) Radiotherapy in low grade gliomas. Abstr Int Meeting on Brain Oncology, Rennes, p 50

100. Kumar ARV, Renaudin J, Wilson CB, Boldrey EB, Enot KJ, Levin VA (1974) Procarbazine hydrochloride in the treatment of brain tumors. Phase 2 study. J Neurosurg 40: 365–371

101. Kunze P, Hoppe W, Riedel C, Döge H (1980) Primäres malignes Lymphom des Zentralnervensystems. Psychiat Neurol Med Psychol 32: 373–381

102. Lee Y, Bigner DD (1985) Aspects of immunobiology and immunotherapy and uses of monoclonal antibodies and biologic immune modifiers in human gliomas. Neurol Clin 3: 901–917

103. Letendre L, Banks PM, Reese DF, Mill RH, Scanlon PW, Kiely JM (1982) Primary lymphoma of the central nervous system. Cancer 49: 939–943

104. Levin VA, Crafts D, Wilson CB, Kabra P, Hansch C, Boldrey E, Enot J, Neely M (1975) Imidazole carboxamides: Relationship of lipophilicity to activity against intracerebral murine glioma 26 and preliminary phase II clinical trial of 5-[3,3-bis(2-chloroethyl)-1-triazeno]imidazole-4-carboxamide (NSC-82196) in primary and secondary brain tumors. Cancer Chemo Rep 59/2: 327–331

105. Levin VA, Crafts DC, Wilson CB, et al. (1976) BCNU and procarbazine treatment for malignant brain tumors. Cancer Treat Rep 60: 243

106. Levin VA, Hoffman WF, Pischer TL, Seager ML, Boldrey EB, Wilson CB (1978) BCNU-5-fluorouracil combination therapy for recurrent malignant brain tumors. Cancer Treat Rep 62/12: 2071–2076

107. Levin VA, Wilson CB, Davis R, Wara WM, Pischer TL, Irwin L (1979) A phase III comparison of BCNU, hydroxyurea and radiation therapy to BCNU and radiation therapy for treatment of primary malignant gliomas. J Neurosurg 51: 526–532

108. Levin VA, Edwards MS, Wright DC, Seager ML, Schimberg TP, Townsend JJ, Wilson CB (1980) Modified procarbazine, CCNU, and vincristine (PCV 3) combination chemotherapy in the treatment of malignant brain tumors. Cancer Treat Rep 64: 237–241

109. Levin VA, Hoffman WF, Heilbron DC, Norman D (1980) Prognostic significance of the pretreatment CT scan on time to progression for patients with malignant gliomas. J Neurosurg 52: 642–647

110. Levin VA, Vestnys PS, Edwards MS, Wara WM, Fulton D, Barger G, Seager M, Wilson CB (1983) Improvement in survival produced by sequential therapies in the treatment of recurrent medulloblastoma. Cancer 51: 1364–1370

111. Levin VA, Edwards MSB, Gutin PH, Vestnys P, Fulton D, Seager ML, Wilson CB (1984) Phase II evaluation of dibromodulcitol in the treatment of recurrent medulloblastoma, ependymoma, and malignant astrocytoma. J Neurosurg 61: 1063–1068

112. Levin VA (1985) Chemotherapy of primary brain tumors. Neurol Clin 3: 855–866

113. Levin VA, Wara WM, Davis RL, Silver P, Resser KJ, Yatsko K, Nutik S, Gutin PH, Wilson CB (1986) NCOG Protocol 6G91: Response to treatment with radiation therapy and seven-drug chemotherapy in patients with glioblastoma multiforme. Cancer Treat Rep (in press)

114. Levin VA, Wara WM, Davis RL, Vestnys P, Resser KJ, Yatsko K, Nutik S, Gutin PH, Wilson CB (1985) Phase III comparison of BCNU and the combination of procarbazine, CCNU, and vincristine administered after radiotherapy with hydroxyurea for malignant gliomas. J Neurosurg 63: 218–223

115. Loeffler JS, Ervin TJ, Mauch P, Skarin A, Weinstein HJ, Canellos G, Cassady JR (1985) Primary lymphomas of the central nervous system: patterns of failure and factors that influence survival. J Clin Oncol 3: 490–494

116. Mackintosh FR, Colby TV, Podolsky WJ, Burke JS, Hoppe RT, Rosenfelt FP, Rosenberg SA, Kaplan HS (1982) Central nervous system involvement in non-Hodgkin's lymphoma: An analysis of 105 cases. Cancer 49: 586–595

117. Mahaley MS jr, Urso MB, Whaley RA, Blue M, Williams TE, Guaspari A, Selker RG (1985) Immunobiology of primary intracranial tumors. J Neurosurg 63: 719–725

118. Mahaley MS (1986) Neuro-oncology review: Radiotherapy, chemotherapy, immunotherapy. (Unpublished manuscript)

119. Maral J, Poisson M, Pertuiset BF, Mashaly P, Weil M, Jacquillat C, Grillo-Lopez AJ (1985) Phase II evaluation of diaziquone (CI-904, AZQ) in the treatment of human glioma. J Neuro-Oncol 3: 245–249

120. Markesbery WR, Brooks WH, Gupta GD, Young AB (1978) Treatment for patients with cerebral metastases. Arch Neurol 35: 754–756

121. Marton LJ, et al. (1979) Predictive value of CSF polyamines. Cancer Res 39: 993–997

122. Mazziotta JC (1985) PET scanning: principles and applications. Discussions in Neurosciences 2/1

123. McKeran RO, Thomas DGT (1980) The clinical study of gliomas. In: Thomas DGT, Graham DI (eds) Brain tumours. Butterworths, London, pp 194–230

124. Mende S, Bleichner F, Stoeter P, Meuret G (1983) Erfolgreiche Behandlung von Hirnmetastasen bei Mammakarzinom mit nicht liquorgängigen Zytostatika und Hormonen. Onkologie 6: 58–61

125. Mertens HG, Bogdahn U, Dommasch D, Krüger H, Wodarz R, Wünsch D (1983) Diagnostik und Therapie cerebrospinaler Manifestationen von Leukosen und malignen Lymphomen. In: Seitz D, Vogel P (Hrsg) Hämoblastosen, Zentrale Motorik, Iatrogene Schäden, Myositiden. Springer, Berlin Heidelberg New York. (Verh Dt Ges Neur 2, S 49–69)

126. Nagai M, Arai T, Kohno S, Kohase M (1980) Interferon therapy for malignant brain tumors. In: Kono R, Vilček J (eds) The clinical potential of interferons. University of Tokyo Press, Tokyo, pp 257–273

127. Nagai M, Arai T (1984) Clinical effect of interferon in malignant brain tumours. Neurosurg Rev 7: 55–64

128. Nagai M, Arai T (1985) Clinical studies on interferon therapy for malignant brain tumors—special reference to the effect of gamma-interferon. Abstracts ann meeting interferon system (TNO/ISIR), Clearwater Beach, p 147

129. Nakagawa Y, Hirakawa K, Ueda S, Suzuki K, Fukuma S, Kishida T, Imanishi J, Amagai T (1983) Local administration of interferon for malignant brain tumors. Cancer Treat Reports 67/9: 833–835

130. Nakagawa Y (1984) Interferon therapy for primary brain tumors (Part I + II). Neurologia Medica-Chirurgica (Tokyo) 24: 83–89, 90–96

131. Neuwelt EA, Glasberg M, Frenkel E, Clark WK (1979) Malignant pineal region tumors. J Neurosurg 51: 597–607

132. Neuwelt EA, Balaban E, Diehl J, Hill S, Frenkel E (1983) Successful treatment of primary central nervous system lymphomas with chemotherapy after osmotic blood-brain barrier opening. Neurosurgery 12: 662–671

133. Newlands ES (1985) Chemotherapy for brain metastases. Prog Exp Tumor Res 29: 167–176

134. Nishio S, Korosue K, Tateishi J, Fukui M, Kitamura K (1982) Ventricular and subarachnoid seeding of intracranial tumors of neuroectodermal origin—A study of 26 consecutive autopsy cases with reference to focal ependymal defect. Clin Neuropathol 1: 83–91

135. Nishio S, Fukui M, Ohta M, Tateishi J, Kitamura K (1983) Spinal subarachnoid seeding from glioblastoma multiforme of the brain stem. Neurol Med Chir 23: 566–570

136. Obbens EAMT, Feun LG, Leavens ME, Savaraj N, Stewart DJ, Gutterman JU (1985) Phase I clinical trial of intralesional or intraventricular leukocyte interferon for intracranial malignancies. J Neuro-Oncol 3: 61–67

137. Ommaya AK (1963) Subcutaneous reservoir and pump for sterile access to ventricular cerebrospinal fluid. Lancet ii: 983–984

138. Otsuka S, Handa H, Yamashita J, Suda K, Takeuchi J (1984) Single agent therapy of interferon for brain tumours: Correlation between natural killer activity and clinical course. Acta Neurochirurgica 73: 13–23

139. Owens G, Javid R, Belmusto L, et al. (1965) Intra-arterial vincristine therapy of primary gliomas. Cancer 18: 756

140. Paoletti P (1980) Therapeutic strategy for central nervous system tumors: Present status, criticism and potential. J Neurosurg SCI 28: 51–60

141. Paoletti P, Knerich R, Butti G, Adinolfi D, Locatelli D, Robustelli della Cuna G, Cordero di Montezemolo L, Schiffer D, Soffietti R, Nicolato A, Giunta F, Buoncristiani P, Scamoni C (1983) Italian cooperative study on malignant glial tumor therapy. In: Krauseneck P, Mertens HG (Hrsg) Therapie maligner Neoplasien des Gehirns. Perimed, Erlangen

142. Pasquier B, Pasquier D, N'golet A, Panh MH, Couderc P (1979) Le potentiel métastatique des tumeurs primitives du systeme nerveux central. Rev Neurol 135: 263–278

143. Patronas NJ, di Chiro G, Brooks RA, et al (1982) Work in progress: (18 F) Fluorodeoxyglucose and positron emission tomography in the evaluation of radiation necrosis of the brain. Radiology 144: 885–889

144. Pierangeli E, Levin VA, Marton LJ (1983) Relationship of brain diffusion and capillary permeability of putrescine (Pu) to CSF levels in brain tumor patients. In: Krauseneck P, Mertens HG (Hrsg) Therapie maligner Neoplasien des Gehirns. Perimed, Erlangen, S 151–153

145. Posner JB (1980) Chemotherapy and the nervous system. In: Ongerboer de Visser, Bosch DA, van Woerkom-Eykenboom WMH (eds) Neuro-oncology. M Nijhoff, Boston, pp 124–132

146. Posner JP (1982) Treatment of leptomeningeal metastases from solid tumors. In: Hildebrand J, Gangji D (eds) Treatment of neoplastic lesions of the nervous system. Pergamon Press, Oxford New York, pp 57–58

147. Pouillart P, Mathe G, Thy TH, Lheritier J, Poisson M, Huguenin P, Gauthier H, Morin P, Parrot R (1976) Treatment of malignant gliomas and brain metastases in adults with a combination of adriamycin, VM 26, and CCNU. Cancer 38: 1909–1916

148. Reuther P, Dommasch D, Fuhrmeister U, Krauseneck P, Mertens HG (1983). Intrathekale DTIC-Therapie bei leptomeningealer Melanommetastasierung. In: Krauseneck P, Mertens HG (Hrsg) Therapie maligner Neoplasien des Gehirns. Perimed, Erlangen, S 135–138

149. Rhodes CG, Wise RJS, Gibbs JM et al. (1983) In vivo disturbance of the oxidative metabolism of glucose in human cerebral gliomas. Ann Neurol 14: 614–626

150. Robustelli della Cuna G, Paoletti P, Bertolotti E, Knerich R, Bernardinelli L, Butti G, Baldi M (1979) Combined modality treatment of metastatic central nervous system (CNS) tumors with nitrosourea compounds. In: Paoletti P, Walker MD, Butti G, Knerich R (eds) Multidisciplinary aspects of brain tumor therapy. Elsevier, Amsterdam, pp 283–295

151. Rosen ST, Aisner J, Makuch RW, Matthews MJ, Ihde DC, Whitacre M, Glatstein EJ, Wiernik PH, Lichter AS, Bunn PA jr (1982) Carcinomatous leptomeningitis in small cell lung cancer. Medicine 61: 45–53

152. Rosenblum ML, Reynolds AF jr, Smith KA, Rumack BH, Walker MD (1973) Chloroethyl-cyclohexyl-nitrosourea (CCNU) in the treatment of malignant brain tumors. J Neurosurg 39: 306–314

153. Rosner D, Nemoto T, Pickren J, Lane W (1983) Management of brain metastases from breast cancer by combination chemotherapy. J Neuro-Oncol 1/2: 131–137

154. Rubinstein LJ (1975) The cerebellar medulloblastoma: its origin, differentiation, morphological variants and biological behavior. In: Vinken PJ, Bruyn GW (eds) Tumors of the brain and skull, part 3, vol 9. Elsevier/North-Holland Biomedical Press, New York, pp 167–194

155. Rustin GJS, Newlands ES, Bagshawe KD, Begent RHJ, Crawford SM (1986) Successful management of metastatic and primary germ cell tumors in the brain. Cancer 57: 2108–2113

156. Safdari H, Boluix B, Gros C (1984) Multifocal brain radionecrosis masquerading as tumor dissemination. Surg Neurol 21: 35–41

157. Sano K, Nagai M, Takakura K, Mogami H, Nomura K (1982) Effects of Hu IFN-β on gliomas. Abstract, the third annual int congr for Interferon Research, Miami, Florida

158. Sapozink MD, Kaplan HS (1983) Intracranial Hodgkin's disease. Cancer 52: 1301–1307

159. Schindler E (1985) Die Tumoren der Pinealisregion. Springer, Berlin Heidelberg New York Tokyo

160. Schmidt M, Krauseneck P, de l'Espine T, Kappos L (1982) Die Wertigkeit von Lungenfunktionsanalysen in der Diagnostik und Verlaufskontrolle von Zytostatika induzierten interstitiellen Pneumonien. Verhandl Dtsch Ges Inn Med 88: 438–441

161. Schöck LV (1983) Hochdosierte intralumbale Methotrexatgaben. Klinischer Erfahrungsbericht. Onkologie 6/3: 109–112

162. Schold SC jr, Friedman HS, Bjornsson TD, Folletta JM (1984) Treatment of patients with recurrent primary brain tumors with AZQ. Neurology 34: 615–619

163. Seiler RW (1982) Die undifferenzierten Astrozytome des Großhirns. Springer, Berlin Heidelberg New York

164. Shapiro WR (1977) High-dose methotrexate in malignant gliomas. Cancer Treat Rep 61: 753–756

165. Shapiro WR (1980) Chemotherapy of metastatic central nervous system carcinoma. In: Weiss L, Gilbert HA, Posner JB (eds) Brain metastasis. Hall, Boston, pp 328–339

166. Shapiro WR (1986) Therapy of adult malignant brain tumors: What have the clinical trials taught us? Semin Oncol 13: 38–45

167. Sklansky BD, Mann-Kaplan RS, Reynolds AF jr, Rosenblum ML, Walker MD (1974) 4'-demethyl-epipodophyllotoxin-B-D-thenylidene-glucoside (PTG) in the treatment of malignant intracranial neoplasms. Cancer 33: 460–467

168. Sorensen SC, Eagan RT, Scott M (1984) Meningeal carcinomatosis in patients with primary breast and lung cancer. Mayo Clin Proc 59: 91–94

169. Stavrou D, Mellert W, Bilzer T, Senekowitsch R, Keiditsch E, Mehraein P (1985) Radioimmunodetection of gliomas by administration of radiolabelled monoclonal antibodies. Experimental data. Anticancer Res 5: 147–156

170. Stewart DJ, Russell N, Atack EA, Quarrington A, Stolbach L (1983) Cyclophosphamide, doxorubicin, vincristine, and dexamethasone in primary lymphoma of the brain: A case report. Cancer Treat Rep 67: 287–291

171. Stewart DJ, O'Bryan RM, Al-Sarraf M, Costanzi JJ, Oishi N (1983) Phase II study of cisplatin in recurrent astrocytomas in adults: A southwest oncology group study. J Neuro-Oncol 1: 145–147

172. Stewart DJ, Richard MT, Benoit B, Hugenholtz H, Russell N, Dennery J, Peterson E, Grahovac Z, Belanger A, Aitkens S, Young V, Maroun JA (1984) Cisplatin plus cytosine arabinoside in adults with malignant gliomas. J Neuro-Oncol 2: 29–34

173. Takakura K, Sano K, Hojo S, Hirano A (1982) Metastatic tumors of the central nervous system. Igaku-Shoin, Tokyo New York

174. Takakura K (1985) Phase II study of recombinant human interferon alpha A (R0 22-8181) for malignant brain tumors. Abstracts 14th int congr chemotherapy, Kyoto, p 353

175. Takakura K (1985) Intracranial germ cell tumors. Clin Neurosurg 32: 429–444

176. Takakura K, Abe H, Tanaka R, Kitamura K, Miwa T, Takeuchi K, Yamamoto S, Kageyama N, Handa H, Mogami H, Nishimoto A, Uozumi T, Matsutani M, Nomura K (1986) Effects of ACNU and radiotherapy on malignant glioma. J Neurosurg 64: 53–57

177. Talamo TS, Mendelow H (1985) Primary intracranial germinoma with massive ventriculoperitoneal shunt metastases. J Surg Oncol 28: 39–41

178. Taylor SG IV, Nelson L, Baxter D, Rosenbaum C, Sponzo RW, Cunningham TJ, Olson KB, Horton J (1975) Treatment of grade III and IV astrocytoma with dimethyl triazeno imidazole carboxamide (DTIC NSC-45388) alone and in combination with CCNU (NSC-79037) or methyl CCNU (MeCCNU, NSC-95441). Cancer 36: 1269–1276

179. Theodore WH, Gendelman S (1981) Meningeal carcinomatosis. Arch Neurol 38: 696–699

180. Tirelli U, d'Incalci M, Canetta R, Tumolo S, Franchin G, Veronesi A, Galligioni E, Trovo MG, Rossi C, Grigoletto E (1984) Etoposide (VP-16-213) in malignant brain tumors. A phase II study. J Clin Oncol 2: 432–437

181. Tranum BL, Haut A, Rivkin S, Weber E, Quagliana JM, Shaw M, Tucker WG, Smith FE, Samson M, Gottlieb J (1975) A phase II study of methyl CCNU in the treatment of solid tumors and lymphomas: A southwest oncology group study. Cancer 35: 1148–1153

182. Voth D, Hüwel N, Al-Hami S, Kuhnert A (1985) Monotreatment of malignant glioma with a derivate of nitrosourea, ACNU (first results). In: Voth D, Krauseneck P (eds) Chemotherapy of gliomas. De Gruyter, Berlin New York, pp 361–372

183. Vaquero J, Martinez R, Rossi E, Lopez R (1984) Primary cerebral lymphoma: the "ghost tumor". J Neurosurg 60: 174–176

184. Walker MD, Alexander E jr, Hunt WE, Leventhal CM, Mahaley MS jr, Mealey J jr, Norrell HA, Owens G, Ransohoff J, Wilson CB, Gehan EA (1976) Evaluation of mithramycin in the treatment of anaplastic gliomas. J Neurosurg 44: 655–667

185. Walker MD, Alexander E jr, Hunt WE, MacCarty CS, Mahaley MS jr, Mealey J jr, Norrell HA, Owens G, Ransohoff J, Wilson CB, Gehan EA, Strike TA (1978) Evaluation of BCNU and/or radiotherapy in the treatment of anaplastic gliomas. J Neurosurg 49: 333–343

186. Walker MD, Green SB, Byar DP, Alexander E jr, Batzdorf U, Brook WH, Hunt WE, MacCarty CS, Mahaley MS jr, Mealey J jr, Owens G, Ransohoff J II, Robertson JT, Shapiro WR, Smith KR jr, Wilson CB, Strike TA (1980) Randomized comparisons of radiotherapy and nitrosoureas for the treatment of malignant glioma after surgery. N England J Med 303: 1323–1329

187. Wasserstrom WR, Glass PJ, Posner JB (1982) Diagnosis and treatment of leptomeningeal metastases from solid tumors: Experience with 90 patients. Cancer 49: 759–772

188. Wilson CB, Boldrey EB, Enot KJ (1970) 1,3-bis(2-chloroethyl)-1-nitrosourea (NSC-409962) in the treatment of brain tumors. Cancer Chemo Rep 54/4: 273–281

189. Yap HY, Yap BS, Rasmussen S, Levens M, Hortobagyi GN, Blumenschein GR (1982) Treatment for meningeal carcinomatosis in breast cancer. Cancer 49: 219–222

190. Young RC, Waler MD, Canellos GP, Schein PS, Chabner BA, DeVita VT (1973) Initial clinical trials with methyl-CCNU 1-(2-chloroethyl)-3-(4-methyl cyclohexyl)-1-nitrosourea (MeCCNU). Cancer 31: 1164–1169
191. Zülch KJ (1979) Histological typing of tumours of the central nervous system. WHO, Genf

Authors' address: Prof. Dr. Dipl.-Psych. P. Krauseneck, Department of Neurology, University Würzburg, Josef-Schneider-Strasse 11, D-8700 Würzburg, Federal Republic of Germany.

8

Malignant Brain Tumors in Children *

G. Jacobi[1] and *B. Kornhuber*[2]

Division of [1] Pediatric Neurology and [2] Pediatric Oncology and Hematology, Zentrum der Kinderheilkunde, Frankfurt am Main, Federal Republic of Germany

Abbreviations

AICA	anterior inferior cerebellar artery
ARA-C	cytosin-arabinoside
ASCY	astrocytoma
BAER	brain stem acustic evoked responses
BBB	blood-brain barrier
CCA	choriocarcinoma
CCSG	Childrens' Cancer Study Group
CEA	carcinoma embryonic antigen
CHT	chemotherapy
CN	cranial nerve
CNS	central nervous system
CP	cyclophosphamide
CPL	cisplatinum
CSF	cerebrospinal fluid
CT	computerized tomography
CVF	citrovorum factor
ECA	embryonal carcinoma
EEG	electroencephalogram
EPDY	ependymoma
EST	endodermal sinus tumor (yolk sac tumor)
GHRF	growth hormone releasing factor
GLB	glioblastoma multiforme
GPO	German pediatric oncologists
HCG	human chorionic gonadotropin
HGH	hypophyseal growth hormone
ICP	intracranial pressure
IT	infratentorial

* This review is dedicated to Prof. Dr. O. Hövels, former head of the Department of General Pediatrics, on the occasion of his 65th birthday.

IV	intravenous
LTH	luteinizing hormone
ME	melatonin
MBL	medulloblastoma
ML	medial lemniscus
MTX	methotrexate
MTX-HD	high-dose methotrexate
MTX-MHD	middle high-dose MTX
NMR	nuclear magnetic resonance tomography
OLG	oligodendroglioma
PBL	pineoblastoma
PCY	pineocytoma
PEG	pneumencephalography
PF	posterior fossa
PICA	posterior inferior cerebellar artery
PIF	prolactin inhibiting factor
PLP	choroid plexus papilloma
PNET	primitive neuro-ectodermal tumor
RT	radiation therapy
SIOP	Société Internationale d'Oncologie Pédiatrique
ST	supratentorial
VCR	vincristine
VECP	visual evoked cortical potentials
VM	VUMON® (VM-26, teniposide)

Introduction

Frequency and Incidence

Among all children suffering from malignant disease brain tumors take the 2nd place: 12–24% after leukemia (31–42%). They are followed by lymphoma (7–13%), neuroblastoma and Wilm's tumor (8–10% each), and tumors of the bones and the gastrointestinal tract (4–5% each)[223, 281, 435, 451]. Brain tumor incidence shows no differences between white and colored children[451].

The morbidity rate does not show any considerable geographical differences: For the USA, it is 24 per 1 million children per year for the age group 0–15 years[79] and 22–25 per million per year for the age group 0–20 years[120]; for Central Europe: 15–20 (0–16 years)[223], for Eastern Denmark: 24–25 per year from 0–14 years[147], and for Finland: 24 per year between 0–16 years[165]. In adults, the morbidity rate is much higher than in children: 40–50 adults per 1 million per annum[223]. For the neonatal period and the first year of life morbidity rate of 16 per 1 million per annum has been reported[189]. This figure seems realistic, since in the German Democratic Republic autopsy is compulsory for this period of life.

Sex and Age

Most brain tumors show a slight preponderance for males: 1.2 : 1[147, 165], 1.3 : 1[120], 1.4 : 1[184, 223]. The exception are germ cell tumors (germinoma and teratoma) which have a very high preponderance for male subjects. Some brain tumors have an age-

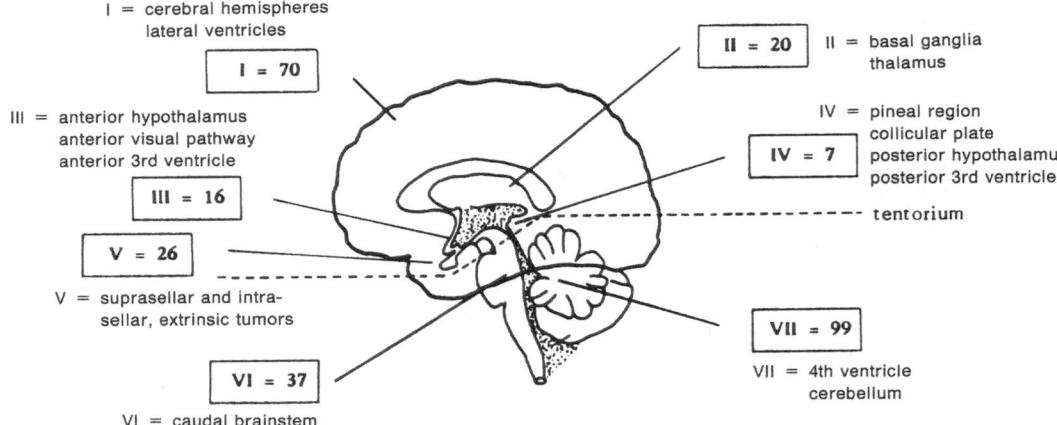

I = cerebral hemispheres
    lateral ventricles

I = 70

II = 20   II = basal ganglia
                thalamus

III = anterior hypothalamus
      anterior visual pathway
      anterior 3rd ventricle

III = 16

IV = pineal region
     collicular plate
     posterior hypothalamus
     posterior 3rd ventricle

IV = 7

tentorium

V = 26

V = suprasellar and intra-
    sellar, extrinsic tumors

VII = 99

VII = 4th ventricle
      cerebellum

VI = 37

VI = caudal brainstem

Fig. 1. Tumor location in 275 children. Children's Hospital, Frankfurt a. Main, 1968–1985

related peak incidence: choroid plexus papillomas and teratomas for the neonatal period and infancy[189], ependymomas of the PF and medulloblastomas for children between 2–5 years, and ST PNETs for the age group 6–12 years. Astrocytomas of the brain stem occur more frequently in younger children than those in the cerebral hemispheres while GLB and OLG have their peak incidence later in life.

Tumor Location

The biological evaluation of a brain tumor depends on 2 important parameters: a) on its benign or malignant morphologic features and b) its location. For the latter reason the site of the tumor growth can be more life threatening than its histological grading, *e.g.* within the caudal brain stem.

Koos and Miller[223] compared ST and IT tumor location in a series of 36 authors. Among 9,960 children there was ST tumor growth in 48.8% and IT location in 51.2%. A Japanese series of 651 children was included in which there was a ST preponderance of 65.4%. In most Western case series there is a preference for IT tumor localization with only some exceptions: Marsa[265] 60%, Tönnis[426] 56.5%, Raimondi[333] 53%, and our own collection (Fig. 1): 50.7%. In the Vienna series of 700 pediatric patients[223] the ratio was 50 : 50. There is some difference in ST and IT tumor location where age is concerned: during the neonatal period and the first year of life ST tumors dominate, whereas there is a reversal during the 2nd to the 12th year of life[189, 223]. During the 2nd decade and in adulthood ST tumors are more frequent.

From the clinical point of view one should be aware of 7 main tumor locations (Fig. 1):

I. Tumors of the cerebral hemispheres and within the lateral ventricles: 20–35%[120, 147, 165, 184, 223, 383, 426, 450].

II. Tumors of the basal ganglia and thalamus: 3–7%[184, 223].

III. Tumors within the 3rd ventricle, the anterior visual pathways and anterior hypothalamus: 8–20%[120, 147, 165, 184, 223, 383, 426, 450].

IV. Tumors in the pineal region, posterior part of the 3rd ventricle, hypothalamus and quadrigeminal plate: 2.5–11% [64, 120, 147, 165, 184, 223, 382, 383, 426, 450].

V. Extrinsic tumors of the suprasellar region and within the sella: 4–15% [120, 147, 165, 184, 269, 383, 384, 426, 450].

Tumors of group I–V are located above the tentorium, whereas the following 2 groups are below the tentorium:

VI. Within the caudal brain stem: tegmentum of midbrain, pons, and medulla oblongata: 4.5–20% [79, 117, 174, 184, 223, 282, 333, 383, 426, 450].

VII. Tumors of the 4th ventricle, cerebellar vermis, and the cerebellar hemispheres: 37–55% [79, 120, 174, 184, 223, 282, 333, 383, 426, 450].

Epidemiology and Genetics

Carcinogenesis might be understood as a "two-hit" or "multi-hit" event [217, 218]. The first step (initiation) is based on germinal (genetic) or somatic alteration of the proliferating cells [79]. Cell proliferation in extrauterine life can be caused by tissue necrosis due to trauma, toxins, or infectious agents. During embryogenesis derivatives of the neural crest seem to be prone to multiple tissue proliferation as a basis for the "neurocristopathies" [53]: pheochromocytoma, neuroblastoma, medullary cancer of the thyroid, intestinal carcinoid, chemodectoma, Hirschsprung's disease, and melanotic progonoma. These diseases were called "simple neurocristopathies" as opposed to complex forms or neurocristopathic syndromes: Neurofibromatosis with an incidence in the normal population of 1 : 3,000 for the peripheral form and of 1 : 30,000 for the central form; 50% of them are thought to be new mutations [79, 178]. Optic glioma has an overall incidence of 1–5% of all pediatric brain tumors [58, 77, 79, 272, 281]. 10–50% of the children with optic glioma have neurofibromatosis [77, 272, 281, 368, 435]. In addition, neurofibromatosis can be linked with the following cerebral disorders: spongioblastoma of the brain stem, glial proliferation in the periaqueductal area with obstructive hydrocephalus (4 personal observations), periaqueductal angiomatosis, heterotopias of the gray matter with epilepsy, congenital defects in the frontal and parietal bones, defects in the anterior cranial fossa with proptosis and lateralization to one bulbe; in adults with calcifying intraventricular meningioma and, most often, with acoustic neurinoma [178]. Another complex neurocristopathy is tuberous sclerosis with an incidence of 1 : 30,000 [405], 85% being new mutations, which clinically present most often with early infantile epilepsy (salaam spasms, Lennox-Gastaut syndrome), multiple leaflet-like white macules, mental retardation, and adenoma sebaceum arising between the age of 3–5 years. These children have subependymal giant cell calcifying astrocytoma infiltrating the lamina affixa of the thalamus which can block the foramina of Monro [457].

Conditions possibly linked with medulloblastoma or glioblastoma are multiple nevoid basal cell carcinoma, autosomally inherited glioma-polyposis syndrome and adrenal cancer, and among peripheral and central tumors: Wilm's tumor, reticulosarcoma, retinoblastoma, and most of the CNS tumors such as meningioma, astrocytoma, pinealoblastoma, etc [75, 162, 216, 273, 405]. In addition, midline cleft formations have been described together with medulloblastoma, *e.g.* exomphalus, malformations of the uterus, spina bifida, agenesis of the vermis cerebelli, and Chiari malformation[75].

The two-hit theory of carcinogenesis[217, 218] means that in those familial hereditary diseases with tissue proliferation the second hit can promote proliferation of malignant cells: *e.g.* promoted by irradiation, oncogenic viruses which may result in malformations when given early during pregnancy and in CNS tumors when administered some days later[79, 189, 212].

Similarities between virus-induced tumors and chemical neurooncogenesis do exist[189, 212]: nitrosureas, triazenes, aromatic hydrocarbons, hydrazines given to an embryo promote malformations interfering with organogenesis, and given to a fetus may produce tumors.

Testosterone in the developing animal decreases the risk of neurooncogenesis as well as does an intact cellular and immunological response[79].

In terms of the two-hit theory this means: deficient DNS repair, lack of cellularly mediated immune-responses or suppressed immunological mechanisms facilitate anaplastic cellular growth promoted by viral, chemical and physical agents. The tissue concerned being in a premalignant state changes to carcinomatous, anaplastic cellular proliferation[79, 405].

Apart from the risk of a child affected by one of the above hereditary syndromes, there are some genetic implications for first degree relatives of children who had tumors of the CNS, particularly for medulloblastoma and glioblastoma: siblings, parents, and their own children have a fivefold risk of getting a tumor at any site: CNS, leukemia, or elsewhere[122].

Clinical Features

Since almost ⅔ of all brain tumors in children are located near the midline, within the ventricles or the basal cisterns thus interfering with CSF flow, they cause early obstruction of the CSF pathways. The child therefore suffers from 2 conditions: a) an active hydrocephalus and b) signs of local involvement of brain function[333].

Symptoms and Signs Due to Raised Intracranial Pressure (ICP)

a) *Symptoms: Headache:* 50–70% of all children with brain tumors complain of headache[147, 183–185, 333, 383]. Cephalea often starts insidiously; it is localized in the front or behind the eyes like in migraine; or is lateralized as in some of the cerebral hemispheric tumors. It can be occipital or bifrontal in PF tumors, bitemporal in suprasellar lesions, or presents as "holocephaly" ("as if the head bursts").

Tumor-headache is related to raised ICP or to stretching and tearing on the dura (tentorium) which may cause head tilt, particularly if the bulk is situated near the foramen magnum or the tentorial opening[51]. Headache in children generally is shorter than in adults[184].

Vomiting, present in 45–75% of the children[147, 183–185, 333, 383] often is misinterpreted: Today in a child with monosymptomatic vomiting for months or even years every disorder of the gastrointestinal tract has been ruled out by refined technical methods before one thinks about the possibility of a brain tumor. A psychologist has been introduced long before the pediatric neurologist has been consulted.

Vomiting due to raised ICP often occurs before breakfast, or the child feels much better after the meal was brought up for the raised ICP was lowered by vomiting. Recurrent vomiting and in some younger children failure to thrive can be a focal sign of the lower brain stem as well, and not be due to raised ICP: The tumor bulk squeezes on the rhomboid fossa or is situated within its structures [34, 57, 60, 127, 223, 238, 364, 369].

Vertigo occurring in 10–25% of children is much rarer than in adults [147, 183–185, 383]. Vertigo is explained by the children as "dizzy feeling" or by elder children sometimes felt as falling downwards or moving along straight converging lines. Mechanical labyrinthine horizontal or altitudinal vertiginous attacks are reported only exceptionally. Vertiginous attacks in tumors of the 4th ventricle are accompanied by nystagmus [34].

Diplopia, present in 15–25% of the children [147, 183, 333, 383] most often is due to unilateral or bilateral VIth CN palsy. In unilateral VIth CN palsy, there is head tilt for the child tries to compensate; the chin is rotated to the nonparetic side, the head tilted towards the paretic abducent nerve. In trochlear nerve palsy the head tilt is to the opposite side, the chin is rotated to the paretic side [51]. Double vision due to acute oculomotor palsies very often make the child feel nauseated. Some of the children have difficulties to differentiate between diplopia, and

blurred vision in 12–15% [147, 183–185, 333, 383]. It is caused by monocular or binocular visual failure. Long standing hydrocephalus (chronic papilledema with insidious optic atrophy) or compression by tumor of the anterior optic pathways are the main causes for visual failure in the child with a brain tumor. Foster-Kennedy syndrome means papilledema with optic atrophy homolateral to a tumor, *e.g.* a meningioma of the olfactory groove or the sphenoid.

To recognize failing vision of one eye sometimes is very difficult for the parents, since it occurs without any pain. The child has lost his ability of foveal fixation, the "bad" eye deviates in a jerky fashion again and again. In bilateral visual failure the child may get closer to the TV-screen or bring his books very near to his eyes. If bilateral fixation is lost in postchiasmal lesions, there is parafoveal alternating fixating: the child presents with changing extraocular (pseudo) palsies. Some of the children with hypothalamic glioma have irregular jerky disconjugated eye movements all the time they are awake. Sometimes this condition is called "amaurotic pendular nystagmus" although this is not nystagmus and the children are not blind; they are able to recognize objects and the pupillary light reaction is preserved.

Disturbances of consciousness are present in 1–16% of the children with brain tumors [147, 183–185, 333, 383]. In general, lowering of consciousness means impaired reticular function a) by increased ICP and b) by tentorial downward or upward herniation. The level of consciousness can fluctuate.

Sudden loss of consciousness occurs in completed tentorial or foraminal herniation; these "cerebellar fits" signal danger for the life of the patient: the child goes opisthotonic, the extremities are extended, the arms adducted to the trunk and the hands pronated. Respiration is slow and irregular, there is skew deviation of the eyes, the pupils might be constricted or more often dilated and there is lack of response to light. The clinical picture can be due to downward transtentorial herniation by a ST lesion or by an IT tumor if there is upward herniation. These cerebellar fits can precede local symptoms even for years and are accompanied by focal or generalized muscle jerks suggesting epilepsy[57, 183].

If the child is atonic, without tendon reflexes, has pinpoint pupils, absent pupillary light and corneal reflexes and apneustic or gasping respiration and neck rigidity there is transforaminal herniation.

Sudden limpness without or with only slight clouding of consciousness may occur in extracerebral tumors of the anterior cranial fossa[119]. Such "cataplexic" attacks are understood as "inhibitory" motor phenomena mediated by mesial frontal and anterior limbic structures. Sudden loss of consciousness without other epileptic phenomena is observed in cystic lesions within the 3rd ventricle[34, 57].

b) Signs: Papilledema, the best known sign indicating raised ICP, is present in 45–70% of children with brain tumors[147, 183–185, 333, 383]. It is seen in 25–40% of children with ST tumors and in 50–85% with IT tumors. One important exception is the intrinsic tumor of the caudal brain stem, where, aqueductal obstruction and papilledema develop late, because the aqueduct of Sylvius and the 4th ventricle are pushed backwards and broadened but remain open until the final stage.

If raised ICP is long standing and papilledema progresses to optic atrophy, the functional loss is heralded by an increase of the central scotoma ("blind spot") and by loss of color vision. Optic atrophy is found in 20–25% of children with brain tumors[147, 183–185, 333, 383]. If there is no rise of the ICP it is caused by compression of the optic nerve or chiasm, *e.g.* by an optic glioma. In monocular blindness due to vetinoblastoma a white appearance of the pupil develops (leukokoria) and the condition is called "amaurotic cat's eye"[223].

Neck rigidity is present in 20–30% of children with brain tumors except those with lesions of the caudal brain stem[147, 183–185, 333, 383]. If there is a unilateral mass lesion in one cerebral hemisphere uncal herniation starts with internal, external or total ophthalmoplegia which is ipsilateral in most cases, and is associated with controlateral pyramidal signs. In children with incipient transforaminal herniation there often is nonocular head tilt, tenderness of the neck muscles, flaccidity of the limbs, hypoactive tendon reflexes and inability to stand and/or to sit up. If these signs are due to increased ICP, they disappear some days after a shunting procedure has been performed[331, 333], own observations).

Increase of head circumference is noted in 10–25%, not only in infants in whom the fontanel may be enlarged and bulged, but sometimes in older children, too. Head enlargement might be due to tumor bulk or hydrocephalus, or both. Its presence in an older child with a brain tumor suggests a lesion of long standing and therefore a benign condition. In a few children with long-standing raised ICP the diastatic sutures are even palpable. A tumor or a cystic lesion situated near the vault can cause the bone to bulge and provoke thinning of the tabula interna radiologically. In an extreme case there is a soft swelling as the whole osseous covering of the vault has been eroded by local tumor pressure and the dura bulges out. If the osteolytic lesion is located on the roof of the orbit there is pulsating exophthalmus (*e.g.* in neurofibromatosis). In long-standing hydrocephalus, caused by a PF tumor, the floor of the 3rd ventricle is dilated and pushed down towards the sphenoid bone; the intraventricular pulsations can cause resorption of the bone; the dura how protrudes into the nasopharynx.

c) Mental and behavioral changes: Apart from mild forms of impairment of consciousness observed in 40–50% of the children with raised ICP[83, 207] there are: irritability, aggressive or agitated behavior, or, withdrawal, fearfulness, feeling depressed in about 25%[183, 184]. This is more often seen in children with central (= bilateral) tentorial herniation than with an uncal syndrome[79].

Loss of higher brain functions clinically presents differently at varying ages[83, 144, 164]: a) retardation under 3 years, b) regression in performance in children between 4–12 years, c) developmental crisis during puberty and adolescence. The younger the child the more vulnerable are his higher brain functions. In addition to brain damage by raised ICP there may be local injury by the tumor pressure or infiltration, by peritumoral edema, circulatory or ictal damage, and additional iatrogenic impairment of functions by the operation, radiation and CHT[79, 83, 144, 223].

In the older child local brain syndromes with psychic symptoms can be observed: euphoria, temper outbursts in tumors of the frontal lobe[83, 164], and, in our experience, in tumors of the medulla oblongata, too. Epilepsy can occur in all cortical sites of a lesion, and Gerstmann's syndrome or dysphasia is present in 5% of lateralized hemispheric tumors[183, 184]. Memory loss and defective recall for recent events is well known in temporal lobe tumors[83, 183], and emotional lability and selective mutism in 25% of all tumors of the brain stem[183, 186]. Akinesia and Korsakoff syndrome are found in diencephalic lesions[164], the Korsakoff syndrome being attributed to bilateral lesions of the fornix or of the mammillary bodies[374]. In limbic-midbrain damage auditory hallucinations are observed[373, 374], and in lesions of the upper cerebellar vermis[207], of the dorsal parts of the superior corpus quadrigeminum and of the posterior thalamus visual hallucinations and visuo-spatial destruction may occur[83, 183].

d) Head injury and brain tumor: Head injury as an immediately preceeding event is reported in a number of patients: in our own series of 275 children there were 23 with head injuries giving rise to further investigations: 6 had bruises of the skull only, 14 had signs of cerebral concussion and 3 of contusions. Similar results were given by other authors: Head injuries were reported in 13 of 90 children with brain stem tumors[34]; in 9 of 27 children with ependymomas[35] and in 4 of 90 patients with medulloblastoma[39], and in 7 of 76 children with brain tumors[349]. All were in critical conditions. This means that even mild head trauma in a child with an undetected brain tumor can lead to decompensation due to edema formation within and around the tumor and impairment of cerebral circulation resulting from increased ICP.

Symptoms and Signs of Supratentorial Tumors

I. Cerebral Hemispheres and Lateral Ventricles

According to Koos and Miller[223] hemispheric cerebral tumors in children are located in the frontal lobe in 36%, in the parietal area in 32%, the temporal lobe in 19%, in the occipital lobe in 5%, and in the lateral ventricles in 8%.

During the first phase of tumor growth the skull compensates by suture separation which is possible until about the 12th year of life. This is one important reason why ST tumors in children often reach an excessive size before a diagnosis is achieved[54, 79, 282]. The huge tumor bulk plus CSF pathways obstruction often results in papilledema: 45–87%[54, 184, 255, 282, 426]. Headache is reported in 35–50% of these children and vomiting less often: 25–45%[54, 184, 255, 282].

Local symptoms include: a) mental symptoms, present in 60% of children with hemispheric tumors, develop insidiously[83, 184, 207], b) hemiparesis and the hemisyndrome have a variable incidence ranging from 23%[282], 25%[223], 35%[54], 40%[184, 282] to even 83%[426]. The incidence of hemisyndromes is linked with the frequency of raised ICP and epilepsy. Unilateral motor, sensory or hemianopic deficits can be postictal, due to compression or infiltration of the motorsensory cortex or the internal capsule, or to unilateral brain stem compression[223]. In about half of the cases it is combined with a supranuclear facial nerve palsy[183, 184]. Hemisensory deficit is found in 7–15%[183, 255], hemianopic inattention in 10–25%[183, 223, 255], and dysphasic symptoms in 10–18%[54, 183, 223, 255]. Truncal ataxia (13–45%) is explained by impairment of the fronto-pontine bundle[54, 183, 255, 282]; c) seizures are reported in tumors of the cerebral hemispheres with an incidence ranging from 35–65%[6, 27, 54, 183, 184, 223, 426]. Based on the literature one should make 3 statements: 1) seizures are more often found with benign than with malignant gliomas[184, 223, 255, 305]. On the other hand: a long history of seizures does not indicate benignity of the tumor; for seizures lasting even for years might precede the detection of either benign or malignant gliomas[27, 147, 184, 305, 385]. 2) About 50% of epilepsies due to tumor in children are generalized, 25% partial elementary and 25% partial complex[6, 27, 154, 183]. In favor of epilepsy due to tumor is: changing profile of seizure presentation with spreading clinical symptoms[6, 183], postictal signs such as dysphasia, hemiparesis or long-lasting amnesia. Normal intelligence, no plausible cause for the epilepsy as (birth) trauma, infection or hereditary incidence, and a persistent delta wave focus in the EEG[49]. 3) Although among children with any form of seizure a tumor is detected in only 1–2%[6, 27, 183, 305], it is stressed by many authors that in $\frac{1}{3}$– $\frac{1}{2}$ of all children presenting with tumor epilepsy the fits are the only clinical symptoms for years[6, 27, 49, 147, 154, 183, 255, 426]. Therefore, in every child with elementary or complex partial seizures and in secondarily generalized epilepsy a cerebral lesion should be excluded: this holds true above all if the fits are therapy-resistant, change their profile and are unexplained by the past history of the child.

Tumors of the lateral ventricles often produce headache, enlarged head, apathy, and seizures. Some of them bleed thus promoting signs of meningeal irritation[151, 223, 366].

II. Basal Ganglia and Thalamus

These tumors represent 3–7%[184, 223]. Grade III or IV gliomas are more frequent compared to benign tumors of the anterior visual pathways or of the anterior hypothalamus[79]. The history often is short and symptoms of increased ICP are present: headache and vomiting in 80% and papilledema in 40%[79]. Hemiparesis, dysphasia, hemisensory changes and mental symptoms, *e.g.* confusion, memory loss and emotional instability are consistent with a tumor in this location. The mental symptoms are related to an involvement of the median thalamic nuclei which project to the frontal granular cortex[79, 144, 223]. An extension of the tumor into subthalamic and mesencephalic structures has to be considered if cerebellar symptoms are present.

III. Tumors of the Third Ventricle, (Anterior) Hypothalamus and Visual Pathways

a) *Third ventricle and intrinsic tumors of the anterior hypothalamus*: Tumors in this site include low grade ASCY and other gliomas, hamartomas, mixed gliomas, EPDY, and malignant tumors as germinoma or GLB, too. The most prominent clinical sign in a young child with a tumor at this site is failure to thrive. The diencephalic syndrome of emaciation in infancy and childhood[360] is featured by loss of fat tissue, shrinkage of the subcutis and therefore they look prematurely aged. Bone age is accelerated, there is a trend for hypoglycemia, hypotension, and hyperkinetic behavior[79, 281, 349]. Occasional vomiting and hyperkinetic behavior does not explain the loss of body fat and weight; their caloric intake and body length are normal. Lipolysis is explained by an activation of pituitary peptides, increase of HCG and lack of somatostasin if there is destruction of brain parenchyma in the preoptic area[79]. Some of these children look quite cheerful despite their miserable nutrional condition; this is explained by supranuclear upper eyelid retraction: Collier's sign[281].

Symptoms and signs associated with tumors of the 3rd ventricle and anterior hypothalamus are endocrinological and visual, and raised ICP. Optic atrophy is observed in tumors compressing one or both optic nerves or the chiasm from above and searching pendular movements of the eyes described in retrochiasmatic lesions (p. 402).

In older children with tumors of the hypothalamus, endocrine dysfunction often dominate the clinical picture: monosymptomatic diabetes insipidus for years (in germinoma), genital hypoplasia, precocious puberty, obesity, growth retardation and other symptoms of hypopituitarism.

In the advanced stage of hypothalamic tumors there are decerebrate posturing, rigidity, and autonomous seizures. Some children have episodes of "central" fever explained by neurogenic hypernatremia and hypovolemia due to damage of the hypothalamic osmoreceptors[281]. On the other hand: after operations affecting this region of the brain sometimes a central hyponatremia is observed with abundant loss of sodium and diuresis. This condition called inappropriate (= excessive) ADH secretion syndrome develops 2–4 days after surgery and is self-limited, but needs excessive amount of intravenous fluid and sodium replacement based on an exact input and output balance. It has to be differentiated from diabetes insipidus by measurement of sodium content of the urine and its specific gravity.

b) *Tumors of the anterior optic pathways*: most of them are optic gliomas growing within one or both optic nerves, the optic chiasm, or both, and sometimes extend into other parts of the diencephalon[59, 77, 79, 223, 272, 368, 435]. Optic glioma accounts for 0.5–5% of all pediatric brain tumors. About 8% of the gliomas of the optic pathway undergo malignant transformation before the age of 10 years[368].

Some children with neurofibromatosis have optic glioma without any visual impairment but with a thickening of the optic nerve in its orbital part demonstrated by CT, and with an impairment of VECPs[79].

If the tumor grows within the orbital part of the optic nerve there are visual failure, optic atrophy, proptosis, and paresis of extraocular muscles[59, 77, 79, 368, 435]. Sometimes at fundoscopy, a reddish mass is seen protruding into the ocular fundus[281]. If the tumor grows within the chiasm its bulk can progress to the foramen of Monro and block it. If its growth is directed more posteriorly, there can be hypothalamic dysfunction, e.g. obesity and diabetes insipidus. Some of the children with optic glioma have bilateral failing vision or are virtually blind in both eyes which clinically manifests itself by rapid, oscillating eye movements with long and short excursions[77, 79, 281]. Late clinical symptoms associated with optic glioma are mental retardation and epilepsy[59]. Mean survival in glioma of the optic nerve is longer (21 years) as for those with the primary site in the chiasm (15 years)[59]. Survival for the whole group of anterior optic pathway tumors is 80% for 5 years and 50% for 10 years[272].

IV. Tumors of the Pineal Area, the Posterior Part of the Third Ventricle and Quadrigeminal Plate

The pineal area harbors tumors of developmental origin, e.g. germ cell tumors, neoplasms derived from the parenchyma of the pineal gland, gliomas and other rare tumor entities.

The history of most children with pineal area tumors is short: less than 3 months, but it varies between 10 days and 2 years[91, 195]. The reason for this short period of complaints is the close neighbourhood of the lesion to the aqueduct of Sylvius. 70–100% of the children have obstructive hydrocephalus[64, 334]. Headache is reported in 71–89%[1, 64, 195, 223, 413], vomiting in 50–60%[1, 64, 195, 223, 413]. Papilledema can be found early: 74–89%[1, 64, 144, 223, 282, 413].

Alterations in mood and mentality are due to increase of the ICP, midbrain compression or invasion, and to hypothalamic dysfunction. The reported incidence of mental symptoms range from 6%[334], 14%[1], 52%[414] to 70%[195].

Postoperative personality changes can be impressive and may continue for weeks: the patient is obtunded, disoriented, indifferent to his surroundings. There is lack of motor drive, spontaneous movements are few and slow, the face without expression. The response to food is inadequate: closure of the mouth. Some of the children are incontinent and do not react to painful stimuli. Sometimes autonomic vegetative functions such as blood pressure, body temperature, salivation are overactive. Some patients develop decubital ulcers very quickly[342, 374, 415].

Aside from tissue damage provoked by the tumor itself and the procedures during operation this transitory clinical state results from interference with the deep venous drainage system[64, 325, 334, 373, 374, 408, 409].

Some of the visual symptoms in pineal tumors are due to obstructive hydrocephalus. Optic atrophy is reported in 8–20%[64, 195, 223], it occurs more often in slowly expanding lesions like teratoma or dermoid. Optic atrophy is promoted by the expanding walls and the floor of the 3rd ventricle which is flattened and pressed downwards to the base of the skull. The optic chiasm can become flattened and encroaches upon such osseous structures as the tuberculum sellae. In advanced states of intracranial hypertension, there is interference with the vascular supply of the chiasm and the optic nerves. The delicate vessels of these structures originating from the posterior communicating artery and the internal carotid artery are stretched.

Important local signs of midbrain dysfunction in pineal tumors include: Parinaud's syndrome, present in 30–50%[1, 64, 195, 223, 325, 334, 342, 449], consists of upward gaze paresis, paralysis of the pupil(s), and paralysis of accommodation and convergence[449]. Upward gaze palsy is due to dysfunction of the corticotectal tract running from 18/19 Brodmann's area to the rostromedial parts of the superior colliculi[325, 334, 449]. There appears to be a second vertical gaze "center" at the pontine level which is responsible for downward movement of the eyes and optokinetic nystagmus[325]. Therefore, up- and downward gaze paresis means advanced involvement of pontine and midbrain structures irrespective of the primary site of the tumor which may be in the pineal area, midbrain or pontine tegmentum or cerebellum.

The *Sylvian aqueduct syndrome*, in addition to vertical gaze paresis shows unequal size of the pupils, sluggish reaction to light, paralysis or spasm of convergence, retractory nystagmus, eyelid retraction, impairment of upward optokinetic nystagmus and lethargy[73, 449]. 27–58% of the patients complain of diplopia or blurred vision[1, 195, 449], particularly when accommodation or convergence are lost. Accommodation can be spastic-paretic: overshooting or impairement as can occur with the reaction to convergence. The patient is not able to converge which produces crossed diplopia[449]. Pupillary changes are present in 50–55% of patients with pineal tumors[195, 373] and disturbed accommodation and convergence in 23%[373]. Paresis of the external eye muscles were reported in 10–50%[195, 325, 373] with decreasing frequency: III, VI, IV. CN in advanced tumors of the pineal area extending into the caudal brain stem and vice versa nearly all fixation and conjugate movements of the eyes are impaired; these patients seem to be blind but really they are not as can be demonstrated by the presence of preserved visual evoked potentials[73]. In 23% of the patients hearing is impaired on one or both sides[373] and tinnitus has been reported when the inferior quadrigeminal plate[91, 144, 223, 281, 334, 342, 373] is involved.

Based on a wide clinical experience with upward gaze paresis in children with malfunction of shunt systems, one can summarize: upward gaze paralysis is merely functional. The more oculomotor phenomena there are, the more tumor compression and invasion of midbrain structure is likely. Upward gaze palsy as the only midbrain sign present may be induced by pressure alone at the entrance of the Sylvian aqueduct or of an elongated suprapineal recess pressing upon the quadrigeminal plate.

Pyramidal symptoms are present in 25–35% of the children[64, 342, 373] which are caused by compression of the cerebral peduncles. In this type of hemiparesis there is predominance of the face and upper extremity[223].

Cerebellar signs are found in about 50% of the children[1, 64, 144, 195, 223, 373, 414]. If they do not disappear after shunt insertion, the upper cerebellar peduncles may be compressed or even infiltrated by the tumor[334].

V. Tumors of the Suprasellar Region and Sella turcica

In children and adolescents craniopharyngiomas constitute the majority of suprasellar tumors which primarily are located outside the diencephalon (= extrinsic growth). In children, adenomas of the pituitary gland are very rare. Other tumors with exophytic growth are germinomas of the suprasellar region. There are 3 groups of symptoms and signs:

a) *Headache* initially is triggered by pressure or traction on the dura. In our experience it is an early integral symptom of a tumor located within the basal cisterns and touching the dura from above or a mass lesion expanding within the sella and piercing the diaphragma sellae from below. Headaches are commented upon by children as being bitemporally located or behind the eyes or the forehead.

A different cause of headaches in a suprasellar mass lesion is CSF obstruction; either by blocking its further flow within the basal cistern or by upward extending as high as the foramen of Monro. Primary extrinsic tumors may thin the floor of the 3rd ventricle, and finally the tumor has penetrated it and appears as an intraventricular mass at a (transforaminal) transventricular operation. Some of the craniopharyngiomas extend posteriorly and finally reach the quadrigeminal cistern having invaded the interpeduncular cistern[281, 2] (personal observations), the cerebellopontine angle[174] or by lateral extension into the Sylvian fissure[269, 281]. In frontal or subfrontal tumors headache may disappear after months or years. This "improvement" is due to further tumor progression involving the frontothalamic fibers. The patient still has "his headaches" but does not complain any longer (3 own observations in craniopharyngiomas).

b) *Visual signs* include pallor of one or both discs, optic atrophy and/or visual field defects. The classical situation in an extrinsic suprasellar mass lesion is heteronymous, bitemporal hemianopia or quadrantic defects. Very rarely there is concentric constriction of the visual fields which generally is functional mainly in older children, but then is fluctuating in intensity at different examinations. Concentric visual field defects in a suprasellar tumor can be explained by tumor growth beneath and above the chiasm (*e.g.* in craniopharyngioma).

c) *Endocrine signs and symptoms* include those of hypo- and hyperfunction: Those of hypoactivity predominate in children: short stature, hypothyroidism, lagging sexual development, adrenal insufficiency, sometimes panhypopituitarism. If the tumor is expanding within the sella itself the symptoms are induced by destruction of the pituitary gland with lack of the respective hormones: human growth hormone, thyrotropic hormone, adrenocorticotropic hormone (HGH, TSH, ACTH) whereas hypogonadism is due to lack of gonadotropines: FSH, LH, LTH. If on the other hand, there is impingement of the extrasellar tumor on the diencephalon there will be lack of the respective releasing factors of the hormones of the pituitary gland. In case of prolactin (LTH) the situation is different: hyperprolactinemia can exist in prolactinomas of the adenohypophysis. These tumors consisting of chromophobe cells were previously called "chromophobe adenomas" of the pituitary. They produce ACTH, HGH and α-chains of the glycoprotein hormones within one type of cells—and prolactin[190]. Growth retardation in prolactinomas is explained by increased dopaminergic inhibition of HGH secretion[198]. On the other hand, hyperprolactinemia is observed in extrasellar tumors and then explained by the missing PIF produced in the hypothalamus. Hyperprolactinemia also was found in intrasellar germinoma[306]. Clinically excessive production of prolactin presents with growth retardation in the younger child and hypogonadism in the (pre)pubertal age. The most important sign of an impaired hypothalamic function in germinoma is diabetes insipidus. In craniopharyngioma it may occur as a late symptom or develop some days after surgery[269].

Signs of hyperactivity in tumors of the hypophysis itself are very rare in children and adolescents[223, 269]: they occur with the Cushing syndrome or acromegaly. Acromegaly means excessive production of HGH (eosinophilic adenoma) and Cushing's syndrome increased ACTH levels (basophilic adenoma). Cushing's syndrome in children nearly always is caused by cancer or hyperplasia of the adrenal gland, but not by hypophyseal adenoma.

Symptoms and Signs of Infratentorial Tumors

VI. Tumors of the Caudal Brain Stem

Brainstem tumors in children are a very heterogeneous group with regard to grading (I–IV) and histology.

Among the tumors growing primarily within the brain stem, gliomas are most frequent. They include fibrillary and pilocytic ASCY, mixed gliomas, MBL and GLB. The grading I for brain stem gliomas seems inadequate since 60–70% of all "benign" pontine glioma harbor islets of glioblastomatous cell proliferation in their substance[280, 281], according to Schmitt and Zeisner[376] even up to 90%. The GLB of the brain stem are preferentially located in the pontomedullary region[134, 262, 337], whereas gliomas of the cervicomedullary junction are often benign tumors located primarily within the cervical spinal cord showing a cephalad extension[117]. Epstein[117] gave a staging system for tumors of the caudal brain stem:

Intrinsic tumors
a) diffuse (= greater than 2 cm, apparent edema),
b) focal, circumscribed, smaller than 2 cm,
c) in the cervicomedullary junction.

Exophytic
a) anterolateral towards the cerebellopontine angle,
b) posterolateral into the brachium conjunctivum,
c) posteriorly into the 4th ventricle.

Brain stem gliomas often (20% or more) metastasize into the spinal subarachnoid space[118, 300].

The history is short, 1–3–5 months in average[134, 236, 236, 237, 243], exceptionally as long as a year[79, 445].

Headache is present in 35–50%[147, 183, 236, 237, 383], whereas vomiting is more frequent: 35–91%[127, 186, 337, 383]. Vomiting for months and even years without any other symptoms of raised ICP is a very important sign in favor of a tumor situated within or pushing from behind on the lower part of the rhombencephalon[186]. In younger children this causes failure to thrive[34, 51, 60, 127, 186, 223, 238, 264, 395], which is a very important sign in a long-standing tumor in this location. Intractable hiccup[125,

[238] which can be caused by head shaking[51], oral or endotracheal hypersalivation followed by apneic spells in infants[127, 395], reflux esophagitis[34, 125] and bladder disturbances[22, 34, 127] are further signs which might herald a brain stem tumor. Aside from these symptoms and signs which are very often overlooked or explained as psychogenic, there are neurological signs, *e.g.* diplopia and head tilt in 30–40%[147, 183, 383, 411], and gait disturbances caused by truncal ataxia or hemiplegia: 50–65%[147, 186, 223, 243, 337, 383, 411]. Mental and personality changes are observed in 35%[183, 337]. The classical triad in brain stem tumors is: multiple CN involvement, long tract signs, and cerebellar signs[236, 237, 238, 251, 262, 281, 435]—usually with no evidence of raised ICP.

ad 1) *Multiple CN involvement:* a) there are few neurological conditions in children in which so many CN are affected: the very rare cerebellopontine angle tumors in children, tumors of the base of the PF invading the dura or protruding through foramine, *e.g.* the foramen jugulare, after basal skull fracture or, in the context of dysrhaphism, Chiari malformation with position of the medulla oblongata low in the cervical canal.

b) although there are no hints of raised ICP, there is bilateral CN involvement in about 25% of all cases, particularly involving the abducent nerve, followed by the facial and auditory nerves[22, 34, 60, 127, 223, 236–238, 249, 310].

c) whereas the CN most often involved is differently given by the authors: VI[22, 51, 183, 223, 186, 243, 249, 445], VII[60, 127, 147, 236, 310, 337, 411, 430, 435], there is very often trigeminal nerve involvement[79]: decreased or absent corneal reflex, diminished sensation in one half of the face which is confined to the triangle: bridge of the nose, internal angle of the eyelid, and nasolabial fold. If the motor part of the trigeminal nerve is affected there is skew deviation of the mandible in mouth opening to the paralyzed side and sagging of the chin if there is bilateral involvement[223].

The CN less frequently affected are the motor part of the IX/Xth clinically presenting as dysarthria and dysphagia. Nuclear involvement of the hypoglossal nerve (unilateral shrinkage of the tongue, fasciculation and deviation to that side if protruded) means that the tumor is located within one half or on one side of the medulla. Paresis of the accessory nerve is not brain stem tumor sign. It was present only in our patients with cerebellopontine angle tumors or tumors outside the cranial cavity[186]. Unilateral deafness in a child is a very open sign in the differential diagnosis; bilateral acquired deafness on the other hand is consistent with brain stem tumor[127].

ad 2) *Long tract signs:* hemiplegia is present in 38–80%[22, 60, 147, 186, 237, 310, 387, 430]. It can be of acute onset, particularly in GLB of the brain stem[351, 410], personal observation). Often bilateral pyramidal signs are present; in contrast to tumors within the 4th ventricle the extremities affected by the paresis are hyp*er*tonic; in fourth ventricle tumors they are hyp*o*tonic[51, 57]. The paresis is more pronounced in the lower limb since in the pontine course of the pyramidal tract, the arm fibers are located more ventrally[237, 238]. Signs indicating damage to the medial lemniscus are found in 10%, mainly in older children[34, 60]. Sometimes brain stem gliomas insinuate themselves between normal structures, fiber tracts and nuclei[79]. There seems to be a selective vulnerability to direct pressure exerted by the tumor: the medial lemniscus seems to be more resistent than the lateral lemniscus, whereas the medical longitudinal fascicle is more sensitive[60, 127]. In addition, in some slowly progressing tumors of the pontomedullary region there is widespread damage to the white substance, particularly of long fiber tracts, whereas the brain stem nuclei are spared[34, 127].

ad 3) *Cerebellar signs*, found in 70% of the children, include gait (truncal) ataxia with loss of supportive head control and/or dysmetria/ataxia of the extremities[22, 51, 60, 134, 237, 310, 387, 430]. Dysarthria and dysphagia are present in 30–40% of the children and are frequent in patients with progressive tumor growth[51, 60, 127, 183, 223]. These two signs suggest mixed motor and cerebellar involvement the motor dysfunction being due to nuclear and supranuclear involvement. Tremor is rarely found in children with tumors of the caudal brain stem[147, 183, 186]. Upward gaze paresis is seen less often than downward and horizontal gaze impairment; this can be preceded by vertical or horizontal gaze (paretic) nystagmus; the incidence of nystagmus is 60–80%[60, 186, 237, 411] but it can disappear with the progression of extraocular muscle palsies. In this stage of the disease there is no longer hope for recovery.

ad 4) *Mental symptoms* in brain stem tumors of children are present in 30–50% of cases[22, 60, 147, 183, 430]. There seem to be two patterns of personality changes, often alternating in the same patient: fatigue, drop in school performance, unwillingness to play, depressed, anxious, withdrawn behavior[57, 60, 79, 183]. On the other hand the same child may behave aggressive, hyperkinetic, with temper tantrums and nightmares[237, 294, 310, 411]. In younger children mental regression and dementia may occur in the last phase of the disease[237, 294]. One sign in brain stem disease of younger children is progressive diminution of speech which may lead to selective mutism[57, 79, 183, 186, 237]. Mutism can resolve completely if there is improvement of neurologic symptoms during and after RT. Some of the older children have unintelligible handwriting[79, 237].

The *diagnosis* is established in most cases by CT[204, 384]: the prepontine and perimesencephalic cisterns are obliterated, the 4th ventricle is deformed, broaded in its floor and pushed dorsally. The basilar artery may be walled in bilaterally by the expanding tissue of the pontine basis and is pushed posteriorly, too. This is best demonstrated by contrast enhanced CT or, by angiography[332]. About 50% of the primary brain stem tumors are hypodense, some are isodense, and only a few are hyperdense in the unenhanced scan. After intravenous contrast there is diffuse or patchy enhancement in more than 50% of brain stem tumors. NMR will be the method of the future in delineating the anatomical structures of the caudal brain stem withoutt osseous superimposition, but sometimes the tumor contour is magnified unrealistically as compared with the true anatomical situation[303, 384].

Angiography[332] in most cases does not give additional information except for intrapontine angioma[243]. In solid glioma shifts of branches of the PICA and AICA, and anterior displacement of the pontomesencephalic venous system are seen.

In any case of doubt in the diagnosis of a brain stem tumor, particularly when an isodense mass is suspected but not proven by the CT scan, fractional lumbar PEG is the diagnostic method of choice by which posterior displacement and elongation of the 4th ventricle and Sylvian aqueduct is demonstrated. The reliability of PEG is superior to CT as the measured distance between the dorsum sellae and the floor of the 4th ventricle depends on how parallel the slope of the scan is to the orbito-meatal line[42].

Treatment: In general, surgery is not indicated, with two exceptions: exophytic growth or a large cyst within the tumor so that evacuation of its content can reduce the tumor bulk. Following biopsy of brain stem tumors the clinical condition of the patient often is worsened: There can be postoperative increase in the intensity of nystagmus of gaze paresis, hemiplegia and hemisensory deficit[337, 430]. Manipulation within the caudal part of the posterior fossa may need tracheostomy and gastric tube feeding for swallowing difficulties[337, 430].

In 15–20% there is advanced posterior displacement of the 4th ventricle and the aqueduct of Sylvius causing obstructive hydrocephalus. Sudden deterioration of speech and swallowing might herald this situation. Shunt insertion is then indicated.

The treatment of choice is RT: 50–60 Gy to the PF[22, 47, 243, 265, 299, 445]. There is improvement in most children in whom symptoms had not progressed too far. However, cure of a child suffering from a brain stem tumor today is still impossible if the diagnosis was correct. The signs will recur after months, in some patients after a few years. If for instance a VIth nerve paresis was the first clinical sign its reappearance after RT means recurrence of the tumor. RT can double the mean survival time from 8 to 16 months[47, 117, 236–238, 243, 265, 281, 299, 430, 445]). The use of MTX-HD prior to RT[346] shows promise. More patient benefit has been achieved compared with other combined treatment schedules[134, 388].

Prognosis: Tumors of the caudal brain stem have a poor prognosis. Some points are to be mentioned:

a) the shorter history makes the prognosis worse[80],

b) the more CN are affected the worse is the prognosis[337, 411, 430],

c) clouding of consciousness, sudden temperature fluctuations or vegetative release phenomena worsen the prognosis considerably[147, 411],

d) calcifications within the tumor demonstrated by CT or exophytic tumor growth sometimes indicate slow tumor progression, whereas marked hypodensity in the center of the tumor or ring enhancement signify rapid growth[80],

e) only a short survival can be expected in children with early development of hydrocephalus[147, 337, 430],

f) the more caudal the tumor site in the brain stem the worse is the prognosis: medulla oblongata worse than pons and pons worse than midbrain[147, 237, 238].

VII. Tumors of the Fourth Ventricle and the Cerebellum

Tumors in this location account for almost half of all brain tumors in childhood, although the PF as a volume accounts only for $1/_{11}$ of the whole cranial cavity[435]. About 80% of PF tumors are situated within or near the midline, only 20% within the cerebellar hemispheres or, rarely, in the cerebellopontine angle. Midline location in a small cavity means early CSF flow obstruction. Therefore, the history of many children with PF tumors is related to signs and symptoms of increased ICP.

65–70% of the children complain of headache[20, 183, 185, 333], 50–75% have vomiting, and of these ⅓ before breakfast. Headache, vomiting and papilledema are the "triad" of PF tumors. However, choked discs are not seen in all children who have headache and vomiting due to raised ICP; for there are some individuals who do not get papilledema at all. Papilledema is found in 70% of all PF tumors[20, 183, 185, 333].

Head tilt, present in 7–25% of the children may be due to double vision, but not every child is able to explain that. It may also be due to pressure and/or traction on the dura. Neck stiffness is found in 30% of the children[183] and can be mistaken for sciatic pain (positive Kernig's sign).

Signs and symptoms less often reported are: tinnitus due to involvement of the inferior quadrigeminal plate or the cerebellopontine angle. Paroxysmal vertigo, sudden hemiparesthetic or quadrant anesthesia, paroxysmal bad taste within the mouth or intermittent bladder urgency can be found when there is tumor pressure within the 4th ventricle[34, 57]. Lightening paresthesia in both arms or all four limbs in a person who bends his head forward constitute the dominant sign of a mass situated at the foramen magnum.

Cerebellar signs and CN involvement are the two most important signs in tumors of the 4th ventricle and the cerebellum:

a) *cerebellar signs:* ataxic gait is found in 32–55%[20, 183, 185, 333]. It is often accompanied by hypotonia and generalized muscular weakness which in advanced cases is so severe that the child is no longer able to sit up or even to support head. Lateralizing signs are seen more often (30–50%) than any real localization of the tumor within the cerebellar hemisphere[20, 183, 185, 333]: dysmetria, ataxic movements of the limbs, dysdiadochokinesis. Intention tremor means involvement of the cerebellar nuclei (*e.g.* dentate nucleus) or of the superior cerebellar peduncle. Lateralizing signs indicate ipsilateral tumor, but sometimes there is false localization. The clinician may try to differentiate three cerebellar syndromes[63, 79, 175]:

a) inferior vermian syndrome: ataxic gait, muscular hypotonia, nystagmus and pendular tendon reflexes,

b) superior vermian syndrome: broad based gait without nystagmus and without hypotonia,

c) syndrome of the cerebellar hemisphere: unilateral limb hypotonia, dysmetria and coarse nystagmus to that side.

b) *Cranial nerve involvement:* This is less often found than in tumors of the caudal brain stem. Multiple CN lesions in a cerebellar tumor indicate secondary infiltration of the brain stem.

Most often, in 40–50%[183, 185, 186, 333] the abducent nerve is paretic, in nearly half of the cases bilaterally. Next is the facial nerve: 20%. If both the VIth and VIIth are affected raised ICP is unlikely[333]. To the clinician this does not necessarily stand for brain stem involvement, for a tumor within the 4th ventricle or even within one cerebellar hemisphere[57] might induce these nuclear palsies by direct pressure. A combination of peripheral facial nerve palsy and nystagmus indicate a MBL of the brain stem[57, 175]. The other CN are involved with diminishing frequency: oculomotor nerve: pupillary changes included 13%, fifth: 10% (motor and sensory part), the acoustic, glossopharyngeal and vagal nerve: 7.5% each, the vestibular and hypoglossal nerves 5%[186]. Gaze palsy is found in 9%[186], and all forms of nystagmus in 20–40%[186, 333]. The slow component of nystagmus indicates the site of the lesion within the brain stem or the cerebellar hemisphere.

Secondary Involvement of the Brain Stem in Posterior Fossa Tumors

In every tumor primarly location within the 4th ventricle (EPDY, PLP), cerebellar vermis or hemisphere, there may be adherence to or invasion of the brain stem, the superior, middle, or inferior cerebellar peduncles; this means that total removal by surgery will not be possible. Although modern imaging techniques, as high resolution CT scanning, subtraction or magnification angiography[284, 332], are able to give a very precise outline of the tumor in size and location, there is no method superior to the analysis of clinical signs and symptoms[186]. Both the technical methods and the clinical examination are essential in order to arrive at the correct diagnosis.

An analysis of important clinical signs and symptoms in 140 children with PF tumors show[186]: primary brain stem tumors have an overall involvement of 4.9 CNs, in secondary involvement there is an incidence of 2.5 and in cerebellar tumors without any anatomical relationship to the brain stem it is 0.75. The only exception are cerebellopontine angle tumors which have a mean incidence of CN of 4.25%.

This clinical analysis indicates that if 2 symptoms/signs of the following list are present brain stem involvement is likely and if 3 are found clinical diagnosis can be made with certainty:

a) symptoms: vomiting for months/years without other signs of raised ICP— permanent yawning—extrapyramidal fits—selective mutism and depressed and withdrawn behavior without overt plausible causes;

b) signs: pupillary changes—internuclear ophthalmoplegias—trigeminal nerve involvement—vertical, dissociated or rotatory nystagmus—nuclear involvement of some of the caudal CN (IX, X, XII) and marked dysarthria/dysphagia[147]. Vertical downward gaze paralysis and unilateral horizontal gaze paralysis have to be added as well as hemiplegia and hemisensory deficits.

The importance of this statement made by the clinician preoperatively is that parents and the neurosurgeon should be aware of these findings and therefore cannot expect total removal of the tumor.

Diagnostic Tests

Some procedures are "simple", *i.e.* not invasive and inexpansive.

a) *Fundoscopy*, testing of visual acuity and the visual fields: There is need for an expert opinion before surgery, because the visual acuity may dramatically deteriorate after shunt insertion or operative decompression in long standing cases with high ICP.

b) Test of *hearing* and *labyrinthine function*: The clinician has the opportunity to make rough testing of hearing by the Weber test: a tuning fork is put on the vertex; if there is lateralization this means possible hypoacusis on the nonlaterialized side. Each ear can be tested separately by whispering some words or numbers giving a guide to hearing loss for high, medium or low frequency tones. If unilateral acquired deafness is found, there always arises the possibility of a cerebellopontine angle tumor, *e.g.* acoustic neurinoma. This is hardly ever found in a child as angle tumors are rare. Unilateral acquired deafness is much more likely due to a postinfectious mononeuritis of the VIIIth CN, *e.g.* as sequelae of epidemic parotitis. If there is bilateral impairment of hearing, brain stem involvement by a neoplastic condition is highly probable[127].

Vertigo or labyrinthine attacks are not very often reported by children. Therefore only in some of them has this function to be tested accurately. We had loss of labyrinthine function on one side or unilateral preponderancy only in 6 out of 140 children with PF tumors[186].

c) *X-rays of the skull:* Suture separation, increased convolutional markings, circumscribed expansion of the skull may indicate a longstanding condition. Enlargement of the sella turcica, demineralization of the anterior and posterior clinoids are much better noticed in the lateral skull X-ray than by CT. The same is true for J-shaped deformity of the sella in optic glioma which means that the lateral part of the chiasmatic sulcus lies beyond the anterior clinoid process [77, 368]. Enlargement of the optic foramen can be visualized by thin layer CT or special X-ray views: the upper limit of normal is a diameter of 7 mm. Tumor calcification is shown by CT much earlier than by conventional X-rays. This is important when looking for signs of tuberous sclerosis.

d) *EEG*, generally, a test of cerebral cortical functions may give insight into brain involvement, *e.g.* in a child with symptomatic vomiting for months before other clinical developments occur. An unusual rhythmical tracing may indicate a midline lesion. On the other hand the opinion sometimes held by pediatricians that in a child with normal ocular fundi, normal plain X-rays and EEG, a brain tumor has definitively been excluded, cannot be supported.

In a child with focal epilepsy and a persistent delta-wave focus a brain tumor has to be suspected until it has been excluded by CT scan or NMR[49].

Initially, in tumors of the cerebral hemispheres there are nonspecific alterations on the side involved: broadening of the alpha-frequency band, some 0.5–1.5/sec loss of α-index or some diffuse slowing. Later there may be some intermittent theta-, subtheta- or delta-wave activity, particularly over the posterior regions[110, 170]. Later, this focus becomes more constant and shifts anteriorly. Slow wave foci can be rhythmic or polymorphous. Finally, mainly if seizures have occurred, this slow wave focus is characterized by local low voltage and double phase reversals both anteriorly and posteriorly. In the CT this low voltage slow wave sometimes is attributed to peritumoral edema. In ST midline tumors sometimes very rhythmic alpha-, theta- or delta-activity is present and dominates the whole tracing[183]. This can be found in PF tumors or before there is raised ICP and in recurrence of PF tumors before they present with clinical signs. In some ST midline tumors the rhythmic slowing is lateralized[79].

In PF tumors EEG alterations are not dependent on the dynamics of raised ICP. Apart from generalized rhythmicity of the tracing bilateral posterior rhythmic slow waves may be seen. Both upward tentorial herniation and downward herniation due to obstructive hydrocephalus can reduce the blood flow within the posterior cerebral and the anterior choroidal arteries. This and an anterior shift of midbrain structures is thought to be the cause for slow wave dominance over the whole cortical cerebral area[170]. In 20% of the children with PF tumors there are "projected slow rhythms" seen over both frontal regions which run parallel with the widening of the 3rd ventricle[266]. In some PF tumors false lateralization of rhythmic slow wave activity might be found which has waned during the same or the next investigation.

EEG is an important method to guide postoperative CHT and RT. It is very sensitive in the postirradiation syndrome [130, 138, 161, 309]: slowing of 1st or 2nd degree is seen before the clinical symptoms of fatigue and lethargy appear. Furthermore EEG might anticipate possible adverse reactions as leukoencephalopathy or seizures in children who are under combined chemotherapeutic treatment or MTX-HD. With regard to local tumor recurrences, EEG alterations, mainly slowing of

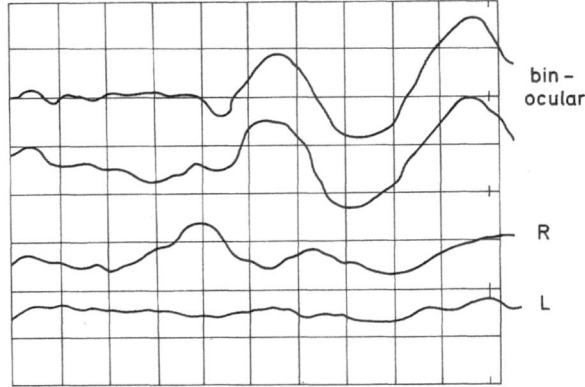

Fig. 2. VECP in a boy, aged $5^{10}/_{12}$ with glioma of both optic nerves, and chiasma: binocular: N2: 86 ms, P2: 103 ms monocular: left: none, right: N2: 92 ms, P2: 128 ms t: 250 ms, filter: $5/_{100}$ Hz, sensit. 25, displ. mult. 1

the background activity, may antedate clinical manifestation and may help to detect "silent" reexpanding lesions throughout the operative defect. This holds true for PF tumors, too.

e) Evoked potential studies should be routinely performed before surgery. Alterations of VECP are mainly found in suprasellar lesions, *e.g.* CRP or optic glioma. In some early stage of optic glioma the VECP are altered before any clinical evidence is found. In tumors of this site VECP are one parameter of high sensitivity. If there is involvement of the posterior parts of the visual pathways peak latency delays and/or decreased amplitude for N2/P2 wave may be found (Fig. 2).

BAERs and SEPs are objective tests to demonstrate involvement of the lateral (auditory) and medial (somatosensory) lemniscal pathways. It is possible to differentiate between medullary, pontine and mesencephalic level of a lesion by the BAERs (Fig. 3). In addition both kinds of brain stem evoked potentials are able to afford guidance about a patient who is in coma.

f) Examination of the CSF is placed at the end of the "simple" methods of investigations, since a lumbar puncture should not been done as a routine if there is suspicion of a tumor and if neck stiffness and head tilt are present. On the other hand, CSF samples obtained by ventricular tap during shunting or postoperatively should be investigated carefully.

Tumor cells can be found as single cells and in clusters; they can be concentrated by sedimentation or centrifuging and stained by different methods[29, 221]. Tumor cells can also be found in the content of tumor cyst[29]. If there is evidence of tumor cells in the follow-up of a patient, this always indicates local recurrence or subarachnoid (spinal) dissemination[100, 113, 221, 230, 292, 378].

Determination of the protein content is very important as a guide for CHT: if the total protein value is constantly raised over 100 mg% in the posteroperative phase there is danger of accumulation of high levels of antimetabolites, *e.g.* by MTX-HD[43]. These toxic levels can cause paraplegia[136, 257, 313, 363, 399] within the following 48 hours.

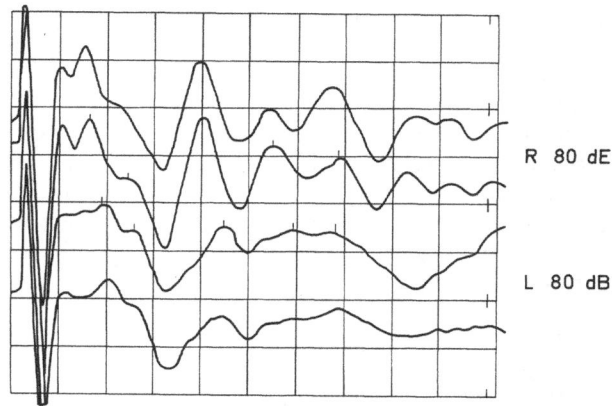

Fig. 3. BEAR in a boy, 11 months old, huge midline MBL of the whole vermis cerebelli (same patient as in Figs. 14 *a* and *b*). Bilaterally peak latency delay for III, IV, and V. No wave V on the left (= inferior colliculus). t: 10 ms, filter: 150/1,500 Hz, sensit. 10, displ. mult. 16, rate: 12.3, duration: 100 ms

Immunoglobulines in the healthy are found in only a small percentage as compared to the plasma levels, *e.g.* IgM in 3%. An increased ratio: IgM-CSF/IgM-plasma means local production of IgM in cells neighbouring the subarachnoid space, *e.g.* in CNS lymphoma. Raised IgM-levels in the CSF may cause polyneuropathy, as they act as paraproteins on the nerve roots[123].

β-glucoronidase normally exists intracellularily within the lysosomes and microsomes of the piaarachnoid and the choroid plexus. Its level is found raised in leptomeningeal dissemination of metastasizing tumors, but more often in bacterial meningitis[123, 378]. One isoenzyme of lactate dehydrogenase (LDH-5) is elevated in meningeal carcinomatosis[123].

Some patients with MBL have been reported to have elevated polyamine levels: putrescin, spermin, spermidine[133, 267]. During and after combined CHT/RT their decline was observed; therefore, repeated determination of the polyamines in the surveillance of patients with MBL is recommended[100, 113, 133, 230, 267, 292]. Polyamines are not of value in the surveillance of patients with malignant gliomas, *e.g.* GLB[133, 267].

CEA is not detectable in the normal CSF by the ELISA technique[123]. Its presence in the CSF means local production by tumor tissue or that the tumor has infiltrated the subarachnoid space[196]. CEA in the CSF is detected in a few patients with germinoma[295], but more often in patients with meningeal carcinomatosis or brain metastases[113, 123, 378].

Neuroradiological Investigations

a) *CT* today takes the first place: A tumor can be isodense, hypodense, hyperdense or mixed. Within the lesion cystic areas, calcification, or hemorrhages can be found which in some cases meander through the tumor tissue into the subarachnoid space or into the ventricular systems causing acute symptoms. Most tumors, particularly those with anaplastic growth present some alteration after IV jodine compounds. This "enhancement" does not indicate the presence of tumor vessels but alteration of the BBB. It is possible to reduce that alteration by about 85% by giving steroids for some days[87]. In ST tumors edema of the fingerprint type can be demonstrated[42, 204, 454]. Edema is quantified as grade I: perifocal edema, grade II: within the ipsilateral hemisphere causing a mass effect upon the midline structures and grade III: within both cerebral hemispheres[204]. Obliteration of the subarachnoid cisterns after contrast can be demonstrated when herniations occur or if tumor dissemination has taken place[36, 42, 116, 244, 454]. In some small lesions located within or near the cisterns (cerebellopontine angle, periquadrigeminal cisterns, chiasmatic cistern) CT 4 hours after intrathecal contrast application (2–5 ml) yields excellent information[36, 384, 445, 455]. Shifts of the midline structures can be seen in the CT, but more precisely by angiography or one-dimensional echoencephalography. Furthermore, enlargement of one cerebral hemisphere, bulging of the bone overlying the lesion and thinning of the osseous lamella is demonstrated by CT.

CT has a very import place in the follow-up of patients with brain tumors[36, 111, 116, 135, 230, 244, 384, 454]. As in the immediate postoperative phase during the first 3 months there might be artefacts in the operative field it therefore is wise to repeat the investigation within the 1st postoperative week or to wait for 3 months[67, 384]

b) *Cerebral angiography* may give very important additional informations to the CT results. Pathological tumor perfusion can be demonstrated in 20% of pediatric brain tumors[183], in 29% signs of herniation and in 55% hydrocephalus are demonstrated by shifts of the arterial and deep venous system[183]. Sometimes, it is important to exclude an angioma or other vascular malformation, *e.g.* in suprasellar lesions, pineal area tumors and in lesions of the caudal brain stem. In addition it may be important for the surgeon to know about huge anastomotic veins (vein of Troland and Labbé) in cerebral tumors, and to be familiar with the presence of a large occipital sinus or peridural veinectasia if he has to decompress the PF. Cerebral angiography with all its technical refinements—magnification angiography, angiotomography and digital substraction angiography—adds so many positive features in brain tumor diagnosis[284, 332, 416] of children that it not should abandoned.

c) NMR is a neuroimaging technique with higher sensitivity but less specifity than CT[228, 303]. There is no superimposition of bone structures in NMR which is important in tumors of the basal temporal lobe and the occipito-cervical region; normal anatomical structures can be better demonstrated by NMR so that tumor infiltration particularly of the caudal brain stem is better shown by NMR. Less specifity of NMR means: the size of the tumor often is amplified, tumor tissue may not be distinguished from surrounding edema. There is no intravenous contrast available with NMR; much important information gained by CT cannot be achieved by NMR; this refers chiefly to the question of tumor dissemination throughout the subarachnoid space[36, 228, 230, 303].

Principles of Pediatric Neurooncology

In the diagnosis and treatment of children with brain tumors a close interdisciplinary cooperation between the pediatric neurologist, neurosurgeon, pediatric oncologist and radiotherapist is mandatory. Coordination of all diagnostic and therapeutic steps of action should be achieved.

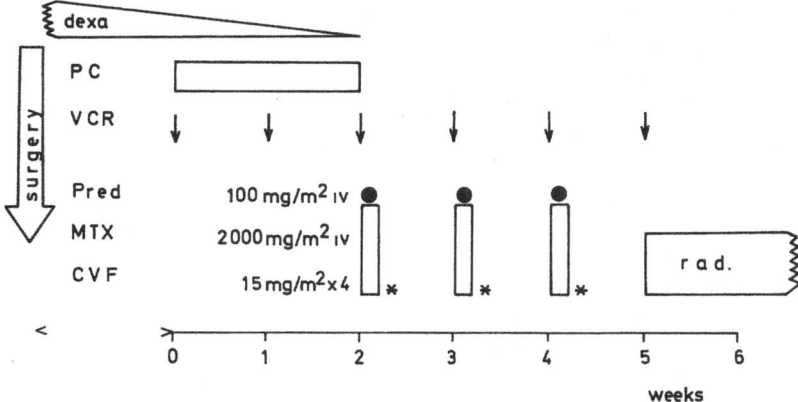

Fig. 4. "Sandwich" CHT used by the GPO and SIOP since 1984. Sandwich refers to the use of CHT between surgery RT

Chemotherapy (CHT) should be placed between operation and radiotherapy (RT) according to the "sandwich" principle (Fig. 4). At present, this opinion of most German pediatric oncologists is shared by some important authors[12, 48, 304]. Candidates for CHT are children with high grade malignomas, GLB, ASCY III/IV, EPDY III/IV, germinomas, PLB, MBL, and all anaplastic tumors of the meninges or the choroid plexus. CHT also is indicated in the highly malignant germ cell tumors: ECA, CCA, EST, malignant teratomas, and brain stem gliomas.

Evaluation of Therapeutic Results

Assessment of the results of therapy should be done based upon the same criteria which are used in pediatric oncology: partial remission, in general, means only a abeyance in a progressive morbid condition for which the patient sometimes has to pay dearly suffering the side-effects of that therapy. The number of partial remissions therefore is not important for the evaluation of a combined therapy. More important points are: lack of tumor progression, quality of life, and particularly cure. As cure definitively can only be stated after many years, it seems reasonable to comment on the time lag between the starting point of the therapy and the definitive statement of further tumor progression. Prospective randomized studies with a considerable number of patients were carried out by the following groups: SIOP, CCSG, and GPO.

The Blood-Brain Barrier (BBB)

If drugs are administered systemically they can penetrate the BBB if they are lipophilic, have low molecular weight, and are nonionized. Drugs having these three properties may be present in the CSF in an adequate concentration although this rarely reaches plasma levels.

Brain tumor tissue is distinct from normal brain parenchyma in some ways: within the center of a tumor the BBB must be disrupted[253]. Endothelial capillary cells are abnormally shaped and there are shunting vessels in the periphery of the tumor. Cell proliferation in the peripheral parts of the tumor is higher than in the center.[171, 298, 432]. Recent findings make it more likely that the BBB is not impaired, at last in some areas of the tumor.

In primary intracranial germ cell tumors, cisplatinum[348] and bleomycin are effective although these are not lipophilic and do not have low molecular weight[145]. Vinblastine, the 3rd component of the "Einhorn regime" used in germinomas of the CNS (Gummerlock/Neuwelt, this volume)[12, 139, 145, 295, 304, 339] does not penetrate the BBB[145], but is effective. This is in accordance with our own findings (Fig. 5). These results suggest selection of CHT for brain tumors even though these drugs are not lipophilic and do not have low molecular weight.

Since the BBB has protective properties for the brain parenchyma, it seems unjustified to break it up by cytotoxic substances[246] if drugs exist which can diffuse into parts of the tumor itself without embarassing the brain in its whole. The data available do not entitle one to exclude drugs from CHT of brain tumors which do not have the property to penetrate the BBB. If one selects medication for cytostatic treatment in patients with brain tumors one should do this less according to BBB-permeability than to tumor specifity and susceptibility.

There are some very important points which are in favor of giving (combination) CHT between surgery and RT (sandwich principle): a) Immediately after an operation the BBB and the blood-tumor barrier are impaired more than before; thus a more effective CHT may well be anticipated[12, 48, 291, 292, 304, 339]. b) Some of the tumors seed along the CSF pathways: MBL, PNETs, EPDY, GLB, germ cell tumors, PBL. The standard RT then is irradiation of the whole neuraxis. After such extensive RT which covers 40–60% of the bone marrow in most cases it is impossible to give a full course and adequately timed CHT because of bone marrow depression[12, 246]. c) Leukoencephalopathy after CHT has been observed only in those children in whome larger doses than 20 Gy were used[35, 326]. In every case of

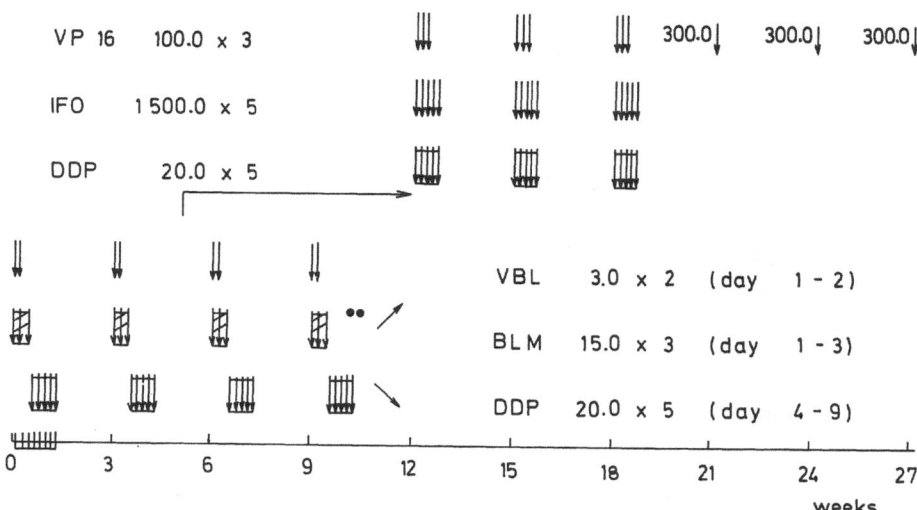

Fig. 5. "Einhorn" regime which was inaugurated 1979 by Neuwelt[295] for CHT of intracranial germ cell tumors. *VP 16* etoposide, *IFO* ifosfamide, *DDP* cisplatinum, *VBL* vinblastine, *BLM* bleomycin

malignant brain tumor the radiation dose given has to be greater than 20 Gy. Today one has to anticipate that the main reason for leukoencephalopathy following CHT (particularly MTX) is due to an impairment of the BBB. This again mainly is due to RTH[8, 25, 54, 61, 89, 166, 203, 296, 327, 359, 421, 422]. It has been shown that during prophylactic irradiation for leukemia using 18–24 Gy there are high concentrations of proteins, which cause clotting, within the CSF indicating transport of the plasma through the BBB[443]. d) Bone marrow depression after CHT is reversible more quickly than after RT.

Iatrogenic BBB Disruption

The BBB can be impaired by perfusion of the feeding arteries (carotid, vertebral) with 25% mannitol solution; such damage to the BBB is reversible (see, Gummerlock/Neuwelt, this volume). An alternative way to overcome the BBB is to perfuse the tumor by the cytostatic drug(s) using a similar technique[436].

There was an incidence of seizures in 12% and clinically symptomatic embolization/infarction in 0.6%. The rise in drug tissue concentration was 10–50fold as compared to intravenous administration of the cytostatic. Steroid administration controls this BBB disruption considerably[87].

According to our opinion this very aggressive therapy with bimodal BBB disruption is experimental and should be practiced in pediatric neurooncology with great caution only. This method as we understand it bears the risk of local, toxic brain tissue damage with resulting in neurological deficit although there is no hope of ultimate cure. The developing brain is more vulnerable to physical and toxic mechanisms than that of an adult. This does not mean that in selected cases, particularly with recurrences, local treatment as outlined above should not take place; reports on this topic are highly desirable.

Treatment of Brain Tumors by Interferon

We only have experiences in treating patients with the benign, virus-induced juvenile papilloma of the larynx. Treatment by α-interferon is effective in tumor control during the period the patient is under medication.

β-interferon which is produced from fibroblast cultures has some *in vitro* effects on human cultured brain tumor cells[81]. There are some anecdotal reports of tumor size reduction as measured by serial CT scanning. But, as definitive and permanent cure is concerned this cannot be expected by interferon monotherapy[350].

Cytostatic Drugs

The drugs most often used are the nitrosoureas (carmustine and lomustine) and procarbazine. These substances penetrate the BBB. Procarbazine often is used 3 weeks following operation in order to avoid more aggressive drugs and not to bring danger to the healing of the operative wound.

The selection of the antineoplastic drugs depends on the grading of the tumor (grades III/IV) and the distinctive property of the drug chosen to penetrate the BBB.

Cytostatic monotherapy, in general, is not recommended in pediatric oncology: cyclophosphamide[10], BCNU[247], carmustine[66]. This topic was reviewed by one of us[226]. High-dose cyclophosphamide (80 mg/kg or greater) for tumor recurrence was recommended by Allen and Helson[10]; there was better response in children with MBL then in those who had gliomas or germinomas.

The administration of MTX-MHD (500 mg/m^2 plus intrathecal) or of MTX-HD (up to 12 g/m^2) (Fig. 4) demands some supportive measures: Large quantities of fluid have to be given by intravenous transfusion, alcalization has to take place and there must be citrovorum factor rescue (CVF-rescue)[226, 289, 292, 346, 347]. The duration of this supportive therapy results from the level of MTX in the plasma and the CSF. In general, there is need for infusion therapy and CVF-rescue for 72 hours. If the MTX-plasma levels are still in the toxic range, there is need to extend this phase of the therapy for another 1–2 days. MTX-MHD or MTX-HD therapy, therefore, should only be undertaken in places where MTX-plasma levels can be checked around the clock. MTX-MHD is infused within 24 hours, MTX-HD within 1–6 hours[289, 347]. CVF rescue starts within 6–24 hours according to the different protocols. Efficacy and toxicity increase together with delayed onset of CVF rescue. The time interval from day 1 of the protocol to the next cycle of the therapy is 1–2 weeks. There are only few protocols in which more than 6 cycles of MTX-MHD or MTX-HD therapy have been recommended[289, 347].

Combined therapies have been recommended by some working groups for MBL, GLB, high grade ASCY, EPDY, OLD, and the germ cell tumors: first surgery—RT—CHT[12, 48, 290, 291].

Since 1977 we carried out CHT in all patients with malignancies of the CNS: MTX-HD with CVF rescue. From 1980–1984 we used the protocol of the GPO: sandwich—CHT by procarbazine, vincristine and MTX-MHD 2–3 weeks after operation, since 1985 by MTX-HD (Fig. 4). The only exception was germ cell tumors in which we used the Einhorn regime (Fig. 5) like other authors [12, 139, 145, 295, 304, 399]. In tumor recurrences the "8 drugs in 1 day" protocol was administered with some success (Fig. 6).

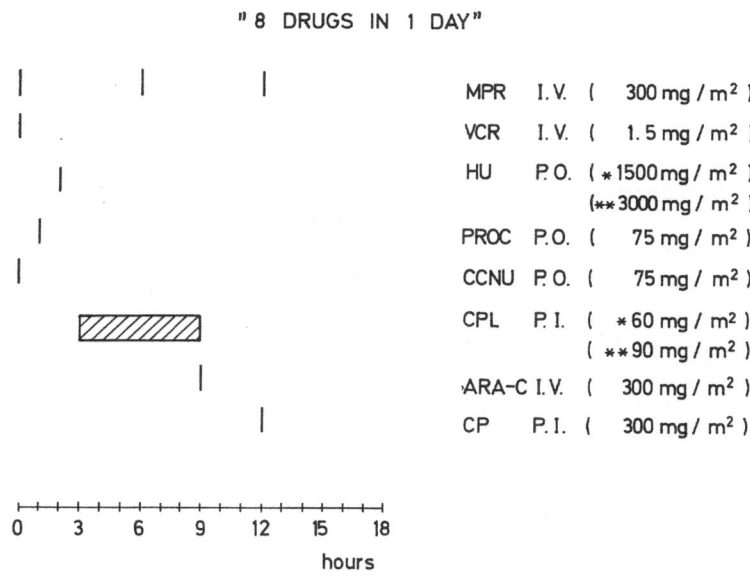

" 8 DRUGS IN 1 DAY"

MPR	I.V. (300 mg / m²)
VCR	I.V. (1.5 mg / m²)
HU	P.O. (*1500 mg / m²)
	(**3000 mg / m²)
PROC	P.O. (75 mg / m²)
CCNU	P.O. (75 mg / m²)
CPL	P.I. (*60 mg / m²)
	(**90 mg / m²)
ARA-C	I.V. (300 mg / m²)
CP	P.I. (300 mg / m²)

hours

Fig. 6. "8 drugs in 1 day"—Bleyer 1983[44]

One limiting factor in the CHT is bone marrow depression. Hochberg[173] reported on an interesting way to avoid it: some 100 ml of blood from the bone marrow were withdrawn and stored at + 4 °C 4–6 hours before an infusion of 600–1,400 mg/m² BCNU. Some 24–36 hours later the bone marrow blood was reinfused. There was no delayed impairment of myelopoesis at all as it usually occurs 28–32 days after BCNU-HD. In all patients there was only leucocytopenia and thrombocytopenia 10–15 days after the cycle for about 10 days. All the patients had vomiting. In 9 out of 10 treated by this regime a tumor regression was shown by CT scanning. Autologous bone marrow rescue was used in the CHT of brain tumors[208]. This therapeutic experimental model can be used in only those patients who have no bone marrow tumor infiltration.

The administration of radiosensitizers (misonidazole, metronidazole)[46–48, 246] did not considerably improve the results of RT. The same applies to cytostatic drugs which are effective in the late G_2 phase of the cell cycle as is RT (anthracyclines and anthracenes).

Side-Effects of Combined Therapy

1. Radiotherapy

After RT there is an increase of risk for infectious diseases to the child during the following 6–12 weeks which is not dependent on the leucocyte count or the number of circulating lymphocytes[50, 79]. This already can be observed after prophylactic radiation for leukemia of the whole cranium with doses of 18–24 Gy. During the course of RT for brain tumors a doubled dose is administered to the neuraxis which compromises 40–60% of the bone marrow in a young child[79]. Myelodepression is observed then, first leucocytopenia, later thrombocytopenia, which can be followed 1–2 months later by anemia. This myelodepressive effect observed during some weeks, is dose dependent and reversible. During this period CHTH must be completely witheld.

In the developing organism growth deficit may be observed after neuraxis RT. There can be damage to the proliferating cartilage of the upper and lower borders of the ossification centers of the vertebral bodies in young children which have an upper dose tolerance of 30 Gy[353]. These children impress as truncal dwarfs years later[157, 328]. Defective skeletal growth can be due to damage to the posterior hypothalamus. The relevant nuclei (ventromedialis and posterior) are within the radiation field in PF tumors which extends to just in front of the posterior clinoids[79, 109]. These hypothalamic nuclei might be damaged by the expanding walls of the 3rd ventricle as well as by obstructive hydrocephalus and by an infiltrating tumor. Radiation, tumor growth and hydrocephalus can interfere with the secretion of GHRF. Low values for HGH were found after insulin-stimulation following RT by 25–29 Gy[386] and after arginine or L-dopa loading[340]. After cranial RT there can be hypothyroidism, too[109, 340]. Either the thyroid gland was within the field of radiation or by damage which was brought on to the pituitary gland or the hypothalamus. Thus, primary, secondary, or tertiary hypothyroidism might result: the basal values for T3/T4 can be decreased with increase of TSH or there is lack of TSH and TRH as shown by the respective tests. Lethargy in a child after combined therapy for brain tumor is due to neuronal damage or to endocrine dysfunction or both. Damage to the adrenal or gonadal axis (lack of ACTH, FSH, LH, LRH) is more often found in adults and adolescents after cranial RT than in children[14, 79, 340].

2. Chemotherapy

CHT can impair skeletal growth, which is only transient and will be balanced later by catching up at the conclusion of chemotherapy.

Bleomycin can cause transient fever which responds well to paracetamol. Its prophylactic administration is recommended so as not to restrict the child subjectively by the fever.

Interstitial pneumonitis[93, 258] is highly specific for bleomycin. Its toxicity is dose dependent: in cumulative doses less than 450 mg/m^2 this side-effect is rare. Functional tests of the pulmonary capacity are more sensitive than clinical symptoms and radiological alterations. Pneumonitis induced by bleomycin clinically cannot be differentiated from interstitial pneumonia due to pneumocystis carinii or cytomegaly virus infection. But bleomycin pneumonitis passes on into interstitial fibrosis. Occasionally the exact diagnosis is only possible by open pulmonary biopsy. Pulmonary fibrosis following bleomycin therapy can develop even without previous pneumonitis.

Cisplatin (CP) causes alopecia, myelosuppression, mucositis, nausea and vomiting, and there is nephrotoxicity and ototoxicity[150, 260, 352]. The damage to the kidney is caused by distal tubular necrosis. This risk can be reduced by forced diuresis: pretherapeutic hydratation for 6 hours with mannitol or frusemide. There is need for replacement of magnesium loss prophylactically and for measuring magnesium levels of the serum during the therapy. High-frequence hearing loss in children under CP therapy is observed in ⅓ and not fully reversible in all[352]. It can be monitored during the therapy by BEAR and/or audiometric testing.

Nausea and vomiting are subjective a side-effects of CHT: whilst MTX-HD does not prompt sick-feeling and vomiting, nitrosureas and CP very often do. After the 1st cycle of the therapy "anticipative" vomiting may occur as an additional psychological factor: some patients already feel sick and start vomiting before they have reached the hospital if CHT was planned for that day.

Like combination CHT in brain tumors is superior to monotherapy this is with antiemetic treatment, too. It was shown that none of the antiemetics available today is able to block all the receptor sites within the "vomiting center" of the medulla oblongata[316].

Based on animal experiments an "intensive-5-drug antiemetic regimen" was introduced[321]: it was given mainly to those children who were under cisplatinum. This combination therapy consisted of: metoclopramide, diphenylhydramine, dexamethasone, diazepam, and thietylperazine. 13 out of 17 patients did not have any vomiting at all; 3 vomited once. None had complaints on nausea the day after cisplatinum. The same patients had vomited before 5 times on average during the CHT. As side-effects sleep was induced in 16 of the 17 patients, and one patient had urine retention.

Of all the side effects during CHT in children, nausea and vomiting are the worst. An effective antiemetic treatment therefore ranks as the first priority as seen from the patient's point of view. Our own practice backs the content of the publications just quoted[321], but one limiting factor should be mentioned here. Some children over 10 years old are against this antiemetic regimen for it makes them sleep. They feel it badly when they no longer have control over themselves. Metoclopramide has an impact on the motility of the intestine. In adults it is a very potent antiemetic. Children often respond to the drug by extrapyramidal symptoms of the axial-dystonic type. Sometimes these spasms are very painful, and often there is anxiety about cerebral seizures. Biperiden (IV) or diazepam (rectal, IV) should be ready for immediate administration.

3. Side-Effects of Combined Treatment

The following neurological sequelae can develop during and after CHT/RT[161]:
     MTX: arachnoiditis—acute paraplegia—leukoencephalopathy,
     VCR: neuropathy—inappropriate ADH-secretion syndrome—convulsions,
     ARA-C: arachnoiditis—acute paraplegia—convulsions,
     CP: water retention—water intoxication—brain edema.

a) Neuropathies: VCR polyneuropathy is dependent on the doses and the time intervals the drug had been given. Initially cramps and pains in the thigh muscles and the jaw are reported. There is loss of tendon reflexes starting with the ankle jerk, motor weakness of the legs followed by the upper extremities and the trunk. Motor nerve conduction velocity may be slowed or even nonmeasurable at all. There may be some muscular wasting of the small muscles of the hand. Paresthesia can develop but there are some children with severe motor polyneuropathy who have no sensory involvement at all. Autonomic neuropathy may be present giving rise to bladder and bowel distensions, paralytic ileus, or orthostatic hypotension.

The cranial nerves can be involved, too: there can be hoarse voice (recurrent laryngeal branch of the vagus nerve), myopathic facies, ptosis, and paresis of all extraocular muscles: Fisher's syndrome[126]. Some children complain of photophobia due to paresis of the sphincter pupillae. Cerebellar symptoms such as gait ataxia, tremor, muscular hypotonia are not infrequent at all, mainly in toddlers[161] (personal observations).

VCR-induced neuropathy is caused by disturbance of the axonal flow with increase of neurofilaments and loss of microtubuli which are replaced by paracristalline substances[11, 161, 231]. The presence of neurofibromatosis, a preexisting (hereditary) neuropathy or liver dysfunction may enhance and prolong VCR polyneuropathy. Clinically most children recover within months completely after discontinuation of the drug; in some of them slow motor conduction velocity and decreased tendon jerks can be present years later without any functional impairment.

Other CNs affected by the combined therapy are the optic nerves which can be damaged by high dose RT for cancer of the nasal cavity or the ethmoid sinus[393]. The lower CNs (X, XI, XII) are damaged by high dose RT of the neck or after radiation of the PF for local recurrences[231]. High frequency hearing loss in children under cisplatinum has already been mentioned[352].

b) Spinal cord: In some of the children who had irradiation of the spinal axis there is an "early delayed effect" as the result of transient demyelination of the posterior columns[390]: positive Lhermitte's sign which means tingling and paresthesia of the limbs bilaterally on neck flexion[79]. This syndrome is limited to within the first weeks after RTH and disappears after some months[412].

Delayed radiation myelopathy is rare in children with acute or remitting symptomatology developing months after completion of RT. On myelography, obliteration of the spinal subarachnoid space may be seen caused by cord swelling or intensive fibrotic changes of the meninges[231, 412]. Apart from meningeal thickening a variably of vascular, neuronal and glial alterations have been described in this condition which is radiographically revealed as a "tight" cord.

In some children 12-48-72 hours after intrathecal injection of MTX or ARA-C a syndrome was observed which clinically has to be grouped with the anterior spinal artery syndrome: acute pains in the groins, thighs or between the shoulders, followed by flaccid paralysis of the legs and by bladder and bowel distension. In some children dissociated sensory disturbance was observed, whereby the level of sensory impairment moved up or down 2–4 segments during the next few days. The signs can resolve after hours or days, or after months, but in some of them spastic paraplegia develops[136, 257, 313, 363, 399]. We observed 6 patients with this syndrome: 2 of whom had quick improvement, 2 were better after some months and 2 remained paraplegic. All these patients had prechemotherapeutic radiation of the spinal axis for different reasons and in different doses (more than 24 Gy). Raised cell and protein levels within the CSF were risk factors. In the 7 autopsy reports available there was no blast cell infiltration of the spinal cord parenchyma, but necrosis, gliosis and scattered demyelination and fibrosis of meningeal vessels[136, 257, 313, 399]. The possibility of reaction to the solvent (parabene, benzoate) has been discussed[161].

c) Cerebral symptoms: 1. In about ⅓ of all children who receive chemotherapeutic drugs intrathecally (MTX, ARA-C), a "chemical" meningitis develops: headache, neck rigidity, vomiting, pleocytosis (50–100 lymphomonocytes/mm^3), slight increase of CSP (50–100 mg/dl), decreased cyclic AMP and elevated values for acid phosphatase and lactic acid dehydrogenese[8, 11, 161] were found. The symptoms clear within 36–48 hours.

2. 1–2 weeks following MTX-MHD or MTX-HD administration there may be convulsions, hemipareses, dysarthria and confusion of sudden onset. These symptoms which are transient even more often come on after L-asparaginase treatment for leukemia[231]. In the EEG generalized slowing of the background activity is seen, focal slow wave or focal seizure activity[79]. Similar symptoms may be observed after VCR; probably here they are due to inappropriate ADH-secretion[161].

3. In about 30–40% out of all children who had radiation of the cranium by more than 20 Gy, a few weeks later a syndrome of fatigue, lack of initiative and anorexia is observed: the postirradiation apathy syndrome (postradiation somnolence syndrome)[54, 130, 138]. The clinical symptoms clear within 1–3 weeks. This syndrome was also observed after prophylactic RT of the cranium for leukemia and after radiation for brain tumors[50, 421]. The EEG-recordings show marked slowing of the background activity[79, 138] with rhythmic generalized or focal theta- delta-wave activity. It was claimed[309] that this patchy slowing of the EEG can be found before RT is given in some of the children with leukemia. This would mean that there had been disseminated infiltration of the meninges by blast cells. The postirradiation somnolence syndrome probably is caused by the interference of ionizing rays with myelin metabolism of the oligodendroglial cells[161].

4. Price and Jamieson[326] reported upon the postmortem findings of 13 out of 238 children who had been treated for leukemia and who had had prophylactic radiation of the cranium. There was leukoencephalopathy with multifocal demyelination, widely spread in the centrum semiovale, putamen, and the cerebellar cortex. Loss of oligodendroglia and astrocyte proliferation were noted. Similar neuropathological reports on patients with leukemia[166, 203, 359] and brain tumors[25, 61, 296] after combined therapy are available. The radiation dose in the children with

leukemia had been 20 Gy and more[326] and the cumulative dose of MTX was not very high in the individual case: 112.5 mg–2.687 mg. Some had single doses between 20–80 mg/m². Intrathecally given MTX accumulated in 42 to 1,131 mg. Different factors like malnutrition, bacterial or fungal infections or blast cells within the meninges did not add to the prevalence of leukoencephalopathy which also was observed after MTX-HD (8–15 g/m² [346, 347]) for osteosarcoma in patients who had had no RT of the cranium before[8, 161].

Clinically this MTX related leukoencephalopathy starts insidiously weeks to several months after treatment with forgetfulness, withdrawn behavior, apathy[8, 50, 161, 422]. Seizures may come on, spasticity (hemiplegia or tetraparesis) develops. There may be ataxic symptoms, tremor, dysarthric speech, dysphagia and decorticate posturing. Some of the patients become obtunded and lapse into coma. The patients die or become severely demented and are left with grave residual symptoms. Most of the children are under 10 years of age. This clinical form of leukoencephalopathy was also observed in a few cases after ARA-C and CCNU[231].

It has been proposed that a breakdown of the tightly knitted network of astrocytes which forms the anatomical basis of the BBB is the fundamental mechanism of MTX-induced leukoencephalopathy[8, 161, 231]. RT in most cases disrupts the BBB, but increased intraventricular pressure might act in the same way[8, 61, 231, 296].

5. Price and Birdwell[327] described a noninflammatory, mineralizing microangiopathy within the lenticular nuclei and cerebral cortex in 28 out of 163 brains of children with lymphoblastic leukemia who had been treated by combined schedules. Some of the children had been given only 15 Gy and all were younger than 10 years. These dystrophic calcifications develop after 10 months. Relapses of the meningeal form of leukemia and systemic and/or intrathecal MTX administration were contributing factors[327]. There is no clear clinical correlation for these findings which can be demonstrated by CT follow-up studies, and may also be present after combined therapies for brain tumors, particularly MBL[50, 161, 231, 274].

Simultaneous treatment by CHT and RT brings about some other acute problems. The results of the study group on MBL of the GPO[289, 292] and our own experiences do favor CHT prior to RT. This bears some risks but leukoencephalopathy is not part of that risk.

d) *Residual neurological signs and symptoms:* It appears reasonable that neurological deficit is unlikely to disappear if the tumor has been eradicated by combined therapeutic efforts: operation—CHT—RT. Despite this common statement many symptoms wane, because they were pressure-related and not due to tissue destruction. Nevertheless, if one compares the degree of neurological impairment after treatment for MBL with cerebellar ASCY one has to admit that handicaps in the children with MBL are more pronounced[158, 172, 177]. Ataxic symptoms and incoordination of movement are more frequent and more prominent in children who suffered from MBL. In some reports it has been stated that none of the long-term survivors was symptom-free[157]. In cerebellar ASCY the history more often is longer than in MBL; therefore any obstructive hydrocephalus in quite a number of these children had been present for a longer period, and the difference in the outcome cannot be related to raised ICP[330]. The more extensive neurological damage therefore has to be attributed to both the invasive nature of the malignant tumor and the side-effects of combined therapy. In addition, age comes into the question of outcome: the younger the child was at the time of treatment the worse were the results[79, 177, 189].

e) *Mental and personality changes:* After cranial irradiation for leukemia mental changes were reported[114, 275]. Similar alterations were not observed in those children with leukemia who had not been irradiated or in whom it had been done with temporary delay[114]. The conclusion therefore was that mental deterioration in these patients is not related to meningeal leukemia or CHT but to prophylactic cranial irradiation using an exposure of 24 Gy. In these children the performance part of their tests was more often affected than the verbal items: general memory scale, visual motor integration and the solving of psychomotor problems[275].

Children who had RT for malignant brain tumors in whom much higher doses for the cranium are needed (40–60 Gy) are likely to be much worse off as compared to children who had RT for leukemia. In commenting on several series[89, 107, 172, 330] it was stated by Cohen and Duffner[79] that 17–54% of the children after RT for brain tumors have an IQ less than 70 and only 11–56% 90 and more. CHT as one further possible cause of this mental deterioration might be discounted although RT plus actinomycin D are supposed to act synergistically in causing diffuse brain damage[301].

From these reports[79, 89, 108, 157, 172, 177, 330, 437, 438] one can draw the following conclusions: formal intelligence may be in the low normal or borderline range. A decline of 20–25 points in a standard IQ test has to be accepted in nearly all children who had full cranial RT[107, 109]. The main findings were: profound impairment of memory, mainly visual retention, speech in part due to dysarthria and general motor slowing, and in the dynamics of the personality: short attention span, emotional instability, anxiety, withdrawal after the child had fully realized his difficulties in performance. These test results were worse in a 2nd set after two years[107, 109]. On the whole, there are four risk factors for changes in personality and mental capacity to a child in this situation: young age, brain stem involvement, hypothalamic damage, and RT[79, 89, 107, 171, 186, 330].

f) *Neooncogenesis:* From the data available is has been calculated that a child who had had RT for a malignant brain has a 12% risk of having a second tumor at any site within the next 20 years[79, 129, 157, 344]. Frederick[129] collected data from 414 children who had different treatment for cancer and survived 5–24 years, 13 years in the mean. 19 had developed malignant and 11 benign tumors, 2 had intermediate forms: Except for two, the site of the neoplasm was related to the site of radiation. Since only 288 of the 414 children had been irradiated, there was an incidence of a secondary neoplasm of 10.1% after 13 years.

It is well known that after radiation for "status thymicolymphaticus" or for tinea capitis there is an increased risk to get brain tumors, particularly meningioma, and tumors of the thyroid or parotid gland. The radiation doses that had been used were very low: 1.4–1.7 Gy. Therefore, after every RT which touched the thyroid gland even by very low doses an increased risk of thyroid adenoma or carcinoma has to be accepted: the doses were calculated by Roggli[344]: 0.2–15 Gy; Whilst higher does (over 20 Gy) bring damage to the thyroid cells in their proliferative capacity. The time lag between RT and diagnosis was 7–18 years. Secondary brain tumors observed after RT for cranial neoplasms were: meningioma, GLB and high grade

ASCY[79] with time intervals of 5–26 years. We observed 3 patients with secondary intracranial malignancies: 1 boy had no RTH for adrenal carcinoma, aged 1 year and developed MBL 10 years later. 1 girl had prophylactic RT of 18 Gy aged 2 years for lymphoblastic leukemia and developed GLB of the cerebellum 8 years later. A boy aged 16 had cerebral GLB 11 years after prophylactic irradiation of the cranium for leukemia, with a dose of 18 Gy.

Special Pediatric Neurooncology

I. Astrocytoma (ASCY)

In our own series of 274 children with brain tumors there were 28.5% ASCY of all sites (Table 1). In the cerebellum there were low grade ASCY only, and anaplastic transformation of ASCY in this site are rare[213, 214, 216]. ASCY of the brain stem are often more high grade tumors: 2 out of 12 in our cases. Meningeal spread of brain stem ASCY has been described[112, 140, 300, 452].

Supratentorial ASCY have an incidence of 15–35% of all ST pediatric brain tumors[79, 120, 148, 165, 223, 184, 279, 282, 450]. They originate anywhere within the white matter of the cerebral hemispheres or the brain stem. Often they show radial growth between normal structures. This is the reason why despite complete infiltration of a

Table 1. Histology and location of 275 brain tumors in children

Histology	Site of the tumor							N	%
	I	II	III	IV	V	VI	VII		
Astrocytoma	21	3	8	2	—	12	32	78	28.4
Oligodendroglioma	2	—	—	—	—	—	—	2	0.7
Ependymoma	4	—	—	1	—	1	9	15	5.4
Glioblastoma	10	—	—	—	—	1	1	12	4.4
Choroid plexus papilloma	3	—	—	—	—	—	2	5	1.8
Gangliocytoma	3	—	—	—	—	1	—	4	1.4
Primitive neuroectodermal tumors (PNET)	4	1	—	—	—	6	38	49	17.8
Germ cell tumors	—	1	5	3	—	—	2	11	4.0
Meningioma	3	—	—	—	—	—	—	3	1.1
Sarcoma	7	—	1	—	—	1	4	13	4.8
Hamartoma—phacomatosis	5	1	1	—	—	—	—	7	2.6
Angioma/angioblastoma	3	—	—	1	—	2	5	11	4.0
Brain metastases	5	3	—	—	—	—	4	12	4.4
Nonclassified	—	11	1	—	—	13	2	27	9.8
Craniopharyngioma	—	—	—	—	23	—	—	23	8.3
Pituitary adenoma	—	—	—	—	3	—	—	3	1.1
Total	70	20	16	7	26	37	99	275	

given area (*e.g.* optic nerve, basal ganglia, thalamus, hypothalamus) there is only CSF obstruction but no or almost no functional loss[60, 280]. The closer to the midline and the more rostral the location is, the more likely it is that the ASCY will be of a low grade[148], but will usually show infiltrating growth. According to the WHO classification they usually correspond to grade II[228, 457].

The more laterally the tumor is located, the more often it will present with epileptic seizures as the first and only symptom: ⅓ of all cases present with epilepsy. The longer the history the more likely it is that the tumor will be benign[385]. However, 35% of pediatric patients with GLB have seizures as the 1st symptom[97] and their history is short.

The *histological classification* (not grading) of an ASCY implies some prognostic features. ASCY can be of the:

a) fibrillary type, mostly affecting the brain stem or cerebellum,

b) protoplasmatic type, often with poorly defined borders, can infiltrate the leptomeninges,

c) pilocytic type (syn. "spongioblastoma"[456]), often cystic or multicystic, with predominant site in the upper brain stem, pons, cerebellum, and spinal cord. Remaining tumor tissue can form new cysts and recurrences often are very large:

d) gemistocytic type; often with high cellularity, pleomorphism, and mitosis,

e) anaplastic type with high cellularity, cellular pleomorphism, and mitoses. This type can degenerate into GLB[79, 361].

Symptoms: Long-standing epilepsy is present in 30–60% of children with ST. ASCY[6, 49, 79, 148, 184, 255, 282, 305, 426]. Seizures can be the only symptom for years. 50–69% of the children with ST ASCY show seizure activity recorded in the EEG even in the absence of convulsions[79, 435]. The EEG localizes the tumor in 90% of cases. The seizures can be partial elementary, complex, or secondarily generalized. If absence-like features are reported in the history[146, 148], one always has to record an ictal EEG by which the focal nature of this "absence" is easily unmasked. Headache and vomiting is present in 40–50% of the children[79].

Signs: 40–70% of the children have papilledema[79, 146, 154, 165, 183, 255, 349, 426]. Frequency of hemiparesis/hemiplegia ranges from 35 to 60%[54, 183, 185, 383, 426]. Hemiparesis is much more often seen in children with focal seizures. ⅓ of the children with hemiparesis have dysphasic features, too. Mental changes are present in 25–40%, particularly in children with ASCY of the temporal lobe. Aggressive behavior associated with therapy-resistent complex partial epilepsy is a clinical situation where an ASCY has to be excluded by modern neuroimaging techniques (3 personal observations). In a child with unexplained focal epilepsy and abnormal EEG a glioma (ASCY) should be excluded. If CT is negative, NMR is indicated and if both are negative, they have to be repeated within 4–6 months. If NMR is not available, angiography has to be performed.

Diagnosis: Diagnosis is currently established by CT with contrast enhancement, but an isodense or slightly hypodense lesion can be detected earlier by NMR[36, 228, 303], 3 personal observations). Grade II ASCY most often are hypodense or isodense lesions without an enhancement and without peritumoral edema[204, 384]. The gemistocytic and anaplastic types have a positive enhancement which may be patchy, annular or festoon-like and in 65% there is peritumoral edema grade I/II[204]. Grade III/IV ASCY are hypodense lesions in 32%, isodense in 15%, hyperdense in 20% and mixed in 32%[204]. The differential diagnosis lies between recent cerebral infarction, cerebral abscess, spontaneous hemorrhage and brain metastasis[204].

Plain X-rays may show nonspecific signs of raised ICP, shift of the pineal gland in children over 12 years old and local bulging of the calvarium probably thinned at that site. An underlying hypodense lesion without enhancement may mimick an arachnoidal cyst. Calcification within an ASCY on plain X-ray is exceptional: 1/34 in our series of ST ASCY.

Angiography should be done in every case of ST ASCY: spider-like tumor vessels may be demonstrated in the depth of the temporal lobe (3 personal cases) even in false negative CT. Apart from this direct tumor sign, shift of arteries and veins can be seen, particularly of the anterior cerebral, posterior communicating, and anterior choroidal arteries, the two latter indicating uncal herniation. If the posterior communicating artery is stretched and depressed there may be involvement of the oculomotor nerve.

Tumor blush in the late arterial, capillary or early venous phase with arterio-venous anastomotic vessels is highly suggestive of high grade ASCY, i.e. GLB.

Therapy: In ST hemispheric ASCY, surgery is the treatment of choice except for lesions within the centro-temporal region of the dominant side. In the latter situation, dominance tests for handedness and writing should be performed and a careful family history of handedness in other family members must be checked. Before the age of 6–8 years, a shift of dominance can take place and may have already occurred in a long-standing lesion[164]. ⅓ of ST childhood ASCY are high grade tumors[79, 146, 148, 184, 279, 281], about 20–30% undergo anaplastic transformation, as OLG may do[79, 286]. In some children with ASCY there is tumor recurrence within a few weeks after subtotal removal. In 3 of our patients the whole tumor bulk had regrown after resection and the site of craniotomy was bulging. Histologically, all these lesions had been labelled as benign. The reasons for this rapid tumor regrowth are not clear. One might consider mechanical irritation/alterations in the vascular supply within the marginal tumor zone/increase of the reduplication rate or shortening of the reduplication time.

Local RT is recommended in grade III/IV ASCY and in tumors of the midline which could only be subjected to biopsy[46, 47, 265, 299, 388, 441]. In grade II ASCY RT is indicated if there are neurological symptoms, such as visual failure in optic glioma, emacication syndrome of infancy, hemiparesis, or increase of ICP[46, 47, 265, 281, 368, 388, 390, 391, 435]. In children with fibrillary or pilocytic ASCY who had "total" removal of the tumor, one can afford to watch with CT control holding RT. The same in reserve holds good for children without neurological deficit, e.g. a thickened optic nerve in neurofibromatosis or a hyperdense lesion without space occupying characteristics in the same condition. Here one can wait unless further tumor growth is evident on CT or anaplastic transformation has been shown by biopsy.

There are some reports on fast neutron beam RT of malignant hemispheric gliomas[47, 169, 389]. A dose of 1,300–1,560 rad induced tumor control in 69%[47], but no longer survival was achieved. The morbidity was worse for these patients became progressively demented due to white matter degeneration and slowly died[47, 169]. This kind of therapy therefore has been abandoned. Steroids should be given to all children preoperatively who present with perifocal edema in the CT or whose level of consciousness is depressed[385, 434]. Steroids also offer some help in the terminal phase of the disease when further RT/CHT is no longer indicated. Most authors recommend CHT only for recurrent GLB or high grade ASCY in order not to burden the short period between RT and the date of recurrence of symptoms[10, 47, 385, 387]. The chemotherapeutic agents used are: the nitrosoureas, BCNU, CCNU, methyl-CCNU, VM 26, VCR, MTX, and procarbazine[46, 47, 79, 226, 322, 385, 387]. High dose cyclophosphamide (80 mg/kg or more) may induce some improvement in recurrent gliomas[10].

When nitrosoureas are given before RT[322], one has to postpone RT for many weeks until delayed myelosuppression (28th to 32th day after administration) has improved[86, 387].

The radiosensitizer misonidazole acts synergistically with some chemotherapeutic agents: MTX, VCR, fluorouracil, and mephalan. Its administration in children with ST and brain stem ASCY achieved no better results than RTH alone[46, 47].

To sum up: if one decides to administer CHT in cases of tumor recurrence, one should do it prior to RT and in the same way as for MBL (*vide infra*).

Prognosis: The 5-year-survival rate is 30–60% for children with low grade ST ASCY[79, 120, 146–148]. The question of total or subtotal tumor removal is important: if subtotal removal of the tumor bulk was possible, there is only a 25% hope for survival for all childhood brain tumors, whereas it is 80% if there was complete exstirpation[146, 148]. According to Shapiro[388] hope for survival longer than 5 years after surgery in low grade ASCY is poor: 25% for grade I and 0 for grade II. After RT, the 5-year-survival rate increases to 58% for grade I and 25% for grade II. Other authors make no distinction between grade I and II Marsa[265]: 41% (N: 40), Onomaya[299]: 50%, Wara[441] 100% (N: 6). According to recent studies, low-grade ST astrocytomas after RT show 5-year-survivals of 30–60%[48, 79], while for grade III/IV the 5-year survival is 0–4% without and 15–20% with RT[46, 47, 169, 364, 388–391].

The quality of life is variable: 25% had fully recovered, 38% had moderate and 15% severe sequelae[147, 148]. In particular, there was epilepsy in 25%, hemiparesis in 17%, visual impairment of one or both eyes in 12% and 14%, respectively, and ataxic symptoms in 20%[148]. Similar findings in children were given by Mercuri[279].

Surveillance: Our proposal for follow-up in children with ST tumor is:

a) Neurological examination including EEG every 4 months after completion of therapy for the next 2 years. In children with high grade glioma the set of appointments is every 2 months. For the next 3 years examination is performed every 6 months and then once a year.

b) Check CTs are performed at 3 months and than every 6 months, if there are no signs of remaining tumor or recurrence. After 3 years one CT examination per year is recommended. All CT control examination require contrast enhancement. CT controls may be replaced by NMR, in midline tumors this seems preferable.

c) Continuation of anticonvulsive treatment for at least 2 years and discontinuation only if there is 1) no tumor recurrence, 2) there have been no more seizures, and 3) if there is no focal or generalized epileptic discharge in the EEG nor any constant slow wave focus.

II. Glioblastoma multiforme (GLB)

GLB are highly malignant tumors in all age groups. In larger pediatric series their incidence ranges from 1%[426], 3%[165, 450], 4–5%[120, 223] (own series, Table 1) 8%[97], 11%[255] to 14%[451]. In series with high figures some other malignant tumors like PNET's or high grade ASCY may have been included. 75–80% of GLB are located within the cerebral hemispheres, 20–25% within the brain stem (caudal parts more often than rostral regions), and only very few within the cerebellar hemispheres and vermis[97, 131, 256, 424]. According to Kopelson[224] there were only 50 GLB reported in the world literature with primary cerebellar site.

Besides a high cellularity, mitoses are present in 70%, necroses in 52%, hemorrhages in 60%. There is much endothelial proliferation and only rarely are cysts and/or calcifications found within the tumor[79].

Symptoms: The history in most children is short: 2 weeks to 4 months. There are a few exceptions in the giant cell type with epilepsy as presenting symptom for years, in one of our cases 2½ years after head injury[97, 223, 268, 305]. In addition, we observed one child in whom GLB developed 5 years after a significant head injury at the site of the contusion[423]. In this child residual symptoms and the EEG focus had persisted throughout all the years. The time of onset of symptoms related to the brain tumor was not clear. Headache and vomiting is present in 70–80% of children with GLB[97].

Signs: Hemiparesis, sometimes associated with seizures and clouding of consciousness are the prominent clinical signs. In GLB of the frontal lobe the seizures most often are of the grand mal type or even initial status epilepticus (3 personal observations). Further signs include ataxic gait, other cerebellar signs, nystagmus, gaze paresis or other brain stem signs[97].

Diagnosis: The EEG often shows a slow wave focus with phase reversal and low voltage runs at its maximum[79, 100]. This slow wave focus has localizing value, but the low voltage runs may be related to peritumoral edema.

In the CT (mixed pediatric and adult series) GLB presents as a hypodense lesion in 9%, isodense in 11% hyperdense in 9% and mixed in 71%[204]. In a few cases GLB may be undetected in the first CT examination even by high resolution technique[384]. Nearly all patients have positive contrast enhancement which intensifies after 10–20 minutes[204]. Peritumoral edema is present in most of the ST GLB, of grade I in 24%, grade II in 58% and grade III in 18%[204]. Grade I edema CGN be of the fingerprint type[79] which resembles embarassment of the subcortical white matter. Enhancement show irregular annular, festoon-like, or even cystic formations[204, 384].—The differential diagnosis must be made from: (multiple) brain abscess/brain metastases/brain infarction 2–4 weeks standing.

Cerebral angiography often gives evidence of an avascular mass with shifts of arteries and veins which sometime indicate herniations. In only a few pediatric patients—contrary to adults—are there pathological vessels, both arteries and veins which may have arterio-venous short circuits or give rise to a tumor-blush[204, 424]. Those new-formed vessels, mainly veins, have to be differentiated from small angiomas with space-occupying intraparenchymatous bleeding in adolescents presenting with hemiplegia of sudden onset. The final diagnosis of the nature of these lesions may be possible only at operation[143].

CSF examination is contraindicated in a high-grade expanding cerebral lesion such as GLB. Despite this statement, some patients have a lumbar puncture to exclude meningitis after spontaneous hemorrhage has occurred. In contradistinction to patients with MBL, determination of the polyamines (putrescine, spermine, spermidine) has not been helpful in anaplastic gliomas; some correlation between the level of polyamines in the CSF and tumors situated near the ventricles was present. However, there were many false negatives due to tumor necroses and hemorrhage as well as tumor recurrence, polyamine determination as a routine for follow-up is open to discussion[133].

Treatment: Nearly all GLB are inoperable, surgery as palliation in the form of an "internal decompression" is undertaken when possible[223]. In tumors of the upper brain stem, biopsy (open or stereotactic) may be indicated whereas in those of the lower brain stem (vide supra) only a shunt is inserted if indicated. RT without adjuvant CHT doubles the survival time from 14–28 weeks (mixed series of children and mainly adults)[387, 388].

Steroids in children with GLB appear not only to have an effect on peritumoral edema, but also on the survival time which is lengthened from 4, 6, to 13.6 months[97].

Adjuvant CHT did not improve life expectancy in patients with GLB[97, 385]. CHT should be given prior to RT as outlined under ASCY (*vide supra*).

CHT in our own opinion should be given if a) the surgeon's reports "total removal" and b) in the giant cell variant of GLB. This subtype in children sometimes has a better prognosis[223], and we had two survivors, one without recurrence for 8 years.

Course: Malignant gliomas often recur at the primary site but spread both within the adjacent ventricular ependyma throughout the leptomeninges[118, 223, 300, 302, 314, 424, 452]. The ventricular seeding may be nodular and the spinal seedlings may thicken the nerve roots even without causing clinical signs and symptoms. On the other hand, back pain, paresthesia, segmental pain and transverse lesions of the cord are on record[300, 452]). Myelography may reveal multiple filling defects, nerve root thickening and wrapping and even spinal block. In general, one has to assume spinal seedlings in malignant glioma in 20–30% of cases[118, 300]. Considering the grade and primary site of the tumor, this question can be answered more precisely: in low grade ST glioma, spinal dissemination is present in 4%, in high grade lesions in 48%, in high grade gliomas of the brain stem in 20% of cases[302].

Extraneural metastases may determine the final outcome of a child with malignant glioma. The extraaxial deposits have a different predilection of sites than in MBL: the lungs/pleura, followed by lymph nodes, bones, and liver, are involved, rarely the heart, kidney, adrenal, or pancreas[79, 82, 106, 112, 176, 252, 312]. The site of origin can be the bone flap with continuous extraneural spread (2 personal observations). Bone lesions can be osteoplastic or osteoclastic[112]. Serum calcium[82, 312] acid or alkaline serum phosphatase can be elevated[112, 307, 312]. Survival time after diagnosis of extraneural tumor spread varies from 1 months to 13 years[312], but in most patients rapid deterioration occurs: 50% die within the first year and 70% within 2 years after diagnosis[252, 312].

Diffuse glioblastomatosis with spongioblastic infiltration of the white matter, satellitosis in the cortical and subcortical grey matter and marked cellular increase within the superficial cortical layers is a different form of anaplastic transformation[201, 372]. Clinically these children present with megalencephaly and either acute symptoms of raised ICP and visual failure or the chronic psychiatric syndrome, brain stem and cerebellar signs, and epilepsy. The condition is related to neurofibromatosis, tuberous sclerosis and aplasia of the adrenals[201] and can be understood as glial dysgenesis with blastomatous features.

III. Oligodendroglioma (OLD)

This tumor is rare in children. It accounts for only 1–2% in pediatric series[79, 99, 147, 165, 183–185, 223, 282, 426, 450, 451]. In "mixed gliomas" (= ASCY + OLD), the oligodendrogliomatous part is the more important one which puts the tumor into the malignant glioma variant[281, 435]. OLD are graded as II or, less often, grade III[228].

The outstanding clinical symptom in OLD is epilepsy: 50–70% present with longstanding seizure disorders[79, 99, 223]. In addition many of these children are mentally retarded or have psychiatric symptoms[79, 99], (1 personal observation). 40–50% have raised ICP: headache, vomiting, and papilledema[79, 99]. The tumor is mostly located within the frontal, temporal or parietal lobes. Therefore the kind of clinical seizure presentation is characterized by the primary site of the tumor, as are the mental and psychiatric symptoms particularly if the tumor is located in the temporal lobe.

At surgery the brain parenchyma seems to be infiltrated in a festoon-like fashion, multifocal growth within the ventricular ependyma can be observed[223]. Often there are microcalcification, mucoid degeneration, and hemorrhages. Next to the cerebral hemispheres the brain stem is the preferential site of OLD[99, 223, 281].

Diagnosis: In the plain X-rays often delicate calcifications are detectable, sometimes years after the beginning of a seizure disorder. The CT shows hypodense lesions in 26%, isodense ones in 5%, hyperdense in 14% and mixed hypodense/hyperdense ones in 55%[204, 431]. Enhancement after contrast is seen in 46%, and focal edema is present in 38% of cases which is delicate in most cases at the beginning. Calcification within the tumor is demonstrated by CT in 90%. According to Vonofakos et al.[431] positive enhancement in an OLD probably indicates malignancy, whereas annular or cyst formation within an OLD prooves anaplastic transformation. This statement is controversial[384].

OLD have a tendency for local recurrence and for anaplastic transformation which occurs in 30–50% of the cases[285]. This may happen after many years with a relatively slow or nonevident tumor progression. Therefore the tumor may show rapid growth on CT and these children may die quite rapidly[79, 285, 377]. Meningeal infiltration and distant seedlings are well known[79, 223].

Treatment: This includes radical surgical removal as far as possible, and recurrences may be reoperated upon several times[223].

The effects of RT are controversial. According to some authors[79, 97], the postoperative survival time in children is 39–45 months and is not influenced by RT at all. Müller et al.[285] found 42 months for low grade and 22 months survival for high grade OLDGL. Sheline[392] reported a 85% 5-year survival rate in irradiated and only a 31% in a nonirradiated group of patients, whereas Marsa[265] recorded a 5-year survival rate of 74%; both groups of patients were not differentiated according to histological grading.

IV. Ependymoma (EPDY)

Ependymomas constitute 7–10 (–14%) of all brain tumors in children[79, 120, 146, 165, 223, 444, 450]). Both sexes are equally affected[151, 320]. The peak incidence of intracranial EPDYs is between 4–6 years, 60% of whom are diagnosed before 6 years[120, 444] and only 5% after the age of 15 years[98]. A considerable number of EPDYs is located primarily within the spinal cord or the filum terminale: 10%[98], 25%[341], 36%[35], 49%[206], 52%[283]. Their most frequent clinical presentation is within the 2nd and 3rd decade of life[283, 444].

Kernohan and Fletcher-Kernohan[206] described 3 histological subtypes of EPDY: the epithelial, myxopapillary, and cellular variants. No prediction can be made from these subtypes with regard to two important biological questions, *i.e.* the risk for local recurrence and seeding throughout the leptomeninges. The myxopapillary type more often has its primary location in the cauda equina[283, 341], (2 personal observations), and the cellular type more often has anaplastic features[341].

Subependymoma, another variant of EPDY, has been reviewed by Scheithauer[371]: This mixed type of tumor consists of astrocytic and ependymal cells and structures. Amongst 95 reported cases 27% were located in the lateral ventricles and septum pellucidum and 71% in the Sylvian aqueduct or 4th ventricle, 2% in the cervicothoracic spinal cord. Subependymomas of the 4th ventricle often are asymptomatic except those adherent to its floor. The tumor may gain considerable size, 6 cm$\emptyset$ and more, and then invades surrounding structures. The presenting signs and symptoms are: mental changes, including memory loss, brain stem signs, and parkinsonian features. The operative mortality in subependymomas of the 4th ventricle is about 80%. 4% of IT tumors had subarachnoid spread. The tumor therefore is to be graded only guardedly as grade I[228].

Mabon *et al.*[259] published a grading system for EPDY and is presented here for its general applicability to brain gliomas[79, 382].

Grade I: normal ependymocytes with cilia and blepharoblasts; perivascular actiniform cell arrangement, pseudorosette formation, and papillary pattern well recognizable. No anaplasia or mitotic figures present.

Grade II: Early anaplastic transformation in some cells; moderate pleomorphism of cytoplasma and some nuclei with hyperchromatism. No mitoses.

Grade III: Anaplastic features of about 50% of the cells; some mitotic figures are present (at least one per high-power field).

Grade IV: Only remnants of the architectural pattern; normal appearing ependymocytes sparse. Anaplastic features prominent. Several mitoses per high-power field.

Mei Liu *et al.*[277] proposed a slightly different grading: I: regular tissue pattern: II: increased pleomorphism, cellularity and endothelial proliferation; III: anaplastic features with giant cell formation; IV: ependymoblastoma which cannot be differentiated from MBL or other PNETs. Cyst formation and calcification is present in 50–60% of all EPDYs; but gives no guidance in grading the tumor. In 25% of patients with EPDY the CSF contains tumor cells and sometimes even in clusters which tends to confirm the diagnosis[29, 221].

1. Supratentorial Ependymomas

⅓ of intracranial EPDYs are situated above the tentorium[35, 79, 84, 98, 128, 141, 151, 210, 229, 283, 317, 320, 394, 444]. They often grow to an enormous size. Their origin is thought to be from the ependymal lining of the ventricles or from remnants of the infolding neural tube which leaves them in a paraventricular site completely separated from the ventricular lumen. About 50% of ST EPDYs lie within one of the ventricles I–III[151]. From the septum pellucidum they protrude into the ventricular cavity as nodules or plaques; in a paraventricular situation they may distend cerebral convolutions[223, 341]. 10% have a biventricular location[151].

Signs and symptoms: The duration of the history varies from 2 weeks to 3 years[79, 84]. Signs of raised ICP prevail: headache, vomiting, increase of head circumference, palpable suture separation in some children[35, 79, 98, 151, 317]. Neck stiffness can be due to tentorial herniation or to recent spontaneous subarachnoid/intraventricular hemorrhage. Later this may lead to "sterile" meningitis[98, 151].

Many children with signs of raised ICP have papilledema; some of them with advanced hydrocephalus and even with visual failure and/or optic atrophy[35, 79, 84, 98, 151]. Hemiparesis and hemisensory deficit may be found, and seizures were reported in 25%[79, 84]. More often than the classical hemiparesis syndromes pseudocerebellar signs are found: gait ataxia and unilateral tremor of the limbs[151]. High grade EPDY more often present with seizures than low grade tumors because they invade the cerebral cortex earlier[98]. 38% of the patients with ST EPDY suffer from postoperatively epilepsy[35].

Diagnosis is established by plain X-ray of the skull which in 50% of the patients show increase of ICP and calcifications in 35%[79, 84, 204]. Angiographically there is more shift of the internal cerebral veins than displacement of the arteries[151]. A tumor blush may be seen in the early venous phase and newly formed vessels as in GLB[204]. Angiography can contribute much in the diagnosis of supratentorial EPDY prior to operation. CT often shows a tumor mass located near the foramen of Monro producing uni- or bilateral hydrocephalus. When the tumor is located within the trigone, its bulk often shifts the quadrigeminal plate from behind and laterally. The tumor by itself is not well delineated from the thalamus. Most of the ST EPDYs are hyperdense or mixed, only a few are isodense or hypodense; 80% have patchy enhancement after intravenous contrast[151, 204, 384]. Perifocal edema more often is seen in low grade than in high grade EPDY. Subependymomas are most often hypodense and enhance very little[204].

The grading of these ST tumors varies widely in different series which implies that uniform grading will be mandatory in the future: Diagnosis of high grade ST EPDY ranges from 15 to 86%[44]. In some pediatric series high grading of ST EPDYs prevails[79, 98, 151, 320]. In 20–60% they are associated with *leptomeningeal spread* which raises the question of prophylactic RT of the whole neuraxis. *Spinal subarachnoidal seeding* in children with ST EPDYs is found less often than with tumors in the IT location: 8–10%[79, 230]. Some authors give even lower figures or nil[151, 320, 435]. If postoperative myelography is performed routinely the percentage of positive findings rises to 23%[79].

Treatment

a) *Surgery:* In most cases of ST EPDY only subtotal removal of the tumor is possible owing to its size and high operative mortality: 15–20%[35, 84, 98, 223, 320, 341] which in intraventricular sites is even higher than in paraventricular locations[151].

b) *Radiotherapy:* Whole brain RTH is recommended by most authors irrespective of the grading[47, 265, 364, 390, 392]. Spinal axis irradiation in high grade ST tumors is an open question. In malignant ST EPDY the risk of seeding within the spinal canal is given between 20 and 50%[210, 230, 444]. Since most patients are in the young age group, growth deficit may occur after whole neuraxis RT. Spinal irradiation seems to be justified only in children who are symptomatic and/or have positive myelographic findings[281, 320, 435]. Therefore, in these children a close surveillance follow-up program is needed by doing myelography in 6, 18, and 36 months after the operation[230].

c) *Chemotherapy* in ST EPDY seems justified in high grade lesions[79], but its efficacy has not been proved[47]. Procarbacine, CCNU, VCR and MTX have been recommended by some authors[79, 320], whereas Shapiro[387] reported on positive results with BCNU and VM26. Our recommendation is to use the same protocol as in MBL. In recurrences, when reoperation or a 2nd course of RT are not possible, the "8 in 1 drug" regimen can be considered[44].

Prognosis in children with ST EPDYs is much worse than in adults[79, 165, 320]: Mean survival is 32 months[120]. 5-year-survival time was 20% for all grades in the Connecticut series[120] or is less[444]. In grade III/IV tumors it was 14%[98] or even nil[84]. Increase of malignancy was found in 50% in those patients who underwent a second operation[3]. Therefore in tumor recurrence the prognosis is much worse than initially. RT increases 5-year survival to 40–50% for all grades[47, 444], but this optimistic view is not shared by all authors[98].

2. Infratentorial Ependymomas

⅔ of intracranial EPDYs are located within the PF. Among IT tumors EPDYs therefore take the 3rd place after MBL and cerebellar ASCY[35, 79, 84, 98, 128, 141, 151, 210, 223, 229, 283, 317, 320, 394, 444]. In a combined series of 301 children with PF EPDYs low grading was given in 61% over/against a high grading in 39%[79, 98]. However, there is a great need for uniform neuropathological classification criteria of EPDYs, to be established[444].

EPDYs of the 4th ventricle are adherent to its floor in the caudal part of the rhombencephalon. In one series[84], 23% were adherent to the roof of the 4th ventricle. Most EPDYs grow by expansion and hide within the 4th ventricle in cauliflower-like fashion which can be demonstrated radiologically. A few tumors infiltrate the whole floor of the rhombencephalon. EPDYs may protrude rostrally into the aqueduct of Sylvius or caudally into the foramen of Magendi. The tumor may extend anterolaterally throughout the lateral recessus of the 4th ventricle towards the cerebellopontine angle[79, 84, 223, 281, 435]. Some EPDYs invade the cerebellar hemisphere(s)[84]. In a few cases the tumor protrudes through the foramen of Magendi to the cisterna magna and subarachnoid space and may fill the cervical canal or exceptionally even extend as far as the cauda equina[281, 319, 341, 435, 456].

Kricheff et al.[229] gave a surgical staging for IT EPDYs:

T 1 = tumor limited to the 4th ventricle,

T 2 = tumor reaches the cisterna magna,

T 3 = tumor has extended beyond the cisterna magna into the cervical subarachnoid space or into the cerebellopontine angle as well,

T 4 = gross invasion of the brain stem or cerebellum,

M = distant metastases throughout and/or outside the CNS.

Operative mortality increases from 6% in T 1/T 2 to 19% in T 3/T 4 while 5 years survival decreases from 90% to 19%[229].

Symptoms: The history may range from a few days to 3 years[35, 79, 223, 319], but extremes up to 6 years[84] or even 10 years[283] have been reported. Leading symptoms are headache and vomiting. Marked neck stiffness and/or tenderness of the neck muscles indicate extension of the tumor into the cervical canal[84, 223]. Visual failure is reported in 35% of the patients due to long-standing hydrocephalus and associated damage to the visual pathways[35].

Signs: Papilledema was seen in 40–63%[84, 98, 317], other CN involvement in 39–59%[84, 98, 317]. The CN most often involved are the VIth and VIIth, sometimes bilaterally. This occurs due to pressure of the tumor bulk exerted on the floor of the 4th ventricle at its intermediate portion (facial colliculus) where internally part of the facial nerve loops around the nucleus of the abducent nerve[79, 223, 319]. Next are the VIIIth (acoustic and vestibular parts) and the oculomotor nerves[84, 319]. CN impairments might be induced by pressure or by tumor invasion of the rhomboid fossa. Cerebellar signs and nystagmus are found in 30–40%[35, 79, 84, 98], and long tract signs in 20–30%[98]. Many of these children have muscular hypotonia and difficulties in supporting their own body weight.

Diagnosis: In children in whom a lumbar puncture was done for neck stiffness raised protein was found ranging from 50–2,000 mg/dl[35]. There may be a raised cell count, particularly in those children who had hemorrhage(s) within their tumor[98]. In 25% of children with EPDYs, tumor cells can be demonstrated in the CSF, in ST EPDYs more often than in IT lesions[29, 221]. In IT EPDYs plain X-rays of the skull show signs of raised ICP in about half of the cases, and in 10% tumor calcification is seen[84, 204].

In the unenhanced CT scan 13% of the lesions are hypodense, 9% isodense, 37% hyperdense, and 40% mixed. 50% have calcifying areas within the tumor, and in 83% there is marked enhancement after contrast[204, 384]. This might be patchy, less often homogeneous. A characteristic CT for an EPDY is a tumor with calcifications within the PF which is hard to distinguish from the brain stem and extends from the floor up to the quadrigeminal plate[204]. In 50% of these tumors there is a rim of fluid still to be seen around the tumor mass[384]. Ventriculography using positive contrast media is only necessary in very few cases: thereby the cauliflower-like structure of the mass within the 4th ventricle can be demonstrated,

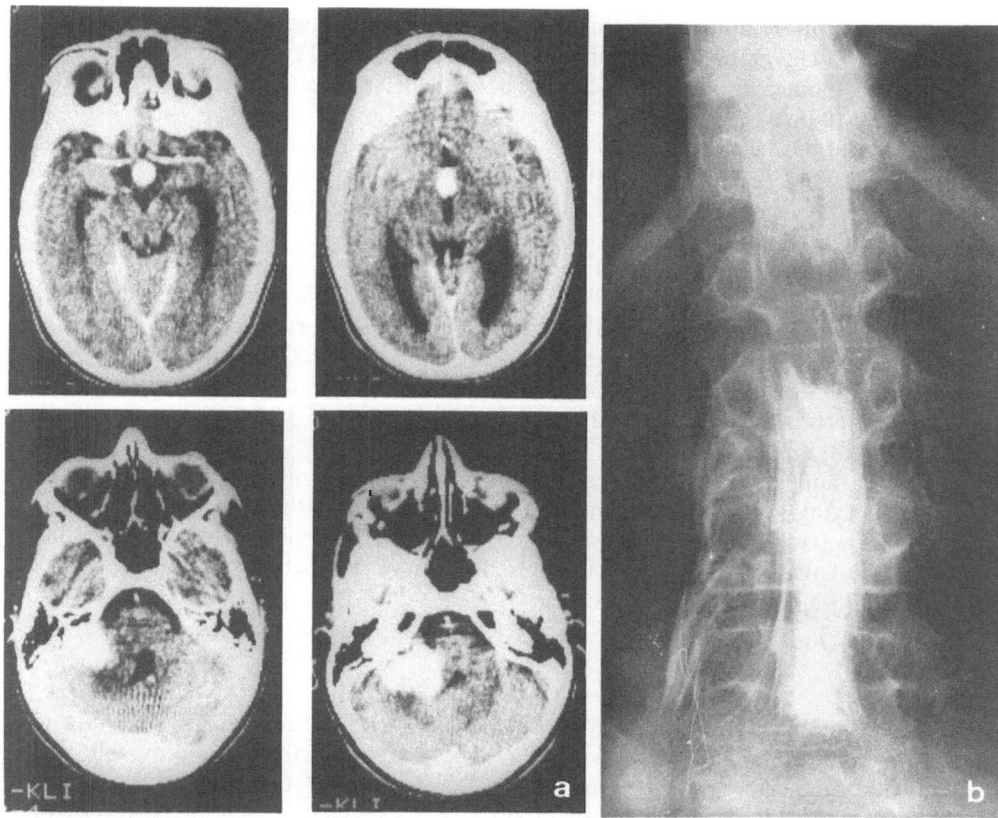

Fig. 7. Metastatizing myxopapillary EPDY in a girl, aged 11, who clinically had bad hearing and facial numbness for 1½ years and later developed hypothalamic obesity and severe back pain. Enhancing tumor mass in the left cerebellopontine angle, the hypothalamus (***a***) and in the lumbar subarachnoid space (***b***). The cerebellopontine angle-mass and the lumbar tumor was confirmed by separate surgical approaches

adherent to its floor or roof. If the rhomboid fossa is infiltrated, its wavy appearance is seen[204].

Displacement of vessels can be shown by vertebral angiography. The basilar artery is bowed anteriorly and pressed down upon the clivus, whereas the PICA is bent downward towards the occipital bone and the choroidal branches of the PICA may be stretched or even hypertrophied. Tumor vessels can arise from the medullary arteries[341]. The precentral cerebellar vein and the supraculminate venous system is shifted upward and anteriorly[284, 332].

Subarachnoid and extraneural seeding (Figs. 7 a and b): Like MBL and other highly malignant ST tumors IT EPDYs can seed along the entire neuraxis. The incidence of seeding is reported from zero[35] to 60%[444]. The frequency of their detection depends on the length of survival, and increases with the care with which one looks for it by routine postoperative lumbar punctures myelography, and routine CT-follow-up. In an autopsy series spinal seeding was reported in 30% of cases[444]. Clinical detection of spinal metastases in IT EPDYs ranges from 25%[230] to 34%[210]. If one compares the incidence of metastases according to the grade of the tumor the figures are:

Grade I/II: 12.5%[210]—15%[320]—20%[230].
Grade III/IV: 38.5%[210]—50%[320]—80%[230].

The incidence of seeding in EPDYs also depends on the extent of the RT[45, 47, 160, 265, 299, 392].

CSF metastases after treatment for PF EPDY can be found in the ST compartment as well[210, 230, 320, 444]. In 80% of the children with recurrence at the primary site of PF seeding in different compartments of the subarachnoid space can be demonstrated by CT after intravenous contrast[116]: They occur in the infratentorial compartment over the cerebellum, in the quadrigeminal and Sylvian fissure cisterns, and in the lateral ventricles. These radiological findings do not all have clinical correlation.

MBL and germ cell tumors[176, 252] most frequently metastasize outside the central nervous system. Next come the EPDYs. The sites of these deposits are: lungs and pleura, lymph nodes and bones[106, 149, 176, 252, 320]. The time of survival from the detection of an extraaxial metastasis until death may vary between 2 months and 10 years[252].

Treatment

a) *Surgery:* Before 1950, the perioperative mortality was as high as 50%[317, 341], but in modern series still is 20–36%[79, 84, 320]. Therefore, in many cases only subtotal removal of the bulky tumor is possible[223]. Total or subtotal removal of the tumor has no significance for the length of survival[283]. In some cases, if the tumor is adherent to the roof of the 4th ventricle or at the level of the aqueduct, operative problems may arise[84, 223]. Extraneural metastases are facilitated by systemic shunts[176, 435]; in some situations an internal shunting by a Leksell drain seems to be preferable[234, 369].

b) *Radiotherapy:* The major cause of death in EPDYs are local recurrences[210, 230], which may occur in 50% after 2 years and in 80% of cases after 4 years[230]. Therefore in this radiosensitive tumor high local irradiation (using more than 55 Gy) is recommended[210]; This applies to tumors of all grading and does not depend on the question of total or subtotal removal.

The question under discussion: is RT of the whole neuraxis indicated? Many of the children suffering from an IT EPDY are very young. Therefore RT of the whole brain and the spinal cord bears some impact on the further mental development and growth of the child. Some authors only recommend whole neuraxis RT in grade III/IV IT EPDY or if seeding to any location had been demonstrated by CT, myelography or CSF analysis[79, 223, 319, 394, 435]

On the other hand, the figures given above clearly are in favor of whole neuraxis RT in all IT EPDYs irrespective of grading and positive CSF or neuroradiological findings[141, 210, 320, 382]. Therefore only those low grade tumors within the 4th ventricle, in which total removal was achieved and close surveillance of the child is guaranteed as outlined for MBL, should local RT only be employed.

Perhaps, studies of the subtypes of EPDYs or of tissue tumor markers, *e.g.* neuron-specific enolase[444] will shed more light on the biological behavior of EPDYs and thereby offer more defined forms of combinations of CHT and RT.

c) *Chemotherapy: cf. CHT prognosis of MBL:* In general, the prognosis for IT EPDYs in children is worse than in adults. Without RT, after 5 years, only 25% of all grades are still alive, in high-grade lesions only 10%[79, 84, 98, 444].

After RT in adequate doses 5-year-survival rates will rise considerably: namely to 40–50%[210, 277, 283, 441] and, according other radiotherapists, even to as high as 70–80%[265, 435].

The surveillance for children with EPDYs of the PF will be discussed under MBL.

V. Tumors of the Pineal Region

Tumors of this area constitute 2.7% (Table 1), 4.5%[223], 9.4%[334], 10%[382], or even 11%[64] of all brain tumors in children. This different incidence in Western pediatric series may reflect local interests in the surgery of these tumors[64, 334]. However, this different incidence is also influenced by environmental and genetic factors. It is well known that germ cell tumors which are representative of tumors of this region, have a much higher incidence in Japan as compared to Western countries[15]. This is also true for craniopharyngioma[15].

According to Rubinstein[355] tumors of the pineal region are divided into 4 groups:

a) Derivatives from multipotential germ cells: these can differentiate into germinoma and embryonal carcinoma (ECA). This tumor again may form alternatively choriocarcinoma (CCA), endodermal sinus tumor (EST = yolk sac tumor) or mature teratoma, formed from the 3 germinal layers.

b) Tumors which stem from the true parenchyma of the pineal gland: the differentiated pineocytoma (PCY) and the anaplastic pinealoblastoma (PBL) which belongs to the PNETs.

c) Glioma and ganglioneuroma of all grades of malignancy.

d) Others: dermoid and epidermoid, chemodectoma, meningioma of the tela chorioidea or the tentorial hiatus, cysts, lipoma, or vascular tumors.

Most authors do not or only slightly diverge from this concept[78, 79, 91, 92, 193, 195, 282, 284, 301, 339, 373, 374, 427, 442, 455].

Two facts seem to be important if the clinician makes the diagnosis of a tumor within the pineal region:

a) There are some benign tumors, but more often they are highly malignant: all germ cell tumors are grade IV except mature teratomas. PBL are grade IV tumors, as are some dedifferentiated gliomas. Some of the malignant tumors are highly radiosensitive, others are not.

b) Germ cell tumors are usually "mixed": the germinoma may harbour islets of CCA or EST, teratoma often embody highly malignant germ cell tissue as well, according to Jellinger[191] in up to 30%[301, 373, 417, 427]. This peculiarity of a teratoma makes it quiescent for many years but, at a certain point, the lesion explodes[92, 334]. Some authors claim that 80–90% of pineal tumors are germinomas[382, 456, 457]. In order to confirm or refute this we collected 457 cases of pineal area tumors from 16

Western series [64, 71, 91, 193, 195, 282, 295, 301, 334, 342, 364, 373, 409, 442, 449, Table 1] compared with
the histological findings of 216 patients of 2 Japanese series [367, 427]. Nearly all
patients were mixed groups of adults and children.

Histology	Western S. N.: 457	Japanese S.N.: 216
Germinoma ("2 cell type")	174 (= 38.0%)	132 (= 61.1%)
Teratoma and teratoid tumors	104 (= 22.8%)	46 (= 21.3%)
Pineal parenchyma tumors: PCY, PBL	69 (= 15.0%)	9 (= 4.2%)
Glioma group	90 (= 19.7%)	23 (= 10.6%)
Others	20 (= 4.5%)	6 (= 2.8%)

From these figures one draws 3 conclusions:

a) Only $2/5$ (Western series) or $3/5$ (Japanese series) of all pineal region tumors
are highly radiosensitive (= germinomas). 60% (30%) of the patients need no RT
or RT in higher dosage and with more extended fields of irradiation (PBL).

b) If one makes the diagnosis of a tumor of the pineal region one's aim should
be to have adequate histological confirmation of the diagnosis.

c) True pineal parenchyma tumors are rare, in Japan even more so than in
Western countries [15, 220, 427]. Germ cell tumors are found more often in Japan than in
Europe and in the USA.

Biological function of the pineal gland: There is still some controverse about the
neuroendocrine function of the pineal gland. Its end product, melatonin (ME), is
derived from serotonin. The final step in this biochemical process is catalyzed by the
enzyme hydroxy-indole-O-methyl transferase (HIOMT). Barber *et al.*[32, 33] found
elevated ME-levels in the serum of patients with tumors of the pineal parenchyma
(PCY and PBL). The HIOMT activity measured in the tumor tissue of one of their
patients was very low, 5–7fold lower than that of controls. The diurnal rhythmicity
for ME formation was retained with low values during day-time and high levels at
night. However, elevated levels of ME in the serum also were reported in patients
with pineal germinoma and ectopic germinoma [220, 335]. In addition, high ME levels
were also seen in the serum of patients with different cerebral conditions, like brain
malformations or chronic extracerebral hematoma [23]. In the patients, the diurnal
rhythmicity was retained, but the physiologic ME peaks were shifted from 24 hours
to 3–6 a clock AM.

All these findings are difficult to interpret: It is not clear that ME has an
antigonadal function as suggested by some authors [281, 234]. If it had, hypogonadism
should be present in a ME-producing tumor and vice versa hypergonadism or
precocious puberty in susceptible ages when the pineal parenchyma has been
destroyed. A different hypothesis [281, 334, 373] suggests that if a disease process (tumor,
hydrocephalus, inflammation, trauma) has isolated the pineal gland from its
sympathetic innervation namely from the superior cervical ganglion there will be
enhanced ME secretion.

An interesting aspect of ME function is that in the first years of life there are
high ME levels which decrease up to puberty. By this decrease testosterone levels
are controlled [338].

The clinical symptoms and signs of pineal area tumors already have been discussed (see p. 406). If a pineal tumor is suspected the following *diagnostic* procedures need to be undertaken:

1. *X-rays of the skull:* The pineal gland is only rarely calcified in young children: 0–4 years: 0%, 5–8 years: 3%, 9–12 years: 12.7%, 13–16 years: 18.9%, 17–20 years: 43%[455]. In colored people the pineal never calcifies except in disease[334].

For these reasons, a calcified pineal gland in a child under 10–12 years old *per se* is a finding which needs closer investigation. Tumors in the pineal region in children calcify in 25–75%[79, 250]. The size of the field of calcification within tumors varies from 2×2 to 16×22 mm[250]. Values exceeding 10×10 mm are always pathological[153]. In addition, in many of the tumor calcifications there is shift anterior-inferiorly[250]; an inferior shift means that obstructive hydrocephalus is likely to be found[153]. All kinds of pineal tumors can calcify: germinomas, teratomas, gliomas[79, 153, 204, 284, 332, 334, 455].

2. *Cerebral angiography:* The neurosurgeon needs to have information of the deep venous system and the posterior choroidal arteries. Knowledge the displacement of these vascular structures helps him to decide which approach he will select[284, 332, 334, 408, 309]. Arterial feeders to pineal tumors can be the posterior choroidal arteries, branches of the superior cerebellar arteries, and the perforating mesencephalic vessels[79, 284, 301]. The posterior choroidal arteries can be shifted or kinked anteriorly, dissociated in the lateral views or pushed posteriorly[223, 284, 332]. The tip of the basilar artery can be pressed downward towards the posterior clinoid processes. Sometimes, the superior cerebellar arteries are bowed inferiorly and the 2 P 2 segments of the posterior cerebral arteries are widened forming an arch around the distended mesencephalic part of the brainstem. The vein of the splenium of corpus callosum can be elevated and/or bowed (due to hydrocephalus) and stretched. A blush is sometimes seen in PBL and malignant teratoma. These are highly vascularized tumors which can be diagnosed by means of angiography[195] (Figs. 8 a and b).

CT: Pineal tumors are either hypodense, rarely isodense, and in most cases mixed hyperdense lesions[79, 135, 204, 301, 373, 455]. The tumor can embody small cysts[455]. Nearly all pineal tumors have diffuse or irregular contrast enhancement, and in some of them infiltration of the walls of the 3rd lateral ventricles, and also the subarachnoid space in both the ST and IT compartments may be seen[111, 153, 195, 204, 301, 373, 384, 455]. This is most often encountered in germinomas, but also in PBL and other highly malignant germ cell tumors[195, 284, 301]. Calcifications within the tumor and marked hypodense areas are in favor of a teratoma[135]. Germinoma can be demonstrated by NMR[301], (personal observation), but the altered BBB within the tumor itself and its surrounding tissues cannot be studied by this method until there is the possibility of using contrast enhancement.

4. *CSF:* Increased cell counts are found in many patients with pineal tumors particularly in those with germinomas[29, 79, 334, 382]. According to some authors[29, 373] positive findings were made preoperatively in germinomas in 60–90%. They are more often positive when ventricular CSF is examined than lumbar. In germinomas, isolated cells or clusters of them are found with lymphocyte-like cells and cells which are rich in plasma and have prominent nucleoli; these cells have good orange staining in their cell plasma indicating high RNA activity as shown by

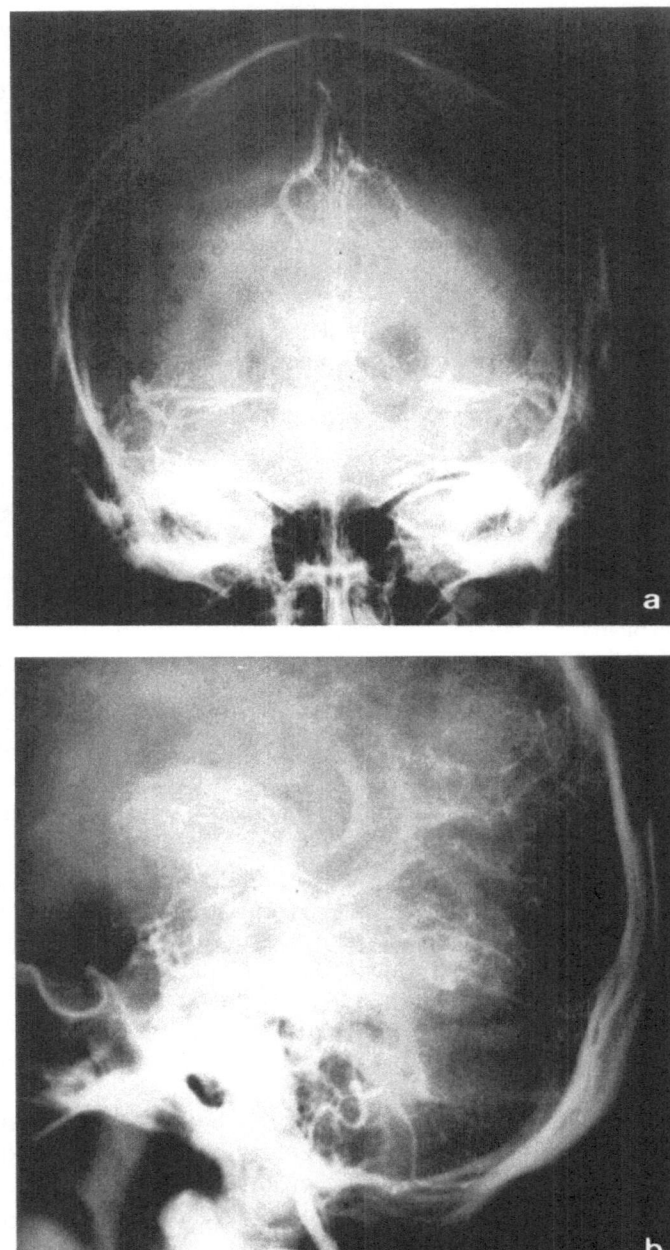

Figs. 8 a and **b.** Malignant teratoma in a $14^{10}/_{12}$-years-old girl. The pineal area tumor blushes in the late arterial phase

acridine orange fluorescence microscopy[113, 221]. In PBL, giant cells, nuclear pleomorphism in cell clusters, and mitotic figures may be seen; protoplasmatic extensions are demonstrated by interference phase microscopy[221].

5. *Tumor markers:* In pineal and suprasellar region tumors two tumor markers are known: β-HCG (= beta fraction of the human chorionic gonadotrophin) and AFP (= alpha-fetoprotein). The statement that CSF concentrations of these markers are superior than serum levels makes it very likely that tumor tissue producing these substances is close to the subarachnoid space. It rather indicates: primary tumor of the CNS and not extraneural tumor seeding within the CNS.

β-HCG is synthetized by the giant cells of the syncytiotrophoblast[4, 297, 301, 306, 417]. β-HCG is produced by ECA and CCA tissue elements and if those are present in germinoma[64, 79, 189, 195, 196, 295, 427]. AFP droplets were demonstrated in Schiller-Duval bodies of EST[31, 288, 297, 406, 417]. They were found with malignant teratomas, ECA, and EST. If the 2 tumors markers β-HCG and AFP are raised markedly in the CSF, a malignant teratoma will be the most likely diagnosis[79, 297, 301].

The percentage of patients with germinomas and elevated β-HCG values in the CSF is given as 14%[4]. The question remains unanswered whether these patients harbor "pure" germinoma or whether they belong to the "mixed" group in whom germinoma tissue embodies ECA and or CCA tissue components as well[191]. Some authors had negative findings in germinoma for β-HCG[9, 220]. The practical value of elevated β-HCG levels in the CSF (as well as AFP measurements) is that this finding means increased resistance to RTH[31, 301, 335, 373].

To sum up these controversial findings with regard to tumor markers for germ cell tumors of the CNS: raised β-HCG levels in the CSF indicate that this tumor contains elements of ECA or CCA[9, 79, 113, 132, 139, 334, 335, 373] and for AFP that yolk sac elements or ECA tissue will be within this tumor and that germinoma is not likely to be the diagnosis[4, 9, 31, 64, 79, 113, 288, 297, 301, 334, 335, 417, 427]. Previously high levels of the tumor markers normalize 2–3 weeks after RT[306]. In extraneural metastases of germ cell tumors the markers can be greatly elevated in the serum[139, 389] but may even be normal[137].

In suprasellar or double-midline germinoma there can be prolactinemia and/or raised prolactin values in the CSF. This is explained by destruction of brain tissue which produces PIF (= prolactine inhibiting factor). In the future, therefore prolactine may be another marker for some germinomas or other intrinsic suprasellar tumors[113, 306].

Clinical Remarks on Tumors of the Pineal Region

1. Germ Cell Tumors

All germ cell tumors[420] have a male preponderance but this varies with some authors: 2/1[442], 3–3.5/1[220, 334, 456, 457], 4.25/1 for EST[31], 7/1[15, 90, 301], and even 13/1[427] or 14/1[367]. In suprasellar germinomas the sex ratio is quite different: about 1/1[68, 219, 418], and only Dayan[90] had a 3/1 ratio.

a) *Germinoma:* This is the tumor most often encountered in the pineal or suprasellar region. Most tumors lie in a midline position and can secondarily invade the structures of the rostral brain stem[228]. In order to ascertain the different sites of intracranial germinomas we collected 656 germinomas from 9 series of the literature[4, 90, 193, 219, 220, 323, 367, 414, 427]:

Primary site	Number of germinomas N: 656	(%)
Pineal area	443	(67.6)
Suprasellar region/3rd ventricle	159	(24.2)
Double midline (suprasellar and pineal area)	27	(4.1)
Thalamus/basal ganglia/lateral ventricles/hemisphere	27	(4.1)

Exceptional sites are: intrasellar (neurohypophysis)[306, 323].
Cerebellopontine angle[4, 367]—mesencephalon/pons[68, 79, 90].

Germinoma may extend underneath the ependyma of the 3rd ventricle thus producing schizophrenia-like clinical symptoms[90]. In some tumors the primary site may be hidden by its widespread primary radiological presentation. Often there is extensive spread along the CSF pathways with local invasion of caudal structures like the Sylvian aqueduct, midbrain or pons[90]. Within the tumor margin active phagocytosis and T-lymphocytes have been recognized[79, 335]. Marked cellular reaction is sometimes linked with prolonged survival[191].

Germinomas located in the *pineal region* may produce symptoms within 10 days and up to 2 years with a mean of 3 months[91, 92, 195, 414].

Suprasellar germinomas have very important endocrine symptoms: diabetes insipidus present in 45–100% in different series. This might be the only symptom from 4 months up to 4 years[68, 91, 195, 323, 339]. Other endocrine symptoms reported are precocious puberty in 3.5%[373], 7%[68] up to 13% if teratomas were included[414]. If precocious puberty is of central origin, the most frequent causes are a tumor of the hypothalamus, followed by hamartoma of the tuber cinereum, obstructive hydrocephalus and, finally, a pineal region tumor[195, 281]. 25–31% of the children present with retarded growth[68, 79, 339, 414]. Obesity/polyphagia was found in 13%[414] and 32% developed a syndrome of emacication[79, 223, 414].

Suprasellar germinoma may be linked with Klinefelter syndrome[5, 355]. Various other hypothalamic features have been reported: instability to keep the body temperature constant and excessive hypernatremia[68, 79, 91, 223] which can be fatal[195].

A second group of signs in suprasellar germinomas are visual: visual field defects, heteronomous hemianopsias, optic atrophy. Disturbed vision is a complaint[79, 91, 223] in up to 95% of patients[68].

From the surgical point of view[68, 78, 200] it is important to know that suprasellar germinoma can

a) be contiguous with the pineal area and thus fill the whole posterior part of the third ventricle. These tumors infiltrate the hypothalamus, the hypophysis and the optic chiasm from behind,

b) occupy the third ventricle at first. Hydrocephalus, therefore, is an early finding; the hypothalamus and infundibulum are invaded later,

c) originate primarily within the optic chiasm and then expand into the chiasmal cistern or into the interpeduncular fossa.

Germinomas of *other primary sites* present very differently: when located in the thalamus/basal ganglia by slowly progressive hemiplegia, often with dysphasic symptoms and personality changes[68, 219, 367, 402], (1 personal observation);

as frontal or patietal lobe tumor[367] or as a tumor of the lateral ventricle[191, 367] or as an intrinsic tumor of the pons/mesencephalon[68, 79] or the cerebellopontine angle[4, 367].

Seeding of germinomas along the CSF pathways in an autopsy collection of 117 cases was reported in 70%[90]: 53% of these seeded anteriorly into the third ventricle and hypothalamus, 22% into the lateral ventricles, and 13% each into the Sylvian aqueduct/fourth ventricle and into the spinal theca.

Clinically, in suprasellar germinoma spinal seeding was reported in 12% and 5% in the subarachnoid spaces anywhere[68]. The incidence of spinal metastasis seems to be different: in 16 suprasellar germinomas it was 37% and in 61 germinomas of the pineal region only 10%[414]. It was 1.7% in nonbiopsied versus 14% in biopsied series[442]. In another series, the difference between nonbiopsied and biopsied cases was 10% versus 36%[414].

The important question how often germinomas seed along the CSF axis is answered by clinicians in a different way: Sano and Matsutani[367] had only 5% spinal seeds after surgery in 60 patients, Jenkin had 13% among 31 patients[193], Jooma and Kendall[195] reported on 17% with spinal and 12% with supratentorial subarachnoidal dissemination among 35 patients. Abay and Laws[1] had 48% local recurrences and 23% spinal metastases among 27 patients; these authors stress that seeding anywhere in the neuraxis had taken place in all patients who were younger than 6 years. Kun et al.[230] commented on 148 germinomas proven by histology and all treated by RT: There were local recurrences in 16%, subarachnoid dissemination in 24% which split up into 14% within the spinal theca and 10% within the ST leptomeningeal space.

Extraneural metastases from all types of germ cell tumors take the second place after MBL among pediatric brain tumors[176]: 14/114 children with brain tumors and extraneural metastases proven by histology (= *12.2%*). Shunt metastases are possible[137, 295, 334]. Extraneural deposits may occur at the site of craniotomy or are due to hematogeneous spread. Most often they are located in the lungs, next are the lymph nodes, pleura, bones, liver, and bone marrow[79, 91, 106, 137, 139]. In the serum of those patients raised β-HCG levels have been reported[339]. EST metastasize via shunt system in 20%[31, 137] and may raise serum AFP levels. Prolonged survival up to 4–13 years has been reported after extraneural metastases of germ cell tumors treated by combined RT/CHT, but most patients succumb within a few months[137, 339].

Staging: A staging system for intracranial germinomas and teratomas was proposed by James and Edwards[187]:

T 1 = diameter less than 5 cm, tumor located in the pineal or suprasellar region, within the sella (germinoma), or within one of the ventricles 1–4 (teratoma).

T 2 = diameter of the tumor greater than 5 cm.

T 3 = tumor encroaches or invades the third ventricle.

T 4 = tumor extends anteriorly or into the middle cranial fossa—double midline tumor.

Mo = no macroscopic subarachnoid or hematogeneous spread.

M 1 = tumor cells in the CSF.

M 2 = macroscopic seedlings in the lateral ventricles or in the ST subarachnoid space.

M 3 = Nodular seedlings in the spinal subarachnoid space.

M 4 = Extraneural metastases.

The size and location of a germ cell tumor is important for both the length and quality of survival: Small midline tumors have a favorable prognosis, while both double midline and laterally situated large tumors are associated with (early) recurrence and/or poor quality of life[427].

Recurrences in patients with germinomas most often occur 2–5 years after the diagnosis and are followed by death within the next 2 years[139, 295, 339, 442]. Recurrences have been reported up to 14 years[427] and even 15 years[335].

b) *Teratomas:* 50–70% of intracranial teratomas lie in the pineal region[15, 427], other sites are the hypothalamus, sellar region, and posterior fossa[189]. The tumor may contain fat tissue (neutral fat, cholesterol) which gives hypodensity in the CT scan (60–90 Houndsfield units). Malignant teratomas may contain sarcomatous, carcinomatous or highly malignant germ cell tissue elements: germinoma, CCA, ECA, EST[191, 193, 419]. All these malignant parts of a teratoma can grow very rapidly and invasively after a period of dormancy rest[91, 92, 334]. 30%[189] or above[373] of the intracranial teratomas are malignant. Both the pineal germinoma and teratoma have a high preponderance for the male sex[15, 373, 427]. Recurrence after operative or combined treatment can be seen within a few months up to 2 years[230, 339, 427].

c) *Embryonal carcinomas (ECA)* are nondifferentiated embryonic tumors with malignant features: they invade adjacent tissues and seed extensively along the CSF pathways[9, 301, 334, 419]. Recurrences are frequent after a few months[9, 301, 334]. Survival for 2–7 years has been reported after combined treatment: operation—RTH for the whole neuraxis—CHT by MTX-HD, vincristine, adriblastine, and cyclophosphamide[301].

d) *Choriocarcinoma (CCA)* clinically either presents with precocious puberty[9, 132] or spontaneous subarachnoid hemorrhage[132]. Reports on "pure" intracranial CCA are rare.

e) *Endodermal sinus tumors (EST = yolk sac tumor)* most often have been reported as "pure" tumors amongst these "highly" malignant germ cell tumors[9, 31, 137, 191, 288, 373, 406, 419]. EST are very invasive, metastasize along the CSF pathways and extraaxially. 7 out of 10 patients with EST died within days or weeks after operation[288]. Although a positive response to RT can be monitored on the CT follow-up, the tumor soon recurs[71]. Of the 18 patients collected by Tavcar *et al.*[419] 17 died within 20 months after diagnosis. Since the tumor is resistant to RT several chemotherapeutic regimen have been recommended: the "Einhorn" scheme: vinblastine, bleomycin, and cisplatinum[79], a combination of vincristine, actinomycin-D, cyclophosphamide, and 5-fluorouracil[288], vincristine, dactinomycine, and cyclophosphamide[31], and MTX-HD[301]. Unfortunately, actinomycin-D adds to mental retardation in those patients who underwent high dose RT[301].

Altogether, 30%[191] up to 50%[419] of these highly malignant germ cell tumors are mixed just as teratomas and germinomas may be. During lifetime, this only may be recognized by the finding of elevated tumor markers in the CSF, particularly if there was no tumor removal possible. All germ cell tumors of this category are grade IV, but the highly malignant germ cell tumors are less radiosensitive than the germinomas and most aggressive additional CHT may be given.

2. Tumors Derived from Pineal Parenchyma

The phylogenetically old function of the pineal gland in fish and amphibia is that of a photoreceptor organ; in reptilia and lower vertebrates it has an intermediate photoreceptor *and* neuroendocrine function[168]. For this reason combinations of the genetic form of bilateral retinoblastoma (RBL) and pinealoblastoma (PBL) may occur in the same patient[28].

Of patients with unilateral RBL 15% have dominant inheritance, with bilateral RBL it is 100%; therefore 40% of all RBL are autosomally dominant[217]. The inherited RBL manifests itself earlier at the age of 15 months, whereas the noninherited forms are symptomatic by 30 months on average[217]. RBL is a highly malignant tumor which spreads along the visual pathways and seeds along the CSF pathways. It may be impossible to differentiate RBL from ST PNETs or IT MBL without knowledge of the primary site of the tumor[144, 168, 223].

In addition to the "trilateral" RBL[28], bilateral RBL in a baby with PBL diagnosed some years later in the same child revealed also other chromosomal anomalies[197]: trisomy X (47-XXX) and subband deletion of chromosome 13[453]. These chromosomal anomalies clinically manifested themselves by mild or moderate, nonspecific developmental delay[197, 453] and therefore have to be looked for. Even without RTH, there is increased risk for a child to develop hepatoblastoma or osteosarcoma of the orbit after removal of an eye for RBL[2].

a) *Pinealoblastoma (PBL):* These tumors resemble pineal parenchyma of the 28th to the 34th week of gestation[220]; the grade of malignancy is always IV[58, 168, 228, 373]. There may be no[168, 220] or only minimal[58], pineocytic[168], neuronal or ependymal[407] differentiation in PBL. There is agreement that PBL with retinoblastomatous differentiation has a very rapid course[168, 407]. In some of these tumor cells photoreceptor-like processes may be found[407]. All patients with PBL had a short clinical course: they are younger than patients with PCY and have a shorter history ranging from 3 to 24 months, 6 months on average[58]. In 50% or even more cases, these tumors extensively seed along the CSF pathways[58, 71, 91, 168, 230, 334, 407, 427]. Melanin-containing cells in PBL produce the most extensive metastases[168, 407], whereas pineocytic or astrocytic differentiation indicate longer survival but radioresistance and local expansion[168].

b) *Pineocytoma (PCY):* The history in these tumors is longer ranging from 4 months to 8 years[58]. Most patients are adults and only few are children[58, 168]. The tumor resembles the pineal gland at the age of the 2nd to 4th month of extrauterine life and can show neuroblastoma-like and pineal-like structures[220]. If there is no astrocytic differentiation a malignant behavior of the tumor and a short clinical course can be expected[168], whereas other types of tumor with neuronal and neuronal plus astrocytic differentiation have a longer course with much less invasiveness and leptomeningeal spread. These more benign tumors (grade I/II)[58,

[228] displace normal structures and may fill the third ventricle[91, 92]. They clinically may present as progressive dementia[58]. Some PCY invade the subependymal linings[58, 91]. Disseminated growth was found in 4/17 cases ($= 28\%$)[168].

Treatment of Tumors of the Pineal Region

a) *Surgery:* As operative mortality was as high as 30–60%[79, 91, 180, 325], most authors have not recommended surgery in pineal region tumors, until more recently[1, 78, 79, 91, 144, 223, 374, 442]. Only shunt insertion was advocated, followed by RT, since 70% of pineal tumors were found to be radiosensitive[47, 79, 299, 335, 364, 442]. An intermediate position was taken by Jooma and Kendall[195]: first RT up to 30 Gy but, if the tumor was not reduced in size as judged by CT, then surgical exploration was considered. This conservative attitude has changed[232, 408, 409]. Today exposure of the pineal area either by the supracerebellar infratentorial or the occipito-transtentorial approach has a primary mortality of 3–5%[295, 306, 334, 409] or even zero[64, 71, 195, 367]. Hence, the mortality of surgery of the pineal region today is not higher than in other tumor site[373]. Postoperative complications include upward gaze paresis in 13%[64] due to impairment of the corticotectal fibers[325, 334] and transient hemianopsia in 20%[64].

Recommendations for the choice of approach to the pineal are determined by deep venous displacements[334]: in upward displacement IT supracerebellar approach—in downward displacement Dandy's posterior transcallosal parasagittal approach—in dorsal displacement of the supraculminate cerebellar vein: ST occipital transtentorial approach. Already Suzuki and Iwabuchi[415] stressed that steroid administration lowers the postoperative complication rate considerably. This finding has been confirmed by many authors[64, 195, 334, 427]. If removal of a pineal tumor is intended a piecemeal reduction is better than total resection where the deep cerebral veins are in danger of being severed[427].

Two reasons for open surgery rather than stereotactic biopsy have already been mentioned: 20–30% of all pineal tumors are benign lesions which are radioresistant. 30–50% of germ cell tumors are mixed lesions[191, 419].

b) *Chemotherapy:* In our opinion CHT should be given prior to RT in pineal tumors as in other malignancies of the CNS[12]. The choice of the cytostatic drugs is not made according to their prospective permeability of the BBB, since pineal area tumors are not subject to the BBB. In germinoma and other germ cell tumors the "Einhorn" protocol is advocated by most authors: vinblastine, bleomycin, cisplatin[139, 295, 301, 339]. We have used this protocol since 1979 in germinomas of the CNS. Allen[12] recommended ⅓ dose reduction for RT after the use of CHT by cyclophosphamide-HD (60–80 mg/kg body weight.) or by the combination of vinblastine, cyclophosphamide, bleomycin and cisplatin. Reduction of RT dosage should not be made if one of the tumor markers was elevated in the CSF, or the serum (vide supra).

Recurrences of germinoma have been successfully treated by the Einhorn protocol[396]. CHT in PBL as in other PNETs is given before RT using MTX-HD or any other protocol as administered for MBL.

c) *Radiotherapy:* In all malignant tumors of the pineal region, *i.e.* germinomas, malignant teratomas, ECA, CCA, EST, and PBL today whole neuraxis RT is recommended[1, 47, 64, 79, 193, 195, 301, 339, 367, 414, 455]. All these tumors are of grade IV and disseminate in 9–30% of cases into the spinal theca[47]. Irradiation of the spinal theca alone in patients with positive myelographic findings or positive CSP cytology is recommended by a few authors[1, 9, 382] or in patients older than 6 years.

Results of Combined Treatment

Survival rates over 5 years after adequate RT are 70–80% and for more than 10 years 60–70%[47, 79, 193, 334, 339, 364, 414, 442]. Even more optimistic are the figures of 80–90% survival rates for 5 and 10 years, and of 70% for 15 years are given by Rao and Medini[335] and Sano and Matsutani[367].

As far as quality of survival is concerned, in 14% of patients visual failure and 18% some neurological impairment is present[367]. 25% of irradiated patients had recent memory loss in the long-term follow-up[339]. According to Ueki and Tanaka[427] the quality of survival depends on 2 factors: the extent of the tumor and its primary site, and the adequacy of RT dosage.

VI. Primitive Neuro-ectodermal Tumors (PNETs)

Here are included ST MBLs, cerebral neuroblastomas, nondifferentiated small cell neoplasms, unclassified gliomas, medulloepitheliomas[202]. The term PNET was introduced in 1973 by Hart and Early[163] for a variety of tumors consisting of strains of nondifferentiated cells resembling fetal neuroblasts. These cells may undergo differentiation towards ependymoblasts, astroblasts, oligodendroblasts, or even retinal elements[79, 105, 163, 314]. The processes of these cells do not from tight junction[263] which means that they show marked enhancement after intravenous contrast on the CT examination, as their BBB is damaged. PNETs are soft tumors, more or less well demarcated from the brain tissue, often lobulated, hemorrhagic, necrotic and/or calcified[79, 163, 202, 227]. Their common sites are: the cerebral hemispheres, third ventricle, rostral brain stem and spinal cord[163, 202, 227, 263, 314]. They may seed widely throughout the CSF pathways as often as GLB do[314], and produce extraneural metastases to the lungs, lumph nodes and liver[176]. Most patients die from the primary tumor or its local recurrence.

PNETs have been described in stillborn babies and up to the age of 24 years. Most patients were in the first decade of life. The history in most patients is short and ranges from a few weeks to months. However, it was 6 years in one of our patients who had RT for pilocytic ASCY of the rostral brain stem and later presented with progressive neuroendocrinological and mental symptoms, changes in the CT findings revealed a PNET proven by biopsy.

Signs of raised ICP, increased head circumference, uncontrollable seizures, hemiplegia and altered consciousness have been reported as the most frequent clinical findings[79, 105, 163, 202, 227]. At operation, there is marked peritumoral swelling of the brain[202], (personal observation of medulloepithelioma). Postoperative CHT with MTX, VCR, CCNU, and procarbacine[79, 105, 227] and RT have been recommended, and may prolong life up to 2 years. Immunotherapy should be discussed in the future[314].

VII. Medulloblastoma (MBL)

According to most authors MBL takes 2nd place after ASCY amongst brain tumors of childhood: 18–28% the different series[19, 75, 120, 146, 357, 400] (Table 1). Some authors even allocate to MBL the first place: Heiskanen (Finland)[165] 23%, Bertold et al. (GFR)[39] 40%.

The annual incidence is nearly identical given by King and Sagerman (1979) as: 3 : 500,000 in the U.S.A.[211] and by Heiskanen[165] 2–3 : 600,000 for Finland.

Although most MBL seem to occur sporadically, some familial cases have been reported including seven pathologically proved pairs and six clinically diagnosed siblings[75]. Adding some new cases, Tijssen et al.[425] gave the figures of 4 female pairs of identical twins and 14 pairs of siblings, 9 of whom were males. There is no report in the literature that other members of one family were affected except siblings; among these familial reports on MBL some details are worth mentioning: onset of illness in both siblings[31, 41] and twins[152] at an identical age; at different ages however if their development has been different[242, 433]; in these cases the retarded twin[242] had clinical symptoms years earlier. In addition, cases occurring in one family have the tendency to present in the first year of life (congenital neoplasms). They have a high incidence of seeding and high grade of malignancy[37, 41, 152, 433]. In addition to the tendency of MBLs to occur in siblings, there are some further references to genetic factors and associated morbid conditions in the same patient: MBL can be observed in patients with retinoblastoma[211], nephroblastoma, carcinoma of the adrenal (1 personal observation of each), von Recklingshausen disease, Louis Bar's disease, congenital ichthyosis[75, 425]. MBL also occurred in children who had malformation of the CNS: agenesis of the vermis cerebelli, spina bifida, and syringomyelia. MBL and other brain tumors like ASCY, ganglioglioma, optic glioma, meningioma, and intracranial epidermoid were observed to occur in the same individual[75, 425].

MBL are thought to be derivatives of medulloblasts of the velum medullare anterior and posterior[281, 355–358, 361] which migrate to form the external granular layer in the midline position of the vermis cerebelli, of the cerebellar hemispheres laterally. 80% of MBL are situated in a midline position. These cells which are remnants of the neural tube formation, under normal circumstances, disappear by the 12th months of extrauterine life. Why these cell nests do not disintegrate but, in a few individuals, have abundant growth potential, remains unexplained today. In congenital MBL, embryonal medulloblasts proliferate into the molecular layer of the cerebellum[199, 357]. The medulloblastic cells induce a mesodermal proliferation of connective tissue which, according to most authors, is reactive: "desmoplastic reaction"[167], but according to others[156] indicates that the MBL develops from the meninx primitiva.

As the "medulloblast" is a multipotential embryonal cell it is not surprising that in some tumors there are cells differenting along astrocytic, spongioblastic, oligodendrocytic, ependymal, and neuronal lines[167, 261, 308, 315, 356–358]. The differentiation into 2 or even more cell lines is characteristic for PNETs[308, 343, 345, 356].

The clinical importance of differentiation of some cells in a malignant tumor is not fully understood even today: does for instance neuronal differentiation mean prolonged survival[308] or resistance to RT? 4 kinds of astrocytes were found in MBL[343] some of which are tumor cells and others reactive proliferating astrocytes.

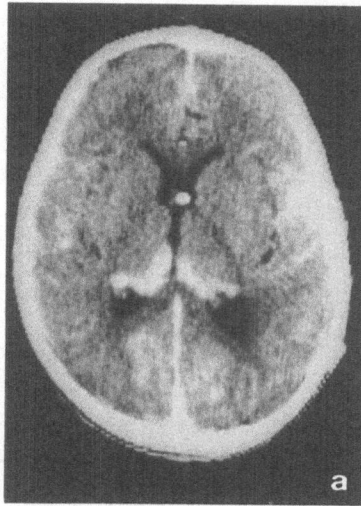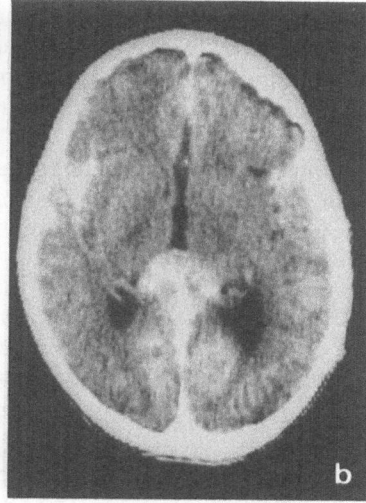

Figs. 9 a and **b.** Explosive tumor spread 3 weeks after operation of the midline of PF in boy, aged 4¹⁰⁄₁₂ for cerebellar MBL, classical type. There is ST spread seen after enhancement in the thalami in the Sylvian and quadrigeminal cisterns

Astrocytic neoplastic proliferation is one problem in modern radio- and chemotherapy which still remains solved, whereas astrocytic reaction can be transient reversible and not a disease condition *per se*. Neuronal differentiation was linked with very unfavorable clinical course in 2 of 3 very young children[315].

MBL have a higher labeling index of H 3-thymidine[181, 182]: 11–14.4% in midline position and 8% within the cerebellar hemisphere. In anaplastic ASCY the labeling index was found 4% and in GLB: 9.3%. Operative decompression sometimes results in explosive tumor regrowth which can be demonstrated clinically by CT scanning and NMR[116, 303, 375, 3] (own observations). This may also happen in ST ASCY (Figs. 9 a and b).

From the clinicians' point of view it seems important that some MBL grow "en plaques": There is wide-spread subpial infiltration of the granular layer and the Purkinje cells throughout the vermis and both cerebellar hemispheres[75, 79]. This more often is found in young children and means a rapidly deteriorating course (personal observations).

An operative *staging system* was given in 1969 by Chang[70]: Tumor size, local tumor extension and dissemination was taken into account. This staging system later was extended by Harisiadis and Chang[162] and by Berry and Jenkins[38]. Better techniques to identify tumor cells within the CSF and the results of postoperative myelography[38, 75, 94, 95, 100, 230, 302] and a check CT on the 4th postoperative day[67] lead to more refined staging systems[95]. A recent proposal for a staging system based on operative and postoperative findings[240] includes:

T 1 = tumor less than 3 cm in diameter, limited to the vermis, roof of the 4th ventricle, and less frequently, to one cerebellar hemisphe.

T 2 = tumor 3 cm in diameter or larger, invading one adjacent structure or partially filling the 4th ventricle.

T 3 A = tumor invading two adjacent structures or filling completely the 4th ventricle with extension into the aqueduct of Sylvius, the foramen of Magendi or the foramina of Luschka, thus producing marked hydrocephalus.

T 3 B = tumor arising from the floor of the 4th ventricle or the brain stem and filling the 4th ventricle.

T 4 = tumor further spreading through the aqueduct of Sylvius to involve the 3rd ventricle or midbrain, or extending to the upper cervical cord.

M 0 = no evidence of gross subarachnoid or hematogenous spread.

M 1 = tumor cells in the CSF.

M 2 = gross (nodular) seeding in the cerebellar, cerebral subarachnoid space, or within the 3rd or lateral ventricles.

M 3 = gross (nodular) seeding within the spinal subarachnoid space.

M 4 = metastasis outside the cerebrospinal axis.

The staging of T 3 A or T 3 B according to our own experience [186] is done on the clinical preoperative assessment, whether there is primary or secondary brain stem involvement. This is then backed by CT and operative findings.

Basically all MBL are grade IV [228]. As far as age is concerned, the younger the child, the worse is the actual prognosis. However, as far as long-term prognosis is concerned, there is not enough experience about 10- and 15-year follow-up in older children and young adults. Some authors still doubt if there is any substantial "cure" for MBL at all [281].

Location: 65% of MBL are found in the midline position, 13% lie paramedian and about 20% are located in one of the cerebellar hemispheres. A few MBL are located within the cerebellopontine angle and 3–4% in the lower brain stem [75]. According to our own observations (Table 1) primary location in the caudal brain stem is more frequent (13%); this is based on autopsy findings.

The tumor may invade the cerebellar peduncles or is adherent to the floor of the 4th ventricle [79]. Parts of it or its whole lumen may be filled by tumor masses causing obstructive hydrocephalus. The tumor can grow between the cerebellar tonsils pushing them aside and downward often far through the foramen magnum, the tumor itself can protrude between the tonsils into the dorsal cervical canal as low as C 2 [244]. Some MBL extend up through the Sylvian aqueduct and invade the third ventricle. In a few cases primary presentation of MBL is as mass lesion within the spinal canal [189, 331, 401], (2 personal observations).

Signs and Symptoms: Most children with MBL have a short history of days to some weeks, on average 1–2 months [223, 446], 2–3 months [18, 75, 184, 274, 357]. Children with a long history up to one year or even more are the exception [274]. Because of the midline position of many tumors symptoms of raised ICP dominate: headache and vomiting (often before breakfast) in 50–80% [18, 39, 75, 183, 184, 241, 357, 383]. Unsteady gait is reported in 20–30%, deterioration in (school or play) performance in 15–20%, and visual symptoms in 15–20% [39, 75]. Stiff neck posturing and truncal en-bloc movements are late signs, as are clouding of consciousness and permanent prostrate body position or seizures. In these children there is tonsillar or tentorial herniation and/or subarachnoid tumor spread into the ST compartments. A temporal lobe sharp wave focus together with a stiff neck indicates spread into the perimesencephalic cisterns and into the Sylvian fissure (3 personal observations).

50–60% of the children with MBL have papilledema, and in 12–36% there is optic atrophy[75]. Abducent nerve paresis was found in 2–30%[75]; VIIIth CN impairment and upward gaze limitation are due to tumor pressure on the lateral parts of the rhomboid fossa[281] as well as nuclear palsy of the facial nerve[57, 174]. CN involvement is seen in 50–60% of patients[39, 75, 155, 183, 184]: next to the VI., VII., and VIII., the trigeminal, glossopharyngeal and vagal nerves are affected, whereas the oculomotor and hypoglossal nerves are the least commonly involved.

Signs of disturbed motor coordination present in 60–65% include truncal ataxia, dysmetria, missing in past pointing, positive pronator sign[39, 75, 155, 183]. Lateralizing cerebellar signs are found in about 25%[75]. Hypotonia and loss of tendon reflexes or muscular hypertonus/clonus may resolve completely some days after shunt insertion; the explanation of this is that incipient herniation has been halted[281, 333], (personal observations).

Diagnostic Procedures

Electroencephalogram: There are pathological findings in 50–60% of the children with MBL but most are nonspecific: posteriorly located slow rhythms or anteriorly projected rhythmic δ-waves. These generalized abnormalities normalize 1–2 weeks after shunt insertion or operative decompression. During and 2–4 weeks after RTH the EEG might become slowed again ("postirradiation somnolence syndrome"). EEG is very sensitive to tumor recurrences. Therefore it is mandatory in the surveillance of children with MBL to do EEG tests at regular intervals.

CSF: Lumbar punctures should not be done preoperatively. A "small" lumbar puncture with only 2–3 ml withdrawal of CSF does not exist: for even after every "smooth" lumbar puncture there is at least some 20–30 ml loss of CSF by leakage through the puncture hole. If CSF was drawn off preoperatively by a ventricular tap, increased cellularity was found in 20–30%[29, 75]. Tumor cells often resemble blasts (= stem cells) in leukemia and are present single or in clusters; some eosinophilic leukocytes may be present[221].

Postoperatively tumor cells can be found in up to 90% of the patients if repeated taps are done[29]. In a few cases positive cell findings are completely absent even if extensive leptomeningeal infiltration was seen at operation and repeated lumbar punctures had been done (own observations).

Preoperative protein electrophoresis of the CSF shows raised α-1 and α-2 values. Postoperatively there is decrease of albumin, β-1- and γ-globuline which indicates disturbance of the BBB[75]. A rise of IgM and IgG in the CSF as compared to the plasma values means local production by immunological processes caused by superficially lying tumor cells, *e.g.* medulloblasts. A marked elevation of IgM in the CSF may induce polyneuropathy since these macromolecules act as paraproteins[123]. This can be clinically relevant in patients under VCR therapy. Under systemic and/or intrathecal therapy with MTX the blasts disappear 2–3 weeks before a decrease of IgM is observed[123].

Determination of the polyamines in the CSF is recommended for the control of the remission phase in MBL patients[79, 100, 292]. There were no false positives among more than 100 children who were in remission[113, 267], and only very few false negatives in those who had tumor recurrence.

CEA only rarely is found as a tumor marker in brain tumors[113, 123]. Normally it is not detectable by the ELISA method in the CSF. The meaning of elevated polyamines or any other tumor markers in the CSF can be twofold: If they do not return to normal values after relevant therapy this, in general, indicates a bad prognosis. When normal values had been found before a rise of polyamines or another marker in the CSF tumor recurrence at any place can be suspected, even if clinical, cytological, myelographic, CT and NMR findings remain negative.

Radiography of the skull: 50–60% show signs of increased ICP[39, 184, 204]. Calcifications are exceptional (1/44 among our own patients).

CT: Most MBL are uniformly hyperdense lesions in the noncontrast CT. Some 10% are isodense, 5% hypodense and 20% are mixed lesions indicating that necroses, old hemorrhages have occurred. Some MBL show small cysts within the tumor[39, 79, 204, 244, 384, 454]. Peritumoral edema grade I and II is seen in 46% of the cases[204]. Homogeneous enhancement after intravenous contrast is present in nearly all patients with MBL which is distinguished clearly from the surrounding brain tissue[39, 204, 244, 384]. By high resolution scanning in about 30% of the patients subarachnoid spread of the tumor within the supra- and infratentorial compartments can be shown at the initial investigation[38, 302, 384].

In healthy individuals the vermis cerebelli may somewhat enhance after intravenous contrast: about 4 Hounsfield units. MBL generally have an enhancement of 10–11 Hounsfield units occurring 10–15 minutes after contrast administration and disappearing after 30–60 minutes[204]. Another point in the differential diagnosis of the CT is: obliteration of one of the lateral recesses of the 4th ventricle. This finding is in favor of a MBL[204].

Diagnosis of tumor recurrence within the PF often is much more difficult than the primary diagnosis. The diagnosis of a local recurrence is made by CT in 40%[116] to 60%[244, 454] of patients with relapses at all locations. After intravenous contrast there may be enhancement in the quadrigeminal cistern, in the Sylvian or the anterior part of the interhemispheric fissure or the supracerebellar cistern. Further enhancement can be seen in the floor of the anterior horns or filling the anterior parts of the inferior horns; or as a mass within the 3rd or one of the lateral ventricles[116, 204, 244, 454]. In case of tumor or search for its recurrence one has to consider that steroids impede enhancement to 17–94% when given longer than one week prior to the scan[87]. Dexamethasone inhibits protein vascular efflux, decreases local lactacidosis and restores vascular autoregulation. A lowered vascular resistance and shunting of tumor vessels is more often in the periphery of any malignant brain tumor[87].

NMR seems to be superior to CT if there is recurrence within the brain stem[303], (*c.f.* Figs. 11 a and b), p. 465). CT, on the other hand, offers more advantage in imaging a subarachnoid tumor spread by contrast enhancement[303].

Myelography: The water soluble dyes available are well tolerated: . Only 12% of the children vomit and 25% have headache after myelography, and only very few suffer fever[100]. Postoperative myelography today is recommended by most authors within the first 1–3 weeks after surgery[38, 75, 79, 94, 95, 230, 302]. 30–50% of the patients have spinal seedlings at the first postoperative mylographic investigation done as a routine[38, 94, 95, 384]. These tumors, in order of frequency are located in the lumbosacral, in the cervico-dorsal, and in the thoracic part of the spinal canal. The lesions may be nodular, a single mass or distend the parenchyma of the cord[94, 100].

Thickening of the lumbosacral nerve roots or posterolateral indentations into the lumen of the spinal canals may be found[75].

Angiography: Preoperative angiography (retrograde brachial or selective vertebral) in most cases is not diagnostic but helpful[75, 281] in the sense that possible diagnostic mistakes are avoided, *e.g.* angioma of the cerebellum or caudal brain stem, or giant aneurysm of the basilar artery[75]. Also venous anomalies not demonstrated by the CT can be seen, *e.g.* a large occipital sinus, or peridural venectasias.

In 60–68% of the patients shifts of arteries and of cerebellar and brain stem veins can be demonstrated[39, 204, 281, 284, 332, 416]. The vermian branch of the PICA is displaced laterally and inferiorly, its supratonsillar segment pressed downwards (with the choroidal branch) and its suprapyramidal segment can form a caudal loop indicating that one or both cerebellar tonsils are herniated through the foramen magnum or even into the spinal canal. The anterior pontomesencephalic vein often is shifted rostrally, the supraculminate vein posteriorly and the precentral vein located anteriorly is angulated[75, 416]. In larger tumors of the inferior vermis or within the 4th ventricle, these shift of veins result in hypovascularity of the middle-inferior parts of the PF in the lateral view. In few children with MBL a tumor blush might be seen[204]. We have recorded this finding mainly in very young children.

Ventriculography: With very few exceptions this investigation is no longer indicated today. When the primary site of the tumor (MBL, EPDY) is within the caudal brain stem it should however be done. In such cases apart from dorsal displacement of the elongated aqueduct and the 4th ventricle irregularities of the floor of the rhomboid fossa are well demonstrated in the lateral exposures. MBL have smooth, clear outlines demonstrated by positive contrast media whereas EPDY and PLP have weavy or cauliflower-like contours[204].

Treatment

a) *Surgery:* If there is marked neck rigidity and/or a depressed level of consciousness caused by obstructive hydrocephalus an external ventricular drainage or shunt insertion prior to direct surgery is required. Ventriculoatrial or ventriculoperitoneal shunt insertion increase the risk of extraneural dissemination; but, we think, if early, preradiotherapeutic chemotherapy is given, the risk of early, postoperative tumor cell dissemination is minimized. This also can be done by using a shunt valve fitted with a filter.

Surgical intervention which should be done under an umbrella of steroid treatment results in a macroscopically "total" tumor removal which nevertheless in the case of an infiltrative tumor like MBL cannot be considered curative. But, removal of the tumor bulk improves the chances of successful CHT and RT later[39, 155].

The mortality of total tumor removal was reported as 80%[75], but by other authors 42%[318] which seems to be more realistic. It is much worse if the neurosurgeon tries to remove all parts of the tumor visible thus severing the floor of the rhomboid fossa or the cerebellar peduncles. This kind of "crippling" neurosurgery should be abandoned in favor of a more cautious approach.

Although the operative mortality is reported to be near zero in some series[75] or 2–5% in big centers[81], it is still 5–30% in collected series[75]: Reports from the seventies give figures of 20%[435], 22%[270], 25%[211], 26%[39], 27%[165] and even 30%[274, 446], but the figures are declining with the beginning of the eighties: 10%[318], 12%[155], 5%[16]. Some authors speculate about these high mortality figures and partially attribute them to air embolism if the operation is done in the sitting position[174], or to unrecognized CSF circulatory failure within the days after the operation[155].

The aim of the operation should be threefold: to remove as much of the tumor mass without adding further neurological damage to the child, to restore the circulation of the CSF, and to enable an exact neuropathological diagnosis to be achieved by removing enough tumor material for investigations by the different modern techniques.

In order to maintain the patency of the Sylvian aqueduct its catheterization by a soft tube (Leksell drain) is possible[75, 233, 234, 369]. This tube is an internal shunt connecting the 3rd ventricle with the cisterna magna at the C 2 level.

Postoperative complications are persistent depression of the level of consciousness, hyperthermia, apnoea, and abrupt alterations of the blood pressure. Secondary depression of unconsciousness may be due to massive hemorrhage within the operative field or purulent meningitis. If seizures or status epilepticus occur days after surgery a ST subdural hematoma or even ST rapid subarachnoid spread of the tumor should be considered.

b) *Chemotherapy:* In accordance with the study group on MBL of the GPO[291] and other authors[12, 48, 292, 304], we suggest CHT is given before RTH. During the 2–3 postoperative weeks procarbazine is given first in order not to risk healing of the operative wound. According to the proposals of the GPO study group three lots of VCR/MTX-MHD are given with intervals of one week. Then, after a break for 2 weeks, the cycle is repeated. The whole of chemotherapy is to be finished 10 weeks after surgery, followed by RT.

c) *Radiotherapy:* Generally, in MBL the whole cranial dose of 35–40 Gy is recommended with additional 15 Gy to the PF, whereas the dose for the spinal axis is 30–35 Gy. The fractions are between 150–180 rad. In children less than 3 years old a dose reduction of 10–20% is recommended[47, 79, 189]. The total period of RT in general is 6 weeks given in fractionated doses daily.

Course

MBL like other PNETs has a great tendency to seed along the CSF pathways and also extraaxially.

1. *Intraaxial metastases:* Involve the ST subarachnoid space and the ventricles (M 2), the IT subarachnoid compartments including local recurrences (M 2), and the spinal part of the neuraxis (M 3). [In addition, positive CSF cytology (M 1) has to be considered.)

a) *Staging M 1:* Preoperatively an elevated cell count is seen in $\frac{2}{3}$–$\frac{3}{4}$ of all CSF specimen, but definitive proof of tumor cells or even cell clusters is only possible in $\frac{1}{3}$[29, 75, 221]. Positive cell findings in the postoperative follow-up vary widely: 3–36%[38, 95, 162]. Balhuizen *et al.*[29] stress that, after repeated investigations, positive cell findings rise to 91% in patients with MBL. On the other hand, discrepancies are possible as for example in patients with leukemia: Negative tumor cell findings in the CSF on several occasions, but dense leptomeningeal infiltration seen at operation, or demonstrated by CT scan enhancement or proven by autopsy[94, 95], (own observations).

b) *Staging M 2:* If there was no preoperative ST involvement, there are 2 possibilities for a later extension of the MBL into the ST subarachnoid or ventricular compartment (M 2): Either residual parts of the primary tumor have seeded or some tumor cells escaped from RT. During and after surgery one has to accept CSF contamination by some tumor cells in every case. Jereb *et al.*[194] found that the region of the cribriform plate and the deepest parts of the middle cranial fossa might get radiation doses as low as 3.5–6 Gy only. In addition, in a person living in an erect position, there is a gravitational effect for CSF cells to the lowest sites, *i.e.* the cribriform plate, the cisterns around the tip of the temporal lobe, and pooling within the lumbosacral cul-de-sac. These considerations lead to the clinicians' plea not to cut off these parts of the anterior and middle cranial fossa from RT[79, 292], since ST tumor spread more often than not may be due to inadequate radiotherapeutic technique than to dissemination from an uncontrolled primary site.

Isolated ST recurrences are found in 6–10%[19, 38, 69, 75, 95, 244, 273]. Together with recurrences within the PF this figure is doubled[38, 39, 79, 270, 329]. In autopsy series total subarachnoid seeding accounts for 50–80%[75, 302, 329, 357]. Tumor seeding is located in the frontal lobe in 50%, in the temporal lobe in 10%, in the parietal lobe in 7%, and wide dissemination is found in 27%[75]. 38% of the lesions are isolated in the ST space, 33% are linked with PF recurrences and 37% with spinal spread[75]. Tumor spread into the ST compartments occurs within the 1st postoperative year in 63% and in 20% after 2 years. Clinically, ST seedlings may produce signs and symptoms like loss of weight, anorexia, asthenia, lack of drive, headache, vomiting and seizures. Hyperphagia and obesity are encountered, similar, to the hypothalamic syndrome caused by meningeal leukemia.

c) *Staging M 3:* Clinically, spinal metastases are heralded by back pain, pains within the groins or legs which can be of the lightening type. In some of the children flaccic paraplegia develops with posterior column loss[223], and bladder/bowel disturbances. Extensive infiltrations of nearly all nerve roots and of the cranial nerves was reported in 3 cases[293]. This "meningiosis blastomatosa" clinically presented as polyneuropathy with a neurogenic pattern of denervation in the electromyogram and high CSF protein values.

The incidence of spinal metastases ranges from 7 to 14%[38, 69, 75, 155, 162, 397] or from 18 to 51%[19, 39, 88, 223, 249, 270, 273, 329, 401]. McFarland *et al.*[273] in 1969 in a collective series of 430 cases reported an incidence of 31%, while Choux and Lena[75] in 1982 only saw an incidence of 16.5%. One has to accept that the quality of RTH had improved in those 20 years. In autopsy series the incidence of spinal seeding is much higher, ranging from 50 to 90%[215, 249, 329, 357].

Local recurrences: Although spinal metastases are tragic for a patient these spinal lesions are only exceptionally fatal. The life of most patients suffering from MBL is threatened by the possibility of local tumor recurrence. The figures for local tumor recurrence vary from 32–87% in clinical series[19, 38, 39, 69, 79, 88, 215, 230, 244, 270, 397] to 100% in autopsy series[329, 357].

2. *Extraneural metastases:* The figures given by the different authors vary between 2–10%[19, 39, 69, 75, 79, 162, 230, 270, 329, 397]; while Berry and Jenkins[38] reported

16%. Lewis and Nunez[248] put forward 3 conditions for the diagnosis of extraneural metastases of a brain tumor: a) identical histology, b) complete autopsy, c) relevant clinical history for extraaxial dissemination. Alvord[13] discussed some factors that might influence extraneural seeding of gliomas: venous channel obstruction exerted by tumor pressure and raised ICP; absence of intracranial lymphatic vessels, resistance of pulmonal parenchyma to glioma cells, resistance of endothelial cells for penetration by glioma cells; inability of glioma cells to induce stroma formation, and immunological factors. Otherwise one has to accept that during surgery tumor cells are channelled into open venous vessels of the bone and the dura. In addition, suboptimal postoperative CHT may damage tissue surrounding malignant cells allowing them now to reenter a cell cycle[79, 106, 400]. Alvord's hypothesis was[13]: extraneural metastasis of clinical significance is most unlikely if the time of survival is short; but it will be come more likely with prolonged survival.

Extraneural secondaries in children suffering from intracranial malignant tumors are rare: Hoffman and Duffner[176] reviewed the English literature on that topic: 40% of the reported 232 cases were children. Of these 112 cases 65 had MBL, 14 germ cell tumors, 13 EPDYs, 5 meningeal tumors, 2 PNETs, 2 PBL and 1 choroid plexus carcinoma. MBL tend to metastasize to bones and the bone marrow, in up to 80–100%. Next are lymph nodes, followed by the lungs/pleura, peritoneum, retroperitoneum, liver, pancreas, adrenals, and kidneys[38, 39, 79, 101, 106, 149, 159, 175, 252, 271, 330, 400]. In larger series the percentages for the different siges are: skeleton 80–82%, pelvis 40–51%, long bones 13–46%, vertebral column 42–62%[65, 75, 215, 252]. The osseous lesions can be osteoclastic (35%) or osteoplastic (65%)[65, 79, 112, 215, 330]. Therefore, raised alkaline or acid phosphatase or raised calcium levels in serum[312] should initiate further investigations: bone scintigram and bone marrow aspiration. An invasion of lymph nodes is present in 29–65% of patients with extraneural MBL metastases, most often in the neck. Figures given for other organ metastases and areas already mentioned vary between 10 and 25%.

The sites of exit for the cancer cells are the bone flap, site of laminectomy, shunting systems, base of the skull via the cranial nerves, the orbit, the spinal canal via the nerve roots[176, 252]. Infiltration of the spinal dura and nerve roots means tumor extension and invasion into the retroperitoneum, the posterior mediastinum, into the vertebral column and the pelvis. The frequency of shunt-induced extraneural seeds is reported to be 10–33%[38, 75, 175, 209, 215, 252, 330]. In Hoffman's and Duffner's review[176] 12% of the patients with extraneural metastases had a shunting system, in 8.5% the metastases had occurred spontaneously, i.e. without any preceding surgery. All the other patients had had some surgery before the metastases were found[175, 176]. Millipore filters do not prevent metastases through systemic shunts in every case[175, 176]. The mean time lag between surgery and the detection of an extraneural metastasis was 2 years with a variation of 4 months to 7 years[79, 106, 252], while others found extremes between 1 month and 10 years[215]. The survival time for patients with extraneural metastases is generally short: 50% die within the first year after the diagnosis of extraneural spread, and 70% within the 2nd year. According to Choux and Lena[75] the figures are even worse: 66% die within the first and 90% within the 2nd year. However, a wide range between the two extremes exists: 1 months and 13 years[312].

Clinically extraneural dissemination has to be suspected if the patient has unexplained anemia, gets anorexic, has pain in his back or the abdomen, or has tenderness and swellings in the neck and in the paravertebral tissue[79, 106, 215], (personal observations).

Prognosis

After exclusion of deaths in the perioperative period (= preoperatively or within the next weeks) the general prognosis in children is dependent upon adequate RT. As early as 1919, Cushing and Bailey recommended local RT of the tumor bed, and in 1927 they advised whole neuraxis irradiation. Despite this early recognition that MBL is a radiosensitive tumor, a first real breakthrough was achieved by systematic application of modern RT in the seventies and the eighties (Table 2). In addition it became evident that a child with MBL treated in a big center has a better chance of survival compared with small neurosurgical units where there is less experience with perioperative management and combined therapy[16, 81, 223, 318].

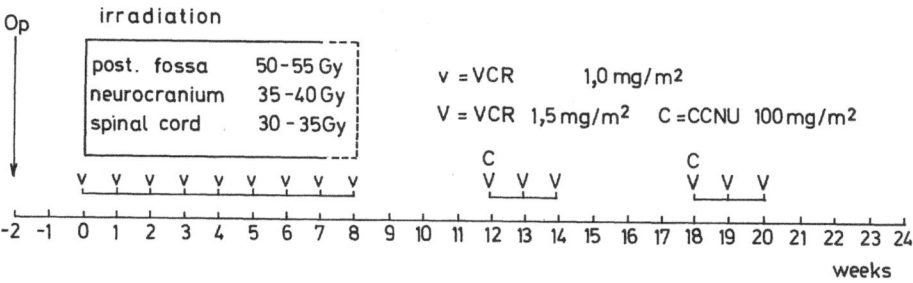

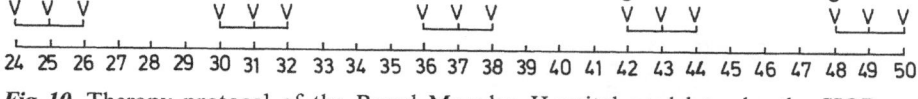

Fig. 10. Therapy protocol of the Royal Marsden Hospital used later by the SIOP and CCSG[47, 290]

According to the collected data given by Choux and Lena[75] a child suffering from MBL has 40–60% chance of survival for 3 years, for 5 years of 20–60% and for 10 years of 10–40% (*cf.* Table 2). The question raised by Bloom[45–80], Neidhardt[289–292] and others[304] is: could these good results achieved by RT alone get markedly improved by a combined modality management? Between 1970 and 1980 37 patients at the Royal Marsden Hospital (RMH)/London had adjuvant postradiotherapy CHT: VCR and CCNU (Fig. 10).

The figures for 3 and 5 year survival were 75% and 71% respectively. These patients were compared with 87 children treated between 1952 and 1970 by RT alone: The respective data were 36% (3 years) and 32% (5 years)[47]. From 1975 to 1980 the SIOP made a comparative study of 280 patients with MBL. One half of the patients received RT only, the other 140 had adjuvant postradiotherapy CHT along the lines of the RMH protocol. The figures for adjuvant CHT are superior: 69/56% (with/without CHT) after 2 years, 62/49% after 3 years, and 60/49% after 4 years.

Table 2. Prognosis in patients with medulloblastoma: length of survival time

Authors	Ref.	Year	Survival	1 year	2 years	3 years	5 years	10 years	N
Smith and Lampe	401	1961	conventional RT			38%	27%		61
Hoffmann	174	1961		32%	14%		7%		72
Bloom et al.	45	1969	conventional RT			35%	33%		72
Koos and Miller	223	1971				50%	30%		60
Chatty and Earle	72	1971	conventional RT	44%		21%	12%	6%	105
Harisiadis and Chan	162	1977	(stage T1/T2) RT			65%	48%	42%	59
			(stage T3/T4) RT			36%	30%	0%	
Quest et al.	329	1978	conventional RT			33%	31%		99
Raimondi-Tomia	331	1979	RT	71%		45%	34%		39
King	211	1979				43%	38%		26
McIntosh	274	1979			32%		14%	38%	87*
Berry et al.	38	1981	CCSG/convent. RT		81%		49%		122
Berthold	39	1981					25%		90*
Mazza et al.	270	1981	cerebrospinal RT + CCNU	67%		43%	27%		35*
Bamberg et al.	30	1982	cerebrospinal RT			55%	53%		22*
Bloom	47	1982	Royal Marsden RT + CHTH (1970–1980)	75%	71%		37*		140
			Royal Marsden RT alone (1952–1970)	36%	32%		87		140
			SIOP RT + CHT		69%	62%	60%	(4 years)	
			SIOP RT alone		56%	49%	49%	(4 years)	
Cohen-Duffner	79	1984	RT + CCNU + UCR			52%	40%		193
Bloom-Glees	48	1985	SIOP—RT + CCNU + UCR			75%	71%		287
Collected series:									
McFarland et al.	273	1969	conventional RT	50%		20%	18%		700*
Farwell	120	1977		70%	29%				117
Castro-Vita	64	1978				33%	33%	23%	700
Wilcke	446	1981					26%	12%	2,500
Müller and Afra	286	1982			40%		22%	9%	202

* Without deduction of the perioperative mortality. In all other series this had been subtracted.

The question remains still unanswered, whether CHT alone could postpone recurrence of the tumor[47].

With regard to the biological behavior of MBL which may influence the outcome in the individual case two questions require discussion:

1. Is there a definite period for a given patient during which he is at risk for recurrence: Collin's rule originally was attributed to children who had Wilm's tumor[47, 79]. This rule later was extended to brain tumors of probable embryogenic origin like germinomas, PNETs, and MBL. This rule states that a child is at risk

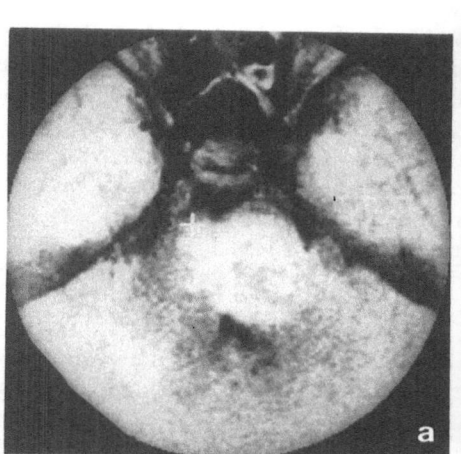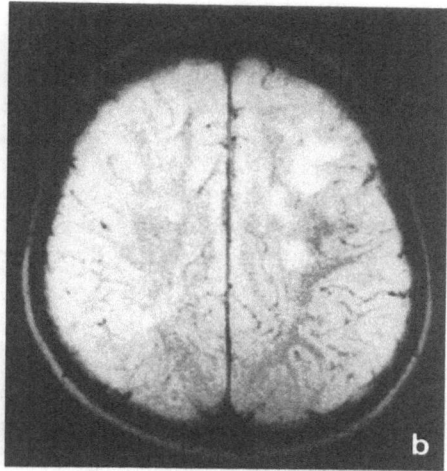

Fig. 11. Tumor recurrence of MBL in a boy aged 11⁸/₁₂: within the pons (**a**) and in the right cerebral hemisphere (**b**). Nuclear magnetic resonance imaging. The diagnosis of MBL was established when the boy was 5⁶/₁₂. Had the recurrence been 1 months later this course would have been an escape from Collin's rule

until he doubled his age at diagnosis plus 9 months. Collin's rule of tumor regrowth states that the tumor needs as much time to become symptomatic again as it did the first time plus 9 months of fetal development (Figs. 11 *a* and *b*). Applied to MBL only a few patients are exceptions to this rule: 22 of 1015 patients[47, 162, 211, 230, 239, 276, 329, 330]. There are exceptions to Collin's rule on the record which occurred later than 8, 9, 10, 11, and even 16 years after the patient was out of the period of risk[75]. On the other hand: ASCY grade III/IV occurring 11 years after completion of RT for desmoplastic MBL in a 11 months old boy seems much more likely to be a new tumor or a radiotherapeutically induced tumor than MBL recurrence[216]. Therefore, generally speaking, a patient who is beyond the period of risk only has a 2% probability to have a recurrence of MBL[239].

2. Of all variables discussed in the natural history of MBL only one parameter seems to be important for the length of survival: The age at diagnosis[287, 446]. Staging is important, T 1/T 2 have better prognosis than T 3/T 4[70, 75, 81, 225]; but not the "classical" or desmoplastic variant, with its location in the midline or in one cerebellar hemisphere[72]. Total versus subtotal removal, short or longer past

history, absence or presence of hydrocephalus only are important for short-term prognosis (= 3 years after operation). Female versus male[72, 75] is not relevant either[81, 225, 287].

Quality of Survival

Comparisons were made between children who had been treated for cerebellar ASCY and for MBL[157, 172] and who had undergone surgical treatment in the same center along the same general lines: Children with MBL came off much worse in the long-term follow-up, they often had neurological deficits for example cerebellar ataxia, dysarthria or slow speech, some were blind or had epilepsy. Many of the MBL patients needed special schooling and/or had emotional problems[89, 107, 109, 157, 172, 330]. In addition, nearly all the younger children who had had RT of the whole neuraxis, finally showed some growth deficit[55, 62, 273, 330, 401]. According to German authors[39] 60% of the patients with MBL have minor problems and deficits only, 20% need special schooling and 20% are dependent on help for their multiple handicaps. In addition, it seems very important to note that learning problems even increase 3–5 years after completion of treatment[108, 109] which in a few cases was found to be due to borderline hypothyroidism.

Medical Surveillance

The observations made here for patients with MBL are similar for those who were treated for EPDY[151, 319], germ cell tumors, PNETs, PBL, and high grade gliomas. The only exception is myelographic control and repeated CSF investigations are not necessary in ST malignant gliomas if there are no clinical symptoms favoring spinal spread of the tumor.

In general: If a child with malignant tumor of the CNS becomes anemic particularly after MBL one has to consider bone or bone marrow infiltration and should undertake the following investigations: calcium, phosphorus, acid and alkaline phosphatase in the serum, bone scintigram, and bone marrow aspiration, eventually a bone biopsy.

If there are unexplained pains diffusely spread over the whole body anywhere, the same examinations should be done. Endocrine function tests should be done every 2 years after the completion of treatment examining the thyroid, adrenal gland and in adolescents the gonadal axis.

From summarizes the recommendations made by different authors[75, 230, 292] the following suggestions emerge

a) clinical/neurological examination after 2, 4, 6, 9, 12, 15, 18, 21, 24, 30, 36, 42, 48 months.

b) CT scan: 5 days after operation/after CHT/after RT, 12, 18, 24, 36, 48 months after diagnosis.

CSF: Several times after operation according to individual demand 6, 12, 18, 24, 36 months after operation. Cytology should be available, determination of the polyamines (in MBL) if possible.

d) Myelography: 1–3 weeks postoperatively, after 6, 18, 36 months. Myelography implies an exact CSF examination. CT scan of the spine should supplement abnormal myelographic findings. The contrast within the subarachnoid lumbar space can be used for outlining of the cranial cisterns some 4–6 hours later if the clinical question of intracranial tumor has arisen.

In nearly all children with malignancies of the CNS who were on combined treatment, psychological testing and counselling is mandatory. Mental deterioration may occur some years after RTH has been completed.

VIII. Miscellaneous Tumors

1. *Meningioma:* In adults they account for 14–21.6% of all intracranial tumors[189, 294, 355, 361, 456, 457], but in children are rare: 1.0–2.8%[189, 223, Table 1]. In general, meningiomas are grade I tumors[79, 228], but some are grade II or even III. Reports on malignant meningiomas in children are anecdotal[79].

Symptoms of intraventricular meningioma are early signs of raised ICP: headache, vomiting, papilledema. There may be early optic atrophy, ataxic gait, seizures, akinetic spells, sometimes "narcoleptic" attacks[79, 119], and polyuria.

Other locations of meningioma are: parasagittal, convexity, sphenoid wings and tuberculum sellae, posterior fossa. These children have[79]: visual loss or field defects, involvement of other CN (mainly in sphenoidal and PF location), seizures (8–31%), focal neurological signs (23–36%), and changes of behavior. The plain X-ray of the skull can show calcifications, local hyperostosis or bone destruction. In the CT the lesions are hypodense in 1%, 14% are isodense, 75% hyperdense, and 10% mixed[204]. Nearly all meningiomas readily enhance after intravenous contrast[79, 204]. The tumor shows up as a curvilinear or slightly lobulated, densely enhancing mass. If the outline of the tumor is poorly defined an anaplastic transformation has to be suspected[204]. Meningiomas may seed along the CSF pathways[79, 255, 261], and the angioblastic variant outside the neuraxis[307]. The CT diagnosis of a meningioma has to be complemented by angiography; 17 blush, sometimes with the feeding vessel can be demonstrated[284, 332].

The treatment of meningioma is surgical removal. This is curative in about half of the cases. If complete removal is not possible or if the lesion was of a high grade of malignancy, high doses RT are indicated. This achieves a 5-year relapse-free interval in 73% and for 10 years in 60% of the patients[47].

2. *Choroid plexus papilloma (PLP):* In children 90% of all PLP are located in one of the lateral ventricles, more often in the left one[79, 281]. In adults most PLP occur within the 4th ventricle, whereas in children 3rd and 4th ventricular location is 5–8% for each site[189]. Differentiation from EPOYs is sometimes only possible under the electron microscope where blepharoblasts are demonstrated which are not a feature of PLP. Biologically, PLP behave like EPDY because they seed along both the spinal axis and into the ventricular system. This seeding in PLP is not only observed after surgery; shearing of tumor villi might occur spontaneously.

The CSF contains elevated protein, is sometimes xanthochromic or even may contain fresh erythrocytes suggesting intracranial bleeding in the newborn. In the CT, PLP of the lateral ventricle is a hyperdense lesion which is sometimes lobulated[204] and gives homogeneous contrast enhancement. Sometimes movement of the tumor is demonstrated by CT[384] or by ultrasound. Angiography should be performed before operation; the feeding vessels are the anterior and the posterior

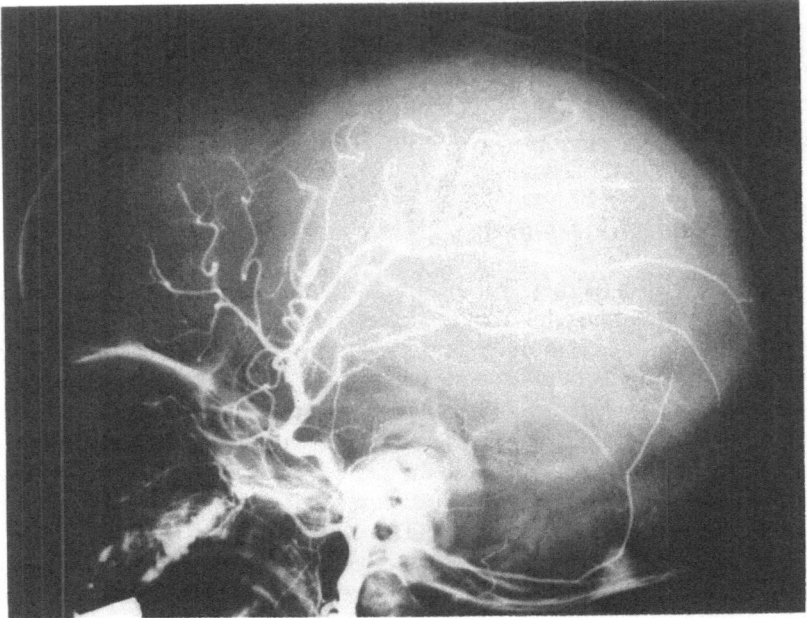

Fig. 12. "Sunbust" staining in the late arterial phase in a 1⁸/₁₂-years-old girl with huge PLP of the left lateral ventricle. The feeding anterior choroidal artery is hypertrophied

choroidal arteries, and sometimes a hypertrophied pedicle is demonstrated. The PLPs of the 4th ventricle are fed by vessels arising from the superior cerebellar or the vermian and medullary branches of the inferior posterior cerebellar arteries[79, 281].

In ST PLP there may be staining in the late arterial or in the venous phase[281] (Fig. 12).

Shunt insertion after tumor removal is necessary in 50%[79, 189, 281]. Shunt insertion bears a high risk of infection within the shunting system[268]. 20% of PLP may undergo malignant change[79] which in most cases occurs before the age of 2 years[384].

3. *Brain metastases:* The seeds of extraneural tumors can be solitary, multiple, or diffuse, infiltrating the leptomeninges (Fig. 13).

Dissemination can be due to hematogeneous spread. In this cases the child has lung metastases[428], (2 personal observations) abdominal, skeletal, or widespread general disease (4 personal observations).

The other way for CNS involvement is by direct spread into the cranial cavity: Tumors of the nasal cavity, the paranasal air sinuses or the base of the skull may directly progress through or along the great vessels, cranial nerves, the cribriform plate, foramen ovale or jugulare, or may extend through the bone and the dura. Orbital tumors may extend into the intracranial cavity via the optic canal or through the orbital roof[223, 281, 428], (personal observations).

Brain metastases in children are rare: In 723 autopsies with extraneural tumors Schreiber *et al.*[379, 380] saw no CNS involvement in an individual less than 20 years of

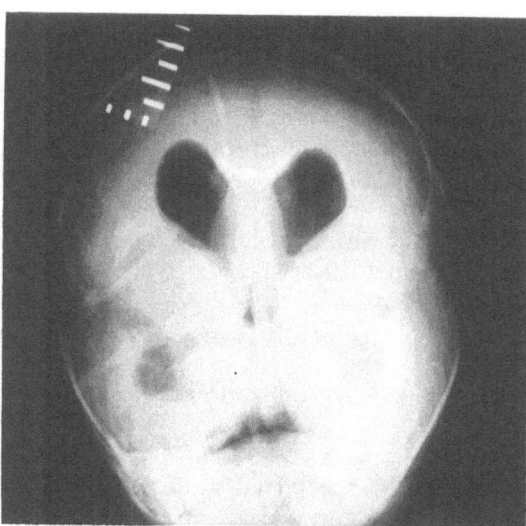

Fig. 13. Calcification of the corpus callosum in a 3-month-old boy with malignant reticulosis of the Letterer-Siwe-type. There is thickening of the falx cerebri 3 cm in width by the malignant metastasizing disease

age. In the Vienna series of 700 pediatric brain tumors there was only one patient with cerebral metastasis[223]. Among 275 children we observed 12 patients with metastatic brain involvement (= 4.3%, Table 1) 6 of whom had hematogeneous spread and 6 continuous tumor propagation from the primary sites.

Pediatric tumors that metastasize are Wilm's tumor, neuroblastoma, hepatoblastoma, malignant melanoma, fibrosarcoma, systemic diseases like M. Hodgkin, malignant lymphomas, or disseminated histiocytosis X (Letter-Siwe syndrome), osteogenic sarcomas, Ewing sarcoma and rhabdomyosarcoma. These malignant osteogenic tumors spread by the blood stream as well as by local extension. Local spread into the cranium is observed in chemodectoma, chordoma, chondroma, cylindroma, and in juvenile fibroma of the nasopharynx[183, 281, 428], (personal observations).

The symptoms and signs in brain metastases of children vary considerably: Mental symptoms, depressed consciousness, visual loss and papilledema are frequently found. Focal seizures, followed by hemiparesis and dysphasic symptoms are findings in favor of a solitary lesion. Local involvement of the CN I, II, and III or of the lower cranial nerves on one side (IX–XII) are in favor of local invasion. In bilateral impairment of the abducent nerves, of the facial nerves, and in multifocal myoclonic epilepsy a widespread and subarachnoid dissemination must be suspected. In 50% of the children with brain metastases there is an increase of cells in the CSF consisting of blasts or lympho-/monocytes.

Diagnosis is made by EEG, CT scan with contrast enhancement and, if a solitary lump is suspected, by angiography. Radionucleotide scanning should be done if a multiplicity of lesions cannot be excluded by CT.

In our 12 patients we observed a mean period of 8 months between the diagnosis of the peripheral tumor and the 1st central symptoms, whereas in Vanucci's series of hematogenous tumor spread the time lag was longer and seemed dependent on the presence of lung metastases[428].

The mean survival after manifestation of CNS involvement is short, ranging from some days to months[428]. In 11 of our patients it averaged 6 months with a range of 1–13 months. The decision for treatment should include assessment of the whole situation of the patient: Surgery is only indicated in solitary metastases and if the clinical condition of the patient warrants it, whereas RT and CHT are given according to the principles governing the behavior of the tumor in question.

IX. Tumors of the Neonatal Period and of Infancy

Brain tumors which present in the first half year of live in most cases are located in the ST compartment[79, 189]. In the second half of the 1st year the incidence equalizes and in the 2nd year more IT tumors are diagnosed[79, 121].

Brain tumors of infants often are huge and comprise more than one lobe of the brain, sometimes the whole brain, they tend to bleed and to obstruct the flow of CSF[17, 79, 189, 278, 413]. The tendency for bleeding was mainly found in babies with PLPs, EPDYs, and PNETs. CSF protein can be markedly elevated and tumor cells are seen in the CSF when the inference is that subarachnoid seeding has already taken place[37, 40, 278, 311].

The neuropathology of the tumors of this age group is different from that in later life[192]. Some of the tumors are highly malignant, and some present with excessive growth which prompts developmental anomalies of the CNS and definit brain tissue destruction in others. Every kind of diagnosis and treatment is more delicate and needs more sophisticated approach as compared to older children and adults.

Tumors of the neonatal period and the first two years of life can be subdivided into 3 subgroups[121, 124, 188, 189, 192, 222, 223, 413]:

a) Those presenting at birth or within the neonatal period (first 4 weeks of extrauterine life). Today the diagnosis of hydrocephalus is possible even during the fetal period, but only very few of congenital cases of hydrocephalus are caused by a tumor. These undoubted "neonatal" tumors account for 2.2% of all brain tumors in childhood[188, 189].

b) The diagnosis is established until the end of the 1st year.

c) The first symptoms can be traced backwards to the neonatal period or the first months of life, but the diagnosis is not made until the end of the 2nd year.

The rate of stillbirth or even antenatal death is quite different among the different groups of tumors. Most frequent are teratomas: of 73 teratomas collected by Jänisch et al.[189] 64% had hydrocephalus at or before birth; this resulted in 22 of them in intrauterine death (= 30%) and in 24.6% in stillbirth. Of 115 babies with ASCY there was "congenital" hydrocephalus in 22 (= 19.1%) and stillbirth in 5.2%. Of 59 babies with MBL, 9 had increased head circumference at birth, of 40 children with EPDY 6, and of 103 babies with PLP 12, of these 27 children with hydrocephalus present at birth only 1 was stillborn. The conclusion reached is that in hydrocephalus caused by a tumor the stillbirth rate is very high in teratoma, followed by ST ASCY, whereas it is unlikely in all other tumors[142, 188, 189].

Symptoms and Signs of Tumors in the First Two Years of Life

a) Hydrocephalus is present in 30–40% of the cases[381]; its pathophysiology is threefold: by CSF obstruction, by blocking the subarachnoid cisterns and the villi by tumor cells or blood, or both, and by increased rate of arachnoid CSF formation which in PLP of the lateral ventricle can be increased fivefold[189, 223, 281]. The blocking of the subarachnoid spaces is important[24, 40, 74, 79, 115, 189, 192, 199, 222, 223].

b) Vomiting is present in 20–30%[381]. In this age it might give rise to many questions in the differential diagnosis if there is no increased head circumference; most of the infants had extensive radiological and absorption tests of the intestine before a morbid condition of the CNS was considered.

c) Seizures are reported in 10–20%[79, 381] which may present as generalized, focal, multifocal, motor, or autonomic. Sometimes these fits are resistent to any therapy[124, 189, 413]. The EEG shows generalized or focal slowing, wandering epileptic focal discharges or even status epilepticus, with multifocal discharges of hypsarrhythmia[79, 124] (personal observations).

d) Failure to thrive can develop during the first months. Some of these babies do not vomit. Their food intake is plenty as assessed by the energy quotient; ¾ of these infants suffer from an ASCY of the hypothalamus[79, 189, 278].

The following signs can be found at the beginning or during the further course in 10–20% of the patients[79, 381]: hemi- or tetraparesis, muscular hypotonia which in cases of tumors of the PF may be so severe as to prompt apnoic spells and difficulties in sucking and swallowing, blindness, other CN palsies, nystagmus, mental and motor developmental retardation.

In some series of neonatal tumors ASCY prevail[381, 398], in others EPDY[79, 124, 222] or PLP[192] or MBL[121, 268]. In a few western series and those from Japan, teratomas are present in about 50%[79]. In their collection of 742 cases Gerlach et al.[142] reported 18.2% ASCYs, 16.3% PLPs, 11.0% teratomas, 9.5% MBLs, and 6.7% EPDYs. Important clinical features of these groups of tumors of the neonatal period are:

a) *ASCY:* Most of them are very huge (5–8 cm in diameter)[189] and are located supratentorially. The clinical presentation can be that of hydrocephalus, seizures, failure to thrive, and pendular ocular movements. ASCY of the brain stem and huge hydrocephalus was found in a premature stillborn infant of the 31st weeks of gestation[103]. Glioma of the brain stem without hydrocephalus can cause apnoic spells as the only symptom[238]. The AFP value can be elevated in both CSF and serum, but in this age it is not diagnostic[324].

b) *Teratomas* are generally located in the midline: in the pineal or suprasellar region, at midbrain-aqueductal level, or in the place of hypoplastic inferior vermis cerebelli. Others have grown out extradurally and present as epignathus within the oral cavity, or are lying in one orbit or in one lateral ventricle in close contact with the choroid plexus[74, 102, 144]. Some may exceed 8 cm in diameter[189]. An extension from the posterior fossa through the whole lumen of the spinal canal down to the sacrum is possible[189]. Malignant parts can develop within the tumor very early[189, 381].

In many children with teratoma—like those with lipomas, dermoids or epidermoids—there are associated malformations of the midline[192], anencephaly[381], agenesis of the corpus callosum, cerebellar agenesis, rostral or parietooccipital meningoencephalocele or signs of spinal dysrhaphism: spina bifida occulta, aperta, dermal sinus or persistent canalis neurentericus[189]. The treatment of teratoma is always operative. If malignant parts are proven by histology (or positive tumor markers like raised AFP, β-HCG or CEA are found), combined treatment is necessary.

c) *MBL:* At this age it presents with vomiting, hydrocephalus, seizures, hemiplegia[189, 381], neck retraction and decerebrate posturing[311]. The tumor grows out of the vermis cerebelli and often fills the 4th ventricle infiltrates the cerebellar peduncles, and cerebellar hemispheres and thickens fivefold the outer granular layer of the cerebellar folia[199]. In ⅓ of the cases the tumor reaches the ST space and in another ⅓ there is leptomeningeal seeding like "candle wax"[79, 189]. The first presenting symptom can be flaccid paraplegia with bowel and bladder disorders due to spinal metastasis.

MBL of true congenital origin was observed in monocygotic twins[152, 433] and in siblings[37, 41]; it can occur together with renal malignoma (personal observation).

Diagnosis of MBL is established in infants by CT and vertebral angiography (Figs. 14a and b). It is important to stress this as the findings sometimes are very extensive[284, 332]. Intravenous contrast and sometimes high resolution CT scanning is necessary in order not to overlook the subarachnoid seedlings already present.

Prognosis in infants with MBL is poor[79], as it is for those with IT EPDY in that age group: 40% of the children die within 6 months after the diagnosis, many of the survivors are tetraspastic, mentally retarded, blind, suffer from epilepsy and need home or foster care. Prognosis (without RT) is hopeless[189].

d) *EPDY:* 3/5 of EPDY in infants are located intra- or paraventricularly above the tentorium; the tumors are high grade (III/IV) and often are of considerable size up to 5–8 cm in diameter[189, 370]. Diagnosis was made in very premature babies as early as the 29th week of gestation[254]. In that particular case there was tumor spread throughout the brain stem and the whole spinal cord. Hydramnion of the mother may be observed as a nonspecific phenomenon. The history of infants with EPDY generally is longer than in those who suffer from PLP, teratoma, or MBL. The presenting symptoms are: hydrocephalus, vomiting, papilledema, and often optic atrophy[79, 189]. Prognosis is similar to children with MBL.

e) *GLB* in infants located in the cerebral hemispheres or the caudal brain stem accounts for 2–4% of the tumors of the first 2 years of life[144, 398, 413]. Some have remarkable size[362] and spread widely throughout the meninges[336].

Other congenital malignancies like *PNETs* spread widely. They can grow from the base of the PF up to the rostral end of the brain stem[40], (1 personal observation). Like MBL, they have been reported in monocygotic twins[115]. Angiosarcoma, hemangioblastoma, hemangiopericytoma[404] have been described in the neonatal period as well as meningal tumors which might have undergone malignant transformation[79] and are reported even to seed extraaxially at this age[307].

Bonnin *et al.*[56] reported on the simultaneous occurrence of renal and cerebral neoplasms: There were 6 malignant rhabdoid and one Wilm's tumor, and independently in these children the following CNS tumors were diagnosed: MBL in

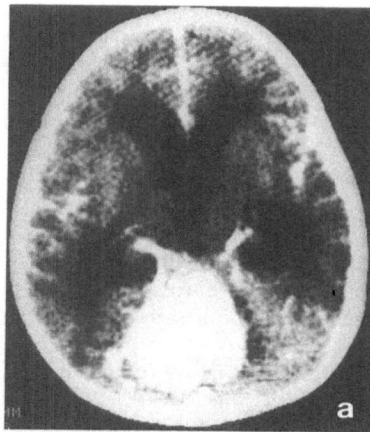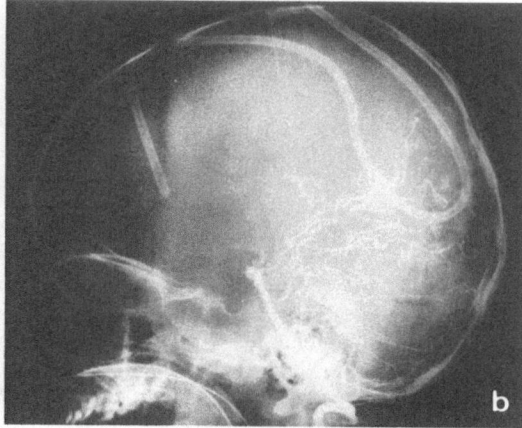

Figs. 14 a and **b.** CT and lateral vertebral angiogram in a boy, 10 months old with MBL of the whole vermis cerebelli

3, PNET in 2, PBL and subependymal giant cell ASCY in one each. In 6 of the patients the renal tumor already had metastasized, and in 2 of them the brain tumor already had seeded within the neural axis.

Treatment of Infantile Brain Tumors

If possible, total or subtotal removal of the tumor is most helpful to the baby, since extensive use of CHT and at this age group is limited. The reasons for giving RT after CHT have already been discussed. It is clear that the later RT is used at this age group the less the risk of interfering with growth will be[197]. Dose reduction in RT for the 1st year of life: 20 Gy and 10 Gy for the 2nd year has been recommended[79].

Acknowledgement

This work was assisted by Gertrud Weiermann, MD, who reviewed our cases and perused the manuscript.

References

1. Abay EO, Laws ER, Grado GL, Bruckman JE, Forbes GS, Gomez MR, Scott M (1981) Pineal tumors in children and adolescents. Treatment by CSF shunting and radiotherapy. J Neurosurg 55: 889–895
2. Abramson DH, Ronner HJ, Ellsworth RM (1979) Second tumors in nonradiated retinoblastoma. Am J Ophthalmol 87: 624–627
3. Afra D, Müller W, Slowik F, Wilcke O, Budka H, Turoczy L (1983) Supratentorial lobar ependymomas; reports on the grading and survival periods in 80 cases, including 46 recurrences. Acta Neurochir (Wien) 69: 243–251
4. Aguila LA, Chou SM, Bay JW (1984) Primary intracranial germinoma presenting as lower cranial nerve involvement: case report and review of the literature. Neurosurgery 14: 475–479

5. Ahagon A, Yoshida Y, Kosuno K, Uno T (1983) Suprasellar germinoma in association with Klinefelter's syndrome. Case report. J Neurosurg 58: 136–138

6. Aicardi J, Praud E, Bancaud J, Mises J, Chevrie JJ (1970) Épilepsies cliniquement primitives et tumeurs cérébrales chez l'enfant. Arch Franç Pédiat 27: 1041–1055

7. Albright AL, James HE (1985) Neurosurgical staging of midline intra-axial (nuclear) tumors. . Cancer 56: 1786–1788

8. Allen JC (1978) The effects of cancer therapy on the nervous system. J Pediatrics 93: 903–909

9. Allen JC, Nisselbaum J, Epstein F, Rosen G, Schwartz MK (1979) Alpha-fetoprotein and human chorionic gonadotropin determination in cerebrospinal fluid. An aid to the diagnosis and management of intracranial germ-cell tumors. J Neurosurg 51: 368–374

10. Allen JC, Helson L (1981) High-dose cyclophosphamide chemotherapy for recurrent CNS tumors in children. J Neurosurg 55: 749–756

11. Allen JC (1981) Neurotoxic potential of methotrexate and vincristine. In: Hanefeld F, Rating D (Hrsg) Aktuelle Neuropädiatrie II. Hippokrates, Stuttgart, S 105–112

12. Allen JC, Walker R, Kim JH (1985) Preradiation chemotherapy for newly diagnosed central nervous system germinoma—an attempt to reduce the radiotherapy dose while increasing survival (abstr). Ann Neurol 18: 404–405

13. Alvord EC (1976) Why do gliomas not metastasize? Arch Neurol 33: 73–75

14. Andler W, Roosen K, Clar HE (1982) Endocrinological investigations in 68 children with brain tumors. In: Voth D, Gutjahr P, Langmaid C (eds) Tumours of the central nervous system in infancy and childhood. Springer, Berlin Heidelberg New York, pp 415–419

15. Araki C, Matsumoto S (1969) Statistical reevaluation of pinealoma and related tumors in Japan. J Neurosurg 30: 146–149

16. Arnold H, Franke HD, Langendorf G, Olotu R, Grosch-Wörner J (1982) Medulloblastoma. Relationship of histologic type to survival. In: Voth D, Gutjahr P, Langmaid C (eds) Tumours of the central nervous system in infancy and childhood. Springer, Berlin Heidelberg New York, pp 404–409

17. Arnstein LH, Boldrey E, Nafziger HC (1951) A case report and survey of brain tumors during the neonatal period. J Neurosurg 8: 315–319

18. Aron BS (1971) Medulloblastoma in children. Am J Dis Child 121: 314–317

19. Arseni C, Ciurea AV (1981) Statistical survey of 276 cases of medulloblastoma (1935–1978). Acta Neurochir (Wien) 57: 159–162

20. Artiles GN (1968) Tumores de la fossa posterior. Arch Pediatria (Barcelona) 19: 240–242

21. Ashley JB (1969) The two "Hit" and multiple "Hit" theories of carcinogenesis. Br J Cancer 23: 313–328

22. Atac MS, Blaauw G (1979) Radiotherapy in brain-stem gliomas in children. Clin Neurol Neurosurg 81: 281–290

23. Attanasio A, Borelli P, di Rocco E, Marini R, Cappa M, Cambiaso P, Crino A, Gupta D (1985) Clinical significance of melatonin in children. In: Gupta D (ed) Pediatric neuroendocrinology. Croom Helm, London Sydney, pp 203–219

24. Auff E, Schuster H (1980) Konnatales Riesengliom. Neuropädiatrie 11: 91–95

25. Aur R, Hustu HD, Simone J (1976) Leukoencephalopathy in children with acute lymphocytic leukemia receiving preventive central nervous system therapy. Proc Am Soc Clin Oncol 17: 97

26. Axelrod L (1977) Endocrine dysfunction in patients with tumors of the pineal region. In: Schmidek HH (ed) Pineal tumors. Masson, New York, pp 61–77

27. Backus RE, Millichap JG (1962) The seizures as a manifestation of intracranial tumor in childhood. Pediatrics 29: 978–984

28. Bader JL, Miller RW, Meadows AT, Zimmerman LE, Champion LAA, Voute PA (1980) Trilateral retinoblastoma. Lancet ii: 582–583

29. Balhuizen JC, Bots GTA, Schaberg A, Bosman FT (1978) Value of cerebrospinal fluid cytology for the diagnosis of malignancies in the central nervous system. J Neurosurg 48: 747–753

30. Bamberg M, Sauerwein W, Scherer F (1982) Methoden und Ergebnisse der Strahlentherapie beim Medulloblastom. Strahlentherapie 158: 71–75

31. Bamberg M, Metz K, Alberti W, Heckemann R, Schulz U (1984) Endodermal sinus tumor of the pineal region. Metastases through a ventriculoperitoneal shunt. Cancer 54: 903–906

32. Barber SG, Smith JA Cove DH, Smith SCH, London DR (1978) Marker for pineal tumors? Lancet ii: 372–373

33. Barber SG, Smith JA, Hughes RD (1982) Melatonin as a tumor marker in a patient with pineal tumour. Br Med J 3: 328

34. Barnett HJ, Hyland HH (1952) Tumours involving the brain-stem. A study of 90 cases arising in the brain-stem, fourth ventricle, and pineal tissue. Quart J Med 21: 265–284

35. Barone BM, Elvidge AR (1970) Ependymomas. A clinical survey. J Neurosurg 33: 428–438

36. Batnitzky S, Segall HD, Cohen ME (1985) Radiologic guidelines in assessing children with intracranial tumors. Cancer 56: 1756–1762

37. Belemaric J, Chau AS (1969) Medulloblastoma in newborn sisters. J Neurosurg 30: 76–79

38. Berry MP, Jenkin DT, Keen CW, Nair BD, Simpson WJ (1981) Radiation treatment of medulloblastoma. A 21 year review. J Neurosurg 55: 43–51

39. Berthold R, Janka G, Lampert F (1981) Kleinhirnmedulloblastom — retrospektive Untersuchung der Wertigkeit von Diagnostik und Therapie. Klin Pädiatr 193: 189–197

40. Bettendorf U (1975) Ein ungewöhnlicher Hirntumor im frühen Säuglingsalter. Monatsschr Kinderheilk 123: 780–786

41. Bickerstaff ER, Connolly RC, Woolf AL (1967) Cerebellar medulloblastoma occurring in brothers. Acta Neuropathol (Berl) 8: 104–107

42. Bilaniuk LT, Zimmerman RA, Littman P, Gallo E, Rorke LB, Bruce DA, Schut L (1980) Computed tomography of brain stem gliomas in children. Radiology 134: 89–95

43. Bleyer WA, Drake JC, Chabner BA (1973) Neurotoxicity and elevated cerebrospinalfluid methotrexate concentration in meningeal leukemia. New Engl J Med 289: 770–773

44. Bleyer WA, Milstein J, Balis F (1983) "8 drugs in 1 day" chemotherapy for brain tumors: a new approach and rationale for preradiation chemotherapy. Med Pediatr Oncol 11: 213

45. Bloom HJG, Wallace ENK, Henk JM (1969) The treatment and prognosis of medulloblastoma in children—a study of 82 verified cases. Am J Roentgenol 105: 43–62

46. Bloom HJG (1975) Combined modality therapy for intracranial tumors. Cancer 35: 111–120

47. Bloom HJG (1982) Intracranial tumors: response and resistance to therapeutic endeavors, 1970–1980. Int J Radiat Oncol Biol Phys 8: 1083–1113

48. Bloom HJG, Glees JP (1985) Chemotherapy of gliomas in adults and of medulloblastoma in children. In: Voth D, Krauseneck P (eds) Chemotherapy of gliomas. De Gruyter, Berlin New York, pp 331–339

49. Blume WT, Girvin JP, Kaufmann JCE (1982) Childhood brain tumors presenting as chronic uncontrolled focal seizure disorders. Ann Neurol 12: 538–541

50. Bode U (1982) Nebenwirkungen antineoplastischer Therapie auf das kindliche Nervensystem. Klin Pädiatr 194: 351–358

51. Bodechtel G, Marguth F, Kollmannsberger A, Kazner E (1974) Hirntumoren, kaudaler Hirnstamm. In: Bodechtel G (Hrsg) Differentialdiagnose neurologischer Krankheitsbilder, 3. Aufl. Thieme, Stuttgart, S 408–410

52. Bogdahn U, Rupniak HTR, Ali-Osman F, Rosenblum ML (1985) Characterization of human malignant brain tumor cells in vitro and comparison of three different in vitro assays to determine their sensitivity to BCNU. In: Voth D, Krauseneck P (eds) Chemotherapy of gliomas. De Gruyter, Berlin New York, pp 321–328

53. Bolande RP (1974) The neurocristopathies. A unifying concept of disease arising in neural crest maldevelopment. Hum Pathol 5: 409–429

54. Boldrey E, Sheline G (1966) Delayed transitory clinical manifestations after radiation treatment of intracranial tumors. Acta Radiol (Ther) 5: 5–10

55. Bongartz EB, Bamberg M, Nau HE, Schmitt G, Bayindir C (1979) Optimal therapy in medulloblastoma. Acta Neurochir (Wien) 50: 117–125

56. Bonnin JM, Rubinstein LJ, Palmer NF, Beckwith JB (1984) The association of embryonal tumors originating in the kidney and in the brain. A report of seven cases. Cancer 54: 2137–2146

57. Borck WF, Rönnis W (1955) Zur Differentialdiagnose infratentorieller Geschwülste. Die Bedeutung von Vorgeschichte und Untersuchungsbefund für die Erkennung und Unterscheidung der Kleinhirntumoren. Bericht über 480 raumfordernde Prozesse. Neurol Psychiatr (Bucur) 23: 123–166

58. Borit A, Blackwood W, Mair WGP (1980) The separation of pineocytoma from pineoblastoma. Cancer 45: 1408–1418

59. Borit A, Richardson EP (1982) The biological and clinical behaviour of pilocytic astrocytomas of the optic pathways. Brain 105: 161–187

60. Bray PF, Carter S, Taveras JM (1958) Brain stem tumors in children. Neurology 8: 1–17

61. Bresnan MJ, Gilles FH, Lorenzo AV, Watters GV, Barlow CF (1972) Leukoencephalopathy following combined irradiation and intraventricular methotrexate therapy of brain tumors in childhood. Trans Am Neurol Assoc NY 97: 204–206

62. Broadbent VA, Barnes ND, Wheeler TK (1981) Medulloblastoma in childhood: long-term results of treatment. Cancer 48: 26–30

63. Brown JR (1967) Cerebellar tumors in Cildren. Mayo Clin Proc 42: 511–516

64. Bruce DA, Allen JC (1985) Tumor staging for pineal region tumors of childhood. Cancer 56: 1792–1794

65. Brutschin P, Culver GJ (1973) Extracranial metastases from medulloblastoma. Radiology 107: 359–362

66. Butti G, Knerich R, Tanghetti B, Adinolfi D, Gaetani P, Buoncristiani P, Paolelli P (1984) Perioperative Carmustine chemotherapy for malignant brain tumors. Cancer Treat Rep 68: 1505–1506

67. Caincross RG, Rexman JHW, Rathborne MP, del Maestro RF (1984) An analysis of post-operative enhancement and other CT artifacts in brain tumor patients. J Neurol-Oncol 2: 273

68. Camins MB, Mount LA (1974) Primary suprasellar atypical teratoma. Brain 97: 447–456

69. Castro-Vita H, Salazar OM, Cova M, Rubin P (1978) Cerebellar medulloblastoma: spread and failure patterns following irradiation. Int J Radiat Oncol Biol Phys [Suppl] 2: 211–212

70. Chang CH, Housepian EM, Herbert C (1969) An operative staging system and a megavoltage radiotherapeutic technic for cerebellar medulloblastoma. Radiology 93: 1351–1359

71. Chapman PH, Linggood RM (1980) The management of pineal area tumors. A recent reappraisal. Cancer 46: 1253–1257

72. Chatty E, Earle KM (1971) Medulloblastoma. A report of 201 cases on the relationship of histologic variants and survival. Cancer 28: 977–983

73. Chatta AS, Delong GR (1975) Sylvian aqueduct syndrome as a sign of acute obstructive hydrocephalus in children. J Neurol Neurosurg Psychiat 38: 288–296

74. Chen HP (1958) Intracranial teratoma of a newborn. Report of an unusual case. J Neuropathol Exp Neurol 17: 599–603

75. Choux M, Lena G (1982) Le médulloblastome. Neurochirurgie [Suppl] 28: 1–229. Masson, Paris

76. Chowdhury C, Roy S, Mahapatra AK, Bhatia R (1985) Medullomyoblastoma. A teratoma. Cancer 55: 1495–1500

77. Chutorian AM, Schwartz JF, Carter S (1964) Optic glioma in children. Neurology 14: 83–95

78. Clar E, Reinhardt V, Gerhard L, Hensell V (1979) Clinical and morphological studies of pineal tumours. Acta Neurochir (Wien) 46: 59–76

79. Cohen ME, Duffner PK (1984) Brain tumors in children. Principles of diagnosis and treatment. Raven, New York

80. Cohen ME, Duffner PK, Heffner RR, Lacey DN, Brecher M (1985) Long-term survivors of brainstem gliomas (abstr). Ann Neurol 18: 395

81. Cook BR, Gutkelch AN (1983) Modern approaches to the treatment of medulloblastoma. Dev Med Child Neurol 25: 245–247

82. Cooper PR, Budzilovich GN, Bergczeller PH, Lieberman A, Battista A (1974) Metastatic glioma associated with hypercalcemia. J Neurosurg 39: 255–259

83. Corboz R (1958) Die Psychiatrie der Hirntumoren bei Kindern. Acta Neurochir (Wien) [Suppl] 5: 1–100

84. Coulon RA, Till K (1977) Intracranial ependymomas in children. A review of 43 cases. Child's Brain 3: 154–168

85. Crafts DC, Levin VA, Edwards MS, Pischer TL, Wilson CB (1978) Chemotherapy of recurrent medulloblastoma with combined procarbazine, CCNU, and vincristine. J Neurosurg 49: 589–592

86. Crist WM, Ragab AH, Vietti TJ, Ducos R, Chu JY (1976) Chemotherapy of childhood medulloblastoma. Am J Dis Child 130: 639–642

87. Crocker EF, Zimmerman RA, Phelps ME, Kuhl DE (1976) The effects of steroids on the extravascular distribution of radiographic contrast material and technitium pertechnetate in brain tumors as determined by computed tomography. Radiology 119: 471–474

88. Cumberlin RL, Luk KH, Wara WM, Sheline GE, Wilson CB (1979) Medulloblastoma. Treatment results and effect on normal tissues. Cancer 43: 1014–1020

89. Danoff BF, Cowchocks FS, Marquette C, Mulgrew L, Kramer S (1982) Assessment of the long-term effects of primary radiation therapy for brain tumors in children. Cancer 49: 1580–1586

90. Dayan AD, Marshall AHE, Miller AA, Pick FJ, Bankin NE (1966) Atypical teratomas of the pineal and hypothalamus. J Pathol Bacteriol 92: 1–28

91. De Girolami U, Schmidek H (1973) Clinicopathological study of 53 tumor of the pineal region. J Neurosurg 39: 455–462

92. De Girolami U (1977) Pathology of the tumors of the pineal region. In: Schmidek HH (ed) Pineal tumors. Masson, New York, pp 1–19

93. De Lena M, Guzzon A, Moǹtardini S (1972) Clinical, radiologic, and histopathologic studies on pulmonary toxicity induced by treatment with bleomycin. Cancer Chemother Rep 56: 343–356

94. Deutsch M, Reigel DH (1980) The value of myelography in the management of childhood medulloblastoma. Cancer 45: 2194–2197

95. Deutsch M, Laurent JP, Cohen ME (1985) Myelography for staging medulloblastoma. Cancer 56: 1763–1766

96. Diksic M, Sako KK Feindel W, Kato A, Yamamoto YL, Farrokhzad S, Thompson C (1984) Pharmacokinetics of positron labelled 1,3-bis(2-chloroethyl)nitrosurea in human brain tumors using positron emission tomography. Cancer Res 44: 3120–3125

97. Dohrmann GJ, Farwell JR, Flannery JT (1976) Glioblastoma multiforme in children. J Neurosurg 44: 442–448

98. Dohrmann GJ, Farwell JR, Flannery JT (1976) Ependymomas and ependymoblastomas in children. J Neurosurg 45: 273–283

99. Dohrmann GJ, Rarwell JR, Flannery JT (1978) Oligodendroglioma in children. Surg Neurol 10: 21–25

100. Dorwart RA, Wara WM, Norman D, Levin VA (1981) Complete myelographic evaluation of spinal metastases from medulloblastoma. Radiology 139: 403–408

101. Drachman DA, Winter TS, Karon M (1963) Medulloblastoma with extracranial metastases. Arch Neurol 9: 518–530

102. Duckett S, Claireaux AE (1963) Cerebral teratoma associated with epignathus in a newborn infant. J Neuropath Exp Neurol 20: 888–891

103. Duckett S, Wilson RR (1964) Fetal spongioblastoma. J Neuropath Exp Neurol 23: 560–564

104. Duffner PK, Cohen ME, Thomas PRM, Sinks LF, Freeman AI (1979) Combination chemotherapy in recurrent medulloblastoma. Cancer 43: 41–45

105. Duffner PK, Cohen ME, Heffner RR, Freeman AI (1981) Primitive neuroectodermal tumors of childhood. An approach to therapy. . J Neurosurg 55: 376–381

106. Duffner PK, Cohen ME (1981) Extraneural metastases in childhood brain tumors. Ann Neurol 10: 261–265

107. Duffner PK, Cohen ME, Thomas P (1983) Late effects of treatment on the intelligence of children with posterior fossa tumors. Cancer 51: 233–237

108. Duffner PK, Cohen ME, Parker MS (1985) Prospective intellectual testing in children with brain tumors (abstr). Ann Neurol 18: 405

109. Duffner PK, Cohen ME, Thomas PRM, Lansky SB (1985) The long-term effects of cranial irradiation on the central nervous system. Cancer 56: 1841–1846

110. Dummermuth G (1958) EEG-Befunde bei Hirntumoren im Kindesalter. Arch Psychiat Zschr Ges Neurol 197: 594–618

111. Dupont MG, Gérard JM, Flament-Durand J, Baleriaux-Waha D, Mortelmans LL (1977) Pathognomonic aspects of germinoma on CT scan. Neuroradiology 14: 209–211

112. Eade OE, Urich H (1971) Metastasizing gliomas in young subjects. J Pathol 103: 245–256

113. Edwards MSB, Davis RL, Laurent JP (1985) Tumor markers and cytologic features of cerebrospinal fluid. Cancer 56: 1773–1777

114. Eiser C (1978) Intellectual abilities among survivors of childhood leukemia as a function of CNS irradiation. Arch Dis Childh 53: 391–395

115. Ende N (1955) Congenital brain tumor in one of identical twins. Cancer 8: 1057–1059

116. Enzman DR, Norman D, Levin V, Wilson C, Newton T (1978) Computed tomography in the follow-up of medulloblastomas and ependymomas. Radiology 128: 57–63

117. Epstein F (1985) A staging system for brain stem gliomas. Cancer 56: 1804–1806

118. Erlich SS, Davis RL (1978) Spinal subarachnoid metastasis from primary intracranial glioblastoma multiforme. Cancer 42: 2854–2864

119. Ethelberg S (1950) Symptomatic "cataplexy" or chalastic fits in cortical lesions of the frontal lobe. Brain 73: 499–512

120. Farwell JR, Dohrmann GJ, Flannery JT (1977) Central nervous system tumors in children. Cancer 40: 3123–3132

121. Farwell JR, Dohrmann GJ, Flannery JT (1978) Intracranial neoplasms in infants. Arch Neurol 35: 533–537
122. Farwell JR, Flannery JT (1984) Cancer in relatives of children with central nervous-system neoplasms. New Engl J Med 311: 749–753
123. Felgenhauer K, Nekic M, Jacobi C, Reiber HO, Frowein RA (1984) Tumormarker im Liquor cerebrospinalis. In: Heyden HW von, Krauseneck P (Hrsg) Hirnmetastasen. Pathophysiologie, Diagnostik, Therapie. Zuckschwerdt, München, S 107–117
124. Fessard C (1968) Cerebral tumors in infancy. 66 clinicoanatomical case studies. Am J Dis Child 115: 302–308
125. Fischer AQ, McLean WT (1982) Intractable hiccups as presenting symptom of brainstem tumor in children. Child's Brain 9: 60–63
126. Fisher M (1956) An unusual variant of acute idiopathic polyneuritis (syndrome of ophthalmoplegia, ataxia, and areflexia). New Engl J Med 255: 57–65
127. Foerster O, Gagel O, Mahoney W (1939) Die encephalen Tumoren des verlängerten Markes, der Brücke und des Mittelhirns. Arch Psychiat Nervenkr 110: 1–74
128. Fokes EC, Earle KM (1969) Ependymomas: clinical and pathological aspects. J Neurosurg 30: 585–594
129. Frederick P, Cassady JR, Jaffe N (1975) Risk of second tumors in survivors of childhood cancer. Cancer 35: 1230–1235
130. Freeman JE, Johnston PGB, Voke JM (1973) Somnolence after prophylactic cranial irradiation in children with acute lymphoblastic leukemia. Br Med J 4: 525–526
131. Fresh CB, Takei Y, O'Brien MS (1976) Cerebellar glioblastoma in childhood. J Neurosurg 45: 705–708
132. Fujii T, Itakura T, Hayashi S, Komai N, Nakamine H, Saito K (1981) Primary pineal choriocarcinoma with hemorrhage monitored by computerized tomography. Case report. J Neurosurg 55: 484–487
133. Fulton DS, Levin VA, Lubich WP, Wilson CB, Marton LJ (1980) Cerebrospinal fluid polyamines in patients with glioblastoma multiforme and anaplastic astrocytoma. Cancer Res 40: 3293–3296
134. Fulton DS, Levin VA, Wara WM, Edwards MS, Wilson CB (1981) Chemotherapy of pediatric brain-stem tumors. J Neurosurg 54: 721–725
135. Futrell NN, Osborn AG, Cheson BD (1981): Pineal region tumors: Computed tomographic-pathologic spectrum. Am J Radiol 137: 951–956
136. Gagliano RG, Costanzi JJ (1976) Paraplegia following intrathecal methotrexate. Cancer 37: 1663–1668
137. Galassi E, Tognetti F, Frank F, Gaist G (1984) Extraneural metastases from primary pineal tumors. Review of the literature. Surg Neurol 21: 497–504
138. Garwicz S, Aronson AS, Elqvist D, Landberg T (1975) Postirradiation syndrome with EEG findings in children with acute lymphoblastic leukemia. Acta Paediat Scand 64: 399–403
139. Gay JC, Janco RL, Lukens JN (1985) Systemic metastases in primary intracranial germinoma. Cancer 55: 2688–2690
140. Geissinger JD, Bucy PC (1970) Astrocytomas of the cerebellum in children: Long-term study. Trans Am Neurol Assoc 49: 178–181
141. Gérard JP (1977) Radiotherapie des Ependymomes. Neurochirurgie (Paris) [Suppl] 1: 39–52
142. Gerlach H, Jänisch W, Schreiber D (1982) Intracranial and spinal tumors in newborns. In: Voth D, Gutjahr P, Langmaid C (eds) Tumours of the nervous system in infancy and childhood. Springer, Berlin Heidelberg New York, pp 53–61
143. Gerlach J, Jensen HP (1959) Zur Differentialdiagnose des Glioblastoma multiforme bei Jugendlichen. Acta Neurochir (Wien) [Suppl] 6: 95–100

144. Gerlach J, Jensen HP, Koos W, Kraus H (Hrsg) (1967) Pädiatrische Neurochirurgie. Intrakranielle Geschwülste. Thieme, Stuttgart, S 459–645

145. Ginsberg S, Kirshner J, Reich S, Panasci L, Rinkelstein T, Fandrich S, Fitzpatrick A, Shechtman L, Comis F (1981) Systemic chemotherapy for a primary germ cell tumor of the brain: a pharmacokinetic study. Cancer Treat Rep 65: 477–483

146. Gjerris F, Klee JG, Klinken L (1976 a) Malignancy grade and long-term survival in brain tumors of infancy and childhood. Acta Neurol Scand (Stockh) 53: 61–71

147. Gjerris F (1976 b) Clinical aspects and long-term prognosis of intracranial tumours in infancy and childhood. Dev Med Child Neurol 18: 145–159

148. Gjerris F (1978) Clinical aspects and long-term prognosis in supratentorial tumours of infancy and childhood. Acta Neurol Scand (Stockh) 57: 445–470

149. Glasauer FE, Yuan RHP (1963) Intracranial tumors with extracranial metastases. J Neurosurg 20: 474–493

150. Gonzales-Vitale JC, Hayes DM, Cvitkovic E, Sternberg SS (1977) The renal pathology in clinical trials of cisplatinum (II)diamedinechloride. Cancer 39: 1362–1371

151. Goutelle A (1977) Les ependymomes intracraniens sous-tentoriels. Neurochir [Suppl] (23) 1: 53–66

152. Griepentrog F, Pauly H (1957) Intra- und extrakranielle, frühmanifeste Medulloblastome bei erbgleichen Zwillingen. Zentralbl Neurochir 17: 129–140

153. Grossman CB, Gonzalez CF (1977) Neuroradiology of the pineal region. In: Schmidek HH (ed) Pineal tumors. Masson, New York, pp 79–98

154. Grote W, Wappenschmidt J (1965) Großhirngeschwülste im Kindesalter. Zeitschr Kinderchir 2: 153–172

155. Grote W, Nau HE, Labers B (1982) Operatives Vorgehen beim Medulloblastom. Strahlentherapie 158: 63–70

156. Gullotta F, Neuman J (1980) Medulloblastome und zerebelläre Sarkome. Eine histologisch-katamnestissche Untersuchung. Neurochirurgie (Stuttgart) 23: 35–40

157. Gutjahr P, Dieterich E, Walther B (1981) Spätstatus Langzeitüberlebender nach infratentoriellen Tumoren im Kindesalter. In: Hanefeld F, Rating D (Hrsg) Aktuelle Neuropädiatrie II. Hippokrates, Stuttgart, S 94–104

158. Gutjahr P, Walther B (1982) Late effects after treatment of brain tumours in childhood. In: Voth D, Gutjahr P, Langmaid C (eds) Tumours of the nervous system in infancy and childhood. Springer, Berlin Heidelberg New York, pp 383–388

159. Gyepes MT, D'Angio GJ (1966) Extracranial metastases from central nervous system tumors in children and adolescents. Radiology 87: 55–63

160. Habermalz H, Stephani U, Riehm H, Hanefeld F (1982) Postoperative chemotherapy prior to radiotherapy in the combined treatment of medulloblastoma, ependymoma and tumours of the pineal region. In: Voth D, Gutjahr P, Langmaid C (eds) Tumours of the nervous system in infancy and childhood. Springer, Berlin Heidelberg New York, pp 338–343

161. Hanefeld F, Riehm H (1980) Therapy of acute lymphoblastic leukemia in childhood: effects on the nervous system. Neuropediatr 11: 3–16

162. Harisiadis L, Chang CH (1977) Medulloblastoma in children: a correlation between staging and results of treatment. Int J Radiat Oncol Biol Phys 2: 833–841

163. Hart MN, Early KM (1973) Primitive neuroectodermal tumors of the brain children. Cancer 32: 890–897

164. Hécaen H, de Ajuriaguerra J (1956) Troubles Méntaux au Cours des Tumeurs Intracraniennes. Masson, Paris

165. Heiskanen O (1977) Intracranial tumors of children. Child's Brain 3: 69–78

166. Hendin B, Devivo DC, Torak R, Lell ME, Ragab AH, Vietti TJ (1974) Parenchymatous degeneration of the central nervous system in childhood leukemia. Cancer 33: 468–482

167. Herpers MJHM, Budka H (1985) Primitive neuroectodermal tumors including the medulloblastoma: glial differentiation signaled by immunoreactivity for GFAP is restricted to the pure desmoplastic medulloblastoma ("arachnoid sarcoma of the cerebellum"). Clin Neuropathol 4: 12–18

168. Herrick MK, Rubinstein LJ (1979) The cytologic differentiating potentials of pineal parenchymal neoplasms (true pinealomas). A clinicopathological study of 28 tumors. Brain 102: 289–320

169. Herskovic A, Ornitz RD, Shell M, Rogers CC (1982) Treatment experience: glioblastoma multiforme treated with 15 MeV fast neutrons. Cancer 49: 2463–2465

170. Hess R (1961) Significance of EEG-signs for localization of cerebral tumors. Electroenceph Clin Neurophysiol [Suppl] 19: 75–110

171. Hirano A, Matsui T (1975) Vascular structure in brain tumors. Human Pathol 6: 611–621

172. Hirsch JF, Renier D, Czernichow P, Benveniste L, Pierre-Kahn A (1979) Medulloblastoma in childhood. Survival and functional results. Acta Neurochir (Wien) 48: 1–15

173. Hochberg F, Parker LM, Takrorian T, Canellos GP, Zervas NT (1981) High-dose BCNU with analogous bone marrow rescue for recurrent glioblastoma multiforme. J Neurosurg 54: 455–460

174. Hoffmann GR, Thiry S, Achslogh J, Brihaya J, Dereymaeker A (1961) Étude statistique de 202 cas de tumeurs de la fosse postérieur de l'enfance. Neurochirurgie 7: 97–107

175. Hoffmann HJ, Hendrick EB, Humphreys RP (1976) Metastasis via ventriculo-peritoneal shunt in patients with medulloblastoma. J Neurosurg 44: 652–666

176. Hoffman HJ, Duffner PK (1985) Extraneural metastases of central nervous system tumors. Cancer 56: 1778–1782

177. Holldack J, Schindler H, Havers W (1985) Neurologische und psychosoziale Störungen bei Kindern mit Hirntumoren. Klin Pädiatr 197: 188–191

178. Holt JF (1978) Neurofibromatosis in children. Am J Roentgenol 130: 615–639

179. Horowitz ME, Kun LE, Mulhern RK, Simmons JC, Sanford RA, Hayes FA, Jacobson M, Igarashi M (1985) Brain tumors in children less than 3 years of age: chemotherapy followed by delayed irradiation. (abstr) Ann Neurol 18: 395–396

180. Horrax G (1950) Treatment of tumors of the pineal body: experience in a series of 22 cases. Arch Neurol Psychiat (Chic) 64: 227–242

181. Hoshino T, Wilson CB (1975) Review of basic concepts of cell kinetics as applied to brain tumors. J Neurosurg 42: 123–131

182. Hoshino T, Kobayashi S, Townsend JT, Wilson CB (1985) A cell kinetic study on medulloblastoma. Cancer 55: 1711–1713

183. Jacobi G (1981) Klinik und Diagnostik kindlicher Hirntumoren. In: Hanefeld F, Rating D (Hrsg) Aktuelle Neuropädiatrie II. Hippokrates, Stuttgart, S 54–69

184. Jacobi G (1982) Intrakranielle Tumoren im Kindesalter. Aktuel Neurol 9: 42–50

185. Jacobi G (1982) Clinical presentation of space-occupying lesions of the central nervous system. In: Voth D, Gutjahr P, Langmaid C (eds) Tumours of the central nervous system in infancy and childhood. Springer, Berlin Heidelberg New York, pp 72–84

186. Jacobi G (1984) Infratentorielle Hirntumoren des Kindes. Klinische Untersuchung zur Frage einer Hirnstammbeteiligung. Therapiewoche 34: 1343–1347

187. James HE, Edwards SB (1985) Systemic staging of supratentorial extra-axial brain tumors in children. Craniopharyngiomas, atypical teratoma and teratoid tumors of the suprasellar region (germinomas), and intracranial teratomas. Cancer 56: 1800–1803

188. Jänisch W, Schreiber D (1966) Neuroektodermale Hirngeschwülste als Todesursache bei Neugeborenen und Säuglingen. Zentralbl Allg Pathol 109: 170–175

189. Jänisch W, Schreiber D, Gerlach H (1980) Tumoren des Zentralnervensystems bei Feten und Säuglingen. VEB Fischer, Jena

190. Jautzke G, Iglesias J (1985) Prolactinomas and mixed adenomas with prolactin cells: an immunohistochemical study of the subcellular localization of hormones. In: Auer LM, Leb G, Tscherne G, Urdl W, Walter FG (eds) Prolactinomas. De Gruyter, Berlin New York, pp 15–25

191. Jellinger K (1973 Primary intracranial germ cell tumours. Acta Neuropathol (Berl) 25: 291–306

192. Jellinger K, Sunder-Plassmann M (1973) Connatal intracranial tumours. Neuropädiatrie 4: 46–63

193. Jenkin RD, Simpson WJ, Keen CW (1978) Pineal and suprasellar germinomas. J Neurosurg 48: 99–107

194. Jereb B, Sundaresan N, Horten B, Reid A, Galicich JH (1981) Supratentorial recurrences in medulloblastoma. Cancer 47: 806–809

195. Jooma R, Kendall BE (1983) Diagnosis and management of pineal tumors. J Neurosurg 58: 654–665

196. Jordan RM, Kendall JW, McClung M, Kammer H (1980) Concentration of human chorionic gonadotropin in the cerebrospinal fluid of patients with germinal cell hypothalamic tumors. Pediatrics 65: 121–124

197. Judisch GF, Patil SR (1981) Concurrent heritable retinoblastoma, pinealoma, and trisomy X. Arch Ophthalmol 99: 1767–1769

198. Jungmann E, Althoff PH, Hermann J, Schöffling K (1985) Evidence for functional impairment of growth hormone secretion in prolactinoma. In: Auer LM, Leb G, Tscherne G, Urdl W, Walter FG (eds) Prolactinomas. De Gruyter, Berlin New York, pp 147–153

199. Kadin ME, Rubinstein LE, Nelson JS (1970) Neonatal cerebellar medulloblastoma originating from the fetal exlternal granular layer. J Neuropathol Exp Neurol 29: 583–600

200. Kageyama N, Belsky R (1961) Ectopic pinealoma in the chiasma region. Neurology (Minneap) 11: 318–327

201. Kahle W (1957) Zum Problem der diffusen Glioblastose. Dtsch Z Nervenheilk 176: 469–499

202. Karch SB, Urich H (1972) Medulloepithelioma: definition and entity. J Neuropathol Exp Neurol 31: 27–53

203. Kay HEM, Knapton PJ, O'Sullivan JP, Harris RF, Innes EM, Stuart J, Schwartz FCM, Thompson EN (1972) Encephalopathy in acute leukemia associated with methotrexate therapy. Arch Dis Childh 47: 344–354

204. Kazner E, Wende S, Grumme T, Lanksch W, Stochdorph O (1981) Computertomographie intrakranieller Tumoren aus klinischer Sicht. Springer, Berlin Heidelberg New York

205. Kemmerling S, Neumärker KJ (1984) Möglichkeiten mehrdimensionaler Therapie der Medulloblastome und Ependymome im Kindesalter unter Berücksichtigung prognostischer Faktoren. Dtsch Gesundh Wesen 39: 1328–1333

206. Kernohan JW, Fletcher-Kernohan EM (1937) Ependymomas. A study of 109 cases. Publ Ass Res Nerv Ment Dis 16: 182–209

207. Keschner M, Bender MB, Strauss I (1937) Mental symptoms in cases of subtentorial tumors. Arch Neurol Psychiatry (Chic) 37: 1–17

208. Kessinger A (1984) High dose chemotherapy with autologous bone marrow rescue for high grade gliomas of the brain. A potential for improvement in therapeutic results. Neurosurgery 15: 747–750

209. Kessler LA, Dugan P, Concannon JP (1975) Systemic metastases of medulloblastoma promoted by shunting. Surg Neurol 3: 147–152

210. Kim YH, Fayos JV (1977) Intracranial ependymomas. Radiology 124: 805–808

211. King GA, Sagerman RH (1979) Late recurrence in medulloblastoma. Am J Roentgenol 123: 7–12
212. Kleihues P, Banborschke S, Kiessling M, Wiestler O (1982) Developmental neuro-oncogenesis in experimental animals. In: Voth D, Gutjahr P, Langmaid C (eds) Tumors of the central nervous system in infancy and childhood. Springer, Berlin Heidelberg New York, pp 19–31
213. Klein DM, McCulloch DC (1985) Surgical staging of cerebellar astrocytomas in childhood. Cancer 56: 1810–1811
214. Kleinman GM, Schoene WC, Walshe TM, Richardson EP (1978) Malignant transformation in benign cerebellar astrocytoma. Case report. J Neurosurg 49: 111–118
215. Kleinman GM, Hochberg FH, Richardson EP (1981) Systemic metastases from medulloblastoma: report of two cases and review of the literature. Cancer 48: 2296–2309
216. Klériga E, Hollenberg Sher J, Nallainathan S, Stein SC, Sacher M (1978) Development of cerebellar malignant astrocytoma at site of a medulloblastoma treated 11 years earlier. Case report. J Neurosurg 49: 445–449
217. Knudson AG (1975) Genetics of human cancer. Genetics 79: 305–316
218. Knudson AG, Meadows AT (1981) Regression of neuroblastoma IV-S: a genetic hypothesis. New Engl J Med 302: 1254–1255
219. Kobayashi T, Kageyama N, Kida Y, Yoshida J, Shibuya N, Okamura K (1981) Unilateral germinomas involving the basal ganglia and thalamus. J Neurosurg 55: 55–62
220. Koide O, Watanabe Y, Sato K (1980) A pathological survey of intracranial germinoma and pinealoma in Japan. Cancer 45: 2119–2130
221. Kölmel HW (1977) Atlas of cerebrospinal fluid cells. Springer, Berlin Heidelberg New York
222. Koos W, Valencak E (1968) Les processus expansifs intracraniens congénitaux présentant l'aspect clinique de l'hydrocéphalie congénitale ou précoce. Neurochirurgie 14: 75–79
223. Koos WT, Miller MH (1971) Intracranial tumors of infants and children. Thieme, Stuttgart
224. Kopelson G (1982) Cerebellar glioblastoma. Cancer 50: 308–311
225. Kopelson G, Linggood RM, Kleinman GM (1983) Medulloblastoma. The identification of prognostic subgroups and implication for multimodality management. Cancer 51: 312–319
226. Kornhuber B (1982) Cytostatic monotherapy of tumours of the central nervous system in children. In: Voth D, Gutjahr P, Langmaid C (eds) Tumours of the central nervous system in infancy and childhood. Springer, Berlin Heidelberg New York, pp 367–377
227. Kosnik EJ, Boesel CP, Bay J, Sayers MP (1978) Primitive neuroectodermal tumors of the central nervous system in children. J Neurosurg 48: 741–746
228. Krauseneck P, Bohndorf W, Bushe KA, Halves E, Mertens HG, Wilms K, Sturm V, Kleihues P (1986) Maligne Tumoren des Gehirns im Erwachsenenalter. Dtsch Ärztebl 83: 686–689
229. Kricheff II, Becker M, Schneck SA, Taveras JM (1964) Intracranial ependymomas: factors influencing prognosis. J Neurosurg 21: 7–14
230. Kun LE, d'Souza B, Tefft M (1985) The value of surveillance testing in childhood brain tumors. Cancer 56: 1818–1823
231. Lacey DJ (1984) Long-term pathologic effects of cancer treatment on the nervous system. In: Cohen ME, Duffner PK (eds) Brain tumors in children. Principles of diagnosis and treatment. Raven Press, New York, pp 328–347
232. Lapras C, Dechaume JP, Deruty R, Capdeville J (1973) Traitement des tumeurs de la région pinéale. Lyon Chir 69: 196–198

233. Lapras C, Lepoire J (1967) Traitement de l'hydrocéphalie non tumorale du nourrisson par la dérivation ventriculo-atriale. Neurochirurgie 13: 209–342
234. Lapras C, Poirier N, Deruty R, Joyeux O (1975) Le cathétérisme de l'aqueduc de Sylvius. Sa place actuelle dans le traitement chirurgical des sténoses des l'aqueduc de Sylvius, des tumeurs de la F.C.P. et de la syringomyélie. Neurochirurgie 21: 101–108
235. Landberg T, Lindgren ML, Cavallin-Stähl EK, Svahn-Trapper GO, Sundbärg G, Garwicz S, Lagergren JA, Gunnesson VL, Brun AE, Cronqvist SE (1980) Improvements in the radiotherapy of medulloblastoma 1946–1975. Cancer 45: 670–678
236. Lassiter KRL, Alexander E, Davis CH, Kelly DL (1971) Surgical treatment of brain stem gliomas. J Neurosurg 34: 719–725
237. Lassman LP, Sarjona VR (1967) Pontine gliomas of childhood. Lancet i: 913–915
238. Lassman LP (1974) Tumours of the pons and medulla oblongata. In: Vinken PJ, Bruyn GW (eds) Handbook of clinical neurology, vol 17. Elsevier, Amsterdam New York, pp 693–706
239. Latchaw JP, Hahn JF, Moylan DJ, Humphries R, Mealey J (1985) Medulloblastoma. Period of risk reviewed. Cancer 55: 186–189
240. Laurent JP, Chang CH, Cohen ME (1985) A classification system for primitive neuroectodermal tumors (medulloblastoma) of the posterior fossa. Cancer 56: 1807–1809
241. Lausberg G (1968) Klinik, Therapie und Prognose des Kleinhirnmedulloblastoms. Zschr Kinderheilk 102: 193–203
242. Leavitt F (1928) Cerebellar tumors occurring in identical twins. Arch Neurol Psychiatry (Chic) 19: 617–622
243. Lee F (1975) Radiation of infratentorial and supratentorial brain-stem tumors. J Neurosurg 43: 65–68
244. Lee YY, Glass JP, van Eys J, Wallace S (1985) Medulloblastoma in infants and children. Computed tomographic follow-up after treatment. Radiology 154: 677–682
245. Leedham PW (1972) Primary cerebral rhabdomyosarcoma and the problem of medulloblastoma. J Neurol Neurosurg Psychiat 35: 551–559
246. Levin VA, Edwards MS, Wara WM, Allen J, Ortega J, Vestnys P (1984a) 1-(2-chloroethyl)-3-cyclohexyl-1-nitrourea (CCNU) followed by hydroxurea, misonidazole, and irradiation for brain stem gliomas: a pilot study of the Brain Tumor Research Center and Childrens' Cancer Group. Neurosurgery 14: 679–681
247. Levin VA, Resser KJ, Grath L, Vestnys P, Nutik S, Wilson CB (1984b) BCNU Treatment for recurrent malignant glioma. Cancer Treat Rep 68: 969–973
248. Lewis MB, Nunes LB, Powell DE, Snider BI (1973) Extracranial spread of medulloblastoma. Cancer 31: 1287–1297
249. Liebner EJ, Pretto JI, Hochhauser M, Kassaraba W (1964) Tumors of the posterior fossa in childhood and adolescence. Radiology 82: 193–201
250. Lin SR, Crane MD, Lin ZS, Bilaniuk L, Plasche WM, Marshall L, Spataro RF (1978) Characteristics of calcification in the tumors of the pineal gland. Radiology 126: 721–726
251. Littman P, Jarrett P, Bilaniuk LT, Rorke B, Zimmerman RA, Bruce DA, Carabell SC, Schut L (1980) Pediatric brain stem gliomas. Cancer 45: 2787–2792
252. Liwnicz BH, Rubinstein LJ (1979) The pathways of extraneural spread in metastasizing gliomas. Hum Pathol 10: 453–467
253. Long DM (1970) Capillary ultrastructure and the blood-brain barrier in human malignant grain tumors. J Neurosurg 32: 127–144
254. Lorentzen M, Hägerstrand I (1980) Congenital ependymoblastoma. Acta Neuropathol (Berl) 49: 71–74
255. Low NL, Correll JW, Hammill JF (1965) Tumors of the cerebral hemispheres in children. Arch Neurol (Chic) 13: 547–554

256. Luccarelli G (1980) Glioblastoma multiforme of the cerebellum: description of three cases. Acta Neurochir (Wien) 53: 107–116

257. Luddy RE, Gilman PA (1973) Paraplegia following intrathecal methotrexate. J Pediatr 83: 988–992

258. Luna MA, Bedrossian CW, Lichtiger B (1972) Interstitial pneumonitis associated with bleomycin therapy. Am J Clin Pathol 58: 501–510

259. Mabon RF, Svien HJ, Kernohan JW, Craig WMK (1949) Ependymomas. Proc Staff Meet Mayo Clin 23: 65–71

260. Madias NE, Harrington JT (1978) Platinum nephrotoxicity. Am J Med 65: 307–314

261. Mannoji H, Takeshita I, Fukui M, Ohta M, Kitamura K (1981) Glial fibrillary acid protein in medulloblastoma. Acta Neuropathol (Berl) 55: 63–69

262. Mantravadi RVP, Phatak R, Bellur S, Liebner EJ, Haas R (1982) Brain stem gliomas. An autopsy study of 25 cases. Cancer 49: 1294–1296

263. Markesbery WR, Challa VR (1979) Electron microscopic findings in primitive neuroectodermal tumors of the cerebrum. Cancer 44: 141–147

264. Maroon JC, Albright L (1977) "Failure to thrive" due to pontine glioma. Arch Neurol (Chic) 34: 295–297

265. Marsa GW, Probert JC, Rubinstein LJ, Bagshaw MA (1975) Megavoltage irradiation of gliomas of the brain and spinal cord. Cancer 36: 1681–1689

266. Martinius J, Matthes A, Lombroso CT (1968) Electroencephalographic features in posterior fossa tumors in children. Electroencephal Clin Neurophysiol 25: 128–139

267. Marton LJ, Edwards MS, Levin VA, Lubich WP, Wilson CB (1981) CSF polyamines: a new and important means of monitoring patients with medulloblastoma. Cancer 47: 757–760

268. Matson DD (1964) Intracranial tumors of the first two years of life. West J Surg Obstet Gynecol 72: 117–122

269. Matson DD, Crigler JF (1969) Management of craniopharyngiomas in childhood. J Neurosurg 30: 377–390

270. Mazza C, Pasqualin A, da Pian R, Donati E (1981) Treatment of medulloblastoma in children: long-term results following surgery, radiotherapy and chemotherapy. Acta Neurochir (Wien) 57: 163–175

271. McComb JG, Davis RL, Isaacs H, Landing BJ (1981) Medulloblastoma presenting as neck tumors in 2 infants. Ann Neurol 7: 113–117

272. McCulloch DC, Epstein F (1985) Optic pathway tumors. A review with proposals for clinical staging. Cancer 56: 1789–1791

273. McFarland DR, Horwitz H, Saenger EL, Bahr GK (1969) Medulloblastoma—a review of prognosis and survival. Br J Radiol 42: 198–214

274. McIntosh N (1979) Medulloblastoma: a changing prognosis. Arch Dis Childh 54: 200–203

275. Meadows AT, Gordon J, Massari DJ, Littman P, Ferguson J, Moss K (1981) Declines in IQ scores and cognitive dysfunction in children with acute cranial irradiation. Lancet ii: 1015–1018

276. Mealy J, Hall PV (1977) Medulloblastoma in children. Survival and treatment. J Neurosurg 46: 56–64

277. Mei Liu H, Boggs J, Kidd J (1976) Ependymomas of childhood. I. Histological survey and clinicopathological correlation. Child's Brain 2: 92–110

278. Meloche B, Sansregret A, LeBlanc P (1964) Tumeurs cérébrales chez le bébé de moins de deux ans. Union Méd Canada 93: 700–705

279. Mercuri S, Russo A, Palma L (1981) Hemispheric supratentorial astrocytomas in children. Long-term results in 29 cases. J Neurosurg 55: 170–173

280. Milhorat TH (1975) Pontine glioma. J Am Med Assoc 232: 595–596

281. Milhorat TH (1978) Pediatric neurosurgery. Davis, Philadelphia, pp 228–332

282. Miller RH, Craig MK, Kernohan JW (1952) Supratentorial tumors among children. Arch Neurol (Chic) 68: 797–814
283. Mørk SJ, Løken AC (1977) Ependymoma. A follow-up study of 101 cases. Cancer 40: 907–915
284. Mori K (1985) Anomalies of the nervous system. Neuroradiology and neurosurgery. Thieme, New York Stuttgart, pp 187–212
285. Müller W, Afra D, Schröder R (1977) Supratentorial recurrences of gliomas. Morphological studies in relation to time intervals with oligodendrogliomas. Acta Neurochir (Wien) 39: 15–25
286. Müller W, Afra D, Schröder R, Slowik F, Wilcke O, Klug N (1982 a) Medulloblastoma: survey of factors possibly influencing prognosis. Acta Neurochir (Wien) 64: 215–224
287. Müller W, Afra D, Wilcke O, Slowik F, Schröder R, Kordas M (1982 b) Data on the biology of medulloblastomas. In: Voth D, Gutjahr P, Langmaid C (eds) Tumours of the central nervous system in infancy and childhood. Springer, Berlin Heidelberg New York, pp 350–353
288. Murovic JA, Ongley JP, Parker JC, Page LK (1981) Manifestations and therapeutic considerations in pineal yolk-sac tumors. Case report. J Neurosurg 55: 303–307
289. Neidhardt M, Habermalz HJ, Henze G, Langermann HJ (1982 a) Medulloblastomstudie der Gesellschaft für Pädiatrische Onkologie. Klin Pädiatr 194: 257–261
290. Neidhardt MK (1982 b) Die Behandlung des Medulloblastoms aus pädiatrisch-onkologischer Sicht. Strahlentherapie 158: 76–81
291. Neidhardt M (1982 c) Report on the medulloblastoma study of the Society of Pediatric Oncology—present position. In: Voth D, Gutjahr P, Langmaid C (eds) Tumours of the central nervous system in infancy and childhood. Springer, Berlin Heidelberg New York, p 349
292. Neidhardt MK (1985) Medulloblastom. Dtsch Ärztebl 82: 3270–3274
293. Neuhäuser G, Schmidt H (1974) Atypischer Krankheitsverlauf beim Medulloblastom. Klin Pädiatr 186: 49–53
294. Neumärker KJ, Neumärker M (1971) Über das psychopathologische Verhalten bei Kindern mit Ponstumoren. Psychiatr Neurol Med Psychol (Leipzig) 23: 509–517
295. Neuwelt EA, Glasberg M, Frenkel E, Clark K (1979) Malignant pineal region tumors. A clinicopathological study. J Neurosurg 51: 597–607
296. Norell H, Wilson CB, Slagel DE, Clark DB (1974) Leukoencephalopathy following the administration of methotrexate into the cerebrospinal fluid in the treatment of primary brain tumors. Cancer 33: 923–932
297. Nørgard-Pedersen B, Lindhold J, Albrechtsen R, Arend J, Diemer NH, Rishede J (1978) Alpha-fetoprotein and human chorionic gonadotrophin in a patient with primary intracranial germ cell tumor. Cancer 41: 2315–2320
298. Oldendorf WH (1974) Blood-brain barrier permeability to drugs. Ann Rev Pharmacol 14: 239–248
299. Onoyama Y, Mitsuyuki A, Takahashi M, Yabumoto E, Sakamoto T (1975) Radiation therapy of brain tumors in children. Radiology 115: 687–693
300. Packer RJ, Allen J, Nielsen S, Petito C, Deck M, Jereb B (1983) Brainstem glioma: clinical manifestations of meningeal gliomatosis. Ann Neurol 14: 177–182
301. Packer RJ, Sutton LN, Rosenstock JG, Rorke LB, Bilaniuk LT, Zimmerman RA, Littman PA, Bruce DA, Schut L (1984) Pineal region tumors of childhood. Pediatrics 74: 97–102
302. Packer RJ, Siegel KR, Sutton LN, Littman PA, Bruce DA, Schut L (1985) Leptomeningeal dissemination of primary central nervous system tumors of childhood. Ann Neurol 18: 217–221

303. Packer RJ, Batnitzky S, Cohen ME (1985) Magnetic resonance imaging in the evaluation of intracranial tumors of childhood. . Cancer 56: 1767–1772

304. Packer RJ, Siegel KR, Sutton LN, Bruce DA, Schut L (1985) Efficacy of combination chemotherapy with lomustine, vincristine, and cisplatin in patients with primitive neuroectodermal tumors—medulloblastoma of childhood (abstr). Ann Neurol 18: 394–395

305. Page LK, Lombroso CT, Matson DD (1969) Childhood epilepsy with late detection of cerebral glioma. J Neurosurg 31: 253–261

306. Page RB, Plourde PV, Coldwell D, Heald JI, Weinstein J (1983) Intrasellar mixed germ-cell tumor. J Neurosurg 58: 766–770

307. Palacios E, Azar-Kia B (1975) Malignant metastasizing angioblastic meningiomas. J Neurosurg 42: 185–188

308. Palmer JO, Kasselberg AG, Netsky MG (1981) Differentiation of medulloblastoma. Studies including immunohistochemical localization of glial fibrillary acid protein. J Neurosurg 55: 161–169

309. Pampiglione G (1974) Somnolence in children with acute leukemia. Br Med J I: 158

310. Panitch HS, Berg BO (1970) Brain stem tumors of childhood and adolescence. Am Dis Child 119: 465–472

311. Papadakis N, Millan J, Grady DF, Segerberg LH (1971) Medulloblastoma of the neonatal period and early infancy. J Neurosurg 34: 88–91

312. Pasquier B, Pasquier D, N'Golet A, Panh MH, Couderc P (1980) Extraneural metastases of astrocytomas and glioblastomas. Clinicopathological study of two cases and review of literature. Cancer 45: 112–125

313. Pasquinucci G, Pardini R, Fedi F (1970) Intrathecal methotrexate. Lancet i: 309–310

314. Parker JC, Mortara RH, McCloskey JJ (1975) Biological behavior of the primitive neuroectodermal tumors: significant supratentorial childhood gliomas. Surg Neurol 4: 383–388

315. Pearl GS, Takei Y (1981) Cerebellar medulloblastoma. Cancer 47: 772–779

316. Perouthka SJ, Snyders SH (1982) Antiemetics: neurotransmitter receptor binding predicts action. Lancet i: 658–659

317. Phillips TL, Sheline GE, Boldrey EB (1964) Therapeutic considerations in tumors affecting the central nervous system: ependymomas. Radiology 83: 98–105

318. Pichler E, Kogelnik HD, Reinartz G, Kärcher KH, Zaunbauer F, Jürgenssen OA, Koos W, Kundi M (1981) Ergebnisse der Therapie des Medulloblastoms in den letzten 15 Jahren. Strahlentherapie 157: 508–515

319. Pierluca P (1977) Les ependymomes de la fosse cérébrale posterieure. Neurochirurgie [Suppl] 23 1: 111–148

320. Pierre-Kahn A, Hirsch JF, Roux FX, Renier D (1983) Intracranial ependymomas in childhood. Survival and functional results of 47 cases. Child's Brain 10: 145–156

321. Plezia PM, Alberts DS, Kessler J, Apro MS, Graham V, Surwit EA (1984) Immediate termination of intractable vomiting induced by cisplatin. Combination of chemotherapy using an intensive five-drug antiemetic regimen. Cancer Treat Rep 68: 1493–1495

322. Poisson M, Pouillart P, Bataini JP, Mashaly R, Pertuiset BF, Metzger J (1979) Malignant gliomas treated after surgery by combination chemotherapy and delayed irradiation. Part I: Analysis of results. Acta Neurochir (Wien) 51: 15–29

323. Pomarede R, Czernichow P, Finidori J, Pfister A, Roger M, Kalifa C, Zucker JM, Pierre-Kahn A, Rappaport R (1982) Endocrine aspects and tumoral markers in intracranial germinoma: an attempt to delineate the diagnostic procedure in 14 patients. J Pediatrics 101: 374–378

324. Pontz BF, Bohl J, Gutjahr P (1984) Konnatales Astrozytom. Kinderarzt 15: 777–781

325. Poppen JL, Marino R (1968) Pinealoma and tumors of the posterior part of the third ventricle. J Neurosurg 28: 357–364

326. Price RA, Jamieson PA (1975) The central nervous system in childhood leukemia. II. subacute leukoencephalopathy. Cancer 35: 306–318
327. Price RA, Birdwell DA (1978) The central nervous system in childhood leukemia. III. Mineralizing microangiopathy and dystrophic calcification. Cancer 42: 717–728
328. Probert JC, Parker BR, Kaplan HS (1973) Growth retardation in children after megavoltage irradiation of the spine. Cancer 32/II: 634–639
329. Quest DO, Brisman R, Antunes JL, Housepian EM (1978) Period of risk for recurrence of medulloblastoma. J Neurosurg 48: 159–163
330. Raimondi AJ, Tomita R (1979) Advantages of "total" resection of medulloblastoma and disadvantages of full head post-operative radiation therapy. Child's Brain 5: 550–551
331. Raimondi AJ, Tomita T (1979) Medulloblastoma in childhood. Acta Neurochir (Wien) 50: 127–138
332. Raimondi AJ, Cerullo LJ (1980) Pediatric cerebral angiography. A descriptive atlas. Thieme, Stuttgart New York, pp 87–136
333. Raimondi AJ, Tomita T (1981) Hydrocephalus and infratentorial tumors. Incidence, clinical picture, and treatment. J Neurosurg 55: 174–182
334. Raimondi AJ, Tomita T (1982) Pineal tumors in childhood. Epidemiology, pathophysiology, and surgical approaches. Child's Brain 9: 239–266
335. Rao YTR, Medini E, Haselow RE, Jones TK, Levitt SH (1981) Pineal and ectopic pineal tumors. The role of radiation therapy. Cancer 48: 708–713
336. Rashkind R, Beigel F (1961) Brain tumors in early infancy—probably congenital in origin. J Pediatr 65: 727–732
337. Reigel DH, Scarff TB, Woodford JE (1979) Biopsy of pediatric brain stem tumors. Child's Brain 5: 329–340
338. Reiter RJ, Esquifino AI, Champney TH, Craft CM, Vaugham MK (1985) Pineal melatonin production in relation to sexual development in the male rat. In: Gupta D (ed) Pediatric neuroendocrinology. Croom Helm, London Sidney, pp 190–202
339. Rich TA, Cassady JR, Strand RD, Winston KR (1985) Radiation therapy for pineal and suprasellar germ cell tumors. Cancer 55: 932–940
340. Richards GE, Wara WM, Grumbach MM, Kaplan SL, Sheline GE, Conte FA (1976) Delayed onset of hypopituitarism: sequelae of therapeutic irradiation of central nervous system, eye, and middle ear tumors. J Pediatr 89: 553–559
341. Ringertz N, Reymond A (1949) Ependymomas and choroid plexus papilloms. J Neuropathol Exp Neurol 8: 355–390
342. Ringertz N, Nordenstam H, Flyger G (1954) Tumors of the pineal region. J Neuropathol Exp Neurol 13: 540–561
343. Roessmann U, Velasco ME, Gambetti P, Autilio-Gambetti L (1983) Neuronal and astrocytic differentiation in human neuroepithelial neoplasms. An immunohistochemical study. J Neuropathol Exp Neuol 42: 113–121
344. Roggli VL, Estrada R, Fechner RE (1979) Thyroid neoplasia following irradiation for medulloblastoma. Cancer 43: 2232–2238
345. Rorke LB (1983) The cerebellar medulloblastoma and its relationship to primitive neuroectodermal tumors. J Neuropathol Exp Neurol 42: 1–15.
346. Rosen G, Ghavimi F, Vanucci R, Deck M, Tan C, Murphy L (1974) Pontine glioma. High-dose methotrexate and leucovorin rescue. J Am Med Assoc 230: 1149–1152
347. Rosen G, Ghavimi F, Nirenberg A, Mosende C, Mehta BP (1977) High-dose methotrexate with citrovorum factor rescue for the treatment of central nervous system tumors in children. Cancer Treat Rep 61: 681–690
348. Rosenblum ML (1983) Stem cell studies of human malignant brain tumors. J Neurosurg 58: 170

349. Rossi LN, Vasella F (1976) Hirntumoren im Kindesalter. Helv Paediatr Acta 31: 211–220

350. Röthig HJ (1982) Interferon and antitumour effects. In: Voth D, Gutjahr P, Langmaid C (eds) Tumours of the central nervous system in infancy and childhood. Springer, Berlin Heidelberg New York, pp 42–43

351. Rothman SJ, Olanow CW (1981) Brain stem glioma in childhood: acute hemiplegic onset. Can J Neurol Sci 8: 63–64

352. Rozencweig M, von Hoff DD, Slavik M, Muggia FM (1977) Cis-diamine-dichloroplatinum. (II): A new anticancer drug. Ann Int Med 86: 803–812

353. Rubin P, Casarett GW (1972) A direction for clinical radiation pathology. The tolerance dose. Front Radiat Ther Oncol 6: 1–16

354. Rubinstein LJ, Northfiled DW (1964) Medulloblastoma and the so-called "arachnoidal cerebellar sarcoma". Brain 87: 379–412

355. Rubinstein LJ (1972) Tumors of the central nervous system. Atlas of tumor pathology. AFIP, Washington DC

356. Rubinstein LJ (1972) Cytogenesis and differentiation of primitive neuroepithelial tumors. J Neuropathol Exp Neurol 31: 7–26

357. Rubinstein LJ (1974) The cerebellar medulloblastoma: its origin, differentiation, morphologic variants, and biologic behavior. In: Vinken PJ, Bruyn GW (eds) Handbook of clinical neurology, vol 18. North-Holland, Amsterdam, pp 167–193

358. Rubinstein LJ, Herman MM, Hanbery JW (1974) The relationship between differentiating medulloblastoma and differentiating diffuse astrocytoma. Light, electron microscopic, tissue, and organ culture observations. . Cancer 33: 890–897

359. Rubinstein L, Herman MM, Long TF, Wilbur JR (1975) Disseminated necrotizing leukoencephalopathy: a complication of treated central nervous system leukemia and lymphoma. Cancer 35: 291–305

360. Russell A (1951) A diencephalic syndrome of emaciation in infancy and childhood. Arch Dis Childh 26: 274–275

361. Russell DS, Rubinstein LJ (1977) Pathology of tumors of the central nervous system. London: Arnold

362. Sacrez R, Juif JG, Friedrich E (1954) Tumeurs cérébrales du nourisson. Arch Franç Pédiatrie 11: 261–263

363. Saiki JH, Thompson S, Smith F, Atkinson R (1972) Paraplegia following intrathecal chemotherapy. Cancer 29: 370–374

364. Salazar OM, Castro-Vita H, Bakos RS, Feldstein ML, Keller B, Rubin P (1979) Radiation therapy for tumors of the pineal region. Int J Radiat Oncol Biol Phys 5: 491–499

365. Salmon S (1980) Clinical correlation of in vitro drug sensitivity. In: Salmon S, Cloning of human tumour stem cells. Alan R Liss, New York

366. Sanford RA, Laurent JP (1985) Intraventricular tumors of childhood. Cancer 56: 1795–1799

367. Sano K, Matsutani M (1981) Pinealoma (germinoma) treated by direct surgery and postoperative irradiation. Child's Brain 8: 81–97

368. Sayers MP (1978) Treatment of optic pathway gliomas. In: O'Brien MS (ed) Pediatric neurological surgery. Raven Press, New York, pp 51–58

369. Schäfer M, Lapras C, Ruf H (1978) Catheterization of the aqueduct in certain lesions of the posterior fossa. Adv Neurosurg 5: 216–220

370. Schatzki PF, Mortati SG, McCain WG (1956) Brain tumor in the newborn infant. New Engl J Med 255: 908–909

371. Scheithauer BW (1978) Symptomatic subependymoma. Report of 21 cases with review of the literature. J Neurosurg 49: 689–696

372. Schenk K, Solcher H (1970) Diffuse Glioblastose im Kindesalter. Neuropädiatrie 2: 98–106
373. Schindler E (1985) Die Tumoren der Pinealisregion. Springer, Berlin Heidelberg New York
374. Schmidek HH (1977) Surgical management of pineal region tumors. Suprasellar germinomas. In: Schmidek HH (ed) Pineal tumors. Masson, New York, pp 99–103 and 115–125
375. Schmidt RC, Engelhardt P (1981) CT und Liquorzytologie bei massiver meningealer Aussaat eines frisch operierten Medulloblastoms. Aktuel Neurol 8: 82–84
376. Schmitt HP, Zeisner W (1982) The diffuse brain stem astrocytoma in childhood: morphology, course, and prognosis. In: Voth D, Gutjahr P, Langmaid C (eds) Tumours of the central nervous system in infancy and childhood. Springer, Berlin Heidelberg New York, pp 149–164
377. Schmitt HP (1983) Rapid anaplastic transformation of gliomas in childhood. Neuropediatrics 14: 137–143
378. Schold SC, Wasserstrom WR, Fleisher M, Schwartz MK, Posner JB (1980) Cerebrospinal fluid biochemical markers of central nervous system metastases. Ann Neurol 8: 597–604
379. Schreiber D, Bernstein K, Warzok R (1982) Tumormetastasen im Zentralnervensystem. Eine prospektive Studie. Zbl Allg Pathol Pathol Anat 126: 41–52
380. Schreiber D, Bernstein K, Schneider J (1982) Tumormetastasen im Zentralnervensystem. Eine prospektive Studie. Zbl Allg Pathol Pathol Anat 126: 64–73
381. Schreiber D, Jänisch W, Gerlach H (1982) CNS tumours in infancy, childhood, and adolescence. In: Voth D, Gutjahr P, Langmaid C (eds) Tumours of the central nervous system in infancy and childhood. . Springer, Berlin Heidelberg New York, pp 62–68
382. Schulte FJ (1984) Intracranial tumors in childhood—concepts for treatment and prognosis. Neuropediatrics 15: 3–12
383. Schwarz ES, Wahlen W, Sitzmann FC (1984) Hirntumoren im Kindes- und Jugendalter. Therapiewoche 34: 1336–1346
384. Segall HD, Batnitzky S, Zee CS, Ahmadi J, Bird CR, Cohen ME (1985) Computed tomography in the diagnosis of intracranial neoplasms in children. Cancer 56: 1748–1755
385. Seiler RW (1982) Die undifferenzierten Astrozytome des Großhirns. Eine Übersicht der aktuellen Therapiemöglichkeiten. Springer, Berlin Heidelberg New York (Neurology, ser 22)
386. Shalet SM (1982) Growth and hormonal status of children treated for brain tumors. Child's Brain 9: 284–293
387. Shapiro WR (1975) Chemotherapy of primary malignant brain tumors in children. Cancer 35: 965–972
388. Shapiro WR (1982) Treatment of neuroectodermal brain tumors. Ann Neurol 12: 231–237
389. Shaw CM, Sumi SM, Alvord EC, Gerdes AJ, Spence A, Parker RG (1978) Fast neutron irradiation in glioblastoma multiforme. J Neurosurg 39: 1–12
390. Sheline GE (1975) Radiation therapy of tumors of the central nervous system in childhood. Cancer 35: 957–964
391. Sheline GE (1975) Conventional radiation therapy of gliomas. Rec Res Cancer Res 51: 125–134
392. Sheline GE (1983) Radiotherapy of adults primary neoplasms. In: Walker MD (ed) Oncology of the nervous system. M Nijhoff, The Hague, pp 223–245
393. Shukovsky LJ, Fletcher GH (1972) Retinal and optic nerve complications in high dose irradiation technique of ethmoid sinus and nasal cavity. Radiology 104: 629–634

394. Shuman RM, Alvord EC, Leech RW (1975) The biology of childhood ependymomas. Arch Neurol (Chic) 32: 731–739
395. Sieben RL, Ishii N (1971) Brain stem glioma causing failure to thrive. Pediatrics 47: 451–455
396. Siegal T, Pfeffer MR, Catane R, Sulkes A, Gomori MJ, Fuks Z (1983) Successful chemotherapy of recurrent intracranial germinoma with spinal metastases. Neurology (Minneap) 33: 631–633
397. Silverman CL, Simpson JR (1982) Cerebellar medulloblastoma: the importance of posterior fossa dose to survival and patterns of failure. Int J Radiat Oncol Biol Phys 8: 1869–1876
398. Simpson DA, Carter RF, Ducru W (1968) Brain tumors of early infancy. Dev Med Child Neurol 10: 190–199
399. Skullerod K, Halvorsen K (1978) Encephalomyelopathy following intrathecal methotrexate treatment in a child with acute leukemia. Cancer 42: 1211–1215
400. Smith DR, Hardman JM, Earle KM (1969) Metastasizing neuroectodermal tumors of the central nervous system. J Neurosurg 31: 50–58
401. Smith RA, Lampe I, Kahn EA (1961) The prognosis of medulloblastoma in children. J Neurosurg 18: 91–97
402. So SC, Ho J (1980) Multiple primary germinomas (ectopic pinealoma of the brain). Neurochirurgia (Stuttg) 23: 147–150
403. Sobin LH (1963) Multiple congenital neoplasms. Arch Pathol 76: 602–608
404. Solitare GB, Krigman MR (1964) Congenital intracranial neoplasma. A case report and review of the literature. J Neuropathol Exp Neurol 23: 280–292
405. Spranger J (1982) Brain tumors and genetics. In: Voth D, Gutjahr P, Langmaid C (eds) Tumours of the central nervous system in infancy and childhood. Springer, Berlin Heidelberg New York, pp 132–141
406. Stachura I, Mendelow H (1980) Endodermal sinus tumor originating in the region of the pineal gland. Cancer 45: 2131–2137
407. Stefanko SZ, Manschot WA (1979) Pinealoblastoma with retinomatous differentiation. Brain 102: 321–332
408. Stein BM (1971) The infratentorial supracerebellar approach to pineal lesions. J Neurosurg 35: 197–202
409. Stein BM (1979) Surgical treatment of pineal tumors. Clin Neurosurg 26: 490–510
410. Stone JL, Zavala G, Bailey OT (1979) Mixed malignant mesenchymal tumor of the cerebellar vermis. Cancer 44: 2165–2172
411. Strange P, Wohlert L (1982) Primary brain stem tumors. Acta Neurochir (Wien) 62: 219–232
412. Sundaresan N, Gutierrez FA, Larsen MB (1978) Radiation myelopathy in children. Ann Neurol 4: 47–50
413. Sunder-Plassmann M, Jellinger K (1972) Großhirn-Glioblastom bei einem Säugling. Z Kinderchir 11: 97–103
414. Sung DI, Harisiadis L, Chang CH (1978) Midline pineal tumors and suprasellar germinomas: highly curable by irradiation. Radiology 128: 745–751
415. Suzuki J, Iwabuchi T (1965) Surgical removal of pineal tumors (pinealoma and teratoma). J Neurosurg 563–571
416. Takahashi M, Okudera T, Tanaka M, Kitamura K, Yonemasu Y (1973) Angiographic diagnosis of cerebellar medulloblastomas. Evaluation of pre- and postoperative vertebral angiograms. Am J Roentgenol 118: 622–632
417. Takei Y, Pearl GS (1981) Ultrastructural study of intracranial yolk sac tumor: with special reference to the oncologic phylogeny of germ cell tumors. Cancer 48: 2038–2048
418. Takeuchi J, Handa H, Atsuka S, Takebe Y (1979) Neuroradiological aspects of suprasellar germinoma. Neuroradiology 17: 153–159

419. Tavcar D, Robboy SJ, Chapman P (1980) Endodermal sinus tumor of the pineal region. Cancer 45: 1646–1651

420. Teilum G (1965) Classification of endodermal sinus tumor (mesoblastoma vitellinum) and so-called "embryonal carcinoma" of the ovary. Acta Pathol Microbiol Scand 64: 407–429

421. Terheggen HG, Rado M (1978) Cerebrale Komplikationen der Leukämiebehandlung. I. Das Apathiesyndrom. Monatsschr Kinderheilkd 126: 693–695

422. Terheggen HG (1978) Cerebrale Nebenwirkungen bei der Behandlung akuter Leukämien im Kindesalter. II. Die methotrexatinduzierte Encephalopathie. Monatsschr Kinderheilkd 126: 696–701

423. Thorbeck R (1981) Hirntumor nach Schädel-Hirn-Trauma. In: Hirt H (Hrsg) Aktuelle Neuropädiatrie III. Thieme, Stuttgart New York, S 192–199

424. Tibbs PA, Mortara RH (1980) Primary glioblastoma multiforme of the cerebellum. A case report. Acta Neurochir (Wien) 52: 13–18

425. Tijssen CC, Halprin MR, Endtz LJ (1982) Familial brain tumours. Nijhoff, The Hague Boston London

426. Tönnis W, Borck WF (1953) Großhirntumoren des Kindesalters. Zentralbl Neurochir 13: 72–98

427. Ueki K, Tanaka R (1980) Treatment and prognosis of pineal tumors—experience of 110 cases. Neurol Med Chir (Tokyo) 20: 1–26

428. Vanucci RC, Baten M (1974) Cerebral metastatic disease in childhood. Neurology (Minneap) 24: 981–985

429. Vick NA, Khandekar J, Bigner DD (1977) Chemotherapy of brain tumors. The "blood-brain barrier" is not a factor. Arch Neurol 34: 523–526

430. Villani R, Giani SM, Tomei G (1975) Follow-up study of brain stem tumors in children. Child's Brain 1: 126–135

431. Vonofakos D, Marcu H, Hacker H (1979) Oligodendroglioma: CT patterns with emphasis on features indicating malignancy. J Comp Ass Tomogr 3: 783–788

432. Waggener JD, Beggs JL (1976) Vasculature of natural neoplasms. Adv Neurol 15: 27–49

433. Waldbauer H, Gottschald M, Schmidt G, Neuhäuser G (1976) Medulloblastom des Kleinhirns und Pinealoblastom bei eineiigen Zwillingen. Klin Pädiatr 188: 366–371

434. Walker MD (1975) Chemotherapy: adjuvant to surgery and radiation therapy. Sem Oncol 2: 69–72

435. Walker MD (1976) Diagnosis and treatment of brain tumors. Pediat Clin North Am 23: 131–146

436. Wallace S, Charnsangavej C, Carrasco CH, Bechtel W (1984) Infusion-embolization. Cancer 54: 2751–2765

437. Walther B, Gutjahr P, Beron CCG (1981) Therapiebegleitende und -überdauernde neurologische und neuropsychologische Diagnostik bei akuter lymphoblastischer Leukämie im Kindesalter. Klin Pädiatr 193: 177–183

438. Walther B, Gutjahr P (1982) Development after treatment of cerebellar medulloblastoma in childhood. In: Voth D, Gutjahr P, Langmaid C (eds) Tumours of the central nervous system in infancy and childhood. Springer, Berlin Heidelberg New York, pp 389–398

439. Wannemacher M, Knüfermann H (1978) Fortschritte in der Therapie des Medulloblastoms. Onkologie 1: 92–96

440. Wara WM, Fellows CF, Sheline GE, Wilson CB, Townsend JT (1977) Radiation therapy for pineal tumors and suprasellar germinomas. Radiology 124: 221–223

441. Wara W, Sheline GE (1978) The role of radiotherapy in the treatment of pediatric brain tumors. In: O'Brien MS (ed) Pediatric neurological surgery. Raven Press, New York, pp 81–86

442. Wara WM, Jenkin RDT, Evans A, Ertel I, Hittle R, Ortega J, Wilson CB, Hammond D (1979) Tumors of the pineal and suprasellar region: Childrens Cancer Study Group treatment results 1960–1975. A report from Childrens Cancer Study Group. Cancer 43: 698–701

443. Welte K, Engert A, Siegert M, Gardner H (1979) Verhalten von Gerinnungsproteinen im Liquor cerebrospinalis bei Kindern mit akuter lymphoblastischer Leukämie (ALL) während der kombinierten Induktionstherapie. Monatsschr Kinderheilkd 127: 262–265

444. West CR, Bruce DA, Duffner PK (1985) Ependymomas. Factors in clinical and diagnostic staging. Cancer 56: 1812–1816

445. Whyte TB, Colby MJ, Layton DD (1969) Radiation therapy of brain stem tumors. Radiology 93: 413–421

446. Wilcke O (1981) Therapie und Prognose der Medulloblastome im Kindesalter. In: Hanefeld F, Rating D (Hrsg) Aktuelle Neuropädiatrie II. Hippokrates, Stuttgart, S 86–93

447. Winkelman NW, Cassel C, Schlesinger B (1952) Intracranial tumors with extracranial metastases. J Neuropathol Exp Neurol 11: 149–168

448. Wisiol ES, Handler S, French LA (1962) Extracranial metastases of a glioblastoma multiforme. J Neurosurg 19: 186–194

449. Wray SH (1977) The neuro-ophthalmic or neurologic manifestations of pinealoma. In: Schmidek HH (ed) Pineal tumors. Masson, New York Paris Barcelona, pp 21–59

450. Yates AJ, Becker LE, Sachs LA (1979) Brain tumors in childhood. Child's Brain 5: 31–39

451. Young LJ, Miller RW (1975) Incidence of malignant tumors in U.S. children. J Pediatr 86: 254–258

452. Yung WA, Horten BC, Shapiro WR (1980) Meningeal gliomatosis: a review of 12 cases. Ann Neurol 8: 605–608

453. Yunis JJ, Ramsay N (1978) Retinoblastoma and subband deletion of chromosome 13. Am J Dis Child 132: 161–163

454. Zimmerman RA, Bilaniuk LT, Pahlajani H (1978) Spectrum of medulloblastoma demonstrated by computed tomography. Radiology 126: 137–141

455. Zimmerman RA, Bilaniuk LT, Wood JH, Bruce DA, Schut L (1980) Computed tomography of pineal, parapineal, and histologically related tumors. Radiology 137: 669–677

456. Zülch KJ (1975) Atlas of gross neurosurgical pathology. Springer, Berlin Heidelberg New York

457. Zülch KJ (1980) Principles of the new World Health Organization (WHO) classification of brain tumors. Neuroradiology 19: 59–66

Authors' address: Prof. Dr. G. Jacobi, Abteilung für Pädiatrische Neurologie, Zentrum der Kinderheilkunde, Theodor-Stern-Kai 7, D-6000 Frankfurt a. M. 70, Federal Republic of Germany.

Subject Index

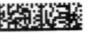